D0983831

Mental Health
Concepts and
Techniques
for the
Occupational Therapy Assistant

Mental Health
Concepts and Techniques

=== *for the* ===

Occupational Therapy Assistant

Second Edition

Mary Beth Early, M.S., OTR

Professor
Occupational Therapy Assistant Program
LaGuardia Community College
City University of New York
New York, New York

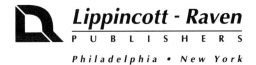

Lippincott - Raven
P U B L I S H E R S
Philadelphia • New York

Lippincott-Raven Publishers, 227 East Washington Square, Philadelphia, Pennsylvania 19106

Made in the United States of America

Library of Congress Cataloging-in-Publication Data

Early, Mary Beth.
   Mental health concepts and techniques for the occupational therapy assistant / Mary Beth Early.--2nd ed.
      p.   cm.
   Includes index.
   ISBN 0-7817-0074-4 (hardcover)
   1. Occupational therapy. 2. Mentally ill--Rehabilitation.
3. Occupational therapy assistants. I. Title.
   [DNLM: 1. Mental Disorders--rehabilitation. 2.
Occupational Therapy. 3. Allied Health Personnel. WM 450.5.02 E12m 1993]
RC437.E3   1993
616.89´165--dc20
DNLM/DLC
for Library of Congress   93-2142

The material contained in this volume was submitted as previously unpublished material, except in the instances in which credit has been given to the source from which some of the illustrative material was derived.

Great care has been taken to maintain the accuracy of the information contained in the volume. However, neither Lippincott-Raven Publishers nor the author can be held responsible for errors or for any consequences arising from the use of the information contained herein.

9 8 7 6 5

Contents

PART 5   Occupational Therapy Methods

PART 6   Professional Development

Preface

Like its predecessor, the second edition of *Mental Health Concepts and Techniques* is designed to provide the occupational therapy assistant student with a basic foundation for the practice of occupational therapy for patients with mental health problems. In addition, the book may be of value to certified occupational therapy assistants who wish to enter psychiatric practice. The book is also a resource for registered therapists with supervisory and administrative roles in mental health settings who wish to explore further the delineation between professional and technical levels of responsibility. It is assumed that the readers of this text have prior coursework in or knowledge of human growth and development, group process, and crafts and other popular occupational therapy activities.

The content is arranged into six main sections. Part 1 establishes a framework, discussing the historical origins of psychiatric occupational therapy and the recent and current theoretical foundations on which today's mental health practice is based. Case examples are included to illustrate how each theory can be applied. The model of human occupation was selected as the primary theoretical structure for the text; the reader is cautioned, however, that this model is still under development. A new chapter has been included on psychiatric diagnosis and the use of the American Psychiatric Association's DSM system, particularly in relation to occupational therapy.

Part 2 addresses the context of the occupational therapy intervention process, and includes chapters on treatment settings, medications, and a new chapter on special populations. The purpose of grouping this material under the heading of context is to draw attention to the effects of these elements on the treatment process.

Part 3 focuses on relationships with patients. There are two reasons why this material is placed here: First, the therapeutic relationship with the mental health worker is a primary force in restoring the patient's motivation and ability to function, and logically should precede any discipline-specific content. In addition, past students have expressed a need to know what to *do* with the patients whom they meet on clerkship, which may run concurrently with the mental health coursework in some curricula. A chapter on safety is also included in this section.

Part 4 describes the occupational therapy process, beginning with an overview and proceeding to individual chapters on data gathering and evaluation and treatment planning and implementation. A separate chapter on documentation describes procedures and contains sample notes for different kinds of settings.

Occupational therapy methods and activities are the focus of Part 5. The first chapter in this section describes the use of groups with psychiatric populations; it is hoped that this chapter will build on previous knowledge of group process. Other chapters detail specific activities in the areas of daily living skills, work and homemaking and child care, leisure, coping and self-expression, and cognitive and sensorimotor skills. The final chapter in this section explains how to analyze and adapt activities to fit the needs of individual patients and groups.

Part 6 contains two chapters. The first, on supervision, provides a perspective on the purpose and use of supervision; it is recommended that this chapter be assigned at the beginning of Level I fieldwork. The second, on being organized, is intended to help students and new graduates structure their work time and work environments more efficiently and effectively.

Appendix A contains several case examples, some of which are referred to within the text. Additional case examples are included in Chapters 2, 3, 4, and 5. Appendix B gives two sample group protocols to supplement the material in Chapter 17.

Masculine and feminine pronouns are used alternately throughout the book. In some chapters the feminine pronoun is used for the registered therapist and the masculine for the certified assistant; in others the pronouns are reversed. The same policy is applied when referring to patients and physicians. The ongoing controversy over whether *patient* or *client* is the more appropriate term for the recipient of occupational therapy services is discussed within the text. Both words (*patient* and *client*) are used selectively throughout.

Acknowledgments

A work of this scope, of necessity, requires contributions by many people besides the author. I am grateful to Dr. Carol Engelbrock-Lee for reviewing the chapter on psychiatric diagnosis, and to Susan Voorhies, COTA, CAODAC, for commenting on the substance abuse section of the chapter on special populations. Susan and her supervisor, Anne Brown, OTR, MS, also provided group protocols, case examples, and other treatment information for substance abuse. I appreciate the help of Kathleen Kannenberg of AOTA's practice division for information on total quality management, and Charlotte Lazaro, COTA, during her days as an occupational therapy assistant student, for research on medications and their side effects. Hermine D. Plotnick, MA, OTR, and Margaret D. Rerek, MA, OTR, created the case study for the new chapter on psychiatric diagnosis. My thanks also to the many occupational therapy technical educators who responded in great detail to my survey questionnaire. All of these contributions were significant, and helped me deal more gracefully with a task that seemed, at times, too daunting to endure. There are many others who helped; they are, unfortunately, too numerous to list by name.

Finally, I appreciate the forebearance and patience of my family, whose love and support are increasingly dear. In particular, I thank my husband Bob, for putting up with my preoccupations and for keeping me better fed than any other author I know, and my son Jeffrey, for waiting all those times for me to finish my work and play with him.

PART 1

History and Theory

1

History and Basic Concepts

Occupational therapy has a great deal to learn from its history. The profession was founded on the visionary idea that human beings need, and are nurtured by, their activity as by food and drink and that every human being possesses potential that can be achieved through engagement in occupation.

ELIZABETH YERXA (26)

People who have mental health problems do not just have trouble controlling their feelings and thoughts. Often they have trouble doing everyday activities, things the rest of us take for granted. Occupational therapy is a powerful resource in the treatment of such problems. Occupational therapists are concerned with how people carry out their daily life activities, how well they do them and how satisfied they feel about them. We define occupation as "man's goal-directed use of time, interest, energy, and attention" (2). Occupational therapy uses carefully selected purposeful activities to help troubled individuals, families, and communities learn new skills, maintain successful and adaptive habits, explore their feelings and interests, and control their own lives and destinies.

MENTAL HEALTH AND MENTAL ILLNESS

Before we consider further the purpose and role of occupational therapy in the evaluation and treatment of mental health prob-

lems, it is useful to explore what we mean by the terms "mental health" and "mental illness." In the words of the American Psychiatric Association, *mental health* is:

> A state of being, relative rather than absolute. The best indices of mental health are simultaneous success at working, loving and creating with the capacity for mature and flexible resolution of conflicts between instincts, conscience, important other people, and reality. (25, p. 89)

This definition views mental health in terms of reasonably successful functioning within a framework of daily life activities (working), relationships (loving), and exploration and growth (creating). Being able to resolve conflicts in a mature (not childish or impulsive) fashion is part of successful functioning. The mentally healthy person has a balanced and satisfying life, his energies divided among work, leisure, self-care, and care of others. He manages the conflicting demands of instincts (such as drives for sex and self-preservation), conscience (internalized moral rules and standards of behavior), significant other people in his life, and the real external world. What is described

3

here is not a state of absolute or perfect mental health, but rather a condition or quality of being able to manage one's daily affairs and respond constructively and creatively to the changing demands and opportunities of real life.

If mental health is relative, defined in relation to changing life conditions, at what point can we say that someone has mental health problems? The term used by the American Psychiatric Association to describe mental illness is *mental disorder,* defined as:

> An illness with psychologic or behavioral manifestations and/or impairment in functioning due to a social, psychologic, genetic, physical/chemical, or biologic disturbance. The disorder is not limited to relations between the person and society. The illness is characterized by symptoms and/or impairment in functioning. (25, p. 89)

Signs of mental illness include abnormal behavior, impaired thinking, disordered emotions, and impaired functioning. The definition suggests that the etiology (causes) of mental disorder may be social, biological, psychological, genetic, physical, or a combination of these. Problems in mental health are not limited to the seriously mentally ill, but are experienced also by those with disorders that are primarily physical in nature and by individuals, families, and communities exposed to chronic or acute stress.

Crucial for occupational therapy is this definition's emphasis on impaired functioning; difficulty in carrying out daily life activities is seen as one of the major symptoms of mental disorder. Occupational therapy is the ideal treatment for such problems, since performance in human occupation and daily life activities is its main concern. Also, since occupational therapy uses activity as its primary treatment tool, the patient must act and perform, and thus prove to himself and to others that indeed he *can* function.

RELATIONSHIP OF ACTIVITY TO MENTAL HEALTH

The notion that involvement in activity can improve mental health is hardly new; it appears in records of ancient civilizations from China to Rome. But it is such an excellent idea that it is continually rediscovered and acclaimed. At the 1961 Annual Conference of the American Occupational Therapy Association, Mary Reilly expressed it this way:

> *That man, through the use of his hands as they are energized by mind and will, can influence the state of his own health.* This is the inherited occupational therapy hypothesis passed on for proof by the early founders.
> The splendor of its vision goes far beyond rating it as an idea conceived once in a lifetime or even once in a century. Rather, it falls in the class of one of those great beliefs which has advanced civilization. Its magnificence lies in the optimistic vote of confidence it gives to human nature. It implies that there is a reservoir of sensitivity and skill in the hands of man which can be tapped for his health. It implies the rich adaptability and durability of the central nervous system which can be influenced by experiences. And more than all this, it implies that man, through the use of his hands, can creatively deploy his thinking, feelings and purposes to make himself at home in the world and to make the world his home. (22, p. 1, emphasis in original)

Every person is born with a drive to act on his environment, to change things, to produce things, to work, and to use his hands and mind. The joy of having an effect and the challenge and pleasure of solving problems give life meaning and purpose. We know that both the unemployed and those employed in routinized jobs suffer from stress and mental disorders because they lack the stimulation of challenging activity. Their drive to act has been frustrated and deadened; an essential part of their humanity has been denied. We know too that many of the mentally ill suffer because they cannot do what they once did; disease has impaired their capacity to act. Unhappiness and inactivity reinforce each other; as the person fails to act, he becomes less able to.

Occupational therapy uses purposeful activity to reverse the negative cycle of inactivity and disease. Purposeful activity requires attention and energy; it has a unique meaning to the individual performing it (14). Activity that engages the entire human being—heart, mind, and body—is powerful therapy. Not every activity is therapeutic— only those that fire the patient's interest and empower his will to do. Helping the patient discover, master, and manage the activities that give his life purpose and direction is the essence of psychiatric occupational therapy.

OCCUPATIONAL THERAPY: HISTORY AND FUTURE TRENDS

Occupational therapy arose out of the moral treatment movement of the 18th and early 19th centuries, and contemporary occupational therapy practice in mental health continues to rely on the ideas and techniques of moral treatment. Although the history of occupational therapy over the past 70 years reveals many digressions from these first principles, it also shows that we have returned to embrace them as essential. Moral treatment was based on ideas developed in France by Pinel and in England by Tukes, and was first practiced in the United States at McLean Hospital in Massachusetts and Frankford Asylum in Pennsylvania in the early 19th century (7). The philosophy of moral treatment included a respect for the individual, and a belief that the mentally ill would benefit most from a regular daily routine and the opportunity to contribute productively to their own care and to the welfare of society in general. Before the advent of moral treatment, the mentally ill were housed in large asylums, where they were largely ne-

glected; observers noted that they were ill fed, unclothed, and often found lying in their own bodily wastes. It was not unusual for mentally ill persons to be subjected to restraint and torture.

In contrast, early moral treatment hospitals provided a prescribed routine of daily hygiene, regular meals (sometimes prepared by the inmates from crops grown on the hospital grounds), and craft work and recreation. Efforts were made to engage as many inmates as possible in regular employment or occupation, such as kitchen, laundry, general cleaning, grounds work, or building repair within the hospital. The effect of such employment was described by Adolph Meyer, a physician and one of the founders of occupational therapy:

It had long been interesting to see how groups of a few excited patients can be seated in a corner in a small circle of two or three settees and kept wonderfully contented picking the hair of mattresses, or doing simple tasks not too readily arousing the desire for big movements and uncontrollable excitement and yet not too taxing to their patience. Groups of patients with raffia and basket work, or with various kinds of handwork and weaving and bookbinding and metal and leather work, took the place of the bored wall flowers and of mischief-makers. A pleasure in achievement, a real pleasure in the use and activity of one's hands and muscles and a happy appreciation of time began to be used as incentives in the management of our patients, instead of abstract exhortations to cheer up and to behave according to abstract or repressive rules. (20, p. 81)

Early occupational therapy practitioners based their work on moral treatment methods and used a variety of activities such as arts and crafts, classroom instruction, manual labor, games, sports, social activities, and self-care activities. These were designed to provide a balanced daily program, which incorporated work, rest, and leisure. Activities were planned and graded for the needs and abilities of individuals. Formation of habits and the development of skills and attention were emphasized. The personality of the occupational therapist was important; kindliness, modeling of correct habits, and an ability to analyze and adjust activities to suit the interests and capacities of patients were valued traits (19).

In the period from 1917 to the 1950s psychiatric occupational therapists continued to provide comprehensive activity programs based loosely on moral treatment principles within institutional settings. The physician prescribed occupational therapy, often ordering specific activities for patients, and the occupational therapist carried out the treatment. After World War II, interest in rehabilitating veterans led to an emphasis on workmanship and vocational readiness.

During the 1940s and 1950s occupational therapy was attacked by the medical profession for failing to have a "scientific basis" for its treatment methods (16, 23). At this time, and in response to this criticism, occupational therapy adopted the vocabulary and concepts of the prevailing psychiatric theory, psychoanalysis. Although occupational therapists continued to work under the prescription of physicians, Gail Fidler and others began to use activities to evaluate their patients' psychodynamics (emotions and psychological defenses). They analyzed activities for their capacity to meet patients' unconscious needs. Activities were matched symbolically to psychic content (for example, clay is like feces and may symbolize anal stage concerns).

Another critical development during the 1950s was the discovery and introduction of the major tranquilizers; this meant that occupational therapists could now work with patients whose behavior had previously been so psychotic and bizarre that treatment was difficult or impossible. The discovery and use of these drugs led indirectly to the passage in 1963 of the Community Mental Health Centers Act, which was designed to establish community-based treatment facilities and to move the mentally ill from institutional settings to community living. Unfortunately, inadequate planning and funding resulted in large numbers of deinstitutionalized mental patients being released into communities that did not have treatment facilities to serve their needs. Nonetheless, the social and political climate of the 1960s promoted increased interest in and funding for mental health research.

Several new theories (gestalt therapy, milieu therapy, behavioral therapy, and family therapy) were applied by occupational therapists during these years. However, as these theories had been developed by other disciplines, primarily psychology, their focus did not always include occupation. Of these new therapies, the behavioral approach was the one most used by occupational therapists. Occupational therapists applied the techniques of *behavioral therapy* in their work with the mentally ill and the mentally retarded in order to diminish acting-out behaviors and promote healthy behaviors. By reinforcing desired behavior through carefully selected rewards, and by enforcing limits on undesirable behavior, therapists felt they were able to improve their patients' functioning. Behavioral approaches will be discussed at length in Chapters 2 and 3.

The 1960s and 1970s brought an explosion of interest in and knowledge about brain chemistry and neurophysiology and their effects on mental functioning. During this time Lorna Jean King applied *sensory integration* theory and methods developed by A. Jean Ayres to chronic psychiatric patients. King proposed that poor functioning and grossly abnormal posture in chronic schizophrenics could be caused by defects in the structure and chemistry of the brain, which might be corrected or at least controlled by carefully designed exercise and relaxation programs. The application of sensory integration techniques remains a major research area in psychiatric occupational therapy today and will be covered in more detail in Chapter 3.

During the 1980s, Claudia Allen outlined

and developed her theory of *cognitive disabilities*. Allen proposes that a patient's performance in a task indicates the quality of his thought. She identifies six levels of cognitive functioning, which can be evaluated through performance of routine occupational therapy tasks, such as leather lacing or mosaics. Diagnosis of cognitive level can contribute to the psychiatric diagnosis, and can be used to predict future functioning and to identify the treatment methods that are likely to be most effective (1). Allen's theory will be described further in Chapter 3.

Both King's and Allen's theories emphasize activity or occupation as a focus for evaluation and intervention. However, most other theories of the 1950s and 1960s have been criticized for the absence of this focus (4). During the 1960s and 1970s Mary Reilly and others criticized the multiple reductionistic (reducing the patient's problems to isolated elements such as insight or behavior) approaches then in use, and argued for a more comprehensive theory for occupational therapy practice, one that would focus primarily on man's occupational nature (6, 22). Kielhofner and Burke and others built upon Reilly's work with the *model of human occupation* (17, 18). This model attempts to organize recent research findings and traditional occupational therapy beliefs for use in all practice areas—physical medicine, developmental disabilities, and psychiatry, among others. The model proposes a three-level hierarchy that describes human response to the environment. The three levels are volition (motivation), habituation (roles and habits), and performance (skills). The relationship between the three levels is dynamic, each level having an effect on the other two. Because it has the potential to embrace so many different aspects of occupational therapy practice, the model of human occupation is explored in its own chapter (Chapter 4).

During the late 1980s and the 1990s Florence Clark and others (9) initiated a new scientific discipline—*occupational science*—to systematically study the occupational nature of humans. It is hoped that research in occupational science will generate data that might validate the model of human occupation and provide more credibility for and scientific understanding of the theoretical underpinnings of occupational therapy.

While occupational therapists have been trying to develop a unique theory and refine their treatment techniques, they have also been increasingly concerned about the rapid proliferation and growth, since the 1950s, of other activity-oriented mental health therapies, all of which share occupational therapy techniques and theories. Vocational rehabilitation counseling and dance, art, music, and poetry therapies each focus on activities previously of concern only to occupational therapists. This trend continued into the 1980s, with nursing, social work, and physical therapy increasingly involved with the daily life activities and occupational functioning of psychiatric patients. One of occupational therapy's greatest challenges today is to maintain its professional visibility, and to make patients, insurance companies, and federal agencies aware of its special expertise in evaluating and treating the problems of the mentally ill. Leaders within the profession urge that we promote a public image of occupational therapy as the only profession with "a comprehensive perspective on human productivity" (12).

The passage of the Americans with Disabilities Act of 1990 (ADA) (Public Law 101-336) may provide increased opportunities for practice in mental health occupational therapy. This law mandates that qualified individuals not be excluded from employment and work activities because of disability due to physical or mental impairments. Occupational therapists and assistants can help to prepare persons with mental disabilities for the world of work through training in work skills, self-advocacy skills, and attitudinal skills and by collaborating with employers to analyze job functions and to determine reasonable accommodations (10). Whether the potential of the ADA to provide increased participation in employment for disabled individuals will ever be realized depends on how the law is actually implemented, how much this costs the public, and how the benefits of the law are perceived (13, 21). Occupational therapy personnel have the training and background to assist employers and disabled individuals to interpret and apply the law in a cost-effective and reasonable fashion.

The future of occupational therapy in psychiatry hinges on the profession's ability to predict and respond to rapidly changing conditions. Among these are a continued movement from hospital-based, disease-oriented practice to community-based, health-oriented models (15). This will necessitate a renewed emphasis on prevention (11), and occupational therapists will be forced to document the health benefits of activity if they expect their services to be reimbursed. Consumers and third-party payers today insist on high-quality care that is effective, reasonably priced, and that includes consumers in decision-making.

THE ROLE OF THE OCCUPATIONAL THERAPY ASSISTANT

Occupational therapy assistant students sometimes question how the registered occupational therapist (OTR) differs from the certified occupational therapy assistant (COTA), since both appear at first glance to perform similar job tasks. Comments such as, "Why are OTRs paid more? They do the same things we do," and "The OTR doesn't even treat patients. She just does paperwork," are typical. Some professional-level occupational therapy students and registered therapists also express confusion about the difference between the professional and the technical level. Understanding the difference between the two levels is essential for both if they are to work together effectively.

Since 1958, when the American Occupational Therapy Association began to plan for occupational therapy assistants, their role in mental health treatment has expanded tremendously. Many factors affect their roles in the United States today; among these are the official educational standards and role delineation provided by the AOTA, the licensing and certification guidelines of the various states, and the local job market availability of OTRs and other activities therapists. In addition, the regulations and needs within mental health treatment facilities and the experience and skill of individual occupational therapy assistants influence their roles.

To identify the role of the COTA, the AOTA has conducted several research projects on *role delineation*. The purpose of these projects has been to outline precisely, or delineate, the roles of entry-level COTAs and OTRs. "Entry-level" refers to new graduates of training programs, as differentiated from experienced therapists. The most recent of the role delineation studies was approved by AOTA's representative assembly in April 1990 and was the foundation for the 1991 Essentials and Guidelines of an Accredited Educational Program for the Occupational Therapy Assistant. These documents provide a framework for describing the role of the COTA in a mental health setting.

First, it is important to understand that the entry-level COTA is trained to collaborate with a supervising OTR to provide occupational therapy services. The OTR and the COTA perform complementary job functions. Both are involved in all stages of patient treatment, from screening and evaluation to discharge planning. Yet there is a difference in their roles and in the areas for which each is responsible. Differences in their educational preparation account for most of this difference.

The COTA, to be certified by AOTA, must successfully complete an assistant-level educational program in a community college or vocational-technical institute.

The course of study includes communication and interpersonal skills, basic biological and behavioral sciences, diseases and conditions treated by occupational therapy, human development, life tasks (work, play, leisure, and self-care), analysis of activities, and instructional techniques. Also included are courses in principles and methods of occupational therapy evaluation and treatment, emphasizing daily living skills and performance components (6) in the sensorimotor, cognitive, and psychosocial areas. The assistant also learns to adapt activities and the environment and is trained in various structured evaluation and treatment techniques and in basic management and supervision of occupational therapy services. At the completion of the program and the required minimum of 12 weeks of related fieldwork, the graduate is eligible to sit for the AOTA certification examination (5).

In contrast, the occupational therapist, to be eligible for registration by the AOTA, must complete an educational program in a university or college that grants degrees at the baccalaureate (B.A. or B.S.) or master's (M.A. or M.S.) level. To enter a master's program, applicants must already have obtained a baccalaureate degree and must have taken prerequisite courses in biology, psychology, other social sciences, and sometimes physics or chemistry. The program of study at the occupational therapist level includes more advanced courses in biological and medical and health sciences (such as anatomy, physiology, kinesiology, neuroanatomy, neurophysiology, medical and surgical conditions, neurological and psychiatric conditions, orthopedic conditions, and congenital and developmental disorders) and in comparative sociology and ethics. Occupational therapy courses emphasize the exploration and comparison of theories that analyze normal and therapeutic use of activities, as well as the application of these theories at each stage of the treatment process. Unstructured as well as structured evaluation and

treatment methods are included, as well as adaptation and environmental modification of activities, advanced management and supervision concepts and skills, and quality assurance and research methods. More than six months of fieldwork is required. After completing the coursework and fieldwork, graduates are eligible to take an examination to be registered and certified by the AOTA (4).

The training of the COTA and the OTR prepares them to work in a complementary fashion, as the following situation illustrates:

> The setting is a back ward of a large state psychiatric hospital. The patients on this ward have been hospitalized numerous times, some over as long as 20 years. Most have an S-shaped posture and rounded shoulders. They are not able even to lift their arms above their heads. Most have very poor self-esteem and show little interest in activities. They prefer to spend their days sitting unoccupied in the lounge.
>
> A COTA has recently been assigned to this and the neighboring unit. The OTR is excited about this, since he has not had the time to provide groups here because he is responsible for evaluation and program planning on six units.
>
> The COTA now runs an excercise group five days a week for a half hour, most often using a parachute and beachballs. One day a week he constructs an obstacle course out of furniture and wastebaskets. On another day he organizes a game of balloon volleyball. These are activities he and the OTR have selected to help the patients develop balance skills, endurance, and coordination. He meets with the OTR once a week to review patients' progress and to discuss new activities to use in the group.

The collaboration between OTR and COTA in this situation is very effective and allows for efficient use of staff time to meet patients' needs. The OTR and the COTA have evaluated the patients, the COTA performing parts of the evaluation as instructed by his supervisor. From the evaluation results, the OTR has identified specific deficits in sensory integrative functioning (a *perfor-*

mance component). The COTA is carrying out a sensory integration treatment regimen designed by the OTR, but the activities employed are selected by both of them. The COTA makes good use of supervision to explore new treatment activities. The patients' progress, as reported by the COTA, is useful to the OTR when he speaks with administrators about the need for more occupational therapy lines. In addition, the treatment program, if carefully documented, can provide data to analyze the effectiveness of the sensory integrative methods used. The COTA and the OTR may even collaborate to write a paper to submit to *The American Journal of Occupational Therapy*. This sort of complementary relationship is only one example of the ways in which COTA and OTR work together.

In the 1990 role delineation study, the job tasks of OTR and COTA were differentiated according to the knowledge required to perform them. The COTA's area of greatest expertise is independent living and daily living skills. These areas of *occupational performance* include self-care, communication and travel, and work and leisure skills. The OTR is trained in these areas but has additional expertise in *performance components* (sensorimotor, cognitive, and psychosocial). The COTA is trained in some of the routine and structured techniques used to evaluate and treat problems in performance component functioning. The COTA is thus able to carry out large segments of the occupational therapy program, with supervision from the OTR, who is better prepared to design the overall program and to evaluate and plan treatment for complex problems involving performance components.

What the COTA working in a mental health setting actually does on a day-to-day basis is quite variable, depending upon the experience of the COTA and the treatment facility and region of the country where she works. Hypothetically, she could plan and carry out a total program of independent living skills, grooming and hygiene, cooking and food management skills, money management, use of public and private transportation, shopping, clothing care and selection, use of telephone and postal services, homemaking, child care, work skills, and play and leisure skills. She might teach coping skills and self-identity skills. She might assist the OTR in evaluating and treating sensorimotor problems, as described previously, or cognitive problems, such as disorientation or impaired concentration, attention span, or memory (3).

In summary, the COTA carries out major portions of the total occupational therapy program, usually under the supervision of an OTR. Supervision will be discussed in Chapter 24. How much supervision is required depends on the regulations of individual states and on administrative patterns within treatment facilities. For example, in New York State, the licensing law for occupational therapists provides specific direction on how the OTR and the COTA shall work together. According to this law, a COTA must be under the direct supervision of an OTR (or a licensed physician) in order to practice. *Direct supervision* has been defined variously by state officials to mean anything from full-time, on-site supervision to monthly cosignature of notes. Other states are less restrictive. Occupational therapy assistants are cautioned to stay current with state regulations and their most recent interpretations.

In practice, the need for supervision will vary with the skills and experience of COTA and OTR. Experienced COTAs may need little supervision, and may be asked to help supervise OTR students, as suggested by the three levels of COTAs (generalist, skilled clinician, and master clinician) outlined by Terry Brittell (8). In situations where patients' conditions are complex or change rapidly, the COTA is likely to require and want more supervision than in a routine situation. The need for supervision, and the quantity and depth of supervision, can be determined only after considering available guidelines and the characteristics of the particular situation.

The future of occupational therapy in psychiatry depends, to some extent, on the ability of OTRs and COTAs to work together and to develop staffing patterns that provide quality services at a reasonable cost. Shortages of qualified applicants for OTR-level positions in mental health settings continue to be reported across the country. In some cases, administrators are filling these lines with other activities therapists. However, COTAs are ideally suited for many of these positions, especially those in chronic care settings such as state hospitals or community mental health centers. The few OTRs who have never worked with a COTA may express misgivings and feelings of defensiveness at the prospect. By openly discussing the possibilities for a complementary and supportive role, COTAs can do much to promote their own future. New OTRs are more likely to appreciate the skills and contributions of the COTA now that the essentials for therapist-level educational programs require content on the management of COTA personnel (4).

REFERENCES

1. Allen C. *Occupational therapy for psychiatric diseases: measurement and management of cognitive disabilities*. Boston: Little, Brown; 1985.
2. American Occupational Therapy Association. *Occupational therapy: its definition and functions*. Rockville, Md: American Occupational Therapy Association; 1972.
3. American Occupational Therapy Association. *Entry level role delineation for OTRs and COTAs*. Rockville, Md: American Occupational Therapy Association; 1990.
4. American Occupational Therapy Association. *Essentials and guidelines for an accredited educational program for the occupational therapist*. Rockville, Md: American Occupational Therapy Association; 1991.
5. American Occupational Therapy Association. *Essentials and guidelines for an accredited educational program for the occupational therapy assistant*. Rockville, Md: American Occupational Therapy Association; 1991.
6. American Occupational Therapy Association Uniform Terminology Task Force. Uniform terminology for occupational therapy, second edition. *Am J Occup Ther* 1989; 43:808–815.
7. Bockoven JS. Legacy of moral treatment—1880's to 1910. *Am J Occup Ther* 1971; 5:223–225.
8. Brittell T. Future concepts of the COTA role, Part II. *Am Occup Ther Assoc Mental Health Specialty Section Newsletter* 1981; 4:1–4.
9. Clark FA, Parham D, Carlson ME, et al. Occupational science: academic innovation in the service of occupational therapy's future. *Am J Occup Ther* 1991; 45:300–310.
10. Crist PAH, Stoffel VC. The Americans with Disabilities Act of 1990 and employees with mental impairments: personal efficacy and the environment. *Am J Occup Ther* 1992; 46:434–443.
11. Diasio K. Occupational therapy in mental health: a time of challenge [editorial]. *Occup Ther Mental Health* 1980; 1:1–10.
12. Fidler G, Fidler J. Doing and becoming: purposeful action and self-actualization. *Am J Occup Ther* 1978; 32:305–310.
13. Frieden L. The issue is—the Americans with Disabilities Act of 1990—will it work? (pro). *Am J Occup Ther* 1992; 46:468–469.
14. Hinojosa J, Sabari J, Rosenfeld M, Shapiro D. Purposeful activities (a position paper of the American Occupational Therapy Association). *Am J Occup Ther* 1983; 37:805–806.
15. Jaffe E. Nationally speaking . . . transition in health care: critical planning for the 1990s, part 1. *Am J Occup Ther* 1985; 39:431–435.
16. Kielhofner G. *Conceptual foundations of occupational therapy*. Philadelphia: FA Davis; 1992.
17. Kielhofner G. *A model of human occupation: theory and application*. Baltimore: Williams and Wilkins; 1985.
18. Kielhofner G, Burke J. A model of human occupation, part I, conceptual framework and content. *Am J Occup Ther* 1980; 34:572–581.
19. Licht S. The early history of occupational therapy—an outline. *Occup Ther Mental Health* 1983; 3:1:67–88. (Originally published in *Occup Ther Rehab*)
20. Meyer A. The philosophy of occupational therapy. *Occup Ther Mental Health* 1982; 2:3:79–86. (Originally published in *Arch Occup Ther* 1921; 1:1.)
21. Nosek MA. The issue is—the Americans with Disabilities Act of 1990—will it work? (con). *Am J Occup Ther* 1992; 46:466–467.
22. Reilly M. The 1961 Eleanor Clarke Slagle lecture: occupational therapy can be one of the great ideas of 20th century medicine. *Am J Occup Ther* 1962; 16:1.
23. Serrett KD. Another look at occupational therapy's history. *Occup Ther Mental Health* 1985; 5(3):1–31.
24. Shannon P. The derailment of occupational therapy. *Am J Occup Ther* 1977; 31:229–235.
25. Stone EM, ed. *American psychiatric glossary*. 6th ed. Washington, DC: American Psychiatric Association; 1988.
26. Yerxa EJ. Some implications of occupational therapy's history for its epistemology, values,

and relation to medicine. *Am J Occup Ther* 1992; 46:79–83.

ADDITIONAL REFERENCES AND SUGGESTED READINGS

Bonder BR. Occupational therapy in mental health: crisis or opportunity? *Am J Occup Ther* 1987; 41:495–499.

Fidler GS. The challenge of change to occupational therapy practice. *Occup Ther Mental Health* 1991; 11(1):1–11.

Fine SB. Looking ahead: opportunities for occupational therapy in the next decade. *Occup Ther Mental Health* 1987; 7(4):3–12.

Fine SB. Working the system: a perspective for managing change. *Am J Occup Ther* 1988; 42:417–419.

Kleinman BL. The challenge of providing occupational therapy in mental health. *Am J Occup Ther* 1992; 46:555–557.

2

Medical and Psychological Models of Mental Health and Illness

Mankind will possess incalculable advantages and extraordinary control over human behavior when the scientific investigator will be able to subject his fellow men to the same external analysis he would employ for any natural object, and when the human mind will contemplate itself not from within but from without.

IVAN PETROVICH PAVLOV (14)

There are many theories about how mental health problems develop and how a therapist might try to help someone deal with them. Many of the theories occupational therapists have used in the past were originally developed by psychologists or psychiatrists.[1] Although most psychiatric occupational therapists today do not use these theories, many use techniques based on them, and occupational therapists and assistants often work in treatment settings where some of the staff use one of these theories. Chapters 3 and 4 will explore theories developed specifically for use in occupational therapy practice.

First, however, why use a theory at all? One very good reason is that a theory gives us ideas about what to do in a situation with a patient. Imagine the following scenario:

Your supervisor on your Level 1 fieldwork has asked you to cover her leathercraft group while she goes to a meeting. Since

you know leathercraft well, you agree to do it. Everything seems to be going fine. All eight patients are busy on their projects. Suddenly one patient, a teenage girl, starts drawing a leather knife across her wrist. She isn't actually cutting herself, but just dragging the knife across her skin.

What would you do? Are you finding it hard to think of an answer? Maybe you would like to think about it for a while, but in a real situation you would not have much time. You would have to respond quickly, and it might help if you had a theory to give you some ideas.

A theory is one way of looking at something, and since there are many ways of looking at how the mind works, we have many theories about it. A theory is one explanation, but there is not yet any one "correct" theory that explains all we want to know about the human mind. Consequently, many theories exist, all trying to explain the same thing. As an occupational therapy assistant, you will use techniques based on these theories, and therefore you will want to know something about them. Techniques are methods or approaches for working with patients.

---

[1]Much of the material in this chapter derives from Early, M.B. *T.A.R. Introductory Course Workbook: Occupational Therapy—Psychosocial Dysfunction* (5).

Five major medical and psychological theories used in mental health treatment will be covered in this chapter. You will learn about the main ideas, special vocabulary, and some of the basic techniques of each theory.

THEORY OF OBJECT RELATIONS

The theory of object relations is a psychoanalytic theory based on the work of Sigmund Freud and his followers, who believed that mental health and mental illness are determined by relationships we have with objects in our environment. These may be physical objects (nonhuman objects) or people (human objects). Our ability to love and respond to other people and to take interest in the things in our environment are seen as expressions of object relations. The way a person relates to things and people gives clues about his lifelong pattern of object relations, which is believed to develop through relationships in very early childhood.

According to object relations theory, the infant develops relationships with objects in the environment in order to satisfy needs, such as hunger or thirst. Humans have an inborn tendency to try actively to satisfy needs. This tendency is called a _drive_. Humans are believed to be born with drives for self-preservation, pleasure, and exploration, and these inborn drives are located in the most primitive part of the self, which is called the _id_. The id is not concerned about other people's feelings, but only with satisfying its own needs. At birth, the entire personality is dominated by the id. It is only through experiences of, and relationships with, objects (human and nonhuman) that other parts of the personality become developed.

As an example, when very young infants are hungry, they cry. This is their way of expressing their drive for food and their terrible frustration at not being fed. As children develop, they are expected to express their needs in ways that are more socially

acceptable. They are put under pressure to adapt to the rules of society. For example, they must learn to talk about their feelings instead of just striking out. If they cry, they might be sent to their room. In the beginning, children's parents make them follow the rules of society, but gradually these rules become part of the children's personalities. Freud called this the _superego._ The superego acts as the conscience or moralizer and "tells" the person what is right and wrong.

As you might imagine, the id and the superego are often in conflict. For example, a woman who is dieting may pass a bakery window and see a chocolate cake. The id part of her wants to eat that chocolate cake. The superego says, in effect, "You shouldn't do that." The conflict between what the id wants and what the superego will allow can create a lot of anxiety. The woman will feel confused and tense, not knowing what to do. Fortunately, a third part of the personality, the _ego,_ controls anxiety by compromising between the warring id and superego.

The word _ego,_ as it is used in object relations theory, refers to something quite different from the everyday meaning ("He's got a big ego"). The ego is the third main part of the personality, and it performs many different mental functions that deal with reality and with the conflicting desires of id and superego. Memory and perception are two important functions of the ego. Another is _reality testing,_ or the ability to tell the difference between reality and fantasy, and to share the same general ideas about reality that most people do. The ego also helps to control impulses and to organize actions. In addition, the ego makes use of many _defense mechanisms,_ which attempt to compromise between the id and the superego and the demands of reality.

One such defense mechanism is _displacement,_ or the transfer of the id drive to another object. In the case of the woman looking in the bakery window, the ego might substitute another object, and the woman would find herself thinking of a bathing suit she saw the other day. All of this would happen without the woman being aware of it, since *all defense mechanisms operate unconsciously.* Some other defense mechanisms are listed in Table 2–1. By understanding the various defense mechanisms, the occupational therapy assistant can often identify why a patient is behaving a certain way and can figure out how to approach him.

Most mental operations, like defense mechanisms, operate unconsciously. Even so, they may dominate behavior. The conflicting demands of the id and superego create anxiety, which the ego attempts to control, usually by unconscious defense mechanisms. Sometimes the ego consciously tries to control the anxiety, through *suppression,* but whether conscious or unconscious defenses are used, occasionally the ego is completely overwhelmed and unable to resolve the conflict. According to object relations theory, the extreme anxiety that results can cause a breakdown of ego functions—in other words, mental illness. *Mental illness occurs when the ego is unable to achieve a successful compromise between the id, the superego, and the demands of reality.* In mental illness, a person's behavior is dominated by tremendous anxiety and

TABLE 2–1. *Selected defense mechanisms*

Defense mechanism	Definition	Example
Denial	Refusing to believe something that causes anxiety.	A mother plans for her retarded child to be a doctor.
Projection	Believing that an unacceptable feeling of one's own belongs to someone else.	A self-isolating patient in a work group says that other patients won't talk to him.
Rationalization	Making excuses for unacceptable behavior or feelings.	A teenager says he didn't do his homework because he didn't have the right kind of paper.
Conversion	Conflicts are turned into physical symptoms. The symptoms are real.	An uncoordinated girl gets a migraine headache when it is time for volleyball.
Regression	Functioning at a more primitive developmental level than previously; going back to a more immature pattern of behavior.	A seven year-old child, hospitalized for major surgery, begins to walk on tiptoes and suck his thumb.
Undoing	Trying to reverse the effects of what one has done by doing the opposite.	A patient accuses the therapist of trying to run his life. Later he brings her flowers.
Idealization	Overestimating someone, or valuing them more than their real personalities and persons seem to merit.	A woman says that the group leader is the most handsome and most kind man in the world.
Identification	Adopting the habits or characteristics of another person.	A teenaged girl begins to wear her hair just like the therapist's.
Sublimation	Unacceptable wishes are channelled into socially acceptable activities.	A child who wants to cut things up to see how they work grows up to become a surgeon.
Substitution	A realistic goal or object is substituted for one which cannot be achieved.	A young man fails the exam for the police department, then takes a job as a security guard.
Compensation	Efforts to make up for personal deficits. (This can also be a conscious effort.)	A woman, blind from birth, learns to travel without a cane or any other aid.

NOTE: All defense mechanisms operate unconsciously, and should not be confused with other mental mechanisms (such as suppression) which are conscious.

by unconscious processes that are out of control.

The fact that mental illness is caused by processes that are unconscious creates problems for therapists. How do you help someone deal with something he is not even aware of? Object relations theory says that in order to change a patient's mental illness the therapist must bring unconscious conflicts to consciousness, and make the patient aware of them. Freud discovered that the *analysis of symbols* in patients' dreams provided clues to their unconscious feelings, and that by talking with patients about their dreams he could sometimes make them conscious of these feelings. Once this consciousness was achieved, Freud believed the symptoms would be relieved.

Analysis of symbols relies on the fact that many symbols are shared by most people, at least in a particular culture. A symbol is something that stands for something else. Some examples of symbols in American culture are the Statue of Liberty, which symbolizes freedom, and the color red, which symbolizes passion or anger. The color red in Chinese culture, however, symbolizes weddings and celebrations, and the color white (which in Western culture symbolizes purity and is used for weddings) is associated with death. Some symbols are believed to be universal to all cultures; the circle, for example, symbolizes unity.

In object relations theory many different symbols are used as keys to the meaning of the unconscious conflicts we experience. For example, food symbolizes the relationship with the mother, who is the first object to satisfy the hunger need. Thus, in our minds, food is often involved with the issues of love and trust. Most of us occasionally overeat, even when we are not hungry. Because food symbolizes comfort and mother love, overeating may be a symbolic way to meet our unconscious needs for love and comfort.

Occupational therapists who follow object relations theory use symbols that can be experienced in arts and crafts and every-

day activities (7). As an example, ceramics can provide an opportunity to explore issues of self-control versus control by others. Because wet clay is so similar to feces in color and texture, it can symbolize the anal period, during which the child learns to control his bowels (and to cooperate with his parents by controlling himself). People have very different reactions to ceramics. Some cannot wait to handle the clay; others shrink back and may try to avoid the activity altogether, as the following situation illustrates:

> The occupational therapist is working alone with a 35-year-old woman, Paula, in the ceramics shop. Paula is rolling out small beads, measuring each against the others. She avoids touching the clay with her hands, using tools and plastic gloves instead. When she finishes with each bead she places it neatly in line with the others.
> The therapist comments, "The beads are very neat and precise."
> Paula answers, "They have to match."
> "Why is that?"
> "It would look like a mess if they didn't."
> The therapist thinks for a few seconds and then responds, "I have seen some necklaces with beads of all different sizes."
> "People who wear those are slobs."
> "Oh?"
> "They don't care about doing things right. . . ."

As this brief dialogue illustrates, there are many ways in which someone can relate to a symbol. A patient's behavior toward an activity may reveal her attitudes and feelings about issues that that activity symbolizes. Because people have their own personal histories, they may also have individual or *idiosyncratic* symbols that are theirs alone. For example, beads may mean something to Paula, because of some previous experience of hers, and although clay is a powerful symbol of anal issues, it may not mean this to everyone, and it has many other uses in occupational therapy.

For a therapist to use the object relations approach successfully, he or she must have an understanding of the theories behind it. This requires years of study and communication with a supervisor who knows the theory well. By focusing on the unconscious meaning of symbols in activities, object relations theory suggests that patients do not need to develop conscious real-life skills. Many occupational therapists feel it has limited usefulness for this reason. In addition, because this approach attempts to analyze and change unconscious processes, it can take a very long time. Consequently, it has been used most often in long-term settings, where patients are expected to remain in treatment for many years. Such settings are rare today.

Kielhofner (9) argues that object relations is inadequate as a basis for practice in psychiatric occupational therapy, as it ignores the essential therapeutic value of individually chosen productive activity, and instead exploits the symbolic elements of activities that are not linked to functional participation in real life. Despite these defects, object relations theory provides a structure for thinking about how the mind works. It is widely studied and used today by other professionals working with psychiatric patients, and for this reason should be known by occupational therapy assistants working in mental health.

◆ Summary of Concepts

1. Humans are born with drives for self-preservation and pleasure. These drives reside in the *id,* the most primitive and childish part of the personality.
2. Children develop control over the id drives by learning the moral standards of society from their parents. These standards become the *superego,* a second part of the personality.
3. The id and the superego often conflict with each other because they desire different things: The id wants to satisfy its own needs, and the superego wants to "follow the rules." Beyond this, reality may not permit either desire to be satisfied, adding to the conflict.
4. The *ego* is a third part of the personality, which attempts to resolve the conflicting demands of the id, the superego, and reality. It does this through ego functions such as memory, perception, reality testing, and defense mechanisms.
5. The id, ego, and superego operate unconsciously. We are not normally aware of their functioning.
6. When the ego cannot resolve unconscious conflict, anxiety becomes overwhelming and ego functions cannot operate normally. This breakdown of ego functions is recognized as mental illness.
7. Ego functions can be strengthened or restored if the patient can become conscious of the unconscious conflict that is causing the anxiety.
8. One method of identifying unconscious processes is by the analysis of symbols.

Vocabulary

Id   The part of the personality that contains the drives toward self-preservation and pleasure. The id is present from birth (or before) and operates unconsciously.

Object   Anything toward which the id directs its energies in order to satisfy a drive. Objects may be human (people) or nonhuman (things).

Superego   The part of the personality that contains standards for behavior. The superego is thought to be a representation of rules learned from parents and other authorities. The superego operates unconsciously.

Ego   The part of the personality that regulates behavior by compromising between the demands of the id and the superego and reality. The ego contains many functions, such as memory, perception, reality testing, and defense mechanisms. These work together in a continuous process of adapting to reality. Many ego functions operate unconsciously.

Reality testing The ability to tell the difference between reality and fantasy, and to share the same general ideas about reality as everyone else. Reality testing is an ego function.

Defense mechanism Any of several methods used by the ego to control anxiety and conflict. All defense mechanisms operate unconsciously (see Table 2–1).

Conscious Mental functions of which we are aware. Suppression is one example.

Unconscious Mental functions of which we normally are not aware. These include the id, the superego, and the defense mechanisms.

Conflict Opposition between simultaneous demands, such as those of the id and the superego, or of the self and of reality.

Anxiety An uncomfortable feeling of tension that may arise from unconscious conflict.

Symbol Something that represents something else. Symbols may be universal, cultural, or idiosyncratic.

Analysis of symbols One of the methods used in object relations therapy. The therapist analyzes symbols in the patient's dreams or artwork in order to discover their unconscious meanings.

Suppression An attempt to control anxiety and conflict by *consciously* controlling or denying it. Suppression is conscious, unlike the defense mechanisms, but it may serve the same purpose with regard to anxiety.

DEVELOPMENTAL THEORY

There are several versions of developmental theory. The best known are those of Erikson, Piaget, and Gesell. In this section we will explore Erikson's theory of psychosocial development, but first we need to outline the main concepts common to all developmental theories.

The first of these is that *a person matures through a series of stages, which occur in a fixed sequence.* At each stage the individual encounters specific *developmental tasks,* which when mastered serve as a foundation for later development. For example, a child learns to stand before learning to walk. The standing stage must come before the walking stage. Physical, social, and intellectual growth all occur simultaneously, but in a fixed sequence in each area. In other words, a child can develop social skills at the same time that she is learning to walk, but she cannot walk before she stands. In the normal growth process, development is gradual and spontaneous and results (after a number of years) in a mature and functional adult.

However, many factors can interrupt the growth process. Physical disease, poverty, malnutrition, trauma, or emotional or social deprivation can keep a person from mastering the developmental tasks of a particular stage. When this happens, a *developmental lag* may result. A developmental lag is a discrepancy (difference) between a person's behavior and the behavior one would expect of a typical individual of that age. In other words, a person who has a developmental lag has fallen behind in development, and is not as mature as his or her peers.

Take, for example, the case of David:

David is a 29-year-old man who has attended several different colleges, majoring in a variety of subjects, but never graduating. He has had a succession of jobs that seem unrelated to each other: dishwasher, produce clerk, busboy, crewman on a sailboat, handyman, horse groomer, waiter, messenger, house painter. David has acquired a lot of skills over the years but knows that he doesn't "stick to anything," and he doesn't know what to do about it. He sees that friends his own age are establishing themselves in careers, and settling down with marriage and family life. David feels increasingly distant from his friends. He is extremely depressed and has twice attempted suicide.

A therapist using Erikson's theory of psychosocial development would first analyze where David was lagging in development.

According to Erikson, at around three years of age, the child enters a developmental stage termed *initiative versus guilt*. In this stage, the developmental task is for the child to establish a sense of purpose and direction (initiative) in his activities. The child experiences a feeling of pleasure and power at his own ability to affect the world around him. This stage lays a foundation for setting goals and working toward their accomplishment in later life, but this can happen only if the child is permitted to follow his own direction.

However, the child's direction may be unacceptable to the parents, who may have their own ideas about what the child should be doing. For example, in reviewing David's history, the therapist discovered that David's parents pushed him to read at an early age, and constantly compared him to his older brother (who could read at age two and a half). David was an active child and good at sports and games, but his parents discouraged these interests and stressed reading as the preferred activity.

Because David was not permitted to pursue his own interests as a child, his sense of purpose (initiative) remained confused and vague. Later, during adolescence, this confusion was reactivated when he attempted to choose a career. Because he had little previous experience in setting his own direction and following it through to success, he was unsure of himself, uncertain of his direction and of how to proceed. This pattern repeated itself over the years. For example, David felt guilty when he enjoyed crewing on the sailboat; he thought he should be doing something "more important" with his life and went back to college, but dropped out after one semester.

According to Erikson's theory, mental health problems occur when developmental tasks are not successfully mastered. Failure at one stage of development does not prevent the person from continuing to develop, but problems may result because the foundation is weak. To help a person who has problems because of a developmental lag, the therapist designs situations that will facilitate growth in the deficient area. In other words, if a person has failed to develop adequately in a given area, the therapist can make it easier for the development to occur by creating conditions that encourage growth. For example, in David's case an occupational therapist might expose David to a variety of activities that fit his skills and interests. She would help him to choose and get involved in an activity that needs fairly consistent effort over a fairly long period of time (for example, woodworking). The therapist would encourage David when he became disheartened and would try to sustain his interest in the activity (by showing him new challenges or problems to solve). She might help him find new ways to use his skills, by producing objects for sale or by having him instruct others. She would have to be careful not to push him too hard; after all, it's *his* sense of purpose that needs developing, not hers.

This example has focused on one of the eight stages of psychosocial development proposed in Erikson's theory. The word psychosocial refers to the interaction between the self (*psyche*) and society, an interaction that Erikson believed was the core of successful human functioning. Table 2–2 defines and illustrates these eight stages. Erikson suggested that each stage is organized around a central crisis, which has two possible but totally opposite resolutions. For example, the crisis of purpose and self-direction can be resolved as either *initiative* or *guilt*. Erikson argues that a continuum of resolutions exists between these two extremes at any stage, and cautions students not to think of the outcome in good/bad, either/or terms. He also notes that human development is continuous, and that any individual facing a problem in the present must rely on the interconnected matrix or network of feelings about earlier developmental events. When a new crisis arises, a person may regress and reexperi-

TABLE 2–2. *Erikson's eight stages of psychosocial development*

Approximate age	Psychosocial stage	Explanation
Birth–18 months	BASIC TRUST versus MISTRUST	The infant needs nurturance from the mother. If he perceives her as reliable, he will develop the capacity to trust others. If not, he will tend to mistrust others, will feel anxious about their willingness to meet his needs, etc.
Two–four years	AUTONOMY versus SHAME AND DOUBT	During this period the child learns to control his bowel and bladder, and becomes more independent in exploring the environment. The child's sense of motivation and will are shaped by the parents' attitudes toward bodily functions and their willingness to allow the child to control himself.
Three–five years	INITIATIVE versus GUILT	The preschool and kindergarten child begins to combine his skills and plan activities to accomplish goals. He begins to imitate adult roles and to try out new ways of doing things. He develops a sense of self-direction.
Six–twelve years	INDUSTRY versus INFERIORITY	During elementary school the child acquires skills and work habits. He compares himself to his peers. Attitudes of parents, teachers, and other children contribute to his sense of his own competence.
Adolescence	IDENTITY versus ROLE CONFUSION	The adolescent experiments with a variety of adult roles. Key issues include vocational choice and gender identification. Rebellion against parents is common, as teenagers try to assert a separate identity.
Young adulthood	INTIMACY versus ISOLATION	The central concern of this period is to find a suitable partner with whom to share one's life.
Middle adulthood	GENERATIVITY versus STAGNATION	The adult looks toward the future and tries to make a contribution to it through work, community leadership, child rearing, etc.
Old age	EGO INTEGRITY versus DESPAIR	Faced with the prospect of death, the older adult reviews and evaluates his life's choices to see if he has done what he meant to do.

ence the conflicts of earlier developmental stages.

Erikson's (and other) developmental theories are consistent with many of the basic ideas of occupational therapy. The concept of gradation, of learning through successively more difficult stages, and the focus on solving problems and acquiring skills make developmental theory an appealing choice for working with patients who have poor social relationships and inadequate skills (24). Similarly, occupational thera-pists have long attempted to meet the patient at his own level, matching tasks to current abilities and interests.

There are three drawbacks to this approach, however. The first is that many psychiatric patients (for example, those diagnosed with chronic schizophrenia) appear to lag in the earliest stage of psychosocial development; they have always had problems trusting others, as their histories show. Attempting to change fundamental and lifelong mistrust is quite a challenge.

Second, like approaches based on object relations theory (which itself has a developmental orientation),[2] application of developmental theory to treatment is possible only in a long-term setting, since developmental change is a gradual process. Third, human development involves many complex and interrelated issues that can be understood only through rigorous study, and therapists must be exceptionally well trained to use developmental theory well. One model used in psychiatric occupational therapy that is related to developmental theory is *development of adaptive skills*. This practice model is described in Chapter 3.

◆ Summary of Concepts

1. Human beings mature through a series of stages, which occur in a fixed sequence. Specific developmental tasks arise at each stage; the individual's experience with these tasks serves as a foundation for later development.
2. Problems occur when developmental tasks are not mastered sufficiently well. This causes a lag in development, which can interfere with a person's attempts to master other developmental tasks in future stages.
3. A developmental lag can be corrected by exposing the person to a situation that will encourage his or her growth in the deficient area. If the proper conditions are created, and the therapist provides corrective guidance, the developmental task can be mastered.

Vocabulary

Development A process of maturation occurring throughout the life span.

---

[2]The alert reader may have noticed that Erikson's developmental theoery is in some respects similar to object relations theory. Erikson's training and background were psychoanalytic, and therefore much of his work is based on the writings of Freud. Freud's work focused on psychosexual rather than psychosocial development.

Developmental stage A specific level of development, generally believed to occur at a specific time in a human being's life span. Different developmental psychologists postulate different theories, each containing a number of developmental stages. Erikson proposed eight stages of psychosocial development. Piaget proposed four stages of cognitive development. Regardless of the particular theory, the stages always occur in a fixed sequence.

Developmental task A problem or crisis that arises during a developmental stage. Solving the problem shows mastery of the task. An example is choosing a career, traditionally a developmental task of adolescence.

Developmental lag A delay in development, demonstrated by failure to master a developmental task.

Psychosocial development The ongoing process in which the individual resolves conflicts between his own needs and what society demands and permits.

BEHAVIORAL THEORIES

The behavioral theories are derived from the work of Pavlov, a Russian physiologist who experimented with dogs, and Skinner, an American psychologist who studied how animals responded to stimulation. The central concept of these theories is that all behavior is learned. *Behaviors that have pleasurable results tend to be repeated.* For example:

> You are in a new class. The professor says something you do not understand, so you ask a question. He says he is glad you asked that question, and gives you an answer that helps you understand. The next time you have a question, you raise your hand.

It seems almost common sense that people will repeat actions that result in pleasure or rewards. Imagine what might happen if the professor had given a confusing answer or had in some way made you feel embarrassed for asking the question. You might feel that you should never ask another question. This illustrates a complementary concept: that *actions that have negative or unpleasant consequences tend not to be repeated.*

According to behavioral theories, each person develops through a process of learning from the results of his behavior. If adaptive behaviors are rewarded, and maladaptive behaviors punished or ignored, then the result should be a mature and responsible human being. Sometimes, however, the wrong behaviors are learned. Mental illness, in this theory, is defined as abnormal behavior that results because normal (or adaptive) behavior was not rewarded, or did not have pleasurable consequences. In some cases, abnormal behavior occurs because maladaptive behavior was reinforced.

As an example, take the case of a two-year-old child who screams and cries when his mother goes out for an evening. Every time he cries, the babysitter gives him a piece of candy. The undesirable behavior (screaming) has had a pleasurable consequence (candy). Very quickly the child will learn that screaming is an effective way of getting candy. In later life he may carry on the pattern, screaming at other people to get what he wants.

Occupational therapists have used a variety of techniques based on behavioral theory. Sometimes this is called an *action-consequence* approach because the therapist tries to change the patient's behavior (action) by changing the consequences of the behavior. The therapist might reward new adaptive behaviors or ignore or punish the maladaptive behavior. Some therapists use both methods. An example might be the case of Eric, who repeatedly interrupts while the therapist is working with other patients. He constantly asks for her opinion of his project. Using the action-consequence approach, the therapist might tell

him that she wants him to work on his own for five minutes, and then she will talk to him. During the five-minute work period she will ignore his disruptive behavior, but after this she will "reward" him with some time and attention.

Identification of terminal behavior is the first step in a behavioral treatment program. Terminal behavior is the normal or adaptive behavior that the therapist wants the patient to perform. In the case of Eric this might be "working on his own for one half hour." Once the terminal behavior has been identified, the therapist determines a baseline by counting and recording the patient's behavior. For example, she might count how often Eric tries to interrupt her during a half-hour period. The baseline is a record of how the patient behaved before the treatment was started.

Next, the therapist selects a reinforcement. Reinforcement is the name given to the therapist's response (consequence) to the client's performance of the desired behavior (action). In Eric's case, the therapist already knows that attention from her will be a good reinforcement. The therapist then decides how often the reinforcement will be given (this is called the *schedule*). The therapist might decide to reward Eric every time he works for five minutes without interrupting her. This would be a continuous schedule of reinforcement, because a reward is given every time the action is performed. Usually *continuous schedules* are used at the beginning of treatment, when the therapist is trying to get the patient to do the desired action. Later, when the behavior is established, the reinforcement might be scheduled intermittently, not every time the action is performed but only now and then. *Intermittent schedules* are believed to be more effective than continuous schedules once the behavior has been learned.

Often the terminal behavior seems very far from the way the patient is acting now. For example, for Eric to sit still and work by himself for a half hour seems like a distant goal. To help Eric reach it, the therapist might use *shaping*. Shaping is a method of working toward a terminal behavior through successive approximations, or small steps. In Eric's case, the therapist might start by expecting him to work on his own for five minutes, at the end of which time she would talk to him. Once the five-minute period of independent work has been established, it would be extended to ten minutes. Then Eric would have to work for ten minutes in order to be rewarded. Gradually the half-hour goal would be reached through a series of steps or approximations, each one closer to the goal than the one before.

When the terminal behavior involves learning a complicated routine with several steps, the technique of *chaining* can be used. Chaining is teaching a multistep activity one step at a time. The patient does the steps he knows, and the therapist does the rest. Gradually the patient learns the whole activity. Chaining can begin with the first step (*forward chaining*) or the last step (*backward chaining*). An example of backward chaining is having a patient fold the laundry (last step) that the therapist has washed. Once he learned folding, the patient would learn how to use the dryer. Gradually, by working backward in this way, he would learn the entire sequence of washing clothes. Mentally retarded adults appear to learn faster with backward chaining than forward chaining (21), and it is likely that other people would too.

Occupational therapists have used behavioral techniques to treat hyperactive (3) and severely mentally retarded (22) children, among others. Unlike therapies based on object relations or developmental concepts, behavioral therapies give quick results, as the following example of a hyperactive child described by Cermak et al. (3) illustrates:

Tom . . . spent a great deal of time lying on the floor kicking his legs and thrashing around. His behavior was disruptive to the group. In the classroom this conduct disturbed the other children and made it dif-ficult for Tom to sit long enough to finish his schoolwork. The therapists decided to give him the attention he wanted. When he was sitting on the bench, the leader or another member of the group sat next to him and put their arm around him. Surprisingly, after one play session of being on the floor 30 times, Tom was on the floor only twice the next session. (3, p. 315)

Like most human efforts, behavior modification programs are only as effective as the thinking and planning that go into them (13). Table 2–3 shows the steps in designing a behavioral treatment program in occupational therapy, as identified by Sieg (16), and gives examples. Sieg's model is a strictly behavioral one. Occupational therapy treatment approaches based on modified behavioral concepts include Mosey's *activities therapy* (12) and the use of social skills training (2). Because these approaches are so widely used today they will be discussed in more detail in the section on "Acquisition of Skills and Social Skills Training" in Chapter 3.

Behavior therapies have been criticized for treating people like machines and for using unhealthy reinforcers (such as candy, coffee, and cigarettes) and aversive reinforcement (punishment). While the idea that people will respond the way a therapist "programs" them to is repugnant, it is also unrealistic. Therapists who set goals with, rather than for, their patients, and who explain the treatment program to them can hardly be accused of taking a mechanistic view. Although therapists at times use unhealthy reinforcers to get chronic patients to respond, other rewards (such as weekend passes and other privileges) are selected wherever possible. Finally, therapists do not use punishment unless there is no other way to stop a patient from harming himself.

In summary, behavioral theories consist of a group of approaches that have in common the idea that people learn from the consequences of their behavior. Understanding how people learn is important to occupational therapists who want to help

TABLE 2–3. *Steps in a behavioral treatment program*

Step	Example
1. Identify the terminal behavior.	The therapist and patient select the treatment goal: Jim will initiate conversation with another patient at least twice in each four-hour work session.
2. Determine the baseline by counting the frequency of the behavior.	Prior to the beginning of treatment, the therapist records how often Jim starts a conversation with another patient during the group. Baseline data is collected over several sessions.
3. Select a method of counting and recording the behavior.	The therapist will note each time Jim starts a conversation and write it on a chart. Jim will check the chart each day to verify that it is correct.
4. Select a reinforcer that is meaningful to the patient.	Jim likes to sit in the hospital coffee shop and drink coffee. The therapist decides that he will be given tokens to use for this.
5. Determine a schedule of reinforcement.	A continuous schedule will help Jim develop the new behavior quickly. The therapist will give him a token every day he shows the desired behavior.

Adapted from Sieg KW. Applying the behavioral model to the occupational therapy model. *Am J Occup Ther* 1974; 28:421–428. Copyright 1974 by the American Occupational Therapy Association, Inc. Reprinted with permission.

patients get rid of maladaptive behaviors and acquire new skills.

◆ Summary of Concepts

1. All behavior is learned.
2. Those actions that have had pleasurable consequences tend to be repeated.
3. Normal behavior is learned if adaptive behaviors are rewarded and maladaptive behaviors are punished or ignored.
4. Abnormal behavior is learned if adaptive behavior is not rewarded or maladaptive behavior is reinforced.
5. Abnormal behavior can be changed if the therapist changes the consequences of the behavior.

Vocabulary

Behavior   Any observable action.

Reinforcement   Consequences of behavior that either encourage or discourage the repetition of the behavior.

Terminal behavior   The treatment goal, the behavior the patient will show at the end of a successful treatment program.

Shaping   A method of approaching the terminal behavior gradually, using a series of steps (successive approximations) that lead to the goal.

Chaining   A method of teaching a complex activity a step at a time, starting with either the first or the last step. The therapist performs the remaining steps until the patient masters the entire sequence.

Backward chaining   Chaining that starts with the last step. This is believed to be more effective than forward chaining.

Forward chaining   Chaining that starts with the first step.

Schedule of reinforcement   The timing of reinforcement. Schedules may be continuous (reinforcement follows every performance of the desired behavior) or intermittent (reinforcement is given only occasionally).

Extinction   Discouraging an undesired behavior by removing any reinforcement.

An example might be a therapist's ignoring a child's temper tantrum instead of responding to it. This is called "planned ignoring."

CLIENT-CENTERED THERAPY

One of several humanistic therapies, client-centered therapy was developed by the psychologist Carl Rogers. Humanistic therapies are concerned with the individual's view of life, and with helping each person find satisfaction in the way that makes most sense to him. Rogers used the word *client,* which conveys a greater sense of self-determination than *patient,* which implies a dependent role within a medical relationship. He believed that the client's personal development is best fostered by a relationship with a warm, nondirective therapist who accepts the patient on his own terms.

A central concept of client-centered therapy is that each human being has within himself the potential for directing his own growth and development. No matter how psychotic or disorganized his behavior may appear, the client is capable of understanding himself and ultimately of changing his behavior.

Another concept is that each person directs his own life. The therapist does not tell the client what to do; the client must choose for himself. By being *nondirective,* the therapist allows the client to take his own direction. The therapist does help the client, however, by making the client more aware of his own feelings, and by helping him explore the possible consequences of contemplated action. Rogers believes that only when the client is aware of how he feels, and of what is likely to happen, is he truly free to choose what to do (15).

For example, a high school student may plan to go to college because that is what his family expects him to do, even though he is really confused and not particularly interested in college. He has suppressed these feelings and is not really aware of them. A client-centered therapist would listen to him and reflect back the hidden feelings that he hears. The student, now aware of the feelings, would be more free to choose not to go to college, or at least to explore other alternatives.

A third and related concept is that mental health problems occur when a person is not aware of his feelings and of the choices available to him. In other words, if a person does not know how he feels about the people and events in his life, he is likely to act in a disorganized, confused, or maladaptive way.

A fourth concept is that a person can become more aware of his feelings and choices by experiencing them in a relationship with a therapist who genuinely accepts himself and the client. The therapist must be aware of his own feelings and attitudes and be comfortable expressing them. He must be able to provide *unconditional positive regard;* that is, he must continue to like the client no matter what the client does. By accepting the client as he is, no matter how bizarre his attitudes or behaviors, the therapist helps him accept himself. Gradually the client's perception of himself changes, and his behavior becomes more organized and more consistent with his feelings. He adapts better to new situations; in short, his mental health improves.

The client's relationship with a warm, empathic therapist is the key to the client-centered approach. Client-centered therapists use several techniques that facilitate the client's awareness and expression of his feelings. Because occupational therapists use some of these techniques when interviewing and conversing with patients, five will be discussed here (8).

One technique is the *open invitation to talk.* This invitation to talk is conveyed through the use of *open questions.* Open questions are designed to require more than a one-word answer. They encourage the client to talk freely and at length. Some examples are:

> "What were your feelings when that happened?"
> "Tell me about your family."

The opposite would be *closed questions,* such as "Are you married?" or "Were you angry when that happened?" Closed questions require only one- or two-word answers and limit self-expression because the person is likely to stop after that; they are not a client-centered technique. Sometimes closed questions are the quickest way to get specific details from a client, but they have little therapeutic value beyond this.

A second technique used by client-centered therapists is the *minimal response,* which shows that the therapist is listening to the client, and that he wants him to go on talking. Some examples are nodding the head, or saying "uh-huh" or "go on." These responses let the client know that the therapist is tuned in to what he is saying.

A third technique is *reflection of feeling.* Through this technique the therapist puts the client's feelings into words and helps him experience the emotional content of what he is saying. For example:

> *Client:* My husband doesn't mean anything by it, by the things he does that, well, you know. (Client looks down to her hands and sighs deeply.) It's just that I feel a certain way that he can't see. Maybe he doesn't want to. But he's really too busy with his work and everything. He works so hard.

> *Therapist:* You're sad that your husband is too busy to see how you feel. You feel that maybe he works so hard so that he doesn't have to see.

Just as reflection of feeling focuses on the emotional aspect of the client's words, a fourth technique focuses on the narrative content or story. Using *paraphrasing,* the therapist restates in different words what the client has said. This lets the client know that the therapist has been listening, and helps the therapist check out whether he

really understood what the client meant. As an example:

> *Client:* So then Jack said he would take care of it, but he never did. You'd think he would do what he said, but no. So *I* had to take time off from work to go to Con Edison and pay the bill.

> *Therapist:* Because Jack was so unreliable you had to lose time from work.

Paraphrasing can help the therapist sort out what the client has been saying, which is particularly valuable when the client speaks for a long time or in a disorganized fashion.

A fifth technique is *withholding judgment.* The therapist refrains from giving an opinion about the client's remarks or behaviors. Sometimes this is difficult to effect, since clients look to the therapist for advice, praise, approval, or rejection. The following is an example:

> *Client:* My mother says I dress too sexy, that's why I have so much trouble. It's none of her business. My clothes are okay, don't you think?

> *Therapist:* What do you think?

Here the therapist is not only withholding judgment, but is also encouraging the client to evaluate the situation herself. If the therapist had said, "Your clothes are okay," or "You dress nicely," or "Maybe your mother has a point there," the client might react to the comment instead of thinking out the problem on her own. The therapist is letting her know that she has to decide for herself.

All five of the techniques described are derived from ones used in object relations therapy. Like object relations therapy, client-centered therapy takes a long time to complete and is most practical in long-term treatment. Client-centered therapy, because it relies on the client's ability to direct himself, seems unrealistic for severely mentally disabled patients, who are often nonverbal and seemingly incapable of making even simple decisions. This issue is at the heart of the debate over the use of the word *client* in occupational therapy practice and literature. Sharrott and Yerxa (17) argue that a client would be capable of choosing and securing occupational therapy services for himself; in contrast, many of the persons served by occupational therapy are so disabled that they are incapable of acting in their own best interests, and for that reason should be called patients.

Despite these criticisms, although it is unusual for an occupational therapist to embrace the entirety of client-centered therapy, psychiatric occupational therapists continue to use client-centered techniques. Client-centered techniques are effective for getting patients to express themselves and for establishing a solid therapeutic relationship. They are often combined with other approaches, such as behavioral techniques, which may give faster results in changing a patient's behavior (4).

Chapter 10, on the therapeutic use of self, describes and illustrates further how Rogers' techniques can be applied by the occupational therapy assistant.

◆ Summary of Concepts

1. Each human being has the potential to direct his own growth and development.
2. Each person is free to choose his own course of action.
3. Mental health problems can occur when a person is not aware of his feelings and of the choices available to him.
4. A person can become more aware of his feelings and choices by experiencing them in a relationship with a warm, empathic therapist who genuinely accepts himself and the client.

Vocabulary

Empathy Understanding the feelings and actions of another person. This is contrasted with sympathy, which includes a sense of *feeling* what the other feels.

Warmth A sense, conveyed by the therapist, that he feels concerned about the patient's well-being.

Genuineness A sense, conveyed by the therapist, that he is really the way he appears, and is not just putting on an act for the patient's benefit.

Unconditional positive regard A sense, conveyed by the therapist, that he accepts, likes, and respects the patient regardless of the patient's feelings or actions.

Nondirective behavior A behavior of the therapist in which he refrains from giving an opinion on anything the patient says or does.

Open invitation to talk An interviewing technique in which questions are worded to require a response longer than one or two words. This encourages the client to talk.

Minimal response A brief verbal or nonverbal action of the therapist, which gives the message that he is listening and wants the client to keep talking. Examples are nodding, saying "go on," and leaning forward in the chair.

Reflection of feeling The therapist's restatement of the *feeling* conveyed by the client's words or nonverbal expression.

Paraphrasing The therapist's restatement of the *story* or narrative content conveyed by the client's words.

Withholding judgment The therapist's deliberate abstinence from giving opinions on the client's behavior, feelings, or intention.

NEUROSCIENTIFIC THEORIES

Neuroscience refers to the entire body of information about the nervous system, what it looks like and how it operates. Understanding neuroscience theories requires knowledge of the anatomy and physiology of the nervous system, content not usually covered in depth in occupational therapy assistant programs. However, since the

COTA may someday find himself working on a psychiatric research unit, and because some students may be curious, we will discuss them briefly.

It is fascinating to speculate that our mental and emotional experience results from physical, biological, and chemical events in the brain. Freud himself explored this possibility during his earliest years in medicine, when he worked on the neuroanatomy of the medulla (23). Research since that time has demonstrated many associations between behavior and brain activity. The central concept of the neuroscience theories is that the phenomena we think of as mind and emotion are explained by biochemical and electrical activity in the brain.

Neuroscience theories are based on the assumption that normal human functioning is possible only when brain chemicals are present in the proper proportions. In addition, the organ of mind and emotion, the brain itself, must be anatomically normal. Neuroscientists believe that many kinds of mental illness can be accounted for by variations from these normal conditions. Some examples are Meltzer's (11) theory of a dopamine mechanism in schizophrenia and Tsai's (20) study showing hemispheric asymmetry in the brains of schizophrenics.

Since neuroscience assumes that mental illness is caused by a bodily defect, logic tells us that treatment must be directed at the body. Treatment of mental illness, according to the neuroscience model, involves changing the abnormal *somatic* (bodily) conditions through somatic intervention. These interventions include chemotherapy (drugs) and psychosurgery, as well as electroconvulsive therapy (ECT). Despite their negative side effects, drugs have been useful in controlling psychotic and affective (mood) symptoms that might otherwise prevent patients from participating in verbal and activity therapies. Psychosurgery (stereotactic and laser surgery on the brain) has been used successfully to stop abnormal rage in patients with temporal lobe epilepsy. Finally, ECT (sometimes incorrectly called "shock treatment") is effective in reversing extreme suicidal depressions that fail to respond to drugs. All of these treatments were discovered felicitously (by accident) and were used for years with little understanding of how they worked; one of the major contributions of recent neuroscience has been to demonstrate some of the mechanisms behind them (19).

Only physicians can prescribe drugs, surgery, and ECT. The role of occupational therapy in the neuroscience approach traditionally has been to monitor the effects on functional performance of the somatic treatments prescribed by the physician. By observing how the patient performs in activities, the occupational therapist or assistant can collect information to help the doctor determine the diagnosis, and later to decide if the treatment is working and if it needs to be increased or decreased. Occupational therapy personnel also help patients adjust their approach to activities to cope with the side effects of drugs and ECT (18). This topic will be discussed in Chapter 8.

Among the exciting new hypotheses in neuroscience are those relating to *neuroimmunomodulation* (6). It is proposed that an interaction among the neurological system, the immune system, and the endocrine system regulates the immune response of the body. Research evidence in support of this idea comes from work with long-term AIDS survivors and others with potentially fatal disorders. Farber (6) suggests that occupational therapy may have a role in strengthening the immune response by reducing helplessness and hopelessness and helping the patient establish positive attitudes.

Two occupational therapy treatment approaches have ties to neuroscience theory. One is Lorna Jean King's sensory integration approach to the treatment of schizophrenia, and the other is Claudia Allen's theory of cognitive disabilities. King (10) showed that games and postural exercises can bring about lasting changes in the sensorimotor functioning of certain types of chronic schizophrenic patients. She argued that these activities stimulate the part of the central nervous system that processes and organizes sensory information. Allen (1) proposes that the problems psychiatric patients have functioning in daily life originate in physical and chemical abnormalities of the brain. She argues that the role of occupational therapy should be to define the patient's functional level very precisely, and to modify the environment accordingly to help the patient function as best he can. She believes that occupational therapy cannot change the patient's level of function, and should instead work on adapting the environment to his disability. Both King's and Allen's approaches will be discussed further in Chapter 3.

◆ Summary of Concepts

1. All mental processes, including behavior and emotion, originate in biochemical and electrical activity in the brain.
2. Abnormal behavior and abnormal emotional states (mental illness) are caused by defects either in the anatomy or in the level of chemicals in the brain.
3. Abnormal mental conditions can be controlled by changing either the anatomy or the chemical and electrical activity of the brain. Treatments include surgery, drugs, and electroconvulsive therapy.

Vocabulary

Neurotransmitter A chemical that transmits nerve impulses from one neuron to another within the central nervous system.

Organic Referring to the structure (anatomy) of the brain, the organ of mind and emotion.

ECT Electroconvulsive therapy: a treatment in which an electrical current applied to the brain causes a brief seizure.

ECT is most often used to treat severe depression.

Chemotherapy A treatment in which chemical substances (drugs) are introduced into the body in an effort to cure a disease or control its symptoms.

Psychosurgery Surgery on the brain in which nerve fibers are cut or destroyed in order to control abnormal behavior or mood disturbances.

Neuroimmunomodulation The proposed interactive regulation of immune responses through the combined actions of the neurological, endocrine, and immune systems.

REFERENCES

1. Allen CK. *Occupational therapy for psychiatric disorders: measurement and management of cognitive disabilities.* Boston: Little, Brown; 1985.
2. Brady JP. Social skills training for psychiatric patients, I—concepts, methods, and clinical results. *Occup Ther Mental Health* 1984; 4(4): 51–68.
3. Cermak S, Stein F, Abelson C. Hyperactive children and an activity group therapy model. *Am J Occup Ther* 1973; 27:311–315.
4. Dunning RE. The occupational therapist as counselor. *Am J Occup Ther* 1973; 27:473–476.
5. Early MB. *T.A.R. introductory course workbook: occupational therapy—psychosocial dysfunction.* Long Island City, NY: LaGuardia Community College; 1981.
6. Farber SD. Neuroscience and occupational therapy: vital connections—1989 Eleanor Clarke Slagle lecture. *Am J Occup Ther* 1989; 43:637–646.
7. Fidler G, Fidler J. *Occupational therapy: a communication process in psychiatry.* New York: Macmillan; 1963.
8. Hays JS, Larson K. *Interacting with patients.* New York: Macmillan; 1963.
9. Kielhofner G. *Conceptual foundations of occupational therapy.* Philadelphia: FA Davis; 1992.
10. King LJ. A sensory-integrative approach to schizophrenia. *Am J Occup Ther* 1974; 28:529–536.
11. Meltzer HY, Stahl SM. The dopamine hypothesis of schizophrenia, a review. *Schizophrenia Bull* 1976; 2(1):19–76.
12. Mosey AC. *Activities therapy.* New York: Raven Press; 1973.
13. Norman CW. Behavior modification: a perspective. *Am J Occup Ther* 1976; 30:491–497.
14. Pavlov IP. Scientific study of so-called psychical processes in the higher animals (1906). In:

Bartlett J, ed. *Familiar quotations.* 15th ed. Boston: Little Brown; 1980:665.

15. Rogers C. *On becoming a person: a therapist's view of psychotherapy.* Boston: Houghton Mifflin; 1961.

16. Sieg KW. Applying the behavioral model to the occupational therapy model. *Am J Occup Ther* 1974; 28:421–428.

17. Sharrott GW, Yerxa EJ. The issue is . . . promises to keep: implications of the referent "patient" versus "client" for those served by occupational therapy. *Am J Occup Ther* 1985; 39:401–405.

18. Smith DA. Effects of psychotropic drugs on the occupational therapy process. *Am Occup Ther Assoc Mental Health Specialty Section Newsletter* 1981; 4:1:1–3.

19. Snyder SH. *Biological aspects of mental disorder.* New York: Oxford University Press; 1980.

20. Tsai LY, Nasrallah HA, Jacoby CG. Hemispheric asymmetries on computed tomographic scans in schizophrenia and mania. *Arch Gen Psychiatry* 1983; 140:171–175.

21. Weber NJ. Chaining strategies for teaching sequenced motor tasks to mentally retarded adults. *Am J Occup Ther* 1978; 32:385–389.

22. Wehman P, Marchant J. Improving the free play skills of severely retarded children. *Am J Occup Ther* 1978; 32:100–104.

23. Winson J. *Brain and psyche.* Garden City, NY: Anchor Press/Doubleday; 1985.

24. Zemke R, Gratz RR. The role of theory: Erikson and occupational therapy. *Occup Ther Mental Health* 1982; 2(3):45–64.

ADDITIONAL REFERENCES AND SUGGESTED READINGS

Andreasen NC. *The broken brain: the biological revolution in psychiatry.* New York: Harper and Row; 1985.

Barris R, Keilhofner G, Watts JH. *Bodies of knowledge in psychosocial practice.* Thorofare, NJ: SLACK; 1988.

Bruce MA, Borg B. *Frames of reference in psychosocial occupational therapy.* Thorofare, NJ: SLACK; 1987.

Hagedorn R. *Occupational therapy: foundations for practice—models, frames of reference and core skills.* Edinburgh: Churchill Livingstone; 1992.

Ornstein R. Thompson RF. *The amazing brain.* Boston: Houghton Mifflin; 1991.

3

Some Practice Models for Occupational Therapy in Mental Health

There are no whole truths; all truths are half truths. It is trying to treat them as whole truths that plays the devil.

ALFRED NORTH WHITEHEAD (33)

In Chapter 2 we learned about some of the many theories of how the mind works. Each theory gives us one way of looking at mental health and mental illness. We can think of theories as similar to eyeglasses with different colored lenses. The world looks different through each one, and we respond differently to what we see when we wear them. Theories are like this; when we look at a patient through the "lens" of a particular theory, we pay attention to the things that theory says are important and we ignore everything else, just as red lenses make green things prominent and make red things fade away. It can be fun trying on these different points of view, but what we must ultimately decide is which one gives us the most useful view of the patient, his problems, and how to solve them through occupational therapy. At the same time, we must appreciate that no one theory is completely sufficient, that each forces us to ignore some aspects that might be important.

Because human activity is the chief concern of occupational therapy, any theory that will be useful to occupational therapists must explain how a person's activity affects his mental health, and how his mental health affects his activity. None of the theories we discussed in Chapter 2 does a

very good job of this. Object relations theory focuses on the symbolic content of activities as a mirror of unconscious processes. Sharrott (30) and others have criticized this approach for failing to take into account the patient's conscious motivation to choose and participate in the activities of human life. Also, this approach works best with those patients who have good insight and good verbal skills—only a small fraction of the patients seen in psychiatric occupational therapy.[1] Finally, object relations and psychoanalytic theory have been criticized for being overly subjective (not suited to observable results), sexist, and unproved through research (6, 9, 12).

As an occupational therapy approach, client-centered therapy has been criticized for being a "talking" therapy and not a "doing" therapy, for lacking the activity core on which occupational therapy is based. Similar to and derived from psychoanalytic therapy, client-centered therapy also works best with patients who are articulate and whose cognitive functions

---

[1]For further discussion of this point, see p. 79 of Bruce MA, Borg B. *Frames of reference in psychosocial occupational therapy.* Thorofare, NJ: SLACK; 1987.

are not greatly disturbed. Thus, it can be applied effectively to only a few of the patients seen in occupational therapy mental health practice (6, 12).

Like client-centered therapy, developmental theories (such as Erikson's) used in mental health are derived from psychoanalytic foundations. They emphasize social and sexual development. Because some of these theories address the development of the motivation, skills, habits, and attitudes that enable full participation in occupation and activity, occupational therapists have used developmental concepts in their practice. Later in this chapter we will look at this more closely, with Mosey's model for development of adaptive skills.

Although the behavioral approach has been used extensively in occupational therapy, primarily with the developmentally disabled and cognitively impaired, it focuses on learning as a consequence of external rewards. In this, behaviorism conflicts with one of the central values of occupational therapy—the internal reward implicit in the intrinsic motivation for activity. Behaviorism has also been criticized for being superficial and for failing to establish permanent changes in behavior (6, 9). Nonetheless, many of the techniques used in behavioral approaches (role modeling, shaping, chaining) have been applied successfully by occupational therapists. We will consider these later in the chapter when we look at social skills training and Mosey's role acquisition model.

Neuroscience theories focus on brain anatomy and chemistry. There is much to be learned about the effects of the brain's structure and metabolism on participation and performance of human activity. Since occupational therapists are not trained to perform surgery or prescribe drugs, our contribution under this theory is our skill in observing and describing the patient's functional behavior as it may be affected by neurosurgical or neurochemical interventions. Another aspect of neuroscience theory, proposed by occupational therapy

leaders since the time of Adolph Meyer, is that participation in activity may affect brain metabolism, thus changing behavior and emotion for the patient. We will look at both of these aspects later in this chapter, with Allen's theory of cognitive disabilities and King's application of sensory integration with chronic schizophrenics.

Although none of the theories considered in Chapter 2 focuses on the relationship of activity to mental health, some of them have been adapted by occupational therapists for use in psychiatry. This chapter will describe four occupational therapy practice models that are derived from or related to the theories of Chapter 2 and that have been used successfully with psychiatric patients. These are

1. *The development of adaptive skills* (also called *recapitulation of ontogenesis*), which is based on developmental concepts;
2. *Role acquisition,* based on developmental and behavioral concepts, used together with *social skills training,* which is based primarily on behavioral concepts;
3. *Sensory integration,* based on neuroscience foundations; and
4. *Cognitive disabilities,* also based on neuroscience foundations.

Each of these models involves occupation or activity as a treatment medium, and each considers functional performance (in daily life activities) to be important to mental health. However, all of these models have features that limit their application to only some of the patients seen in mental health settings.

We will call these practice models rather than theories, because they are really ways to organize our thinking about problems in clinical practice (just as a cardboard or plexiglass model helps an architect organize her thoughts about the design of a physical space). As occupational therapy assistants, you will need to know the evaluation and treatment techniques, or what to do with the patient under each practice model. A brief discussion of treatment principles and a case example will be given with each model. Because the role of the occupational therapy assistant in psychiatry is primarily to carry out treatment, more detailed description of clinical techniques will follow in Chapters 10, 11, 12, and 13 through 23. Although the technical aspects of treatment are most important for you to learn, we hope that you will also appreciate the power of each practice model as a lens that gives us a unique view of the patient.

DEVELOPMENT OF ADAPTIVE SKILLS

The development of adaptive skills model was conceived by Anne Cronin Mosey (23, 24) and has traditionally been referred to as *recapitulation of ontogenesis*. This term means the repeating of stage-by-stage development. Mosey (23) identifies six areas of adaptive skills and lists stages of development within each skill. The skills are[2]

Sensory integration skill: the ability to receive, select, combine, and use information from the balance and movement senses to perform functional activities.

Cognitive skill: the ability to perceive, represent, and organize sensory information for the purpose of thinking and problem solving.

Dyadic interaction skill: the ability to participate in a variety of relationships involving one other person.

Group interaction skill: the ability to participate successfully in a variety of groups.

Self-identity skill: the ability to recognize one's own assets and limitations, and to perceive the self as worthwhile, self-directed, consistent, and reliable.

---

[2]These skills are paraphrased from Mosey AC. *Psychosocial components of occupational therapy.* New York: Raven Press; 1987. In Mosey's earlier work, a seventh skill—drive-object skill—was included. For a discussion of this skill the reader is referred to Mosey AC. *Three frames of reference for mental health.* Thorofare, NJ: SLACK; 1970.

Sexual identity skill: the ability to accept one's sexual nature as natural and pleasurable, and to participate in a relatively long-term sexual relationship that considers the needs of both partners.

Each of these skills is acquired in a series of stages that follows a developmental sequence. Table 3–1 gives the breakdown of stages for some of these skills. Cognitive skills has been omitted because this area is not appropriate for entry-level practice by the occupational therapy assistant. Sexual identity skills has been omitted because this is not a primary emphasis of occupational therapy. In normal development, and in therapy, stages are encountered and mastered in order, and no stage can be skipped. The reader may wish to review the information on the developmental model in Chapter 2 for further detail on this fundamental concept of developmental theories.

According to Mosey, this practice model is suitable for those individuals who have not mastered all of the stages of development appropriate for their chronological age. Mosey specifically states, however, that this model does not directly address performance in occupation. The focus is instead on the general skills and behaviors needed to negotiate one's environment successfully (23); these skills in turn support performance in occupation. The aim of this model is to help the patient master, step by step, those occupation-supporting skills he has not yet acquired. Four basic concepts guide the use of this model:[3]

1. *The therapist must provide an environment that facilitates growth.* The details and features of the environment depend quite specifically on which particular subskill is being addressed. For example, if the self-identity subskill of perceiving the self as self-directed is the focus, then the patient must be given freedom to make her own decisions and to explore a variety of

---

[3]Mosey lists these as three concepts, with the second and third combined into one.

TABLE 3–1. *Stages in development of selected adaptive skills*

Adaptive skill	Age of mastery
Sensory integration skill	
1. The ability to integrate the tactile subsystem	0–3 months
2. The ability to integrate primitive postural reflexes	3–9 months
3. Maturation of mature righting and equilibrium reactions	9–12 months
4. The ability to integrate the two sides of the body, to be aware of body parts and their relationship, and to plan gross motor movements	1–2 years
5. The ability to plan fine motor movements	2–3 years
Dyadic interaction skill	
1. The ability to enter into trusting familial relationships	8–10 months
2. The ability to enter into association relationships	3–5 years
3. The ability to interact in an authority relationship	5–7 years
4. The ability to interact in a chum relationship	10–14 years
5. The ability to enter into a peer, authority relationship	15–17 years
6. The ability to enter into an intimate relationship	18–25 years
7. The ability to engage in a nurturing relationship	20–30 years
Group interaction skill	
1. The ability to participate in a parallel group	18–24 months
2. The ability to participate in a project group	2–4 years
3. The ability to participate in an egocentric-cooperative group	5–7 years
4. The ability to participate in a cooperative group	9–12 years
5. The ability to participate in a mature group	15–18 years
Self-identity skill	
1. The ability to perceive the self as a worthy person	9–12 months
2. The ability to perceive the assets and limitations of the self	11–15 years
3. The ability to perceive the self as self-directed	20–25 years
4. The ability to perceive the self as a productive, contributing member of a social system	30–35 years
5. The ability to perceive the self as having an autonomous identity	35–50 years
6. The ability to perceive the aging process of oneself and ultimate death as part of the life cycle	45–60 years

Used with permission and adapted from Mosey AC. *Psychosocial components of occupational therapy.* New York: Raven Press; 1987:416–417.

options. This is best practiced outside the treatment setting, where the options of real life can be found in ample supply. Requiring the patient to attend an arts and crafts group, regardless of the variety of crafts available, is less likely to produce development of this skill.

2. *The subskills are mastered in order.* This follows from the above example; unless the patient has already come to appreciate and recognize her assets and limitations, she will have great difficulty making choices in a totally unstructured environment. She cannot begin to attempt to develop a sense of self-direction until she understands well her capacities and limitations.

3. *Subskills from different areas may be* addressed at the same time provided they are normally acquired at the same chronological age. Thus, the person needing to develop a sense of his own assets and limitations might also work on cooperative group skills, but not as easily on mature group skills, which are dependent on learning both self-assessment and cooperative skills.

4. *The patient's intrinsic motivation or desire for mastery (of the subskills) must be engaged.* Mosey cautions therapists to be exquisitely sensitive to evidence of the patient's motivation or lack thereof. For example, if the patient is anxious or frustrated, this might suggest that the environment and activities are not motivating or suitable for that patient at this time. When

the proper environment, activities, and sub-skill behaviors are present, the patient will appear engaged, involved, and interested.

Case Example: Judi, a 27-Year-Old Unemployed Single Woman

Judi has been a patient at a suburban community day treatment center for three months. She is a high school graduate and has taken some courses at a local community college but has not declared a major. She has worked in the past, but never for more than a few weeks at a time, and has held many different kinds of jobs—shop clerk, supermarket checker, lifeguard, assembly line worker, and office clerk. She has been hospitalized twice for suicide attempts and has attended several different outpatient programs. Currently, she lives at home with her widowed mother; they are financially comfortable with the pension and life insurance income from Judi's father, a business executive.

Judi is of medium height and weight. Her physical appearance is clean but not very attractive. Her hair is well brushed but not attractively cut. Her clothing is new and stylish but not well coordinated, and the colors are not flattering to her. Judi appears to relate well to other patients in social situations but often says that she feels left out and that others dislike her. She alternately feels superior to everyone else and totally inadequate. She has had problems relating to staff members also. Often she will seem to agree with a staff suggestion, but she fails to follow through. At other times she argues with staff over every detail and has several times left the center in a huff.

After interviewing Judi and her mother, reviewing her record, and administering a task skills evaluation (done by the occupational therapy assistant), the occupational therapist summarized the findings on the Adaptive Skills Developmental Chart (PS COMP). The following subskills were targeted for development in occupational therapy:

1. *dyadic interaction skill:* subskill 3, the ability to interact in an authority relationship;

2. *group interaction skill:* subskill 3, the ability to participate in an egocentric-cooperative group; and
3. *self-identity skill:* subskill 2, the ability to perceive the assets and limitations of the self.

Since the first two of these are normally learned at the same chronological age—5 to 7 years—these were the first to be addressed. Judi was placed in the jewelry production group, an egocentric-cooperative group that meets three afternoons a week for two and a half hours each time. She was also to meet weekly with Paulette, the occupational therapy assistant, to review progress in the group and to discuss expectations and goals. She was expected to sign in each day in Paulette's office on her arrival at the treatment center.

The purpose of the jewelry group is to produce items for sale in the treatment center gift shop. Design and production decisions are delegated to the group members, who needed some assistance to get started. Evelyn, an occupational therapy assistant assigned to lead this group, provided suggestions and guided the group in making their decisions and generating new ideas. Since group members lacked experience with estimating needs, ordering supplies, and pricing items for sale, Evelyn shared resources and experiences with them. As the group became more confident and as members learned more skills, Evelyn began to step back from the group and let them work things out by themselves. As needed, she intervened in a nonauthoritarian way to help group members recognize each other's needs for approval and for respect from other group members. For example, when Judi complained that she never got a chance to participate in design work, Evelyn helped her problem-solve and practice how to ask for this from the group. Judi was surprised and pleased when they agreed to give her a turn.

In her weekly sessions with Judi, Paulette's first goal was to have Judi trust her and want to be with her. Accordingly, she allowed Judi to take candy from a dish kept on Paulette's desk when she signed in each morning, and she was careful to stop what she was doing and pass a few pleasantries with Judi each day. When Judi wore something becoming, Paulette was sure to compliment her. Judi was often late, both for individual sessions and for attendance at the center, but Paulette made little mention of this at first. Once Judi seemed genuinely to look forward to her meetings with Paulette, Paulette introduced the expectation that Judi be more punctual. Initially resentful, Judi gradually became more accepting of this and other demands placed on her. She asked to be placed in a second group, the clerical production group, so that she can work on computer and word processing skills. Paulette feels this is reasonable for Judi at this time, and that it would give her the experience of working with another authority figure. She will recommend this to the occupational therapist.

The case example of Judi shows how the development of adaptive skills model can be applied by the occupational therapy assistant both in individual meetings and in group activities to promote development of adaptive skills. The setting in the example is a long-term community setting, where a patient could comfortably receive treatment for a period of many months and even years. This lengthy period is necessary for the development of these adaptive skills, which are ideally learned over quite a long period of time in the child's life. Therefore, this developmental approach is not well suited to short-term treatment.

The role of the occupational therapy assistant in the development of adaptive skills can be highly influential to the patient's progress. Assistants wishing to apply this practice model should obtain regular supervision and would benefit from further study of Mosey's work (22, 23, 24).

◆ Summary of Concepts

1. The therapists must provide an environment that facilitates growth, as defined by the subskill(s) to be developed.
2. Subskills are mastered in order.
3. Subskills from different skill areas may be addressed at the same time provided

they are normally acquired at the same chronological age.
4. The patient's intrinsic motivation (or desire for mastery of the subskills) must be engaged.

Vocabulary

Recapitulation of ontogenesis Mosey's title for this practice model. This refers to the return to or review of early stages of development.

Sensory integration skill The ability to receive, select, combine, and use information from the balance and movement senses to perform functional activities.

Cognitive skill The ability to perceive, represent, and organize sensory information for the purpose of thinking and solving problems.

Dyadic interaction skill The ability to participate in a variety of relationships involving one other person.

Group interaction skill The ability to participate successfully in a variety of groups.[4]

Self-identity skill The ability to recognize one's own assets and limitations, and to perceive the self as worthwhile, self-directed, consistent, and reliable.

Sexual identity skill The ability to accept one's sexual nature as natural and pleasurable, and to participate in a relatively long-term sexual relationship that considers the needs of both partners.

ROLE ACQUISITION AND SOCIAL SKILLS TRAINING

Role acquisition is the name Mosey has given to the teaching of all daily life, work, and leisure skills as they converge in the ability to participate in a variety of social

---

[4]Mosey's levels of group interaction will be further explained in Chapter 17: Group Concepts and Techniques.

and productive roles. These roles include student, worker, family member, leisure participant, and many others. Although other occupational therapy leaders have elaborated on this model, as discussed in this chapter role acquisition is based primarily on Mosey (22, 23, 24).

Social skills training refers to the teaching of those interpersonal skills needed to relate to other people effectively in situations as varied as dating or applying for a job. These skills support successful role acquisition. Both models focus on here-and-now behaviors; they are concerned with how the patient is functioning in the present, and not with how he came to be that way. For example, Mark, a 52-year-old man, has been hospitalized for much of his life. In the hospital, his needs for food, clothing, and shelter have been taken care of by the staff. To live in the community successfully, Mark needs to learn daily living skills like doing the laundry and shopping for food, and social skills like how to talk to shopkeepers and neighbors.

Since both role acquisition and social skills training use techniques derived from behavioral theory, the reader may find it helpful to review that section of Chapter 2 before proceeding further. It is important to realize, however, that neither of these models relies entirely on behavioral concepts. Unlike behavior theory, which views behavior as conditioned (and for that reason beyond the control of the individual), these models view behavior as motivated from within. The individual's needs, wants, and goals are seen as a starting point for clinical intervention. Role acquisition also relies on developmental concepts to explain the order and manner in which skills that support role behaviors are acquired (23).

Role Acquisition

The aim of treatment under the role acquisition model is to help the patient ac-quire the specific skills needed to function in the occupational and social roles he or she has chosen. Not only does the patient need to develop specific skills, but he needs also to develop an awareness of what he is doing and why. To continue with the example of Mark, while he needs to learn how to care for his clothing, he also has to develop a sense that it is important to do so because it affects how other people see him as a neighbor and member of the community. In other words, what someone believes and understands about what he is doing is just as important as the physical actions he performs.

We have said that role acquisition is based, at least in part, on the idea that all behavior is learned. By extension, what has been learned can be unlearned, and new behaviors can be learned to take their place. What has not been learned previously can be learned for the first time. Occupational therapists have long been concerned with how best to help people learn, and with discovering under what circumstances learning is most likely to occur. Their collected experience and wisdom can be translated into the following set of principles for planning and providing treatment (7, 22, 26).

1. *The patient should be involved in selecting problems and goals for treatment and in evaluating his own progress* (7, 22). This conveys the idea that the patient is ultimately responsible for himself and that his ideas about what he needs are important. Not all patients can participate equally in this. Some will be able to tell the therapist exactly what their problems and goals are, and will spontaneously evaluate their own progress during treatment, but this is rare. Other patients will have such limited awareness of their own deficiencies and needs that developing this awareness will itself be a goal of treatment. An example would be a severely ill, psychotic patient with chronic schizophrenia, who has been living on the street and who has adopted a bizarre costume of twisted and knotted rags. Per-

suading such a patient to give up his costume can be quite difficult. Improving his basic hygiene and grooming is a goal the therapist chooses because the patient is incapable of understanding this need himself. Even so, the therapist should try to explain it to him. This sort of patient is equally rare, however. Most patients fall somewhere between these two extremes.

Involving the patient in identifying problems and setting goals can be structured into the first meetings with him. During the interview and the evaluations the assistant should try to learn what the patient's view of his situation is and what he wants out of the treatment. Evaluations that the patient can complete and score himself are useful. Also, the therapist or assistant can present the results of the evaluation to the patient and incorporate his responses into the treatment plan. An example would be sharing the results of an unemployed man's vocational interest evaluation with him, and discussing the need for further evaluation of skills and aptitudes before a training program is selected. If the patient wants to try a training program before the evaluation is finished, a compromise plan can be arranged.

Some patients may have a general view of what they want to achieve but little sense of the steps they must take to get there. An example is a mildly mentally retarded woman in her early twenties who wants to have a boyfriend. Although she can identify this goal, she needs the COTA to help her understand that she must first learn how to dress appropriately and how to make conversation. Once she appreciates how these skills are connected to her goal of having a boyfriend, she will be eager to learn them.

Other patients may be preoccupied with an idealized role. An example is the harried mother of three preschool children who wants to have a picture-perfect home, picture-perfect children, a trim athletic figure, and dinner on the table at exactly 6:30 every evening. Nothing less will satisfy her image of what a mother should be; consequently she is frequently tense and depressed. In this situation the therapist or assistant helps the patient examine her goals and reason through their implications, perhaps in a discussion group with other patients.

Occasionally, a patient is so apathetic and unmotivated that he cannot identify any goals at all, or chooses ones that present no challenge. An example is a 34-year-old man who wants to live with his parents and collect public assistance rather than return to his own apartment and his job as a clerk in a law office. If the patient cannot think of suitable goals, then the therapist must. Further, the therapist may need to cajole and persuade such a patient to become involved in activities at all. Involving patients in activity when they feel hopeless and incompetent is the occupational therapy equivalent of a doctor's saving someone's life. It is important that the COTA recognize this responsibility and not be afraid of imposing her will on the patient in such a situation.

Getting patients to assess their own progress or lack thereof is equally important. American medicine has accustomed us to seeing the treating professional as all-powerful and the patient as a passive receiver of treatment. In occupational therapy, the patient, by engaging in activities, is really carrying out his own treatment. The therapist is responsible for making sure the patient knows what he is supposed to be doing and why. But the patient needs to learn to attend to his performance of and his feelings about the activities he is involved in, not only because this helps the therapist evaluate the effectiveness of the treatment, but also because being able to think about these things is important. Being able to assess one's own reaction, to reflect on how an activity feels, how competent one feels doing it, and whether it achieves what one set out to do, are skills we all need to maintain a balanced, flexible, and satisfying lifestyle.

2. *Choose goals and activities that reflect the patient's interests, personal and cultural values, and present and future life roles* (7, 22). No two people are alike, and the therapist (COTA or OTR) must avoid the tendency to assume that she can predict what is best for the patient on the basis of her own preferences. Information about the patient's interests and values can be obtained through interview or evaluation (such as the Interest Checklist) and sometimes from the medical record or from family members.

Patients' values may be shaped in part by their ethnicity, social class, and culture. Ethnicity means race and national origin—for example, Native American, Saudi, Polish, Jamaican, Trinidadian, Mexican, or Guatemalan. Social class refers to the person's rank or status within the larger society. This rank is based in part on educational level and family background, and in part on present occupational role and personal wealth. For example, those whose earnings fall below the poverty level are generally considered to be in the lowest social class, but a Harvard-educated farm worker from a wealthy family would be considered upper class, even though his earnings fall in this range.

Culture is a complex and constantly changing concept, which includes the customs, beliefs, and objects associated with specific groups of people (18). Many cultural variations exist within each ethnic group, since family tradition and new customs acquired from association with members of other cultural groups are often quite individual. Consider, for example, the situation of American Jews, who may be orthodox, conservative, or reform in their religious practices; some are so distant from Jewish tradition that they have a Christmas tree in their homes, exchange Christmas gifts, and go to work on Jewish holidays such as Yom Kippur. Likewise, men from the West Indies have expectations of their wives that are different from those of black men born in the United States.

In addition to the specific cultural group to which the patient belongs, the values and trends of the larger culture need to be considered. Traditional occupational therapy media such as weaving, basketry, and copper enameling have risen and fallen in popularity over the years. Other media that may be in fashion for brief periods such as video games, roller blading, and gourmet cooking, although less versatile, should also be analyzed and used wherever possible.

The patient's present and future life roles will also determine the choice of activity. Activities used in occupational therapy should be geared toward helping the patient acquire needed skills and making him competent at something he needs to do in real life. Teaching the patient to do something he will not have the opportunity to do once he leaves the treatment setting is at best of little value, and at worst may confuse or embitter the patient. The best activities are those that, once learned, will enable the patient to handle the everyday demands of his life. For example, a high school student hospitalized for a brief period will probably benefit more from keeping up with his schoolwork and learning better note-taking and study skills than from practicing leather carving and tooling.

3. *Choose goals and activities that provide a realistic challenge but are consistent with the patient's present level of ability* (7, 22). People suffering from psychiatric disorders are often unable to perform their usual activities as effectively as they once did. Their thinking may be slowed or confused; they may see or hear things that are not there; they may have to make a conscious effort just to perform simple motions; and they may be so preoccupied with their own concerns that they have trouble attending to what is going on around them. Nonetheless, they may expect themselves to accomplish tasks that are beyond their capability at the moment; they may see less-demanding tasks presented by the occupational therapy assistant as a sign that

others think very little of them. The assistant should express absolute conviction that the patient will recover and will be able to accomplish more in the future; at the same time he should explain the purpose of the activity and its relationship to the patient's present condition and future goals.

Activities should require some effort from the patient; otherwise he may just go through the motions without really becoming involved. The activities should not be so simple and routine that the patient does not have to pay attention to what he is going. On the other hand, they should not require such intense effort that the patient quickly becomes tired or frustrated.

4. *Increase challenges and demands as the patient's capacity increases.* At the beginning many patients will be capable of working only for short periods, or at only simple activities. Positive support from the therapist or assistant may be needed to encourage their first efforts. After a person feels comfortable and reasonably successful he will be willing and ready to try more difficult tasks. Some patients will improve only slowly, whereas others improve so rapidly that they become bored or tuned out unless given new challenges.

5. *Present skills in their natural developmental sequence* (7). All skills are developed in a predictable direction, moving from simple to complex. This is true of motor skills, which begin as gross, generalized motions and progress gradually to finely coordinated movements. Similarly, the ability to interact in a group starts with being able to tolerate the presence of other people and only gradually develops into a varied repertoire of ways of actually relating to other people. In both cases there are many steps along the way to full mastery of the skill. When teaching skills to patients this principle should be kept in mind. Moving from simple to complex and following a natural, step-by-step sequence strengthens learning because the skills are built on a solidly developed foundation.

6. *The patient should always know what*

he is supposed to be learning and why. The assistant should orient the patient to each new activity, and never assume that the patient sees the connection between the immediate activity and the treatment goal. Orientation should include an explanation of why the activity is being done, what steps are involved, how long the activity will take, and what is required for successful performance. A patient who has never had a job and who is placed in a prevocational treatment group may have little idea of what behaviors are expected in a work situation. Unless the importance of being on time for work is explained to him, he may assume that the assistant's emphasis on punctuality is a personal quirk of hers. Similarly, if asked to perform a task he has never done before, such as filing papers, the patient will need to be told exactly how to go about this.

7. *The patient should be made aware of the effects of his actions* (7). Often a patient will lack the skill or perspective necessary to evaluate his own performance; if so, the therapist or assistant must do this for him. As Mosey (22) states, "The consequence of an action is important." You can appreciate this yourself just by thinking of how eagerly you await the results of tests, especially ones in which you are uncertain of your performance. Similarly, patients need to know whether they have achieved, to what extent, and how they may improve in the future. If the patient seems at loose ends about what to do next, and does not comment on her own success or failure, the assistant has ample evidence that she needs feedback and guidance from someone else.

Severely disabled patients often make slow progress, and improvements may be so slight as to be barely perceptible. With such patients, the assistant will need to be especially alert to small changes in behavior so that she can reward them immediately. Take, for example, the patient whose social skills are so impaired that he keeps his eyes downcast and fails to make eye contact with others. To increase this patient's eye contact the assistant should respond positively to even the briefest and most glancing look from him.

There are many ways of responding to a patient's efforts and giving feedback. One is through the systematic use of reinforcers, as discussed in Chapter 2. The assistant needs to be aware of her emotional reaction to the patient and of the verbal and nonverbal responses she gives. There is no overestimating the value of tolerance, acceptance, positive support, and a sense of humor in motivating patients. On the other hand, the assistant needs to remain in control of the situation and not allow the patient to use her as a doormat. Because of the powerful effects of the assistant's reaction on the patient's motivation and future behavior, it will be discussed separately in Chapter 10.

8. *Skills need to be practiced repeatedly and then applied to new situations* (7, 22). There is truth to the old saying that "practice makes perfect," and although we do not expect our patients to achieve perfection in everything they attempt, we do want to make sure they really know a skill well enough to use it in the future. To ensure this, the assistant must provide opportunities for patients to practice until they become comfortable. A single correct performance cannot be taken as evidence that the patient has learned the skill; if Mark does the laundry correctly today, this does not guarantee that he can do so next week. Performing a skill repeatedly strengthens learning and helps transform skills into habits.

Once a skill or habit is well established through practice, variations and shortcuts can be attempted. It is crucial that the patient be encouraged to practice new skills and habits in his own environment, and that someone monitor his efforts there. When, for example, Mark attempts to do the laundry at home, he may discover that the machines in his local laundromat operate differently from the one on which he learned in the treatment setting. If Mark, like many

psychiatric patients, has trouble asking others for help and is unable to solve problems on his own, he may give up on doing his laundry altogether.

Practicing a skill in a variety of situations helps the patient see that what works in one situation can work in others. This is called *generalization*. For example, assembling needed supplies before beginning an activity is a skill that works just as well in studying for a test as in doing the laundry. People can be helped to apply learning from one situation to another similar one by being involved in varied activities and environments. In addition, this variety can help the patient learn that a given behavior or skill does not work in all situations. This ability to recognize what behavior is appropriate (or not) for a given situation is called *discrimination*. An example is knowing that sneakers and sweats should be worn for athletic activities and not to a job interview.

9. *If a task is too complex or time consuming to learn all at one time, teach one part at a time, but always do or show the whole activity.* Many tasks that patients need to learn are lengthy, involved, multistep operations. Doing the laundry is an example. The major steps are sorting the clothes by color and type of fabric, assembling laundry supplies and money, getting to the laundromat, loading the clothes in the washer (including knowing which laundry products to use and in which order), inserting the coins and running the machine, unloading the washer, loading the dryer, inserting correct change and turning on the dryer, removing the dry clothes, and folding and/or ironing them. Further refinements include using spot removers and fabric softeners, using net bags for lingerie, adjusting water and dryer temperature, and using special cycles on the washer. The patient must also learn which clothes can be washed and which must be dry-cleaned or washed by hand.

Probably the most effective way to help someone learn a complex task like this is to go through the entire process with him many times. However, because there are many other demands on an assistant's time in a treatment setting this is not often possible, and a complex task can seem overwhelming if presented all at once. The recommended approach is to teach only what can be learned in a given time—for example, folding clothes immediately after removing them from the dryer. Taught in isolation this step may not make much sense to the patient, but connecting this step to the rest of the activity will demonstrate why it is important. This may be done in a variety of ways.

One method for showing the relationship of a step or subskill to the larger complex activity of which it is a part to talk it through. In the example we are using this would involve a brief verbal overview of the whole process of doing the laundry, emphasizing why and when and how the clothes should be folded. It is important to keep the overview brief and to the point, to maintain the patient's interest and attention. Since some people have trouble following spoken descriptions and directions, other learning aids such as posters, printed handouts, samples of how a project looks at various stages, photos, or videotapes can also be used. Chaining, as described in Chapter 2, can be incorporated with these techniques.

Another technique is to simplify the activity by removing all but the most basic steps. For example, starting with a load of mixed color wash-and-wear items in a washer with only one temperature setting, using only detergent (omitting all other laundry products), and using a dryer with a single temperature setting focuses attention on the essential key steps of the activity and reduces confusion.

Activities make most sense when they are presented in the context in which they belong. Barris et al. (7) give the example that a makeup class for female adolescents becomes more motivating if it is followed by a dance or other activity in which makeup is appropriate. Similarly, an actual trip to a real destination enhances learning how to use the subway or bus, and doing the laundry when the patient's clothes need washing makes more sense than just washing things to show how it is done.

10. *People learn how to do things by imitating other people.* It is easy to see this in small children, who mimic their parents' actions, words, and even intonations. The tendency to learn through imitation continues throughout life; watching how someone does something and then trying to do the same thing is a familiar process for all of us. This is no less true for psychiatric patients, but with an important difference: Their past experience may have included few good role models. Consider the case of a woman who was abused by her parents when she was a child; when she has children herself she is likely to repeat this destructive pattern, because it is the only behavior she is familiar with. To learn other ways of handling her children, she has to be exposed to better role models. In a child-care skills group, she can learn how to control her own feelings and reduce stress by watching other mothers and imitating what they do.

Patients often look to staff for role models. Being a good role model can be hard work. It requires that the assistant or therapist actually embody the qualities she is trying to get the patient to develop. A tense therapist is not going to be able to help a patient relax, and a shy therapist will have trouble developing assertiveness in her patients because she lacks it herself. This will be discussed further in Chapter 10.

Other patients can also serve as models for imitation. Encouraging a patient to observe and copy the behavior of another patient reaps a double reward, since it increases the confidence of the one being imitated. Patients can also be taught to imitate role models from their past. For example, a childhood teacher or a favorite uncle may possess characteristics useful in a present situation; in this case, the assistant would help the patient remember and focus on the model while attempting the activity.

Social Skills Training

As mentioned previously, social skills training refers to the teaching of interpersonal skills needed to relate effectively to other people. Many psychiatric patients have problems in this area. They may fail to make eye contact or to respond to questions asked of them, or they may say bizarre things. Such behavior is a serious handicap when applying for a job, asking someone for a date, meeting new people, or just shopping for food or clothing. Kelly (16) defines social skills as "those identifiable, learned behaviors that individuals use in interpersonal situations to obtain or to maintain reinforcement from their environment." In other words, social skills help us get what we want from others. Others respond to the way we act, and the more awareness and control a person has over his social behavior, the more successful he will be in dealing with other people.

Social skills have been classified in many different ways. One way is to group together the behaviors that are needed in a given situation. For example, in a job interview the necessary skills include eye contact, emotional expression appropriate to the situation, clear speech at an appropriate volume, listening, responding, sticking to the topic under discussion, stating one's qualifications positively, showing interest, and asking relevant questions.

Another way of grouping skills is by content or purpose. This approach recognizes that the same social skills may apply in a variety of situations; showing interest is important in friendship and dating, as well as on the job. Generically, social skills can be classified into four groups (32): self-expressive skills, other-enhancing skills, assertive skills, and communication skills. Among the many self-expressive skills are stating feelings and opinions, stating positive things about oneself, and stating one's values and beliefs. Other-enhancing skills include such behaviors as giving compliments, smiling and expressing interest, and giving support and encouragement. Assertive skills are varied. Making requests, disagreeing with another's opinion or statement of fact, refusing requests, questioning another's behavior, and setting limits on another's aggressiveness are some examples. Communication skills include controlling the tone and quality of one's voice, articulating words clearly, and choosing the proper words for a situation. There are many skills in each category besides those listed.

The occupational therapy assistant will probably not be involved in the evaluation of patients' social skills; this task is usually performed by the registered therapist, a social worker, or a psychologist. However, the assistant may be asked to participate in social skills training (treatment to remedy social skills deficits) and so should know the methods and techniques.

A social skills training session usually consists of four distinct phases: motivation, demonstration, practice, and feedback. These phases are probably already quite familiar to you, as they are similar to those used in the traditional occupational therapy method of instructing a patient in an activity (31). *Motivation* consists of identifying the behavior to be learned and explaining why it is important. The therapist should give examples of the desired behavior and discuss why it is relevant to the patient's goals. If the patient can state his own reasons why he thinks it important, so much the better.

In the *demonstration* phase the therapist shows the patient how the behavior is performed. Among the many methods that can be used are modeling by the therapist, role play by the therapist and another person, and film or videotape models. Regardless of the method, during this phase the patient watches and observes but does not attempt the behavior himself until the practice phase.

Practice can be structured to improve learning. One way is to ask the patient to rehearse the desired behavior by talking through how he would behave. This can help reduce anxiety before the actual performance. For example, if the target behavior is asking relevant questions on a job interview, the patient would be asked to list some questions first in a discussion with the therapist. Then he might try them out in role play with another patient.

Feedback is given at the end of the treatment session to summarize what the patient has learned and focus attention on what is to be learned next. However, throughout the session, the therapist should also provide immediate feedback on the client's performance. It is important that the feedback be immediate and specific, emphasizing positive aspects of the patient's performance, and providing concrete details about how to improve it. To illustrate, following the patient's role play of interviewing for a job, the therapist might say:

Good, you looked me right in the eye while you were talking. Your answers to the questions were brief and to the point. Now let's work on showing more enthusiasm. How much do you want this job? Convince me.

Training in social skills should involve not only learning the appropriate behaviors, but learning to perceive when and where they are appropriate (8). Social perception requires reading subtle variations in others' behavior and in the immediate environment. For example, if two people are seated in a room conversing with each other and a third person comes in, several things can happen, depending on the situation and who is involved. One of the seated people might look at the entering person, stand up, and greet him. This would be good etiquette in many situations, especially where the entering person has greater authority (e.g., is the boss or an older person). However, if the scene was a student lounge and all three persons were students who knew each other well and had spent all day together, it might be rude or strange for one person to stand up, effectively ending the conversation.

To summarize, social skills training is a structured approach for teaching interpersonal behaviors. It fits within the general framework of role acquisition and uses behavioral concepts and techniques. Both role acquisition and social skills training can be used as treatment approaches within the model of human occupation; both approaches recognize that the therapist must first motivate the patient and that skills and habits are acquired through learning within a social environment. Both approaches assume that if the input from the environment is changed, the patient's behavior will change. The case example of Howard illustrates the application of both role acquisition and social skills training.

Case Example: Howard, a 45-Year-Old Single Man

Howard is a single Jewish man who lives with his widowed mother in a two-bedroom apartment in a rundown neighborhood of a large city. Howard was first hospitalized at the age of 14 and has been in and out of the hospital many times in the intervening years. He has received a dual diagnosis of chronic schizophrenia and mild mental retardation.

Until three weeks ago, Howard had been employed for 25 years by a messenger service. His job was to pick up and deliver packages via the subway and bus system. He had gotten this job following successful vocational rehabilitation during one of his hospitalizations. Recently, however, the old manager (who had been fond of Howard) retired, and his replacement found Howard's hygiene "unbearable." This was given as the reason for dismissal. After being fired Howard began to experience hallucinations and became afraid to leave his apartment. His mother brought him to the emergency room, and he was admitted to the inpatient service.

On meeting Howard, the occupational therapy assistant, Gloria, immediately observed that his hygiene was quite poor. His clothes were ill-fitting, his pants buttoned but unzipped, he had several days' growth of beard, and his hair was uncombed. He had a noticeable body odor and visible food particles stuck in his teeth. He walked with a shuffling gait and kept his eyes downcast. He was, however, able to answer Gloria's questions, although his answers were often long, rambling, and difficult to follow. At the end of the interview, Howard followed Gloria to the door and continued talking and asking her questions even though she had three times told him the interview was over.

During the evaluation of daily living skills it became evident that Howard knew how to perform basic hygiene and grooming routines, but did not always remember to do them, and had trouble keeping his attention on what he was doing. He was easily distracted by the presence of other people and would interrupt whatever he was doing to talk to them. An evaluation of task skills revealed similar patterns: Howard was able to perform simple tasks (such as stuffing envelopes) once instructed, but often stopped in the middle to talk to others, and had to be reminded to return to his task. The content of his speech was egocentric and tangential; he talked mostly about himself, about TV shows he had seen and things he had done. He frequently sought approval of his task performance from staff members.

Ben, Gloria's supervisor, interviewed both Howard's mother and his former employer by telephone. The employer said that he felt badly about firing Howard, but that he didn't know how to deal with his poor hygiene and incessant talking. He agreed to take Howard back on a trial basis if these problems were solved. He also stated that the company's insurance policy, under which Howard was still covered, provided for six weeks of inpatient psychiatric hospitalization and up to six months of outpatient treatment. No new information was obtained from Howard's mother.

Ben evaluated Howard's social skills, using structured role plays in which other patients played the parts of Howard's employer and various customers. The following problem behaviors were noted: interrupting others who are speaking, failure to make eye contact, introducing inappropriate topics, and failure to perceive and act on the other's desire to end the interaction.

Ben and Gloria discussed the evaluation results with Howard. Howard was most interested in returning to work and agreed to the following goals:

1. To perform daily hygiene and grooming routines
2. To learn conversational skills appropriate for a job situation.

Because social contact was so important to Howard, one-to-one meetings with Gloria were selected as the main reinforcer. Gloria also felt this would provide opportunities for her to explore other aspects of Howard's social behavior in different environments like the hospital coffee shop and local stores and parks.

Specific training situations included a day-long job skills group run by Marlene, another COTA, and a daily morning hygiene group run by Gloria and Paul, a nurse's aide. Howard was also scheduled for evening recreation groups. All staff were directed to give Howard feedback on incorrect behaviors and to praise and support any improvements.

The first target behavior in the job skills group was learning not to interrupt others. Marlene explained this to Howard, giving several examples and indicating other patients who had already mastered this skill, and whom Howard could watch as role models. During discussion periods at the end of each day's work, Howard reviewed and assessed his behavior that day and listened to feedback from Marlene and the group members. Other behaviors were taught in the same fashion.

The daily hygiene skills group gave Howard the opportunity to practice his hygiene and grooming under supervision. He gradually learned an entire sequence of brushing his teeth, showering, shaving, using deodorant, and combing his hair. After Howard had practiced the routine daily for several weeks, it became a habit.

Howard was able to return to his job after one month, although he stayed in the hospital at night for the first two weeks of this. Gloria visited him twice at work to observe and give him feedback on his behavior at the job. On discharge he was enrolled in the evening aftercare program, which he continued to attend for three months until space was available in an evening club program near his home.

Throughout the treatment program Howard was involved in selecting his own goals and evaluating his own progress. Since his role as a worker was so important to him, this became the central focus of the treatment plan. New skills and behaviors were taught sequentially, allowing Howard to succeed at easier tasks first before attempting more difficult ones. Each task was explained to Howard and role models were provided. Finally, the newly acquired skills were carried over into the job situation, with staff support and supervision.

This example also shows how various levels of occupational therapy staff can work together with each other and with nursing staff to carry out a treatment plan. Both role acquisition and social skills training are approaches well suited to team effort, since the goals and methods are easily understood and carried out by all levels of staff.

Social skills training has been criticized as limited in effectiveness. It appears that behavioral change transfers best to environments similar to those used for training (13, 14). Although this approach has been thought promising to prepare schizophrenic patients for community living, this has yet to be demonstrated conclusively through research.

◆ Summary of Concepts

1. The patient should be involved in selecting problems and goals for treatment and in evaluating his own progress.
2. Choose goals and activities that reflect the patient's interests, personal and cultural values, and present and future life roles.
3. Choose goals and activities that provide a realistic challenge but are consistent with the patient's present level of ability.
4. Increase challenges and demands as the patient's capacity increases.
5. Present skills in their natural developmental sequence.
6. The patient should always know what he is supposed to be learning and why.

7. The patient should be made aware of the effects of his actions.
8. Skills need to be practiced repeatedly and then applied to new situations.
9. If a task is too complex or time consuming to learn all at one time, teach one part at a time, but always do or show the whole activity.
10. People learn how to do things by imitating other people.
11. Skills should be taught in a four-stage process consisting of motivation, demonstration, practice, and feedback.
12. Feedback should be given throughout the learning process and should be immediate, specific, positive, concrete, and directive.

Vocabulary

***Behavior   Reinforcement   Shaping
Chaining   Extinction***

(The above words are defined in the section on behavioral theories in Chapter 2.)

Skills Basic action patterns that can be combined into a variety of more complex actions.

Social skills Skills used to relate to other people in the variety of situations life presents.

Generalization The ability to apply a skill or behavior to new situations that are similar to the one in which it was learned.

Discrimination The ability to recognize differences in situations that indicate a change in behavior is needed.

Imitation A method of learning by copying or mimicking the behavior of another person.

Target behavior The new behavior to be learned in the immediate treatment situation. The target behavior is a short-term goal, which is distinguished from the long-term goal known as the *terminal behavior,* a desired behavior that will be mastered by the completion of the treatment program.

Motivation The first stage in the cycle of skills training, in which the target behavior is identified and its importance explained.

Demonstration The second stage in the cycle of skills training, in which the target behavior is demonstrated to the patient via role play, videotape, or other example.

Practice The third stage in the cycle of skills training, in which the patient attempts the target behavior and repeats it until he becomes comfortable.

Feedback This word has several meanings. In the cycle of skills training, it is the fourth stage, in which the patient's performance of the target behavior is reviewed and summarized. More generally, however, feedback means information from the environment about the effect of one's action. When given by a person, feedback is most effective when it occurs immediately after the behavior is performed, includes positive aspects of the patient's performance, and gives specific information on what can be done to improve it.

SENSORY INTEGRATION

Sensory integration is a theory and practice model initially developed by the occupational therapist A. Jean Ayres (5) for the treatment of learning disorders in children. It was later applied by Lorna Jean King (17), another occupational therapist, to the treatment of adult patients with chronic schizophrenia. Sensory integration theory is based on neuroscience studies of how the brain operates. Although the underlying neuroanatomy and neurophysiology would be difficult for the entry-level assistant to understand without more knowledge of these fields, the basic concepts and assumptions of sensory integration theory are easy to grasp.

Sensory integration is the smooth working together of all of the senses to provide information needed for accurate perception and motor action. We will explore this concept one step at a time. First, the senses include not only the five that are commonly recognized (sight, hearing, taste, smell, and touch), but also proprioception, kinesthesia, and vestibular awareness.

Proprioception is the sense that helps us identify where parts of our bodies are, even if we cannot see them. For example, you don't have to look under your desk to know where your feet are; you have a built-in sense, proprioception, that keeps you informed of their location and position.

Kinesthesia is a related sense, which gives us information about the muscular effort that accompanies a motion of the body. To illustrate, when you lift a heavy bag of groceries your brain is aware of the work involved, and which muscles are working against gravity. This is something that happens automatically, however; you do not have to think about it.

Vestibular awareness is the sense that detects motion and the pull of gravity during movement. For instance, when you fall while learning to roller skate or ride a bicycle, you know that you have gotten off balance, and you have a feeling for what speed you are going and in what direction you are likely to fall. You get this information from your vestibular system, which coordinates sensations of balance, velocity, and acceleration.

Sensory integration involves combining all of the information from the five basic senses and from kinesthesia, proprioception, and vestibular awareness so that you can accurately interpret what is going on around you, and act on it. For example, suppose that you are about to cross a busy street. You see the traffic and the lights; hear the cars, trucks, and perhaps sirens; smell the fumes. In addition, you feel the pressure of your feet on the concrete and sense where your body weight is centered. You have a sense of how fast you are moving forward, and of whether the surface under your feet is level and smooth. To cross the street safely, you have to receive all of this information, interpret it correctly, and act on it accordingly. If a siren sounds louder, you look for the source of it, to learn whether you can cross safely when the light is with you.

We do not usually give much thought to the complex neurological, sensory, and perceptual processing that goes into everyday actions like this. This is not the case, however, with learning-disabled children and some schizophrenics. King (17) hypothesized that persons diagnosed as having the chronic type of schizophrenia suffer from a proprioceptive deficit, a disturbance in the sense of where the body is in space. She further suggested that this proprioceptive disturbance causes other observable symptoms, such as difficulties in perception, problems with body image, and motor incoordination.

Before discussing the physical signs and symptoms of this proprioceptive defect, it is necessary to appreciate some of the difficulties faced by the patient with chronic schizophrenia. Corbett (10) vividly describes how he imagines the chronic schizophrenic experiences the world when he talks about the patient who walked hunched over with his hands holding his head, because he believed the ceiling was only two inches away.

Imagine for yourself, then, what it would be like to live in a world where sensation and perception are unreliable. All of a sudden things feel very strange. Your clothing hurts. The sidewalk seems to be rising up at you. Ordinary smells seem overpowering. Your fork feels like it's made of some spongy material, and it gets bigger and bigger when you bring it to your mouth. Your tongue feels so large you can't believe it fits inside your mouth. The world moves up and down with every step you take. Memories and ideas come charging at you and feel more real than what is going on around you. When you try to study, the words on the page turn squiggly and you can't make any sense of them. Not only that but the sound of the air conditioner is as loud as a jet plane and you become fascinated by the texture of the paint on the walls and can't concentrate on anything else. You can see that this would be very unpleasant, and it's easy to understand why schizophrenics have so much trouble doing even simple activities.[5]

In addition to these hallucinations and perceptual inconsistencies, schizophrenics in a psychotic episode have problems moving about in the environment, partly because they cannot tell where things really are but also because they have to plan every movement consciously. Nothing seems to happen automatically; every action requires conscious effort. For instance, to climb a flight of stairs, the patient may have to deliberately lift each knee to raise the foot for each step. This phenomenon is known as *decomposition of movement,* because previously automatic motor behaviors become decomposed or broken up out of their pattern. Generalized slowing of movement, known as *psychomotor retardation,* is also common.

King (17) speculated that some individuals with schizophrenia have defects in their reception or processing of proprioceptive and vestibular information, and that these sensory integrative deficits contribute to, or perhaps even cause, the psychotic symptoms they experience. On the basis of several research studies demonstrating poor vestibular reactions in schizophrenic patients, she hypothesized that a defect in the vestibular or balance system might be the cause of the hallucinations and perceptual disturbances these patients experience.

King identified six postural and movement patterns commonly observed in chronic schizophrenics after many years of illness:

1. An S-curve posture, in which the head and neck are flexed, the shoulders rounded, the abdomen protruding, and the pelvis tipped forward (see Fig. 3–1).

---

[5]Based on descriptions given by Corbett (10).

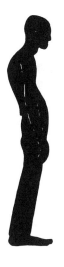

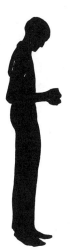

2. A shuffling gait, a style of walking with the feet constantly flat in contact with the floor.
3. Difficulty raising the arms above the head.
4. Inflexibility of the neck and shoulder joints, which prevents the head from rotating or tipping back.
5. A resting posture in which the shoulders and hips are flexed, adducted, and internally rotated.
6. Various changes in the hand, including a weakness of grip, ulnar deviation, and loss of tone and bulk in the muscles acting on the thumb.

King attributed these features to an underlying problem in the central nervous system, and demonstrated that a treatment program of gross motor activities could produce improved mobility in such patients. At the same time, she noted that the patients receiving the treatment also spoke more often and more freely, expressed emotion more spontaneously, and attended better to their grooming. From this she concluded that activities designed to stimulate the proprioceptive and vestibular systems might be useful in the treatment of certain types of schizophrenia. Further, King has stated repeatedly that the improvements gained from sensory integrative treatment are permanent, because they involve a change in the way the central nervous system operates.

Before exploring the treatment principles and activities that King and others have recommended, it should be noted that sensory integrative treatment has been found effective only for patients with certain diagnoses. King recommends its use with all schizophrenias except the paranoid type.

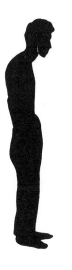

FIG. 3–1. Process schizophrenic postures. From Fig. 1 in King LJ. A sensory-integrative approach to schizophrenia. *Am J Occup Ther* 1974; 28: 529–536. Copyright © 1974 by the American Occupational Therapy Association, Inc. Reprinted with permission.

She has used it with depressed adolescents but does not think it suitable for patients with diagnoses of mania (25). Because of its powerful and occasionally unpredictable effects on the central nervous system, a sensory integrative treatment program must be designed and monitored by a registered therapist. Assistants can help by carrying out the treatment once it is designed.

Two major treatment principles should be kept in mind when choosing activities and carrying out a sensory integrative program. The first is that attention should be focused on the outcome of the activity, or on the objects used in it, rather than on the movements involved. In other words, the patient must move without having to think about how to do it. For example, if a ball is thrown at someone, he will move; he may try to catch it or just to dodge it, but in either case he will move quickly and without much conscious deliberation (17). In contrast, to learn tap dancing, a person must consciously observe, think out, and imitate a motor pattern demonstrated by the teacher. Some activities that focus attention on objects or outcomes include stepping or jumping over ropes placed close to the ground, playing with a parachute or balloons, tossing a large ball overhead, walking a balance beam, spinning in a desk chair, noncompetitive ball games, and obstacle courses (17, 28). These and other activities are discussed in more detail in Chapter 22.

The second treatment principle is that the activity must be pleasurable. The patient should have fun doing it, as evidenced by smiles, laughter, or playful behavior (17). This can be facilitated by staff members themselves showing pleasure in the activity. Patients with chronic schizophrenia have probably failed at many things in their lives, and consequently have fragile self-esteem. Staff should avoid criticizing or trying to improve on patients' performance and should focus instead on helping the patients enjoy themselves, praising their efforts, and having a good time themselves.

The goal of a particular sensory integra-tion program will depend on the needs of the patients involved. In general, however, these programs are directed at five main areas: balance, posture, range of motion, spontaneity of motion, and correction of abnormal hip and shoulder positions. The following are examples of activities that are suitable for or that can be adapted to meet these goals:

Balance   Activities that incorporate hopping, skipping, or standing on one foot. Where available, bicycle riding, cross-country skiing, and roller skating can also be effective, provided the patients are capable of attempting them safely.

Posture   Activities that require straightening the back and lifting the head, such as holding up a parachute or throwing a ball in the air.

Increased range of motion   Many ball games and housework activities (e.g., sweeping) can be adapted to encourage this.

Spontaneity of movement   Activities that are varied, not entirely predictable, and incorporate chance and surprise. Patients can be instructed to take turns being the leader or to make up their own variations.

Correction of abnormal adduction, flexion, and internal rotation   Activities that use the opposite motions are needed. Adduction, extension, and external rotation of the shoulder occur when the parachute is lifted over the head, and increase if the hands are held apart from each other. Shaking out bedclothes and throwing a beachball also involve these same motions.

To summarize, sensory integration is a treatment approach that aims to improve the reception and processing of sensory information within the central nervous system. Vestibular stimulation and gross motor exercises are the preferred treatment activities. To be effective, activities must be pleasurable and not require conscious attention to body movement. Although appealing and exciting, sensory integration

meets only some of the needs of schizophrenic patients, who also need training in
daily living skills, recreational skills, and
vocational skills (25).

Now let us look at a case example that
illustrates sensory integrative treatment:

Case Example: Richard, an 18-Year-Old with Schizophrenia, Undifferentiated Type

Richard is an inpatient in a state psychiatric hospital. He has been hospitalized
since age 14 because his violent temper
tantrums could not be controlled with
medication. Because of this he could not
remain in the community residence for
emotionally disturbed children where he
had lived since age 8. Richard's mother
had placed him there because she could
not control him; he was physically abusive
and frequently threw things. He twice bit
her so badly that she needed emergency
treatment. She says that he was always a
difficult child; even as an infant he was
floppy and unresponsive and had trouble
sucking.

Richard's behavior in the hospital has
been erratic. At times he is fairly calm but
unresponsive to people around him; he
says he is dead and appears to be hallucinating. At other times he makes wild animal noises and attempts to bite and claw
staff and patients. His hygiene is very
poor; nursing staff is somewhat afraid of
him and reluctant to force him to bathe
and groom himself.

Blanca, the occupational therapist in
charge of rehabilitation services for Richard's unit, identified him as someone who
might benefit from a sensory integration
treatment program. A behavior modification program had been attempted over an
eight-month period, with no improvement. Richard was not cooperative during
the evaluation, which consisted of a test
of postrotatory nystagmus, gait analysis,
drawing double circles on a chalkboard,
and imitation of postures.[6] Evaluation
took several sessions. Results showed deficits in bilateral motor coordination, a flat-
footed gait, and rigidity and limited range
of motion in the neck, trunk, hip, and
shoulder joints. Richard refused to complete the test of postrotatory nystagmus or
the imitation of postures. At times he appeared tactile-defensive, jumping when
touched. On the basis of the evaluation,
Blanca selected the following treatment
goals:

1. Increase range of motion in the neck,
   trunk, hips, and shoulders.
2. Increase tolerance of others so that
   Richard can be in a group.
3. Develop other behaviors needed for
   discharge and community placement.

Blanca instructed Alan, the occupational therapy assistant, in the specific
treatment activities, approaches, and techniques she had planned for Richard's program. Alan carried out the program,
which included mirror play, rolling in a
parachute and blankets, tossing a ball
overhead and later into a hoop, kickball,
and swimming. Treatment was one-on-one
and occurred daily for 30 to 45 minutes.
Activities were rotated; some occurred
only once a week (swimming) whereas
others were done almost daily (rolling in
blankets).

After three weeks of treatment, Richard
appeared more alert and seemed calm
enough to be placed in a low-level task
skills group. Although he had one serious
violent outburst, he was able to tolerate
the group situation. He continued his individual treatment with Alan for two more
months, during which time sessions were
gradually tapered off and replaced with
a sensorimotor activities group. In this
group Richard is learning to play various
noncompetitive games with the other 20
patients and the two staff members.

Richard's social worker now believes
that community placement is a realistic
goal, and is trying to locate an appropriate
facility. Blanca has placed Richard in a
prevocational training group, with the goal
of preparing him for employment in a sheltered workshop.

Although this example shows the dramatic improvement sensory integrative treatment can achieve for some patients, not all
patients react so positively or improve so
quickly. Some patients may not respond at
all for several months, but begin to change

---

[6]These evaluations were recommended by L.J.
King in a workshop entitled "Sensory Integration and
Psychiatric Assessments," sponsored by MNYD-
NYSOTA, New York, 1979.

slowly if treatment is continued.[7] Some patients do not improve at all.

The effectiveness of sensory integration with schizophrenic patients has been investigated through several research studies. In a review of the literature, Hayes (13) concludes that little evidence has been found to show improvement in patients' conditions. Reisman and Blakeney (27) however, in a recent study with only five patients, demonstrated significant improvement in measures of ward behavior (social interest and reduction of psychopathology) following sensory integrative treatment of only a few weeks duration. Additional research is needed.

Occupational therapy for sensory integrative dysfunction requires extensive evaluation, which must be selected and carried out by a registered occupational therapist. Additionally, the American Occupational Therapy Association has taken the position that therapists desiring to use sensory integrative techniques should receive advanced training, because sensory integration is based on more advanced knowledge than is provided in entry-level professional education programs (15).

The role of the occupational therapy assistant within sensory integrative treatment will vary depending upon location, availability of registered therapists, and the results of future research within existing treatment programs. Certainly, the assistant is not qualified to initiate a program, but may be trained by a skilled and appropriately trained therapist to carry out treatment activities and to perform structured parts of evaluations.

◆ Summary of Concepts

1. Successful motor output depends upon accurate reception and interpretation of sensory input.

2. Persons with nonparanoid schizophrenia and other types of chronic psychiatric illness may suffer from a defect in reception or processing of proprioceptive and vestibular input.

3. This sensory integrative defect may cause or contribute to other psychiatric symptoms such as hallucinations, lack of perceptual constancy, psychomotor retardation, and decomposition of movement.

4. Certain chronic schizophrenics have visible postural and movement abnormalities such as poor balance, shuffling gait, an S-curved posture, weakness of grip and atrophy of hand muscles, immobility of the neck and trunk, difficulty raising the arms overhead, and a tendency to hold the hips and shoulders in a flexed, adducted, and internally rotated position.

5. Activities that provide increased vestibular, tactile, and proprioceptive input can help reorganize the way the central nervous system organizes and interprets sensory input.

6. Activities selected for a sensory integrative treatment program should not involve conscious attention to movement, but should focus instead on the objects used or on the outcome.

7. Activities selected for a sensory integrative treatment program should be pleasurable to the patient and should be presented in a noncompetitive, unpressured, and cheerful manner.

8. Improvements gained from sensory integrative treatment are permanent, because they involve a change in the way the central nervous system operates.

Vocabulary

Sensory integration   The process of receiving and organizing sensory information within the central nervous system.

Proprioception   The sensory mechanism for locating body parts in space without visual clues.

---

[7]King LJ. "Sensory Integration as a Broad Spectrum Treatment Approach." Symposium sponsored by Continuing Education Programs of America, Philadelphia, 1978.

Kinesthesia   The sensory mechanism for receiving information about gravity and the weight of body parts and other objects during movement.

Vestibular awareness   The sensory mechanism for receiving information about balance, velocity, and acceleration of the body.

Body image   An internalized image of oneself, one's physical size and attractiveness, and other qualities such as coordination.

Perceptual constancy   A learned ability to recognize different objects regardless of their position or context. In other words, the ability to see the world and the objects in it as relatively predictable, based on past experience.

Decomposition of movement   A symptom associated with psychotic illness, in which complex movements are no longer performed automatically and are broken up into their parts.

Corticalization of movement   A symptom associated with psychotic illnesses, in which movement requires conscious effort and deliberate planning, rather than being automatic or involuntary.

Psychomotor retardation   A generalized slowing of movement, seen in some psychotic illnesses.

Vestibular stimulation   Sensory input to the balance system. Such input may include rocking, spinning, and other movement.

Postrotatory nystagmus   Rapid eye movements that normally occur immediately after vestibular stimulation that involves rotation.

Bilateral motor coordination   The ability to skillfully perform activities that involve the use of both sides of the body, particularly when the two sides perform different motions, as in swimming or tying one's shoes.

Tactile defensiveness   A syndrome in which the person has an aversive response to being touched. Touch is perceived as unpleasant (29).

COGNITIVE DISABILITIES

The theory of cognitive disabilities, developed by occupational therapist Claudia Kay Allen, focuses on the effect of impaired thinking (a frequent symptom of psychiatric disorders) on task performance. The central concept is that some psychiatric patients suffer from a disturbance in the mental functions that guide motor actions. (We have already discussed some of the perceptual disturbances that accompany schizophrenia.) Allen states that ". . . just as physical disabilities restrict the physical ability to do a voluntary motion action, a cognitive disability restricts the cognitive ability to do a voluntary motor action" (2). In other words, a patient's mental disorganization can impair performance of tasks such as leather lacing or getting dressed. Allen believes that the reason some psychiatric patients cannot perform these activities correctly is that they have a cognitive disability. She further states that such cognitive disabilities may prevent patients from successfully adapting to life outside a hospital or supervised living situation.

To appreciate the subjective experience of a cognitive disability, think of how you feel when you have a fever. Everything seems extraordinarily difficult; it is hard to make sense of what people are saying; studying for a test may be impossible; even following the dialogue on a television show can be a challenge. This is the sort of experience people with cognitive disabilities have all the time. Cognitive disability can occur to various degrees with different diagnoses such as schizophrenia, affective disorders, dementia, and substance abuse, among others.

Allen has identified six levels of cognitive ability and disability related to task performance. These range from Level 1 (severe impairment) to Level 6 (no impairment). Patients functioning at the lowest four levels will have difficulty living on their own, unassisted, in the community, because they cannot perform the routine tasks that are

TABLE 3–2. *Cognitive levels: motor actions and associated sensory cues*

	Level 1: automatic actions	Level 2: postural actions	Level 3: manual actions
Spontaneous motor actions	automatic	postural	manual (but not goal-directed)
Imitated motor actions	none	approximate imitation	manual or manipulative
Example of motor action	sniffing, walking, swallowing	gesturing, calisthenics	picking up or touching objects, stringing beads
Attention to sensory cues (inferred from observation)	subliminal (dimly conscious awareness)	proprioceptive (movements and position of the body)	tactile (touchable cues)
Examples of sensory cues	hunger, thirst, or discomfort	posture, gesture, motion	texture, shape

Adapted with permission from Table 2–1 in Allen CK. *Occupational therapy for psychiatric diseases: measurement and management of cognitive disabilities.* Boston: Little, Brown; 1985:34.

needed (such as paying bills, obtaining adequate nourishment, and finding their way to an unfamiliar location). The lower the cognitive level, the more difficulty the patient will experience.

Cognitive level is assessed by observing the motor actions the patient performs during a task, and by inferring the sensory cue that the patient was paying attention to at the time. In other words, the therapist watches what the patient does (motor action) and tries to identify what sensory information caused or started that action. The sensory cues progress from internal at the lowest cognitive levels to external and more complex at the higher levels. Motor actions are automatic at the lowest level and become more refined at higher levels. Table 3–2 illustrates the motor actions and associated sensory cues for the six levels.

Identification of a patient's cognitive level involves a careful evaluation, which must be interpreted by a registered therapist, although the assistant may be asked to perform some parts of the evaluation. Evaluation includes the Routine Task Inventory (RTI), which covers 14 tasks in which the patient's performance is to be observed. The tasks are grooming, dressing, bathing,

walking, feeding, toileting, housekeeping, preparing food, spending money, taking medication, doing laundry, traveling, shopping, and telephoning. For each of the tasks, descriptions are given of the behaviors typical of the cognitive levels. To illustrate, for traveling, using a map is typical of Level 6, and not even being aware of the passing scenery when riding in a car is typical of Level 2. The RTI will be discussed further in Chapter 14.

Patients scoring at Level 2 and above on the RTI are then evaluated with the Allen Cognitive Level Test (ACL). The patient is asked to imitate the therapist's demonstration of leather lacing stitches graded in complexity from the running stitch (Level 3) to the single cordovan stitch (Levels 5 and 6). A patient's performance on this test must be interpreted cautiously, since visual deficits and drug side effects can impair performance (2). The Lower Cognitive Level Test (LCL) is used for those patients who cannot perform the ACL; in this test they are asked to imitate the therapist clapping his hands three times.

Allen describes each of the levels in great detail. Only a registered therapist can evaluate the patient and plan treatment under

TABLE 3–2. *(Continued)*

	Level 4: goal-directed actions	Level 5: exploratory actions	Level 6: planned actions
Spontaneous motor actions	goal-directed	exploratory (experimentation and trial and error)	planned
Imitated motor actions	copy or reproduction of an example	new steps are imitated	often unnecessary—action can be initiated without demonstration
Example of motor action	chopping carrots, sanding wood	spacing of tiles, blending of makeup colors	budgeting, building a project from a diagram
Attention to sensory cues (inferred from observation)	visible (what is not in plain sight is ignored)	related (relationships between two visible cues)	symbolic (abstract or intangible)
Example of sensory cues	color, size, or discomfort	overlapping, color mixing, and spatial relationships	evaporation, electrical current, heat, time, gravity

this model. The assistant may actually carry out the treatment, but the principles for this are given in Chapter 23; the curious reader may wish to look ahead to Table 23–3 for more detail. Therefore, the following descriptions, which are brief, only summarize and illustrate the six levels (2):

Level 1: The patient seems totally unaware of what is going on around him. He pays attention for only a few seconds, but carries out automatic habitual motor routines, such as feeding himself when food is presented. The patient does not respond to the therapist's efforts; he will not imitate an action or take an object placed in his hands.

Level 2: The patient seems to be aware of movement and position, her own and that of others. She can imitate the therapist's movements, but the imitation is inexact. She is not aware of how she affects others, and may assume bizarre positions or perform strange-looking movements.

Level 3: At this level the patient is interested in what is going on around him. He is easily distracted by objects in the environment and enjoys touching and manipulating them. He is capable of using his hands in a simple, repetitive craft or other activity but seems unaware of the purpose and is likely to be surprised to see he has produced

something. He has difficulty understanding cause and effect, except in simple actions he performs himself. He may be easily disoriented and may become lost.

Level 4: The patient is able to copy demonstrated directions presented one step at a time. She is interested in making simple two-dimensional projects, such as mosaic tile trays with a checkerboard pattern, but will not plan for such details as spacing between the tiles. She finds it easier to imitate a sample than to follow a diagram or picture. She will not be able to recognize her own errors and may not be able to correct them when they are pointed out. She will not understand that objects can be hidden from view; she may not look for her shoes under the bed. Similarly, she will not notice glue sticking to the bottom of a tile tray.

Level 5: The person shows interest in the relationships between objects. However, the relationships must be concrete and obvious. Some examples are overlapping edges in paper folding or woodwork, space between tiles, and matching colors in makeup or clothing. The person is interested in the effects he can produce using his hands; he may vary the pressure or the speed with which he uses them. He can generally perform a task involving three familiar steps and one new one. New steps must be demonstrated.

The person at Level 5 may appear careless because he sometimes does things without being aware of the possible consequences. For example, he may damage a garment when removing the price tag or label because he pulls too hard or cuts through the fabric. The person who functions at Level 5 may benefit from social skills training to help him learn to attend to the nuances of expected social behavior. Allen believes that Level 5 is sufficient for a person of lower educational and occupational background to function in the community.

Level 6: The person appreciates the relationships between objects even when these are not obvious. Some examples are anticipating that a dark-colored, hand-dyed garment may bleed when washed, and planning ahead to have enough money for infrequent expenses (such as car repairs or doctor bills). At Level 6 the person is able to anticipate errors, reason why they might occur, and plan ways to avoid them. Level 6 is associated with a high level of education, occupational background, and socioeconomic status.

Allen believes that cognitive levels cannot be changed by occupational therapy treatment. Although this statement may at first seem alarming, it is no different from recognizing that we cannot help a quadriplegic walk again on his own or help a person with mental retardation get into law school. Allen believes that the proper role of occupational therapy is to identify the patient's cognitive level through the evaluation procedures described above, monitor changes in cognitive level that may occur as a result of other treatments (such as medications), and adapt the environment to help the patient accommodate to his disability. In other words, occupational therapy can help the person function better but probably cannot change his underlying mental problems.

To illustrate the effect of medication on cognitive level, consider a person who, on admission, is overactive, has trouble concentrating even for brief periods, is distracted by objects in the environment, has little awareness of her effect on others, but is able to do repetitive manual tasks like stringing beads. Such behavior, which is at Level 3, is typical of the manic patient. Such patients are usually given lithium carbonate; when this drug reaches therapeutic levels the patient's cognitive level will return to whatever it had been before the manic episode (probably Level 5 or 6). Occupational therapy staff can observe improvements in task performance, which should be reported to the physician as evidence that the drug is taking effect (2).

As an example of how an environment must be modified to allow a person functioning at a lower cognitive level to succeed, many patients with nonparanoid schizophrenias need supervised living situations, because when they are functioning at their best they function only at Level 4. They may dress oddly because they are unable to match clothing colors, and they do not always recognize what clothing is appropriate for a given situation. Similarly, although they can wash and groom themselves, they may neglect hidden parts such as underarms, the neck, and the back of the head. They may burn themselves on hot cooking equipment and will have trouble budgeting money and paying bills. They may not be able to manage their own medication, forgetting to take pills or to get prescriptions refilled. For all of these and many other reasons they will need assistance and supervision from someone more capable. Depending on what is available, the patient may live in a group home or supervised residence or in an apartment with other similar patients. In the latter case, daily visits from a supervisor are advisable.

Another example of environmental modification or compensation is setting up supplies and tools for activities in a manner that allows for the patient's disability. At Levels 3 and 4 patients are easily distracted by anything visible. Consequently, supplies that are not needed until the later stages of an activity should be placed on a separate table. Also, each patient should have his own tools and supplies. By contrast, at Level 5 a person can be expected to share tools and to focus on only those supplies needed for the current step, although supplies for other steps may be present.

Although occupational therapy may not be able to change a patient's cognitive level, our ability to modify the task environment to allow the patient to succeed despite his disability is a meaningful and valuable contribution. Allen has recently stated that over the long term (years), environmental change (and time) may enable a person to function at a higher level, and may actually result in a change in cognitive level.[8] An extended discussion of how to modify activities, the task environment, and the manner of presentation for patients at each of the six levels appears in Chapter 23.

Allen's theory of cognitive disabilities is summarized in nine propositions. These are quoted from her text, *Occupational Therapy for Psychiatric Diseases: Measurement and Management of Cognitive Disabilities* (2):

1. *The observed routine task behavior of disabled patients will differ from the observed behavior of nondisabled populations* (p. 73). Patients with cognitive disabilities perform less well than other people in activities needed for independent community living.

2. *Limitations in task behavior can be hierarchically described by the cognitive levels* (p. 74). In other words, the degree of disability is more severe at Level 4 than at Level 5, at Level 3 than at Level 4, and so on.

3. *The choice of task content is influenced by the diagnosis and the disability* (p. 92). Although people functioning at Level 6 typically prefer some balance of work, self-care, and leisure activities, those functioning at lower levels may find work too difficult and prefer crafts instead. Crafts allow lower functioning patients to produce something tangible as a result of their efforts; these tangible products may compensate in some way for the loss of self-esteem from not being able to work in competitive employment.

4. *The task environment may have a positive or a negative effect on a patient's ability to regulate his or her own behavior* (p. 93). In general, tasks that are unstructured and creative tend to make lower functioning patients feel worse. Since the directions are not clear, the patient who lacks good internal organization has no way to organize his efforts and may become confused and frightened. An example is asking a schizophrenic patient like Richard (p. 51) to draw a picture of himself. He is likely either to reject the task totally, to perform it in a perfunctory fashion (by drawing a stick figure, for example), or to produce something bizarre that reflects his hallucinations and other symptoms (for example, drawing a huge mouth with jagged teeth). When a patient appears uncomfortable with a task because it is beyond his capabilities, the therapist should adjust the directions or the steps involved, and sometimes should substitute a different task altogether.

5. *Patients with cognitive disabilities attend to those elements of the task environment that are within their range of ability* (p. 98). This is another way of saying that a patient will ignore whatever he does not understand or think he can make sense of. For example, someone functioning at Level 4 or 5 cannot be expected to construct a project from a three-dimensional plan (like a working drawing or mechanical diagram); he will

---

[8]Allen CK. "Cognitive Disabilities: Part One—Measurement and Management." Workshop given by Advanced Rehabilitation Institutes, New York, 1985.

not have the slightest idea of how to proceed from such directions, although this would be a reasonable task for someone at Level 6. Similarly, the patient at Level 4 may not recognize that he can get up and look in a closet or ask the therapist for a tool that he needs; because he cannot see the tool, he assumes it does not exist or is unavailable.

6. *Therapists can select and modify a task so that it is within the patient's range of ability through the application of task analysis* (p. 100). In other words, the therapist can restructure the directions, materials, or nature of the activity so that the patient can perform it. As an example, when instructing patients in sanding of wooden kits, the therapist can expect that the patient at Level 6 will be able to sand with the grain once the concept of grain is explained to him. At Level 5 the person can be told to sand "up and down, the long way" or other similar wording; after a few experiences of sanding and more verbal instruction, he should be able to understand and apply the concept of grain. The patient at Level 4, on the other hand, because he can follow only demonstrated directions presented one at a time, will need to be shown the motion he should use with the sandpaper. He will need to be instructed to turn his project over and sand the other side. The Level 3 patient will be able to sand once the motion is demonstrated, but may sand back and forth as well as up and down and have difficulty learning to sand in just one direction. Similarly, unless the therapist or assistant intervenes, he may continue sanding until he has reduced the project to toothpicks, because he does not recognize the purpose of the sanding or that he should stop at a given point.

7. *An effective outcome of occcupational therapy services occurs when successful task performance is accompanied by a pleasant task experience* (p. 187). In other words, the therapist or assistant should help the patient feel good about what she has done, both during the process

and afterward. In part this is achieved by presenting only tasks that are at the patient's level of ability. When faced with a task that is too difficult, the patient is likely to feel overwhelmed, ashamed, frustrated, or angry. Sometimes it is helpful to select an activity that the patient has performed well in the past and feels good about. When a new task is introduced it should be analyzed and presented at the patient's level of comprehension (see proposition 5).

8. *Steps in task procedures that require abilities above a person's level of ability will be refused or ignored* (p. 190). This is self-explanatory. If a patient cannot do something, he will find a way to avoid it. For example, a Level 4 patient, when shown how to braid the upper edge of a basket, will instead substitute a less involved finishing method such as making simple loops. He will not be able to follow the over-under, multistrand demonstration of braiding.

9. *The assessment of the cognitive level can contribute to the legal determination of competency* (p. 271). Because persons functioning at Level 4 or below have identifiable problems that prevent them making sound judgments about their own welfare, assessment of a person's cognitive level could be useful in a court of law. Persons at Level 1 and 2 typically behave so bizarrely that their disabilities are obvious, but the person functioning at Level 3 or 4 may appear reasonably intact, especially if he has good verbal skills. At these levels of disability there is serious question about a person's competence to manage his own financial affairs or to stand trial for a crime that he may not really understand.

In summary, the theory of cognitive disabilities provides a system for classifying patients' ability to carry out routine tasks needed for successful community adjustment. The theory provides instruments for evaluation of cognitive level and prescriptions for how to modify tasks, environment, and therapeutic approach for patients with varying levels of disability. This theory shares some principles with the model of human occupation. It recognizes that the environment affects task performance, and that changing the environment can allow the patient to function better. However, Allen's proposition that the patient's cognitive level does not really change, except possibly over the course of many years, sharply contrasts with the human occupation concept that change is constant in an open system. This issue needs further exploration.

Now let's look at a case example that illustrates the theory of cognitive disabilities:

Case Example: Marvin, a 45-Year-Old Man[9]

Marvin has been hospitalized twice in the past month. On the last admission his diagnosis was adjustment disorder, based on his report of a recent separation from his wife. During the current admission it was learned that Marvin and his wife have been separated for five years, that his wife lives out of state, and that Marvin is concerned about his two children. He has threatened to harm his wife. The social worker has been unable to locate Marvin's wife or anyone else who can verify his story.

Marvin is tall, overweight, and dressed sloppily. He appears to need a shave. He says that he knows eight foreign languages, which he learned in his 20 years as a business consultant. He is able to speak some of them, according to staff fluent in foreign languages. His current diagnosis is major depressive episode, with suicidal ideation. On the ward he has shown a good appetite at meals, has slept soundly, and does not appear depressed.

Marvin scored at Level 3 on the Allen Cognitive Level Test. He was placed in a basic skills group. During his first week in this group the following behaviors were observed:

1. When asked to cut apart strips of mailing labels, he held the scissors upside down, but was able to perform the task.
2. When asked to cut rags into 7-inch squares, given a sample, he cut pieces of varying sizes ranging from 10 to 18 inches. None of the pieces were square. When this error was pointed out to him, Marvin apologized and his eyes appeared wet. He then tried to correct his error by trimming the edges, but did not attempt to trace the sample size on to the squares or otherwise measure them.
3. After satisfactorily completing a découpage project, Marvin attempted to attach the hanger to the front of the plaque, but had the attachment prongs facing up, and was using the round end of a ball-and-peen hammer.

Based on the misuse of scissors and hammer, and the failure to recognize the proper positioning of the hanger, the registered therapist recommended that the patient be evaluated for organic brain syndrome. Misuse of common tools is not usually seen in depression, but is often a feature of organic mental conditions. Marvin's teary-eyed apology for cutting the rags incorrectly was seen as evidence to support the diagnosis of depression.

The therapist also recommended that Marvin be placed in a supervised living situation, since he was indeed functioning at Level 3.

As this case example illustrates, assessment of cognitive level is very useful for diagnostic and discharge planning purposes.

In the relatively few years since Allen first published her theory, much research and development has occurred which supports this practice model (11, 21). In addition, detailed and specific treatment guidelines for patients at each level have been developed (4, 18, 19). We will explore some of the basic guidelines in Chapter 23.

◆ Summary of Concepts: Allen's Nine Propositions

1. The observed routine task behavior of disabled patients will differ from the ob-

served behavior of nondisabled populations.

2. Limitations in task behavior can be hierarchically described by the cognitive levels.
3. The choice of task content is influenced by the diagnosis and the disability.
4. The task environment may have a positive or a negative effect on a patient's ability to regulate his or her own behavior.
5. Patients with cognitive disabilities attend to those elements of the task environment that are within their range of ability.
6. Therapists can select and modify a task so that it is within the patient's range of ability through the application of task analysis.
7. An effective outcome of occupational therapy services occurs when successful task performance is accompanied by a pleasant task experience.
8. Steps in task procedures that require abilities above a person's level of ability will be refused or ignored.
9. The assessment of the cognitive level can contribute to the legal determination of competency.

Vocabulary

Cognitive disability Lack or impairment of ability to carry out motor actions, caused by a disturbance in the thinking processes that direct motor acts. Cognitive disability can be observed in the way a person performs routine tasks.

Cognitive level The degree to which the mind is capable of responding to task demands. Allen has identified six cognitive levels ranging from Level 1 (severe impairment) to Level 6 (no impairment).

Routine tasks Activities of daily living, such as grooming, dressing, bathing, walking, feeding, toileting, housekeeping, preparing food, spending money, taking medication, doing laundry, traveling, shopping, and telephoning.

Task demands The degree of complexity present in the materials, tools, and skills needed to perform a task. Task demands vary from simple (eating a sandwich) to complex (providing for adequate income at retirement).

Task abilities What the patient can do successfully; those tasks or parts of tasks that the patient can complete adequately in his present state.

Task environment The people, objects, and spaces in which the patient performs a task. Psychological and emotional aspects of the environment must be considered, as well as physical aspects.

Task directions Oral, written, or demonstrated instruction about how to perform a task.

Environmental compensation Modification of the task environment to permit successful task completion. An example would be seating a distractible patient away from other people.

Routine Task Inventory (RTI) A checklist of 84 task behaviors in 14 task categories, used as a guide for observing and classifying a patient's task abilities.

Allen Cognitive Level Test (ACL) An evaluation in which the patient is asked to imitate the therapist's demonstration of leather lacing stitches graded in complexity from the running stitch to the single cordovan stitch.

Competence A legal term meaning having sufficient mental ability to manage one's own financial affairs, safeguard one's own interests, and understand right and wrong.

REFERENCES

1. Allen CK. Independence through activity: the practice of occupational therapy (psychiatry). *Am J Occup Ther* 1982; 36:731–739.
2. Allen CK. *Occupational therapy for psychiatric diseases: measurement and management of*

cognitive disabilities. Boston: Little, Brown; 1985.

3. Allen CK, Allen RE. Cognitive disabilities: measuring the consequences of mental disorders. *J Clin Psychiatry* 1987; 48:185–191.

4. Allen CK, Earhart CA, Blue T. *Occupational therapy treatment goals for the physically and cognitively disabled*. Rockville Md: The American Occupational Therapy Association; 1992.

5. Ayres AJ. *Sensory integration and learning disorders*. Los Angeles: Western Psychological Services; 1972.

6. Barris R, Kielhofner G, Watts JH. *Bodies of knowledge in psychosocial practice*. Thorofare, NJ: SLACK; 1988.

7. Barris R, Kielhofner G, Watts JH. *Psychosocial occupational therapy: practice in a pluralistic arena*. Laurel Md: RAMSCO; 1983.

8. Brady JP. Social skills training for psychiatric patients. I: concepts, methods and clinical results. *Occup Ther Mental Health* 1984; 4:51–68.

9. Bruce MA, Borg B. *Frames of reference in psychosocial occupational therapy*. Thorofare, NJ: SLACK; 1987.

10. Corbett L. Perceptual changes in schizophrenia. In Symposium: *A neuropsychological perspective of sensory integration in psychiatry*. Chicago, Nov. 12, 1981.

11. David SK, Riley WT. The relationship of the Allen Cognitive Level Test to cognitive abilities and psychopathology. *Am J Occup Ther* 1990; 44:493–497.

12. Hagedorn R. *Occupational therapy: foundations for practice—models, frames of reference and core skills*. Edinburgh: Churchill Livingstone; 1992.

13. Hayes R, Halford WK, Varghese FN. Generalization of the effects of activity therapy and social skills training on the social behavior of low functioning schizophrenic patients. *Occup Ther Mental Health* 1991; 11(4):3–20.

14. Hayes R. Occupational therapy in the treatment of schizophrenia. *Occup Ther Mental Health* 1989; 9(3):51–68.

15. Hinojosa J. AOTA position paper: occupational therapy for sensory integrative dysfunction. *Am J Occup Ther* 1982; 36:831–832.

16. Kelly JA. *Social-skills training: a practical guide for interventions*. New York: Springer; 1982.

17. King LJ. A sensory-integrative approach to schizophrenia. *Am J Occup Ther* 1974; 28:529–536.

18. Litterst TAE. A reappraisal of anthropological fieldwork methods and the concept of culture in occupational therapy research. *Am J Occup Ther* 1985; 39:602–604.

19. Levy LL. Activity, social role retention, and the multiply disabled aged: strategies for intervention. *Occup Ther Mental Health* 1990; 10(3):2–30.

20. Levy LL. Psychosocial intervention and dementia. II: The cognitive disability perspective. *Occup Ther Mental Health* 1987; 7(4):13–36.

21. Mayer MA. Analysis of information processing and cognitive disability theory. *Am J Occup Ther* 1988; 42:176–183.

22. Mosey AC. *Activities therapy*. New York: Raven Press; 1973.

23. Mosey AC. *Psychosocial components of occupational therapy*. New York: Raven Press; 1987.

24. Mosey AC. *Three frames of reference for mental health*. Thorofare, NJ: SLACK; 1970.

25. Posthuma BW. Sensory integration in mental health: dialogue with Lorna Jean King. *Occup Ther Mental Health* 1983; 3(4):1–10.

26. Reed K. *Models of practice in occupational therapy*. Baltimore: Williams & Wilkins; 1984.

27. Reisman JE, Blakeney AB. Exploring sensory integrative treatment in chronic schizophrenia. *Occup Ther Mental Health* 1991; 11(1):25–43.

28. Rider BA. Sensorimotor treatment of chronic schizophrenics. *Am J Occup Ther* 1978; 32:451–455.

29. Royeen CB. Domain specifications of the construct tactile defensiveness. *Am J Occup Ther* 1985; 39:596–599.

30. Sharrott GW. An analysis of occupational therapy theoretical approaches for mental health: are the profession's major treatment approaches truly occupational therapy? *Occup Ther Mental Health* 1985; 5(4):304–312.

31. Spackman CS. Methods of instruction. In: Willard HS, Spackman CS, eds. *Occupational therapy*. 4th ed. Philadelphia: JB Lippincott; 1981.

32. Stein F. A current review of the behavioral frame of reference and its application to occupational therapy. *Occup Ther Mental Health* 1982; 2(4):35–62.

33. Whitehead AN. Dialogues with Alfred North Whitehead (prologue). In: Bartlett J, ed. *Familiar quotations*. 15th ed. Boston: Little, Brown; 1980:697.

ADDITIONAL REFERENCES AND SUGGESTED READINGS

General

Barris R, Kielhofner G, Watts JH. *Psychosocial occupational therapy: practice in a pluralistic arena*. Laurel, Md: RAMSCO; 1983.

Hagedorn R. *Occupational therapy: foundations for practice—models, frames of reference and core skills*. Edinburgh: Churchill Livingstone; 1992.

Reed KL. *Models of practice in occupational therapy*. Baltimore: Williams & Wilkins; 1984.

Tiffany EG. Psychiatry and mental health. In: Hopkins HL, Smith HD, eds. *Willard and Spackman's occupational therapy*. 6th ed. Philadelphia: JB Lippincott; 1983.

Willson M. *Occupational therapy in long-term psychiatry*. Edinburgh: Churchill Livingstone; 1983.

The Development of Adaptive Skills

Mosey AC. *Psychosocial components of occupational therapy.* New York: Raven Press; 1987.

Mosey AC. *Three frames of reference for mental health.* Thorofare, NJ: SLACK; 1970.

Acquisition of Skills and Social Skills Training

Brady JP. Social skills training for psychiatric patients. I: Concepts, methods and clinical results. *Occup Ther Mental Health* 1984; 4(4):51–68.

Broekema MC, Danz KH, Schloemer CU. Occupational therapy in a community aftercare program. *Am J Occup Ther* 1975; 29:22–27.

Goldman L. Behavioral skills for employment of the intellectually handicapped. *Am J Occup Ther* 1975; 29:539–547.

Linnell KE, Stechmann AM, Watson CG. Resocialization of schizophrenic patients. *Am J Occup Ther* 1975; 29:288–293.

Mosey AC. *Activities therapy.* New York: Raven Press; 1973.

Sensory Integration

Corbett L. Perceptual dyscontrol: a possible organizing principle for schizophrenia research. *Schizophrenia Bull* 1976; 2:249–265.

King LJ. A sensory-integrative approach to schizophrenia. *Am J Occup Ther* 1974; 28:529–536.

Cognitive Disabilities

Allen CK. Independence through activity: the practice of occupational therapy (psychiatry). *Am J Occup Ther* 1982; 36:731–739.

Allen CK. *Occupational therapy for psychiatric diseases: measurement and management of cognitive disabilities.* Boston: Little, Brown; 1985.

Allen CK, Allen RE. Cognitive disabilities: measuring the consequences of mental disorders. *J Clin Psychiatry* 1987; 48:185–191.

Allen CK, Earhart CA, Blue T. *Occupational therapy treatment goals for the physically and cognitively disabled.* Rockville, Md: The American Occupational Therapy Association; 1992.

4

The Model of Human Occupation

There is a proper dignity and proportion to be observed in the performance of every act of life.

MARCUS AURELIUS ANTONINUS (9)

[handwritten: What a model is for]

In Chapter 3, we explored four practice models that have been used in psychiatric occupational therapy. We compared these to the kind of model a designer might construct before building a project. Each model of the patient and his problems provides a foundation on which to build a program of intervention. While very useful for some aspects of the patient's problems, each feels incomplete. The role of intrinsic motivation and interest in provoking and shaping human activity, a concept which is central to our profession's statement of philosophy, is hardly addressed by any of these models.

During the 1960s through and including the 1990s, one school of occupational therapists has been trying to develop a more comprehensive, over-arching, way to organize our understanding of how activity affects human beings and their physical and mental health. This synthesis, today called the model of human occupation, draws together beliefs and practices from throughout the history of occupational therapy (1, 3, 6). Based on occupational behavior concepts first developed by Mary Reilly and others in the 1960s and 1970s, it addresses specifically the health-maintaining and health-restoring aspects of activity. It emphasizes (to an extent that others do not) the roles of choice, interest, and motivation in human

activity. The model is particularly useful because it can be applied in all areas of occupational therapy practice and can be combined with other theories, such as those described in Chapter 3, used today in psychiatric occupational therapy. The model of human occupation is the focus of this chapter.

BASIC CONCEPTS

The central organizing principle of the human occupation model is that humans have an innate (inborn) drive to explore and master their environments. Occupational therapists have named the process of exploring the environment *occupation*. Man's natural tendency to engage in activity, and the ways in which this tendency can be nourished or thwarted, are what the human occupation model seeks to analyze and explain.

This model views man as an open system. *[handwritten: open system]* An open system can be affected by things around it (the environment) and can also affect things around it. A pond is an example of an open system: It makes the land around it green with vegetation but can be damaged by chemicals in the runoff from the land. In contrast, a closed system cannot affect or be affected by its environment. *[handwritten: closed system]*

63

Consider as an example the cabin of an airplane in flight; it is sealed and pressurized and protected from the pressure of the air outside it; it cannot interact with its environment.

As an open system, man acts on his environment; this is called *output*. The information he receives back from the environment is called *intake* or *feedback*. Intake is the process of taking in energy or information from the environment; feedback is a special kind of information through which man learns about the effects of his actions (see Fig. 4–1).

By constantly reacting to intake or feedback, man changes his actions and adapts to his environment. For example, when attempting to open a bottle of prescription medication, a woman might just try to turn the cap (output), and discover that this does not work (feedback). A family member might tell her to push down while turning (intake), which she would then try (output)

and perhaps find that this does not work either (feedback). Then she might read (output) the directions (intake) printed on the cap. By carrying out the series of actions described in the directions she would finally get the bottle open.

The process by which man turns environmental intake and feedback into action (output) is called *throughput*. Throughput is the process of organizing, evaluating, and reorganizing information from within the self (e.g., memory) and from the environment. In the example of the woman opening the pill bottle, throughput would include her recognizing that simply turning the cap did not work, searching her memory for past examples of similar situations, and thinking about possible actions she might attempt. All of this would occur internally, within the woman's mind, before she tried any new actions. Figure 4–1 illustrates this concept.

Human activity is quite a bit more com-

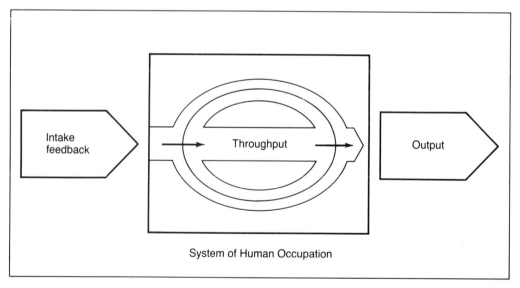

FIG. 4–1. The open system cycle: human occupation and the environment. Adapted from Fig. 1.1 in Kielhofner G. *A model of human occupation.* 4th ed. Baltimore: Williams & Wilkins; 1985.

plex than this, however. People can respond or not respond to feedback or intake from the environment. You have probably seen someone attempt to do something over and over again the same way even when it was not working. People sometimes do things by habit, and sometimes just because they want to. The human occupation model includes these ideas and identifies three levels or subsystems that organize man's capacity for occupation. The three levels of this internal organization, called volition, habituation, and performance, are illustrated in Fig. 4–2.

Volition is another word for motivation; it is considered the highest level of the human system, meaning that the will to act is necessary for the action to take place. *Habituation* refers to habits or routinized behaviors (behaviors that are so automatic they require little attention) and roles; this

is the second level. The third level, *performance,* consists of skills and skilled actions that can be reorganized in different patterns. This is the lowest of the three levels of organization in the human system. Each of the three levels affects the others.

Before considering how the three levels interact with each other, let us examine each of them more thoroughly. *Volition* or motivation is the starting point of any action. The wanting to do is what ultimately makes the action happen. Each person has a different capacity for motivation or volition, because of differences in innate interests and talents and in previous experiences of what happened in the past when the person tried to do things. Everyone wants to do what he is good at; a person is more likely to pursue a career as a singer if he has a good voice than if he cannot carry a tune. This is what is meant by innate interests

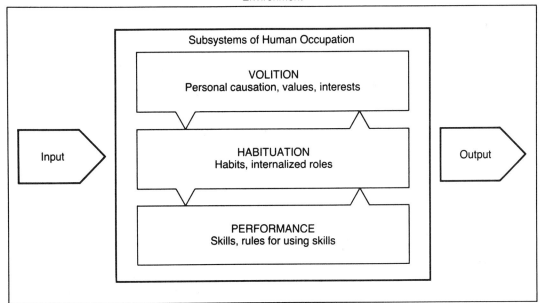

FIG. 4–2. Internal organization of the system of human occupation. Adapted from Fig. 4 in Kielhofner G, Burke JP. A model of human occupation. I: Conceptual framework and content. *Am J Occup Ther* 1980; 34:572–581. Copyright © 1980 by The American Occupational Therapy Association. Reprinted with permission.

and talents. Previous experiences also affect volition. People learn how other people react and what happens when they try certain actions. For example, if our budding singer's mother had listened and applauded when he tried to sing, he would have been encouraged.

The volition subsystem is thought to consist of three elements: personal causation, values, and interests. *Personal causation* refers to a person's beliefs about his ability to have an effect on the world. Does he think he can do things well? Does he think he can control his own destiny? Does he believe he can try new things and succeed?

Values are internalized images of what is good, right, and important (4). Values are commitments to action. Magic Johnson's decision to leave professional basketball so that he could help with AIDS education and research is one example. Not only did he want to further the understanding of and research into AIDS (a value); he also put this value into action.

Interests are "personal dispositions to find pleasure in certain objects, events, or people" (6). In other words, interests are what people *like*. Interests attract a person to new activities and help broaden and diversify the person's occupational pattern. When a person chooses an activity that makes him feel good he feels energized and ready to try other activities. The ability to take pleasure in doing things is just as important to man's motivation or volition as is his belief in his own competence (personal causation) and his sense of the importance of his own efforts (values).

The *habituation* subsystem is the second or middle-level subsystem. Habituation refers to activities that have been done so frequently that they are routine and organized into predictable patterns. The habituation subsystem consists of habits and internalized roles. *Habits* are automatic routines, actions that are carried out often without apparent conscious decision. Some examples are brushing your teeth or making coffee. Because they are so ingrained, habits

can be hard to change, even when life situations demand it. Just think of how difficult it can be to remember to brush your teeth the way the dentist tells you to if it is different from the way you have done it your whole life. Habits help organize time by maintaining day-to-day behaviors (5). This frees time and energy for more complex activities and decisions.

Internalized roles organize actions according to the occupational role the person is trying to carry out. Some examples of occupational roles are worker, student, and homemaker. Each role has certain expected behaviors that go with it. The individual's beliefs and perceptions about these behaviors are the internalized role, which, like habits, helps organize daily activities. Internalized roles involve more active choice and decision making than do habits. As a student, you have certain tasks you want to accomplish every day, but the timing and order in which you do them, and how you do them, are a matter of choice and planning. Consider, for example, studying for a test scheduled two weeks from today. When, how, and how much you study are personal choices in your enactment of your internalized role of student.

Changing from one role to another—for example, from high school student to college student, or from homemaker to college student—can be difficult and complex. Role change involves replacing established habits and skills with new ones needed for the new role. Although role change is exciting, it is also stressful and occasionally causes stress severe enough to require psychiatric treatment. One example is the depression and aimlessness that some women experience when their children grow up and leave home. Sometimes a disability will force a role change upon a patient who might otherwise have continued in his accustomed role.

We have seen that the habituation subsystem consists of habits and internalized roles, which organize actions into daily patterns. When behavior is organized in this way, man's relationship with the social and nonhuman environment is more predictable and requires less conscious effort. Not having to think and decide about every aspect of our daily activity frees energy for new or more complex activities.

The third and lowest level or subsystem is the *performance* subsystem, which consists of skills. Skills are little pieces of bigger actions; they can be combined with each other to form patterns of action. For example, lifting one's hand to one's mouth is a skill. If this skill is combined with other skills, it can become part of a skilled action like brushing one's teeth, eating, or applying lipstick. The performance subsystem also contains rules for using skills—for example, rules about how to bring sharp objects to one's mouth. Another example is that talking to one's boss requires a different verbal content and style than does talking to one's friends on a Saturday night. Skills and rules for using skills are learned throughout life, but primarily in childhood, through playful exploration of the environment.

These skills and the rules about using them are the building blocks of habits and internalized roles. In this way, the performance subsystem supports the functioning of the entire human system. Just as the volition subsystem controls whether an action will occur, the performance subsystem controls whether an action is even possible. For example, a patient with a spinal cord injury will not be able to carry out skilled actions as he could before his injury. All three subsystems interact and respond to changes in the others, so that an injury to the performance subsystem can impair volition and habits; the spinal cord patient may feel negative and unmotivated because he cannot do the things he is used to doing (3).

Similarly, an injury to the volition subsystem can impair the habituation and performance subsystems. A woman who has devoted herself to her husband and has really lived her life through his might, on his death, become very disorganized because her primary motivation has vanished.

The environment also influences the system of human occupation. We already know that intake and feedback come from the environment as information. Obviously, different environments give different kinds of information and should have very different effects on human activity. Even subtle changes in the environment can change the way a person will act; for example, substituting a round table for a long narrow one will increase communication in a group. For optimum occupational performance, the environment should provide the proper level of stimulation. Too little stimulation will lead to apathy and mechanical performance; too much will cause anxiety and withdrawal. People, objects, noise, color, texture, air quality, and temperature are some examples of environmental features that affect occupational performance. To understand how environment affects performance you need only reflect on the many courses you have taken in school. The teacher, the other students, the furniture, the design and layout of the room, the maps and models and learning aids, and the presence or absence of windows and daylight all have influenced your work, although not to an equal extent. Perhaps you can gather from your experience of how environment affected your learning some ideas about how you might change a patient's environment to improve his occupational performance. We will discuss specific recommendations for changing the environment in later chapters.

Improving occupational performance is the goal of occupational therapy interventions. Although many specific recommendations for evaluation and treatment will be discussed in later chapters, none is as important to understand as the underlying principle that unites them. The principle is this: *In an open system, changes in any of the parts will change the whole.* In other words, when treating a patient who has problems in occupational performance, the therapist and the assistant must be aware that the environment and each of the subsystems and their components are influencing what is going on (7). If the treatment is to have a positive effect, it has to create a change in the direction of more adaptive behavior, behavior that helps the person meet his needs and succeed in his life situation. How to create this change is a complex question and requires careful analysis; it is a question best answered by a registered therapist, who will have the educational background to evaluate and analyze the subsystems and their relationship to the patient's present functioning. The assistant can contribute, however, by carrying out selected portions of the evaluation, participating in the analysis and planning, and performing much of the treatment.

Case Example: Rose, a 20-Year-Old Mother of Two

Rose was admitted to the inpatient psychiatric unit with a diagnosis of depression following an unsuccessful suicide attempt. Over the past three weeks she had begun to neglect the housework and the children. She spent long periods of time just sitting around "thinking." She was able to feed and clothe her two children, a boy age four and a girl age two, but she paid little attention to her own grooming. When she was brought to the emergency room by her husband, Larry, her hair was oily and dirty and her clothes food-stained.

Larry and Rose married four and a half years ago, when she was pregnant with their first child. Because both were still in high school, they lived with Larry's parents until Larry got his diploma; they then moved to a one-bedroom apartment nearby. Since then, Larry has been working for his uncle, who installs aluminum siding, and since the birth of the second child he has had a second job pumping gas at night. Rose, who is a year younger than Larry, did not complete her senior year of high school.

Rose's parents, who are extremely religious, totally disapprove of Rose and Larry and the out-of-wedlock pregnancy.

They have not seen Rose since she left their home four and a half years ago; they have never seen their grandchildren.

During the first day of her hospitalization, Rose was quiet and subdued. She isolated herself from other patients, but responded when spoken to by them or by staff. She carried out her morning grooming in a superficial and inattentive manner, and only after several reminders from nursing. She ate little, instead pushing the food listlessly around on the plate.

After a brief discussion with Raquel, the supervising OTR, the occupational therapy assistant, James, reviewed Rose's chart, looking through the admitting information, the history, and the nursing notes for any information about Rose's feelings about herself, her interests, past and present roles, habits, and skills. He then introduced himself to Rose, briefly explained what occupational therapy is and how it might help her, and asked her a series of questions (from the Occupational History Interview) about her childhood, her schooling, and her present life at home. Rose spoke softly, sometimes hesitating, but answered all the questions. She said she was willing to fill out some questionnaires. James left her with the Interest Checklist and the Activity Configuration for her to complete on her own. He also gave her a schedule for general activity groups for the next three days, and scheduled a meeting for the following day to collect and review the two questionnaires. Conveniently, Larry would be visiting at that time, and James planned to schedule an interview with him then.

Later that same day, after reviewing James's interview notes, Raquel met with Rose and explained that she would be working with James to plan the occupational therapy program. She followed up on some points from James's notes, and had Rose complete the Internal-External Locus of Control Scale. She encouraged Rose to talk about her child-care and homemaking responsibilities, and asked her what her goals were for the hospitalization.

Four days later, Raquel and James went over the results of all of the evaluations and arrived at the following conclusions:

1. *Volition subsystem:* Rose feels that she has no control over her life. She is overwhelmed by the responsibilities of

caring for her home and family; she loves her children but feels she cannot handle them. She checked several group sports activities and computer programming on the interest checklist, but says she has no time to pursue these things.

2. *Habituation subsystem:* Rose is having difficulty with the homemaker and child-care roles. She had wanted to study computer science in college and to become a computer programmer, but now sees this as impossible. She performed well in the student role, completing her junior year in high school despite her advanced pregnancy. She manages her time poorly, not completing household chores before attempting others, does not have a routine schedule for housework, and has trouble managing money (pays bills late, buys unnecessary items).

3. *Performance subsystem:* Rose has trouble sticking with a task and complains she cannot concentrate. She is personable and relates well to others but usually waits for them to approach her rather than taking the first step. She seems not to plan things before she does them, which may be one reason why she has trouble managing time and money.

4. *Environment:* According to both Rose and Larry, their home life is very disorganized. Although Rose rarely leaves the home, their small apartment is filled with furniture, dirty clothes and dishes, unanswered mail, and children's toys. The disorder increased when Rose started to become ill three weeks ago. Larry's parents visit about twice a week, and Larry's mother tries to help out but has recently become impatient with Rose, who seems unable to follow through on her advice. Rose and Larry both had friends during high school but have not seen any of them in the past six months. They have no explanation for this.

Since Rose's hospitalization insurance will run out in two weeks, Raquel and James decided to arrange for continued care with a community mental health agency that provides occupational therapy services. They contacted a local agency and scheduled an appointment for Rose to visit the center and meet the therapist. James agreed to accompany Rose on the trip. Then, after a brief meeting with Raquel, James and Rose together outlined a series of goals on which Rose could begin to work while still in the hospital, but which she would continue and complete at home. These were:

1. Increase Rose's sense of self-control by allowing her to choose, with guidance, the occupational therapy groups she will attend during the next two weeks, and by allowing her to participate with James and Raquel and the community occupational therapist in designing the treatment plan. Encourage her to try out computer games or simple word processing on the OT department's computer.

2. Establish a daily routine for self-care, housekeeping, and child care, scheduling only necessary tasks and leaving time for leisure. Later, establish a weekly and finally a seasonal housekeeping and child-care schedule.

3. Review Rose's plans for the future, explore options for her to complete school, and help her plan a way to approach this.

4. Plan for the community occupational therapist to visit Rose and Larry at home after discharge to evaluate the home environment and discuss ways it could be reorganized.

5. Support Rose's past interest in group sports by helping her explore opportunities for volleyball and softball at the local YWCA and community center.

6. Encourage Rose to try streamlined routines for housework and self-care, while providing positive feedback on her present skills.

This case example of Rose illustrates some basic principles for using the model of human occupation. The first is that, in order to get the patient moving, the volition subsystem must be engaged; allowing Rose to choose her own activities, encouraging her to use the computer, and helping her figure out a way to finish school achieve this. Second, in an open system, all parts affect the others; Rose's home environment is critical to her ability to become and stay organized. Similarly, learning simplified housework routines will help her establish efficient habits and will free her time for other pursuits, such as sports or finishing school.

The example also shows the role of the COTA in this model. The assistant carries out the structured parts of the evaluation, gathers data from the medical record, and collaborates with the OTR to develop the treatment plan. The COTA works closely with the patient to set treatment goals and schedule activities. Either in the hospital or in the community agency, the COTA could provide training in household management or leisure planning, could teach child-care and self-care skills, and could help Rose reorganize her home environment.

The model of human occupation gives us a good basic design for understanding man's occupational nature. The description of the model as presented here has been brief and basic, and is intended to help the occupational therapy assistant obtain a general sense of the clinical reasoning a therapist might apply to a patient's problems. The model itself is much more complex; an entire text has been written to explain it (4). In addition, several research studies are currently exploring the effectiveness of the model and attempting to develop it further. We can expect to witness changes and growth in the model in the future.

HUMAN OCCUPATION IN RELATION TO OTHER PRACTICE MODELS

This text will use the model of human occupation as the organizing framework for occupational therapy practice in mental health. Since the four practice models discussed in Chapter 3 can be used together with the human occupation model, we need to understand how and where they are linked to human occupation.

Development of adaptive skills as a practice model relates almost entirely to the performance subsystem of the model of human occupation. Cognitive and sensory-integrative skills can easily be seen as component

skill areas. Dyadic and group interaction seem also to be skill areas, but these overlap with the habituation subsystem. Relating to others individually and in groups can be conceptualized as both a habit and a role. The volition subsystem is not specifically addressed by this model.

Both *role acquisition* and *social skills training* can be used as treatment approaches within the model of human occupation; both approaches recognize that the therapist must first motivate the patient and that skills and habits are acquired through learning within a social environment. Both approaches assume that if the input from the environment is changed, the patient's behavior will change. Role acquisition focuses on the habituation subsystem, and social skills training overlaps the habituation and performance subsystems. The volition subsystem is not addressed except in the choice of roles pursued.

Sensory integration approaches can be used within the model of human occupation to improve skills in moving within the environment and perceiving reality. Again, this addresses the performance subsystem. A possible incompatibility concerns the human occupation principle that the volition subsystem must be activated first; in other words, the patient must be motivated before the treatment begins. King maintains that motivation comes after, not before, the patient is stimulated to move (8). Nonetheless, the prospect of fun and the playful quality of sensory integrative activities can motivate the patient to move and to explore her environment, and perhaps this is a way to reconcile the apparent disagreement between the two models. This question will need further research, and is one illustration of our need for greater understanding of sensory integration.

The *theory of cognitive disabilities* shares several concepts with the model of human occupation. Both recognize that the environment affects task performance, and that changing the environment can allow the patient to function better. Thus, occupational therapy is seen by both to have a role in changing the environment to influence positively a patient's performance of activities. Both acknowledge the importance of interest, choice, and volition, though Allen does not really explain how this relates to her primarily biological orientation. A major difference between the two, then, is in Allen's focus on the biological basis of cognitive level contrasted with Kielhofner's focus on the volitional basis of human occupation. However, this is not so much a true incompatibility as a difference in emphasis. In fact, Katz (2) believes that Allen's biological orientation complements the psychosocial orientation of the model of human occupation.

In summary, the four practice models of Chapter 3 are compatible with the model of human occupation, and can be used to address specific elements of that model. None of the four practice models, however, satisfactorily addresses the volitional subsystem, which Kielhofner and his colleagues view as the starting point for intervention.

◆ Summary of Concepts

1. Human beings have a natural, inborn tendency to act on the environment, to explore and master it.
2. Man is an open system. He interacts with his environment and affects it; he is also affected by it.
3. Man receives information from the environment. This is called intake.
4. Man acts on the environment. This is called output.
5. Man receives information from the environment about the results of his actions. This is called feedback.
6. Man organizes, evaluates, and analyzes his actions and the information he receives from the environment by a process called throughput.
7. The aspect of man that acts in the environment is called human occupation. Human occupation is organized into

three levels or subsystems, each of which affects and is affected by the others.

8. The highest level is volition or motivation, which initiates action.
9. The next level is habituation, which organizes actions into predictable routines and patterns.
10. The lowest level is performance, consisting of the skills and rules for skills from which more complex actions are organized.
11. Because it is an open system, man's system of human occupation is vulnerable to effects from the human and nonhuman environment, which may damage or impair the function of any of the subsystems. This will affect the entire system and can result in problems in occupation. These problems require occupational therapy intervention.

Vocabulary

Open system   Any system that is capable of influencing and being influenced by its environment.

Human occupation   A fundamental aspect of being human, this refers to the process of exploring, responding to, and mastering the environment through activity.

Environment   The human and nonhuman object world in which human occupation is carried out.

Output   An action performed by a person.

Intake   The process of taking in energy or information from the environment.

Feedback   A special kind of information through which man learns about the effects of his actions.

Throughput   The process of attending to, evaluating, organizing, and responding to environmental intake and feedback.

Volition   The highest subsystem within the system of human occupation, this is the same as motivation or the desire to act. Volition is based on personal causation, values, and interests.

Personal causation   The individual's sense of his own competence and ability to be effective.

Values   Internalized images of what is good, right, and important.

Interests   Personal preferences in activity or people. Interests are pleasurable and motivate actions because of this.

Habituation   The second-level subsystem in the system of human occupation, this contains patterns and routines for organizing actions; these are called habits and internalized roles.

Habits   Automatic routines, actions carried out so frequently that they can be done without any conscious effort.

Internalized roles   The individual's personal interpretation of the behaviors required of him in his occupational role.

Occupational role   A pattern for carrying out productive activity. Some examples are playing child, homemaker, worker, retiree.

Performance   The lowest-level subsystem of the system of human occupation, this contains skills and rules for using skills.

Skills   Basic action patterns that can be combined into a variety of more complex motor actions. Three types of skills are communication/interaction skills, process skills, and perceptual skills.

Rules   Internal representations of the effect that skill use will have under different conditions.

REFERENCES

1. Barris R, Kielhofner G, Watts JH. *Psychosocial occupational therapy—practice in a pluralistic arena.* Laurel, Md: RAMSCO; 1983.
2. Katz N. Introduction to the collection (the development of standardized clinical evaluations in mental health). *Occup Ther Mental Health* 1988; 8(1):1–5.
3. Kielhofner G. A model of human occupation. 3: Benign and vicious cycles. *Am J Occup Ther* 1980; 34:731–737.
4. Kielhofner G, ed. *A model of human occupation: theory and application.* Baltimore: Williams & Wilkins; 1985.
5. Kielhofner G, Barris R, Watts JH. Habits and habit dysfunction: a clinical perspective for psychosocial occupational therapy. *Occup Ther Mental Health* 1982; 2(2):1–21.
6. Kielhofner G, Burke JP. A model of human occupation. 1: Conceptual framework and content. *Am J Occup Ther* 1980; 34:572–581.
7. Kielhofner G, Burke JP, Igi CH. A model of human occupation. 4: Assessment and intervention. *Am J Occup Ther* 1980; 34:777–788.
8. King LJ. A sensory-integrative approach to schizophrenia. *Am J Occup Ther* 1974; 28:529–536.
9. Marcus Aurelius Antoninus. Meditations IV, 32 (121–180). In: Bartlett J, ed. *Familiar quotations.* 15th ed. Boston: Little Brown; 1980:124.

ADDITIONAL REFERENCES AND SUGGESTED READINGS

Barris R, Kielhofner G, Watts JH. *Psychosocial occupational therapy—practice in a pluralistic arena.* Laurel, Md: RAMSCO; 1983.

Burke JP. A clinical perspective on motivation: pawn versus origin. *Am J Occup Ther* 1977; 31:254–258.

Burke JP. Commentary: combining the model of human occupation with cognitive disability theory. *Occup Ther Mental Health* 1988; 8(1):xi–xii.

Evans KA. Definition of occupaton as the core concept of occupational therapy. *Am J Occup Ther* 1987; 41:627–628.

Kielhofner G. *Conceptual foundations of occupational therapy.* Philadelphia: FA Davis; 1992.

Kielhofner G. A model of human occupation, part 3. Benign and vicious cycles. *Am J Occup Ther* 1980; 34:731–737.

Kielhofner G, ed. *A model of human occupation: theory and application.* Baltimore: Williams & Wilkins; 1985.

Kielhofner G, Barris R, Watts JH. Habits and habit dysfunction: a clinical perspective for psychosocial occupational therapy. *Occup Ther Mental Health* 1982; 2(2):1–21.

Kielhofner G, Burke JP. A model of human occupation. 1: Conceptual framework and content. *Am J Occup Ther* 1980; 34:572–581.

Kielhofner G, Burke JP, Igi CH. A model of human occupation. 4: Assessment and intervention. *Am J Occup Ther* 1980; 34:777–788.

Neville A. The model of human occupation and depression. *Am Occup Ther Assoc Mental Health Special Interest Section Newsletter* 1985; 8(1):1–4.

Sharrott GW, Cooper-Fraps C. Theories of motivation in occupational therapy: an overview. *Am J Occup Ther* 1986; 40:249–257.

Smyntek L, Barris R, Kielhofner G. The model of human occupation applied to psychosocially functional and dysfunctional adolescents. *Occup Ther Mental Health* 1985; 5(1):21–40.

5

Understanding Psychiatric Diagnosis: The *DSM-III-R* and Proposed *DSM-IV*

The diagnosis of disease is often easy, often difficult, and often impossible.

PETER MERE LATHAM (4)

The occupational therapy assistant in a mental health setting will most often work with patients who have received a psychiatric diagnosis from a physician. Understanding how this diagnosis is reached may broaden the occupational therapy assistant's view of the patient, and assist in his understanding of the viewpoints of other personnel involved in the patient's treatment. While the occupational therapy staff may be most concerned with the patient's ability to function in everyday life and major occupational roles, other staff will focus more on the patient's symptoms and expressed feelings. To appreciate how the occupational therapy assistant fits within the treatment team in a mental health setting, one must first understand the larger framework of psychiatric diagnosis.

 The American Psychiatric Association defines diagnosis as "the process of determining, through examination and analysis, the nature of a patient's illness."[1] This definition implies that diagnosis is an ongoing process rather than a final verdict. As was suggested in Chapter 3, the behaviors and complaints that are grouped together as men-

tal illnesses are not well understood. We still do not know the causes of many conditions, although increasing evidence supports the hypothesis that brain chemistry and structure are involved in at least some psychiatric illnesses. Also, it is widely recognized that the social environment, particularly during development, plays a role. Stress and life circumstances are similarly implicated in causing or contributing to mental illness.

Today's patient entering the mental health system is usually assigned, within the first few weeks, a diagnosis from the *Diagnostic and Statistical Manual of Mental Disorders,* third edition, revised, commonly termed the *DSM-III-R.* The purpose of this chapter is to introduce the reader to the major concepts and overall structure of this manual. As a new edition of the manual is currently in progress, we will also consider some of the proposed changes for the *DSM-IV.* We will review briefly the history of the *DSM*s since the publication of the first *Diagnostic and Statistical Manual* in 1952. The reader will learn some of the underlying assumptions of psychiatric diagnosis. We will explore the structure and organization of the *DSM-III-R,* and the features of some major diagnostic categories commonly encountered in occupa-

---

[1]From Stone EM, ed. *American psychiatric glossary.* 6th ed. Washington, DC: American Psychiatric Press; 1988:50.

tional therapy practice in mental health. Changes proposed for *DSM-IV* will be discussed where relevant to the practice of occupational therapy. For each diagnostic category, we will briefly outline some of the problems typically addressed by occupational therapy.

Throughout this chapter we will refer to the diagnostician, the individual responsible for the psychiatric diagnosis. Depending on the practice setting, this may be a psychiatrist, a physician with another practice specialty, a psychologist, a psychiatric nurse practitioner, or a psychiatric social worker.

HISTORY OF THE DIAGNOSTIC AND STATISTICAL MANUALS

From the 1840s, when all mental disease was categorized as "idiocy," to the mid-twentieth century, when a few diagnostic categories were listed in the *International Classification of Disease (ICD)*, very little information was available to guide the diagnostician in determining the cause and nature of a patient's mental health problems. The *Diagnostic and Statistical Manual, Mental Disorders* (referred to now as *DSM-I*), published in 1952, was an attempt to offer more structure. However, the *DSM-I* and its successor, the *Diagnostic and Statistical Manual of Mental Disorders*, second edition (*DSM-II*), published in 1968, were criticized widely for being too general and vague to serve as reliable guides for diagnosis.

Consequently, the *Diagnostic and Statistical Manual of Mental Disorders*, third edition, published in 1980, was designed to provide more specific and detailed guidelines. These included *operational criteria*, or observable characteristics that could be agreed upon by more than one person. Criteria listed in the *DSM-III* were determined through extensive research evaluations involving large numbers of patients and many independent evaluators. In all, over 150 separate diagnoses were included. The *DSM-III* did not state the causes or etiology of the various disorders but provided a guide to differentiating one disorder from another.[2]

Shortly after the release of the *DSM-III*, work was begun on a revision. This revision, published in 1987, was titled the *Diagnostic and Statistical Manual of Mental Disorders*, third edition, revised, or the *DSM-III-R*. This relatively rapid effort at revision was driven by complaints about some unclear criteria in the *DSM-III* and by the results of new research that contradicted some of the diagnostic criteria of the *DSM-III*. Nonetheless, the *DSM-III* represented a dramatic improvement over the *DSM-II*, and was greeted with much excitement by the psychiatric community.

The authors of the *DSM-III* recognized that the diagnosis alone was not enough to convey adequately the condition of the patient. Consequently, four other *axes* or dimensions were included. It was hoped that these four new dimensions would give a clearer picture of the patient and of her life situation. The five axes were retained in the *DSM-III-R*, the current manual as of the writing of this text. The five axes are:

Axis I   Clinical syndromes and V codes
Axis II   Developmental and personality disorders
Axis III Physical disorders and conditions
Axis IV   Severity of psychosocial stressors
Axis V   Global assessment of functioning

Axis I is the main psychiatric diagnosis (e.g., schizophrenia, depression). The V codes refer to situations that may cause psychological symptoms but that cannot be attributed to a mental disorder. These are

---

[2]The information in this section up to this point is summarized from Bonder BR. *Psychopathology and function.* Thorofare, NJ: SLACK; 1991.

taken from the *International Classification of Disease,* ninth edition (*ICD-9*). Examples include V62.20, an occupational problem, and V62.89, a phase of life problem or other life circumstance problem (1). For some patients, no diagnosis is made on Axis I, with the main diagnosis appearing as a condition classified on Axis II.

Axis II also describes mental disorders, but these are not the "disease entities" of Axis I, but rather the characteristic styles of adaptation that comprise a "personality." Some examples include paranoid, histrionic, and passive-dependent. There has been and continues to be considerable debate as to what constitutes a "personality" and what constitutes a "personality disorder." In other words, since large numbers of people have these personality styles and never make contact with the mental health system, why do we label them as "disorders?" To illustrate, at what point should the person with a suspicious nature be labeled with an Axis II diagnosis of "paranoid personality disorder?" Developmental disorders are also coded on Axis II. These conditions originate before age 18 and cause a handicap or impairment of mental functioning.

Axis III lists physical disorders and conditions. The inclusion of Axis III indicates that physical conditions are stressful and may evoke psychological reactions. Some physical conditions, such as multiple sclerosis, characteristically present with psychological symptoms. The authors of *DSM-III-R* also here acknowledge the interactive relationship between physical and mental conditions, that the mind and the body affect each other's health.

Axis IV describes the severity of psychosocial stressors, or events and life situations that may contribute to mental distress. These are rated on a scale of 1 (none) to 6 (catastrophic), with separate scales used for children and adolescents, and for adults. The code of 0 is used when insufficient information is available to make a rating. Examples of stressors used on the

scale for adults to illustrate the severity of the various levels are marriage (rated as 3 or moderate) and death of a child (rated as 6 or catastrophic).[3]

Axis V provides for the coding of the patient's highest level of functioning within the past month and within the past year. Two separate ratings are made (past month, past year). Since occupational therapy is concerned with the patient's ability to function in daily life roles and activities, Axis V should be an area for occupational therapy involvement. Information from occupational therapy evaluations and observations can assist the physician or other diagnostician in determining the appropriate rating. Axis V is rated from 90 (absent or minimal interference with daily life activities) to 10 or less (severe, indicating persistent danger to self and others). Axis V is rated with the *Global Assessment of Functioning Scale (GAF Scale),* to which the reader is referred for more information.[4]

A case example using the multiaxial (many axes) diagnosis from *DSM-III-R* is shown as Figure 5–1. This case illustrates how psychiatric disorders may be compounded by chemical abuse, social conditions, and physical disorders. Multiaxial diagnoses may also be found in the case examples included in Appendix A.

A new edition of the *Diagnostic and Statistical Manual of Mental Disorders,* to be titled *DSM-IV,* will be released in 1993 or 1994. The work on the new manual began in 1988 and includes extensive reviews of the literature, research evaluations involving many sites, and the use by independent raters of a tentative diagnostic guide with multiple options, titled the *DSM-IV Options Book.* It is beyond the scope of this text to discuss the *DSM-IV* or its options book at any length. However, the reader may be interested in the following proposed changes.

---

[3]The Severity of Psychosocial Stressors Scales are found on page 11 of the *DSM-III-R.*
[4]The Global Assessment of Functioning Scale (GAF Scale) is found on page 12 of the *DSM-III-R.*

A 27-year-old white Jewish male was admitted through the city hospital emergency room to Garden of Eden State Psychiatric Center in New York City two days after the police found him wandering on the street in a neighborhood known for its illegal drug trade. When the police apprehended him, he was naked, shouting, "The ozone layer is gone! God is burning us up for our sins!" and, "I am the son of God. I can heal the ozone layer by my touch."

The patient was restless and required restraint during the initial examination to prevent injury to self and others. The patient was 40 pounds underweight, poorly nourished, unkempt, with open sores on his feet and hands and track marks on his arms and feet (suggesting IV drug use).

A family history reveals a paternal uncle hospitalized for mental disease in late adolescence who never subsequently lived outside the hospital. A cousin on the mother's side has had several acute schizophrenic episodes. The patient's parents and older sister are all professionals. Patient has had 17 admissions to both public and private psychiatric and drug rehab centers; while the family has been concerned, they have not always followed through with treatment recommendations.

Previous records indicate that the patient was a difficult child who argued and fought with playmates from an early age. By the time he entered kindergarten, the pediatrician had recommended a psychiatric consultation because of concern about bed wetting, playing with matches, and near torturing of the family dog. The psychiatrist told the parents that the patient had an above average IQ (133), possessed an ability to take apart and reassemble mechanical devices (clocks, radios) remarkable in a child of his age, and was developing a severe and chronic behavioral disorder. Various therapies during childhood had poor results; the patient was first hospitalized at age 13 when he tore the house apart after a teacher asked him to rewrite a composition. As the patient was already abusing alcohol and marijuana, his parents agreed to inpatient treatment. On discharge after 90 days (extent of insurance coverage), the hospital recommended that treatment be continued at a public hospital. This recommendation was rejected by the family, who found the public facility frightening.

This was the first instance in a repeating pattern of treatment followed by lack of cooperation with treatment recommendations. The patient moved into the hard drug scene in adolescence, dropped out of school in tenth grade and ran away from home many times. He would come home and ask for food, a bath, and money. When refused money, he would try to steal from his parents and sister.

When the patient was 19, the family told him that he could not come home again after their parents-of-addicts support group confronted them with their "enabling" him to continue his drug abuse. He has been living on the street for much of the eight years since. He tried five community residential rehabilitation programs for drug abusers and for MICA (mentally ill chemical abuser) patients, but was unwilling or unable to comply with the rules, and failed each time. He has since been rejected by five other residential programs. At times when the patient has been detoxified and appropriately medicated, his symptoms have been reduced. He states that his problems are really simple: "People should just be allowed to do whatever they want as long as they don't hurt others. I could do just fine if the police would mind their own business."

The patient's Social Security benefits have been discontinued because he failed to report for an annual evaluation. His parents refuse to allow him to return to their home.

DSM-III-R Diagnosis

Axis I:	295.3 Schizophrenia, paranoid type
	305.00 Alcohol abuse
	304.20 Cannibis abuse
	R/O 305.50 Opioid abuse
Axis II:	301.70 Antisocial personality disorder
Axis III:	Malnutrition
	R/O HIV infection
Axis IV:	Severity: 4—Severe (poverty, homelessness)
Axis V:	Current GAF: 0 (inadequate information)
	Highest GAF past year: 25 (unable to function in most areas)

FIG. 5–1. Multiaxial *DSM-III-R* Diagnosis, "Ozone Layer." Adapted from a case example contributed by Hermine D. Plotnick, MA, OTR, and Margaret D. Rerek, MA, OTR.

DSM-IV is targeted for publication around the time of release of the *International Classification of Disease,* tenth edition (*ICD-10*). A treaty between the World Health Organization and the United States obliges the authors of *DSM-IV* to maintain consistency with the *ICD* system. Whether the actual coding (numerical codes for each diagnosis) and organization of the *DSM-IV* will look more like the *DSM-III-R* or the *ICD-10* is one of the major issues under consideration. Many new diagnostic entities have been proposed and are being investigated. In addition, the multiaxial system is being reevaluated. The additional axes of *DSM-III* and *DSM-III-R* have been used relatively little, despite the praise they received initially (2). The many options suggested for the *DSM-IV* range from the elimination of the four additional axes to addition of others.

One problem with the *DSM-III-R* has been the difficulty of classification of disorders within Axes I, II, and III. Of more concern to occupational therapists are the problems with Axes IV and V. Clinicians have criticized the rating system of Axis IV, psychosocial stressors, in *DSM-III-R* as unreliable and not especially helpful for clinical decision-making (2). In *DSM-IV* this axis may be replaced by a *Personal Resources Scale* (which attempts to quantify social and environmental support systems) and/or a *Psychosocial Problem Checklist* (which provides for a descriptive listing of educational, occupational, social, health, legal, and other problems) (2).

Axis V of the *DSM-III-R* has been criticized as cumbersome and difficult to use, as it requires separate ratings for current functioning and for highest level of functioning within the past year. In addition, it mingles psychological symptoms together with social and occupational functioning. Clinicians have suggested that these need to be rated on different scales (2). To illustrate, one person with depression may report extreme feelings of despair and hopelessness and frequent tearfulness, yet be able to carry on with work and family life in a way that appears more than adequate to those around him. Another person with depression may report less painful feelings and yet be unable to get out of bed in the morning and go to work. Using different scales for rating psychological symptoms and social and occupational functioning would permit clearer differentiation of the situations of these two patients with depression.

In summary, the science of psychiatric diagnosis is evolving. It is not yet an exact or definitive process as is the diagnosis of most physical conditions. The *DSM-IV* will no doubt be an improvement over the *DSM-III-R,* and we can anticipate that any further revisions will be incrementally better. The fact that experts debate the exact classification of the variety of mental disturbances experienced by humanity in a manner very different from their classification of physical medical conditions should alone suggest how difficult it has been to understand mental disease.

THE DIAGNOSTIC CATEGORIES OF *DSM-III-R*

Information in this section will follow the organization of the *DSM-III-R.*[5] Selected disorders or categories will be summarized. Selection is based on the prevalence of the disorder and the likelihood that it will be encountered by the entry-level occupational therapy assistant working in a psychiatric setting. Details and descriptive illustrations will be used as needed to provide a clearer picture. Typical problems addressed by occupational therapy will be indicated. For a more scholarly and exact discussion, the reader should consult one of the references listed.

---

[5]Unless otherwise noted, all information in this section is summarized from the American Psychiatric Association. *Diagnostic and statistical manual of mental disorders*. 3rd ed., revised. Washington, DC: American Psychiatric Association; 1987.

The summaries are brief. The reader is cautioned that *duration* and *frequency* of symptoms are considered by the diagnostician and are part of the operational criteria for each diagnostic entity. Duration refers to the length of time the symptoms have been present. Frequency refers to how often the symptoms are experienced. Also, while some of the operational criteria are listed for each diagnosis, space does not permit a full listing. The reader should consult the relevant *DSM* version for detail where needed.

Disorders First Evident in Infancy, Childhood, or Adolescence

Developmental disorders are coded on Axis II. In the *DSM-IV* some or all of these may be reclassified to Axis I. These included mental retardation, autistic disorder, learning disabilities, disruptive disorders, anxiety disorders, eating disorders, gender identity disorders, and some others. Because the treatment of developmental and pediatric conditions in occupational therapy is a separate area of specialization, these disorders will be discussed only briefly in this section.

Mental retardation is characterized by (1) below average intellectual functioning as measured on an IQ test, (2) deficits in adaptive functioning (in daily life activities and roles), and (3) onset before age 18. Generally, the more severe the retardation, the greater the impairment in ability to function. Those with severe and profound retardation are likely to have significant impairment in motor functioning and physical development and may not be able to ambulate or self-toilet. Typical problems addressed by occupational therapy goals for a patient with this condition might include deficits in self-care, impaired social functioning, impaired or absent vocational functioning, and perceptual-motor deficits.

Autism is a rare disorder that is often seen in association with mental retardation. It is characterized by (1) marked impairment in social relationships generally including a lack of awareness of others, (2) marked impairment in communication, both verbal and nonverbal, (3) highly restricted interests and activities, and (4) onset during childhood or infancy. Autistic individuals typically show stereotyped movements, such as flapping the hands. It is difficult and often impossible to obtain and maintain eye contact with the autistic person, or to interest him in a new activity or feature of the environment. It is widely believed that autism is a neurological condition, with underlying organic brain pathology. Problems addressed by occupational therapy goals include impaired sensory processing and sensory integration, perceptual-motor deficits, deficits in social functioning, and delayed or absent vocational functioning. Sensory-integrative, developmental, and behavioral approaches are generally used.

Learning disabilities can be diagnosed for any area of childhood skill development. Thus, academic and language and motor skills are all classified separately. This is a highly specialized practice area for occupational therapy. Problems addressed are specific to the type of learning disability diagnosed. Sensory-integrative assessment and treatment are often applied for this condition.

Disruptive behavior disorders is a category that includes attention-deficit disorder, hyperactive disorder, conduct disorder, and oppositional defiant disorder. These children are "hard to handle" due to their inadequate attention span (*attention deficit disorder*), extremely high energy and activity level (*hyperactive disorder*), deviant and antisocial behavior such as stealing or violence (*conduct disorder*), or argumentative and resentful behavior (*oppositional defiant disorder*). Diagnoses in this category require a pattern of behavior that is sustained for at least six months. Typical problems addressed in occupational therapy include inadequate attention span, poor impulse control, deficient age-appropriate skills (academic, social, occupational), and social skills deficits. The sensory integrative approach is sometimes used with this population.

Eating disorders include several different conditions, the major feature of which is a disturbance in behavior related to the consumption and retention of food. *Anorexia nervosa* is characterized by abnormally low body weight with refusal to gain weight, and a disturbed body image. *Bulimia nervosa* is characterized by binge eating followed by self-induced vomiting or other drastic measures to reduce body size (fasting, use of laxatives). Typical problems addressed by occupational therapy include disturbed body image, low self-esteem and social isolation, and self-care deficits related to eating and exercise. More detail on the occupational therapy treatment of eating disorders can be found in Chapter 9.

All of the disorders first seen in childhood and adolescence are developmental in nature, and thus it is likely that the disorder or its aftereffects will continue into adult life.

Organic Mental Syndromes and Disorders

The category of organic mental syndromes and disorders encompasses the disorders that are associated with temporary or permanent disruptions in the functioning of the brain. The condition is called a "syndrome" when no clear or definitive etiology or cause is known, and a "disorder" when the cause is known, documented, or reliably suspected.

Delirium is characterized by a reduced ability to pay attention, by disorganized thinking (usually evident in rambling or incoherent speech), probable organic cause (e.g., fever, head injury, or recent ingestion of toxic substance), and rapid onset of symptoms. Delirium usually lasts only a week at most, and patients are generally not seen in occupational therapy until the delirium has passed.

In contrast with delirium, the major feature of *dementia* is an impairment of short- and long-term memory as documented by the mental status examination. Additional criteria for a diagnosis of dementia include evidence of impaired thinking or judgment, social or occupational impairment, absence of delirium, and probable organic cause. Dementia is rated mild, moderate, or severe. Patients with dementia are seen in occupational therapy in mental health settings, physical medicine settings, and geriatric settings.

Primary degenerative dementia of the Alzheimer type is a type of dementia in which deterioration of intellectual, social, and occupational functioning is progressive and significant. In other words, the person gets worse and worse, and is less and less able to function in daily life as the disease progresses. On autopsy, the brains of patients with this type of dementia have shown clear and characteristic changes.

Multi-infarct dementia is a type of dementia caused by damage to the cerebrovascular system (blood vessels of the brain). Deterioration in function in this type of dementia is more "step-wise" or "patchy" than in the Alzheimer type, which is more steadily progressive. Functioning varies from day to day, and while there may be significant problems in one area (for example, memory of names) other areas are relatively intact. Evidence of cerebrovascular disease from physical exam or laboratory tests is also needed for this diagnosis.

Organic personality syndrome is a persistent and pervasive change in personality with probable organic cause. Diagnosis is made on the basis of changes in affect or expressed emotion (outbursts, mood swings, apathy) or impaired judgment, in the absence of delirium or dementia, and with likely organic basis.

Intoxication and *withdrawal* are organic mental syndromes that follow the consumption of substances that act on the central nervous system (e.g., alcohol, drugs). Intoxication is due to the presence of the substance in the nervous system. Withdrawal occurs when the individual ceases taking the substance. Patients in these two stages of substance-involved organic disease are generally not seen in occupational therapy.

Occupational therapy treatment of persons with organic mental disorders and syndromes addresses the problems found in this population: memory deficits, limitations in judgment and other cognitive functions, deficits in social skills, and the emotional reaction to one's deteriorating mental state. Since improvement is not generally expected, therapy seeks to maintain maximum functioning as long as possible, through the teaching of compensatory strategies and by careful environmental management. When function declines to a point where independence is no longer possible, the occupational therapy approach includes working with the family or other care giver to assist them in dealing with the patient while encouraging as much independent function as possible. Further detail on these treatment approaches can be found in Chapters 11, 12, 22, and 23.

Psychoactive Substance Use Disorders

Psychoactive substance use is a large category of disorders that are characterized by regular use of psychoactive substances (substances that affect the emotional and intellectual functions) and by the presence of symptoms and maladaptive behavioral changes. The substances listed include alcohol and various drugs (marijuana, cocaine, opiates, hallucinogens, inhalants, amphetamines, phencyclidine or PCP, sedative-hypnotics, and nicotine).

The diagnostician attempts to differentiate between dependence and abuse. *Dependence* implies that the person does not have adequate control over the use of the substance and continues to use it despite clear evidence that it is harmful. Some of the symptoms of dependence include taking

the substance in larger amounts than originally intended (e.g., having more than the promised "just one drink"), attempting unsuccessfully to control or reduce substance use, tolerance for greater amounts over time, social and physical problems such as health problems and family conflicts, and preference for the company of other substance users. A diagnosis of *abuse* is made when there is insufficient evidence for a diagnosis of dependence but where there are clear examples of maladaptive behavior, as in driving while intoxicated or using the substance when it is clearly against one's own interest (causing one to miss a few days of school, for example).

Each of the psychoactive substances has a particular pattern of use and a particular group of associated behavioral features. Many substance-dependent and abusive individuals are involved with multiple substances. Occupational therapy treatment for substance-abusive individuals is directed toward creating new habits of time use and daily life activities to fill the hours once spent on substance-related occupations. Development of social skills and social relationships and training in problem-solving and cognitive reappraisal are other modalities for this group. We will consider some specific treatment protocols for this population in Chapter 9.

Schizophrenia

Although the common usage of the word "schizophrenic" is a catch-all for bizarre behavior, the actual disease of schizophrenia is believed to be a discrete entity. Only a fraction of the people who suffer from psychotic symptoms actually receive a diagnosis of schizophrenia. In many cases, the diagnosis is later revised to another with less serious implications for prolonged dysfunction. Schizophrenia is characterized by several specific psychotic symptoms, a deterioration in functioning from a previously higher level, and a duration of illness of at least six months. If a mood disorder is present, the diagnosis of schizophrenia is not made.

Some of the psychotic symptoms peculiar to schizophrenia include disturbances in the form and content of thought. The individual's thoughts (evidenced by what he or she says) are highly disorganized and unusual, sometimes with the idea that others are inserting and removing one's thoughts, or that one's thoughts are being broadcast or controlled by some external force. The person may shift from one subject to another, linking them with transitions that are not logical to others. Hallucinations are common, with auditory hallucinations being most typical. The person may report that voices are commanding him to perform certain actions. Affect or expressed feeling is often flat (unresponsive) or inappropriate to the situation. Motivation to participate in daily life is usually impaired, as is the ability to interact with others. As discussed in Chapter 3, psychomotor disturbances such as decomposition of movement may also be seen.

The progression of schizophrenia has been divided into three phases: prodromal, active, and residual. In the *prodromal phase* the level of functioning deteriorates. Usually this can be seen in a decline in hygiene and grooming, interaction with others, and overall participation in life. In the *active phase* the psychotic symptoms become apparent. Sometimes a psychosocial stressor appears to precipitate or bring on the active phase. Following the active phase, the *residual phase* consists in the remission of the psychotic symptoms that are most disturbing to others (although the schizophrenic may still hear voices he no longer acts as excited about it) and by a continuation and in many cases worsening of impaired functioning.

Symptoms of schizophrenia are often divided into two classes, *negative* and *positive*. Negative symptoms include apathy, deterioration of hygiene, diminished functioning and participation in daily life, lack

of motivation, social isolation, and psychomotor slowing. These are seen in both the prodromal and the residual phases. Positive symptoms include hallucinations, delusions, and loosening of associations. These symptoms are seen in the active phase of the illness. Though they may be present in the other two phases, they are not severe or prominent.

There are five subtypes of schizophrenia. The *catatonic type* is differentiated by extreme psychomotor disturbance. This may be either a lack of movement, a rigidity of movement, a resistance to movement, an excited and apparently purposeless style of movement, or catatonic posturing in which bizarre postures are held. This type is not commonly diagnosed today in the United States.

The *disorganized type* shows incoherent thinking, ineffective and bizarre communication, and grossly inadequate functioning. The person may grimace, demonstrate strange mannerisms, and otherwise behave oddly. This condition is considered chronic, with a prognosis of continued functioning at a very low level.

The characteristic difference seen in the *paranoid type* is more systematized delusional thinking organized around themes of persecution. Other aspects of thinking are usually unaffected. Affect and behavior are also more normal. Schizophrenics of the paranoid type usually function better, and most are able to live independently. They may participate effectively in many aspects of community life, all the while harboring systematized ideas that others are out to get them.

The diagnosis of *undifferentiated type* is used when the criteria for the other types are not present. The diagnosis of *residual type* is assigned when active psychotic symptoms are not present but residual negative symptoms (impaired functioning) are found. The *DSM-IV Options Book* lists the possible reinclusion of the *simple type* of schizophrenia. Simple schizophrenia is a "less severe" form of a schizophrenic-like

[Handwritten notes at top:]
OT Tx 1. Orientation   6. SI (doesn't work for parinoid)
2. Reduce thought Symptoms
3. Provide social & avocational training (activities)
4. Environment (Family Education)
5. stress mgmt

condition, characterized by deteriorating functioning in the absence of a mood disturbance or organic condition. This diagnosis was included in *DSM-I* and *DSM-II*. The authors of the *DSM-IV Options Book* suggest that simple schizophrenia may not be a schizophrenia at all, and caution that this diagnosis may be used to label improperly as schizophrenic behavior that is merely odd or different. Therefore they recommend that simple schizophrenia be listed in the appendix rather than the body of *DSM-IV*.

Occupational therapy treatment of patients with diagnoses of schizophrenia can be quite varied. Much depends on the person's level of functioning. Some persons with schizophrenia may already function quite well, though this is not the norm. In such cases, occupational therapy treatment is directed at the problems that interfere with functioning or with dyadic or group interaction skills. Social skills training is one approach used to improve the individual's success in relating to others. In many cases, however, the person with a diagnosis of schizophrenia is a long-term recipient of mental health services, and will be seen in both inpatient and outpatient settings for the remainder of his or her life. Many individuals with schizophrenia never attain or regain the ability to function in a job. For this group, participation in family life may also be highly deficient. If a parent, the individual often needs regular intervention and support from mental health professionals to meet the needs of the children. Many schizophrenics also benefit from structuring and guidance in use of the large amounts of leisure time available. Detailed suggestions for specific problem areas (e.g., work, parenting) may be found in chapters on those modalities or areas.

Mood Disorders

Mood disorders are a group of psychiatric disorders with disturbance of mood as the primary feature. The mood is either depressed, manic (high), or alternating between the two. A single incident of disturbed mood is termed a "mood episode." A recurring pattern of mood episodes is termed a "mood disorder."

Mania refers to a mood that is elevated (high), expansive (including everyone and everything), and/or irritable. Sleep is often disturbed. The person may undertake many activities that are inconsistent with her prior behavior (e.g., spending sprees, travel, attention-seeking). Since mania is a symptom as well as a diagnosis, the reader may find additional material on the behaviors associated with mania in Chapter 11.

Depression refers to a mood that is low-spirited, with loss of interest in activities that were previously pleasurable. As with mania, sleep is often disturbed. Appetite may be diminished or increased. Associated symptoms include low energy, suicidal thoughts, feelings of worthlessness, and restlessness or torpor (inactivity). Depression as a symptom, with its associated behaviors, is further discussed in Chapter 11.

Bipolar disorders refer to conditions in which both mania and depression have occurred, alternating with each other. If the episodes have been primarily manic but there has been at least one depressive episode, the diagnosis is *bipolar disorder, manic*. If the episodes have been primarily depressed but there has been at least one manic episode, the diagnosis is *bipolar disorder, depressed*. Where both mania and depression are present, and rapidly alternating with each other, the diagnosis is *bipolar disorder, mixed*. Occupational therapy treatment of mood or affective disorders is primarily directed at symptom reduction during hospitalization. Chapter 11 gives more detail on how the occupational therapy assistant might approach and manage the patient with active depressive or manic symptoms. Following a major episode of either mania or depression, once the symptoms have been reduced, the individual may benefit from occupational ther-

[Handwritten notes at bottom:]
Parachute *vestibular   Posture
Big Ball   *Proprioception Motor planning
            *Tactile   oxygen
            *Visual   Socialization

apy directed at helping her resume previous life routines in self-care, work, and social and family life. Some patients, particularly those with a chronic and lengthy history of illness, will benefit from training in specific skills needed for life roles (e.g., parenting, work behaviors).

Anxiety Disorders

The major symptom of the anxiety disorders is anxiety. The category includes panic disorder, phobias, obsessive-compulsive disorders, and post-traumatic stress syndrome.

In *panic disorder,* the patient suffers repeated and unexpected panic attacks, characterized by such symptoms as shortness of breath, racing pulse, dizziness, and nausea. After suffering many such attacks, the patient becomes fearful of further attacks and for this reason is generally anxious.

In *agoraphobia* (which often accompanies panic disorder), the patient fears being in strange places (where he might have a panic attack). This can become so severe that the person is unable to leave his home.

Phobias are characterized by panic attacks that occur in response to a specific stimulus. In *social phobia,* the patient fears situations in which she might be exposed to ridicule or appraisal by other people (as in, for example, public speaking). Other common phobias are to snakes, airplanes, school, and heights. Phobias, agoraphobia, and panic attacks all impair functioning by interfering with the performance of tasks related to occupational roles. The degree of impairment may be more or less severe, depending on the extent of the phobia. For example, a severe fear of school may prevent a child from attending, but if less severe may just cause anxiety in specific situations at school.

Obsessive-compulsive disorder is characterized by the presence of either or both obsessions or compulsions, which are time-consuming and distressing to the patient

and which interfere with functioning. An *obsession* is an unwanted intrusive thought or impulse (for example, to drive into a wall). The person attempts to rid himself of the obsession but often cannot do so. A *compulsion* is a repetitive behavior performed in response to an obsession. Examples include hand-washing and checking or touching things.

Generalized anxiety disorder is diagnosed when the patient is anxious about two or more unrelated situations, and no other Axis I diagnosis can account for the anxiety. Subjective symptoms are similar to those of panic disorder.

Occupational therapy treatment of anxiety disorders usually involves activities that are relaxing. Often, a conscious effort is made to teach the patient the relaxation response and how to achieve it. Individual assessment is used to identify activities that are relaxing for that person. For example, exhausting physical exercise may be beneficial for some, while others will prefer yoga or a stretch and relax approach. Also, some people may find it helpful to release fears through drawing or other expressive media, but this may frighten others. Where the anxiety is stimulus-specific and impairs function (as in agoraphobia) systematic desensitization may be used to neutralize the anxiety response. This approach requires additional training.

Post-traumatic stress disorder or PTSD is an anxiety disorder that follows a significant stressful event, an event so stressful that it would upset almost anyone who experienced it. Such traumatic events include war (especially combat), natural disasters, and experiencing or witnessing or participating in personal violence. The anxiety provoked by the original trauma is reexperienced by intrusive memories, dreams, and flashbacks. An avoidance response characterized by withdrawal, isolation, psychological numbing, constricted expression of feelings, and lack of interest in previously enjoyed activities serves to reduce contact with the world and psychologically ward off the distressing feelings. Other associated symptoms may include hypervigilance (tense alertness), disturbed sleep, impaired concentration, and feelings of guilt. These patients have a tendency to self-medicate with alcohol and drugs.

Treatment of PTSD aims to reduce these disturbing, function-impairing symptoms by providing support and opportunities to express feelings so that the reaction to the trauma can be explored and integrated (8). A crisis intervention approach such as that described by Rosenfeld (see Chapter 7) is often used. In working with the PTSD patient, Wilson (8) suggests that mental health professionals give unconditional acceptance. While the patient's strong emotional reactions should be tolerated, it is also important to set limits on abusive behavior. These patients may benefit from stress management education and training. Wilson also mentions wilderness experiences and rituals such as the Native American sweat lodge; talking with others who have shared the experience is a particularly helpful aspect of these activities. Yet another approach that can be helpful for the PTSD patient is involvement in an activity that is socially productive and which involves giving help to others. For example, for Vietnam veterans who are also substance abusers, service positions within Alcoholics Anonymous or other 12-step programs (see Chapter 9) give opportunities to work with others and in so doing to achieve status in the eyes of the group (8).

Personality Disorders

As stated earlier in this chapter, all personality disorders are coded on Axis II. To differentiate between personality and personality disorders, the *DSM-III-R* makes the following distinction:

Personality *traits* are enduring patterns of perceiving, relating to, and thinking about the environment and oneself, and are exhibited in a wide range of important social

and personal contexts. It is only when personality traits are inflexible and maladaptive and cause either significant functional impairment or subjective distress that they constitute *Personality Disorders*. (1, p. 335)

The *DSM-III-R* further states that the traits must be of long standing, rather than associated with another disorder, to merit the Axis II diagnosis of personality disorder. This is helpful to distinguish obsessive-compulsive personality disorder from the obsessive-compulsive patterns that are seen in some persons with depression, for example. The latter would not be rated as a personality disorder.

Before exploring further the classification of the various personality disorders, the reader is cautioned to understand that the personality, whether seen as "traits" or a "disorder," is a central and necessary part of the self that cannot be easily changed. Treatment of personality disorders is beyond the scope of this book, and is perhaps not within the scope of practice of occupational therapy today. Suggestions for occupational therapy approaches included in this section should therefore be read as recommended areas for intervention, primarily to reduce the individual's discomfort and not to promote more satisfactory functioning in life and work, and *not* as ways to change the personality to something "more normal."

In the *DSM-III-R*, the personality disorders have been classified into three "clusters." Cluster A disorders include the following types: paranoid, schizoid, and schizotypal. Persons with these disorders may appear odd, eccentric, different, or bizarre to others. Bonder (3) suggests these disorders may have a neurological component and that sensory integrative treatment may be appropriate. Cluster B disorders include the personality types of antisocial, borderline, histrionic, and narcissistic. The commonality in these disorders is erratic, emotional, self-centered behavior. Cluster C disorders include avoidant, dependent, obsessive-compulsive, and passive-aggressive. The common feature here is a fearful, anxious, or avoidant approach to life. The personality disorders have been criticized as having a sexist orientation. In particular, the histrionic and dependent labels are more often assigned to female patients. The behaviors associated with these labels are normal aspects of the social conditioning of women in some cultures.[6]

Paranoid personality disorder is characterized by a tendency to interpret the actions of others as deliberately harmful to the self. Suspiciousness of others, including spouses and others who would normally be trusted, is common. Disturbances in routine may be seen as threatening. For example, if the bus is rerouted, this may be taken personally. Persons with this disorder may have problems functioning at work, due to suspiciousness of the intentions of bosses and coworkers. Occupational therapists may assist the person with a paranoid personality to learn and use new strategies to deal with problems at work. However, no overall change in attitude should be expected, as the paranoid stance is an integrated and necessary aspect of the person's adaptation to life.

A diagnosis of *schizoid personality disorder* is sometimes given to persons who have very limited social involvement with others. These individuals live alone, avoid social contact, and seem disinterested in the social relations on which most people thrive. Occupational therapy treatment of persons with this diagnosis may be directed at assisting them to find and fit into a niche in life that is compatible with their personality structure. For example, a job with limited or no need for interpersonal relatedness and a high opportunity for independence may permit the schizoid individual to be socially productive while attaining a sense of personal competence and avoiding the threatening situation of being with other people.

Schizotypal personality disorder is characterized by the indifference to social involvement seen in schizoid personality disorder, coupled with peculiarities of behavior that are similar to those seen in schizophrenia. In *DSM-IV* this diagnosis may be reclassified with the schizophrenias. The occupational therapy approach is similar to that for the schizoid personality, with additional attention to improvement in self-care and the minimal social skills needed for community survival.

Antisocial personality disorder is diagnosed for individuals who have evidence of *conduct disorder* before age 15 and who show a continuing pattern of antisocial acts after age 18. These acts may include various crimes, deliberate cruelty to animals and people, failure to honor debts, lying, neglect of duties as a parent, and a pattern of impulsivity, among others. Persons with this diagnosis are often seen in the criminal justice system or in the forensic units of hospitals. Because of the developmental aspect of this disorder, these individuals never really have the opportunity to acquire the behaviors, skills, and attitudes needed to succeed in life. Little has been written about occupational therapy treatment approaches to this population. Bonder (3) suggests that a behavioral approach is best suited for use with this group and with other Cluster B personality disorders.

Borderline personality disorder is characterized by a fluctuating sense of personal identity. Moodiness and chronic feelings of emptiness are common. The moodiness is often acted out in impulsive acts such as overspending, substance abuse, sexual relations, and self-mutilating behaviors. Interpersonal relationships are unstable, but highly intense, with the partner in the relationship viewed as alternatively all good or all bad. Occupational therapy treatment is usually directed at symptom reduction, with the aim of increasing the individual's self-esteem and self-identity.

---

[6]For an extended discussion of this point, see p. 36 of Nahmias and Froelich.

The central pattern of *histrionic personality disorder* is one of attention seeking and extreme emotionality. This diagnosis is more commonly given to women than to men. Typically, the individual with this diagnosis dramatizes herself, seeks center stage in all situations, and is uncomfortable when not the center of attention. While the person may express very strong emotions, these often appear overly exaggerated to others. Also, the histrionic individual expresses global approval or disapproval, without the usual details. For example, she might say that her boss is "a very negative person, a very negative channel" but not provide any examples of incidents that led her to this evaluation. This disorder may interfere with functioning in work, especially in positions of any responsibility, since impaired judgment is common. This disorder may be confused with borderline and narcissistic personality disorders.

Narcissistic personality disorder is characterized by extreme self-centeredness, shown in lack of understanding of the feelings of others, exploitation of others, grandiosity, and preoccupation with success. Fantasies of success may lead the person with this disorder to undertake unrealistic goals. Little has been written about treatment of this condition through occupational therapy, but one focus might be the identification of realistic goals after realistically examining the unrealistic goals previously chosen. However, since a sense of "special uniqueness" is central to this condition, the person will resist relinquishing the fantasy, however unrealistic and remote. Forcing a confrontation with reality is counterproductive until the person is ready. Occupational therapy staff should use a gentle and consistent manner with firm limits and expectations.

The essential feature of *avoidant personality disorder* is a fear and avoidance of social contact with others. This is an exaggerated form of the shyness or discomfort many people experience in unfamiliar social situations. Typically, the person has no close friends and is easily hurt by criticism, to the point of avoiding situations in which he or she might be evaluated (however briefly) by others. Understandably, this interferes with functioning in the work world and in social situations. Occupational therapy treatment for this and other Cluster C personality disorders may be directed at social skills training and realistic self-appraisal.

Dependent personality disorder is more commonly diagnosed in women than men. It is characterized by a pattern of submission to the wishes of others and an apparent inability to make decisions on one's own. Persons with this disorder seek guidance, reassurance, and support that is out of proportion to the situation. For example, an adult might let her spouse decide what she will eat when they are dining out, and will permit or even seek recommendations as to what hobbies or social interests should be pursued. These individuals function well on the job except where independent decision-making is needed. Persons with this diagnosis are not usually seen in occupational therapy in the absence of another diagnosis on Axis I or II.

Obsessive-compulsive personality disorder is characterized by perfectionism and is more often diagnosed in men than in women. Typical patterns of behavior include a preoccupation with details (not seeing the forest for the trees), inflexible insistence that others do things a certain way, overvaluing of productivity and undervaluing of social relations, miserliness, and overconscientiousness. These patterns can interfere with functioning at work because of the overall tendency to miss the main point, being sidetracked by the details. Occupational therapy approaches to working with persons showing obsessive-compulsive behaviors are described in Chapter 11.

The central feature of *passive-aggressive personality disorder* is a pattern of resistance to the normal expectations for social and occupational functioning. This may take the form of procrastination, argumentativeness, slowness and general pokiness, scorn and criticism of those in authority, refusal to take suggestions or direction, and rating one's own performance as better than it is rated by others. As might be expected, this condition seriously interferes with functioning in occupational roles. In general, persons with this disorder are more likely to pursue a goal if they believe it is their own idea, rather than the expectation of another person.

APPLICATIONS OF *DSM-III-R* DIAGNOSES TO OCCUPATIONAL THERAPY

Occupational therapists and assistants practicing in mental health settings must appreciate the reality of psychiatric diagnosis and its relationship to reimbursement. Without a *DSM* diagnosis of sufficient severity, insurers (both public and private) will not pay for treatment. Therefore, the psychiatric diagnosis is an inescapable fact of practice today. The diagnosis provides some information that is useful to occupational therapy staff. Each diagnosis has functional implications, and this helps staff in targeting the areas that might need attention (work, social skills, etc.). Ratings on Axis V give a sense of the individual's relative impairment in functioning. But, there are limitations to the diagnosis, and other information is needed to guide occupational therapy treatment and evaluation.

Many psychiatric diagnoses share similar presenting symptoms, particularly in the acute phase of illness, before medication has taken effect. Since reduction of symptoms is a primary concern of all the professions in acute care settings, the information in Chapter 11 provides detail on responding to the various symptoms. However, once the symptoms have remitted, the residual disability becomes the focus of treatment. In some psychiatric conditions, occupational functioning is unimpaired and it is hard to justify giving occupational therapy

treatment to these patients. For most, however, occupational functioning is disturbed or inadequate in some objective and describable way. To focus us in the rehabilitation of these patients, we need clear problem and goal statements that are within our scope of practice.

Too often, occupational therapy staff become sidetracked by the goals and interests of the treatment team leader. The team leader may be a physician, psychologist, or social worker, and may emphasize intrapsychic functioning, family relationships, or social adjustment. Occupational therapy staff who lack a clear sense of their role may find themselves undertaking tasks that are outside their scope of practice (scheduling clinic visits and accompanying the patient to appointments at social service agencies). Worse, the occupational therapy staff may provide a range of activities from which the patient may choose, as in a summer camp or activity center. While this may provide diversion and is clearly helpful for patients with large amounts of unstructured leisure time, it is not enough. Each patient must have clearly written goals that can be met through occupational therapy, and a program of treatment must be designed to meet these goals. The goals and the program must be reevaluated at intervals.

What is most needed, but has not yet been created, is a set of *occupational therapy diagnoses* associated with the various *DSM* diagnoses. These could follow the model used by the nursing profession. Each occupational therapy diagnosis would catalog the impairments in human occupation that are typically found in persons with the corresponding psychiatric diagnosis. All occupational therapy diagnoses would derive from occupational therapy's scope of practice. For example, the occupational therapy diagnoses for schizophrenia might include impaired volition, absence of major occupational roles, disorganized or inadequate habits related to self-care and use of time, and skills deficiencies in many areas. Some of these diagnoses (for example, impaired volition) would be listed for other *DSM* diagnoses, such as depression. A separate manual of protocols for addressing each occupational therapy diagnosis would provide details on how to use activities and the social and physical environment to approach each diagnosis. Something similar to this was attempted by Kielhofner (5) but has not been further developed or integrated into practice.

In conclusion, while all staff working with psychiatric patients should be acquainted with the *DSM* system currently in use, each profession must have its own focus of energy for its work with the patient. When we as occupational therapy professionals venture outside our scope of practice we open ourselves to criticism from those better prepared for these areas.

SUMMARY

This chapter has provided a brief overview of the structure and contents of the *DSM-III-R,* the current version of the American Psychiatric Association's diagnostic manual for psychiatric disorders. The history of the prior versions of the manual and information on the forthcoming revision were included. Information on the focus of occupational therapy intervention for each diagnosis was provided. The author has attempted to assess and give direction to the use of psychiatric diagnosis in the development of occupational therapy problem and goal statements. This is seen as an undeveloped area, to which the oc-

cupational therapy assistant might contribute clinical recommendations.

REFERENCES

1. American Psychiatric Association. *Diagnostic and statistical manual of mental disorders.* 3rd ed., revised. Washington, DC: American Psychiatric Association; 1987.
2. American Psychiatric Association, Task Force on DSM-IV. *DSM-IV options book: work in progress.* Washington, DC: American Psychiatric Association; 1991.
3. Bonder BR. *Psychopathology and function.* Thorofare, NJ: SLACK; 1991.
4. Latham PM (1789–1875). Collected works, bk. I, ch. 25. In: Bartlett J, ed. *Familiar quotations.* 15th ed. Boston: Little Brown; 1980:463.
5. Kielhofner G, ed. *A model of human occupation: theory and application.* Baltimore: Williams & Wilkins; 1985.
6. Nahmias R, Froelich J. Women's mental health: implications for occupational therapy. *Am J Occup Ther* 1993; 47:35–41.
7. Stone EM, ed. *American psychiatric glossary.* 6th ed. Washington, DC: American Psychiatric Association; 1988.
8. Wilson JP. *Trauma, transformation and healing: an integrative approach to theory, research and post-traumatic therapy.* New York: Brunner Mazel; 1989.

ADDITIONAL REFERENCES AND SUGGESTED READINGS

Pacquette M, Neal MC, Rodemich C. *Psychiatric nursing diagnosis care plans for DSM-III-R.* Boston: Jones and Bartlett; 1991.
Perry S, Frances A, Clarkin J. *A DSM-III-R casebook of treatment selection.* New York: Brunner Mazel; 1990.
Spitzer RL, Gibbon M, Skodol AE, et al. *DSM-III-R case book.* Washington, DC: American Psychiatric Association; 1989.

6

Human Occupation and Mental Health Throughout the Life Span

Madness is always fascinating, for it reveals the ungluing we all secretly fear: the mind taking off from the body, the possibility that the magnet that attaches us to a context in the world can lose its grip.

MOLLY HASKELL (10)

The desire to act upon the environment, and to have an effect, is a force that drives and shapes human behavior from birth to death. Occupation, or the expression of this urge through activity, is essential for human growth and development. Without occupation, growth is frustrated and impaired. The focus and specifics of occupation change throughout life as the playing child matures into the working adult, who later retires and occupies himself with nonwork activities. The foundation of occupation-related skills formed in childhood profoundly influences all later development.

This chapter will consider how occupation develops and changes as the person matures and ages. We will also look at some of the more common mental health problems that arise in different life stages, with a particular emphasis on the role of occupational therapy in evaluation and treatment. It is important to remember that mental health problems do not always impair a person's ability to engage in occupation, or to use occupation to further his own growth and development.

MOTIVATION TOWARD OCCUPATION

To understand how occupation develops and changes throughout life, we must first consider why humans engage in occupation at all. What are the reasons? And are the reasons always the same? Reilly (19) identified a sequence of three levels of motivation for occupation or action: exploration, competency, and achievement.

Exploration motivation is the desire to act, to explore, for the pure pleasure of it. This is the primary or first motivation for action. Infants and small children do things because they are exploring what will happen, but adults do the same thing when they encounter new situations that arouse their interest.

Competency motivation is the desire to influence the environment in a specific way, and to get better at it. When motivated by competency, the individual will practice the action over and over again, and seek feedback from the environment (including other people) about the effects of his action. Competency is the second level of motivation and helps sustain actions that were initially motivated only by exploration.

Achievement motivation is the desire to attain, compete with, or surpass a standard of excellence. The standard may be an external one or may be generated by the individual. Achievement is the third and highest level of motivation for occupation. Once the person becomes competent at the action, he continues to perform it in order to achieve success according to a standard.

These three levels of motivation—exploration, competency, and achievement—form a continuum, which gradually transforms playful exploration into competent performance and ultimately into achievement and excellence. The skills that the child learns through play are later practiced and refined, and finally polished and combined with other skills to enable more sophisticated and complex behavior to emerge.

Whenever the individual encounters novelty in the environment he reexperiences these three levels of motivation, in sequence. New situations and unfamiliar environments bring out the urge to explore, and then to become competent, and then to achieve. This is as true of the working adult and the retiree as of the preschool child.

Kielhofner (11) argues, also, that different levels of motivation predominate at different stages in the life span. He suggests that the child engages in occupation primarily because of a motive to explore, that the adolescent does so to become competent, and the adult to achieve. He states that the older adult is motivated by an urge to explore his past and his own life's accomplishments, and to explore his present capabilities through leisure. Let us now take a closer look at this view of how occupation evolves as the individual grows and matures.

CHANGES IN OCCUPATION OVER THE LIFE SPAN

Human occupation is traditionally divided into two main categories: work and play. Play consists of activities that man engages in for pleasure, relaxation, self-exploration, or self-expression. Work includes all those activities through which man provides for his own welfare and contributes to the welfare of the social group to which he belongs. For the child, play is the dominant form of occupation; for the adult, work is the dominant form; the balance and relationship between work and play change throughout life in certain predictable ways. These are illustrated in Fig. 6–1.

The patterns of work and play illustrated in Fig. 6–1 are based on a Western (American) notion of normal human life and activity. Although anthropological studies show many similarities in patterns of work and play across different cultures, it is important to remember that individuals who come from different cultural backgrounds may have different expectations and experiences than those illustrated. Keeping this important caveat in mind, let us now look at the different life stages.

Childhood

Play is the main occupation of the child. The chart shows that in early childhood the child performs no work at all. Gradually, as the child is assigned chores and other responsibilities in his home and in school, he spends some of his time in activities that must be classified as work. The purpose of play and work in childhood is distinctive. As the child plays, he explores his environment, learns about reality, and develops rules that he uses to guide his actions. For example, he learns that objects fall to the floor when he drops them, that a stove is sometimes hot, that his uncle will let him

Levels of Organization of the Occupational Behavior Career

	CHILDHOOD	ADOLESCENCE	ADULTHOOD	OLD AGE
Waking Hours Occupied By Work & Play	Time spent in play		Time spent in work	
Play Yields	Reality is explored via curiosity for rules of competent action.	Competent behavior is learned and experienced in games, personal hobbies, and social events.	Relaxation and recreation support the worker role. Exploration of novel situations allows new roles to be taken on.	Play allows the exploration of past achievements and the unknown future, and maintenance of competence through leisure pursuit of interests.
Relationship of Play & Work	**Exploration** Skills for productivity are acquired and work roles explored through imitation and imagination.	**Competency** Personal and interpersonal competency are developed in a matrix of cooperation yielding habits of sportsmanship & craftsmanship.	**Achievement** Play supports the worker roles by providing an arena of retreat and rejuvenation. Exploration in novel situations allows the ongoing development of new competency for work.	**Exploration** Retirement leisure signals that the productive obligation to society has been fulfilled. Past work has earned for the person the right to leisure. Leisure replaces work as the major source of life satisfaction.
Work Yields	Productive behaviors are practiced through chores and in school.	The work role is practiced and the commitment process of occupational choice takes place.	There is entry into worker roles with the requirement of establishing and maintaining a productive and self-satisfying career.	Retirement brings reduced expectations for productivity and personal capacities for productive action are waning.

The Balance of Work and Play

FIG. 6–1. The balance and interrelationship of work and play during the life span. From Fig. 3 of Kielhofner G. A model of human occupation. 2: Ontogenesis from the perspective of temporal adaptation. *Am J Occup Ther* 1980; 34:657–663. Copyright © 1980 by the American Occupational Therapy Association, Inc. Reprinted by permission.

do things that his mother will not. These rules about motions, objects, and people (20) are tools that the child uses to guide future action and to develop skills. The child needs to learn as much as he can about how the world works because this knowledge is a foundation upon which later accomplishments are built. Thus, the playing child acquires knowledge and develops rules and skills that underlie and support the work of the student and the adult worker.

Recent research (1) confirms that play is essential for later development. Studies of many species show that important neurological connections such as cerebellar synapses and long fiber tracts are formed in their greatest numbers during the same period that play is most vigorous in the young animal. These connections establish a foundation for skillful, responsive motor actions. Another important function of play for young animals is to practice and rehearse the subtle social behaviors they will need to survive as adults (1). Thus, imitation and exploration of future occupational roles are enacted in play. Through fantasy and imitation the child investigates and experiences various adult roles (mommy, doctor, teacher, etc.). This experience, known as the fantasy period of occupational choice, is the first step in the three-stage process of choosing a career or adult occupation (9).

During play, the child also learns the joy of having an effect on the world and on other people. This helps her see herself as personally effective and powerful, thus developing and enhancing her sense of personal causation. The pleasure that she experiences in one activity over another helps her form interests that will motivate her throughout life.

Although the child is not expected to do much work, the productive activities that he does engage in are very important for later development. Studies have shown that industriousness in childhood is associated with greater job success and better personal adjustment in adult life (24). Chores and schoolwork are the major productive activities of childhood. By engaging in these tasks over time, the child acquires habits of industry and responsibility and learns to schedule his activities so that he still has time for play. Although play remains the major occupation throughout childhood, as the child matures he spends increasingly more time in activities that prepare him for his future as an adult worker.

Adolescence

The adolescent continues, like the child, to spend more time in play than in work. However, he is now motivated more by the desire to become competent than by the urge to explore; the activities he chooses are ones in which practice and the habits of sportsmanship and craftsmanship make the difference between success and failure. Whether the activity is the track team, the chess club, or video games, the adolescent approaches it with a determination to master and succeed. The biological changes of puberty interact with the adolescent's use of occupation to motivate a growing interest in social activities that provide opportunities to explore and practice social and sexual behaviors.

The work of the adolescent consists, like the work of the child, of school and chores. Schoolwork becomes more rigorous and more time consuming, in keeping with the adolescent's growing cognitive capacity and discipline. Depending on the parents and the family situation, the chores may also be increasingly challenging. Many adolescents take on part-time jobs, which provide important experiences of what life is like in the adult working world, and which give feedback about the adolescent's readiness for work.

The adolescent is concerned about what he will do with his life as an adult, and occupational choice is generally viewed as one of the most important developmental tasks of adolescence. The process that began in the fantasy period of childhood enters a new stage, known as the *tentative period*. During this time, the adolescent considers possible adult occupations that interest him. He evaluates whether he is capable of succeeding in them as well. Finally, he weighs his choices in terms of his personal values and his place in the social system. From this overwhelming mass of factors he finally makes a decision about a career, a decision that he may make again several times in his life.

Once the decision is made, the adolescent begins to work toward it, by (for example) enrolling in a training program or looking for a job. At this point he enters the *realistic period,* in which he examines whether his choice of career really meets his needs for achievement, satisfaction, status, and economic security. For example, if the chosen career is one in which jobs are scarce (e.g., acting) or where the pay is low, he may reconsider his decision, and then must come up with alternatives and choose among them.

Thus, occupational choice is crystallized and acted upon during adolescence, although for adolescent children of affluent parents the choice may be delayed into early adulthood. By contrast, adolescents from disadvantaged backgrounds may encounter overwhelming obstacles to realizing their occupational choice. In times of high unemployment, the adolescent with few skills may be denied employment or forced into a job that he finds demeaning and unsatisfying. Ultimately, the process of occupational choice may be repeated by the adult who decides or is forced to change careers later in life.

Adulthood

The adult spends many hours in work, leaving little time for play. The work of the adult is centered around the occupational role selected through the process of occupational choice. This work, which is not necessarily salaried (e.g., consider the homemaker), consumes much of his time and energy and allows him to express and gratify his urge to achieve. For many adults there is the additional work of parenthood.

The adult works in order to provide for his own needs and those of his family. Beyond this, he also works in order to produce something of value to the rest of society. Having a productive work role is important for the self-esteem of the adult; it gives him a sense of identity, a place in the social hierarchy, and a reason for being. Adults who are unemployed or underemployed (working at jobs that are beneath their capacities) often have negative views of their own abilities and worth. They may experience themselves as incompetent and helpless, rather than as competent and achieving members of society.

Despite the fact that working adults have less time for play, the time they spend in leisure and recreation serves an important function: it restores and refreshes their energies to work again. The word *recreation* actually means the creation (again) of the laboring capacity. Different people feel different degrees of need for recreation; some people spend almost all their time working, leaving only negligible amounts for play, and appear to be quite satisfied and happy. Others limit their work to a specific number of hours, precisely because they want to make time for leisure pursuits.

In middle and later adulthood, the individual looks toward the future and retirement, and begins to explore and plan for this next stage. He reevaluates his interests and develops new hobbies and goals. Without this preparation, the transition from full-time work to retirement can be stressful, even devastating.

Old Age

During the latter part of life, and certainly after retirement, the number of hours spent in work dramatically decreases. Thus, vast quantities of time suddenly become available, and decisions must be made about how to fill the hours. Leisure replaces work as the primary occupation, although many "retirees" continue to serve productive social roles (e.g., as volunteers) that can only be classified as work.

The loss of a work role (or the role of parent/homemaker) represents not just the loss of activities that once filled one's day, but also of status and social identity. To adjust, the older adult needs to have goals and occupations that provide satisfaction and opportunities for success, and that support a sense of self-worth. In the words of the 18th-century poet William Cowper,

> Absence of occupation is not rest,
> A mind quite vacant is a mind distressed.

Thus, one of the important tasks of this stage of adult life is to identify and develop interests and challenges for oneself that will sustain one's sense of independence and self-worth.

SUMMARY

Since occupational therapists and assistants are concerned primarily with a person's ability to develop and maintain occupational patterns that he finds satisfying, it is helpful to understand the functions and typical patterns of occupation during the major life stages.

The child samples and learns about the world through playful exploration, laying a foundation of motor and social skills. The adolescent, acting on the drive to become competent, practices and refines these skills and consolidates them into habits and roles. The adult, wishing to achieve and contribute, makes choices about career and life goals and selectively continues to develop and elaborate the skills and habits cultivated earlier in life. In later life, once career patterns are established, and especially after retirement, the older adult may

wish to integrate the long-abandoned interests of her younger self. Thus, strands of favored activities may be renewed and repursued in later life. New occupations can be discovered and old interests reexplored.

We know that the ability to engage in occupation is one of the signs of mental health, and we also know that mental illness can interfere with a person's ability to carry out daily life activities and to fulfill occupational roles. Let us look now at other significant factors in mental health at various ages, and the kinds of mental health disorders that tend to occur at different stages of life.

MENTAL HEALTH FACTORS THROUGHOUT THE LIFE SPAN

This section will provide an overview of the mental health needs of patients of different ages, and the ways in which occupational therapy intervenes to help them. The section is divided according to six major life stages: infancy and early childhood, middle childhood, adolescence, early adulthood, midlife, and late adulthood and aging. The material for each stage will briefly describe normal development and the kinds of mental health problems that sometimes arise. The general goals and methods of occupational therapy will be identified, and, where relevant, special treatment settings and evaluation and treatment methods will be described. More detail on specific diagnoses and treatment settings can be found in Chapters 5, 7, and 9.

Infancy and Early Childhood

A baby starts life with incredible needs and wants, and absolutely no ability to satisfy them on his own. His parents have to be able to figure out what he wants, whether he is hungry or thirsty or needs to be burped or cuddled or changed, and then provide these things for him. To be able to relate to other people later on, and to engage in activities that involve others, infants and small children need to learn to trust their parents and then people in general. In addition, they need to learn how to communicate their needs and feelings and how to control their impulses. Thoughtful interaction and consistent discipline by the parents help the child to acquire these skills. A stable, secure, and predictable environment is one of the most important factors in helping the child (at any age) to develop trust in himself, other people, and the world in general.

While all of this psychosocial development is going on, the child is developing in other ways too. His sensory abilities are becoming more refined, his motor skills more coordinated, and his perceptual and cognitive abilities more complex. He constantly uses and refines his developing abilities to learn more about the world and how to interact with it.

It is unusual for mental health problems to be diagnosed in infancy and the preschool years. Often, problems that are brought to the attention of psychiatric professionals are quite severe. Some of these problems are believed to have biological causes, meaning that the behavioral or emotional disorder is caused, at least in part, by something physical within the body or the brain.

Attention deficit disorder and infantile autism are in this category. Hyperactivity is another term sometimes used to describe attention deficit disorder. The child with attention deficit disorder has a shorter attention span than is normal for a child his age; he jumps from activity to activity, often with a high level of energy, but with an apparent inability to concentrate long enough to finish many of the tasks he attempts. It is not hard to imagine how this would interfere with learning.

Infantile autism is a disorder in which the very young child fails to respond to other people, often ignoring them completely. Autism is believed to have an underlying biological component. Recent research supports this view (18). The child is usually slow to develop language skills (the learning of which seems to rely upon interactions with others). In addition, children with autism may exhibit strange mannerisms (such as wiggling their fingers in front of their eyes) and bizarre interests (for example, in bright lights or spinning objects).

Occupational therapy for children with these disorders often focuses on sensorimotor or sensory integrative treatment approaches, which are believed to have an effect on the underlying biological problem. Occupational therapy assistants may carry out such treatment only under the direct supervision of registered occupational therapists who have special training in these approaches. Psychoanalytic (object relations) methods are sometimes used instead, but these also require direct supervision and special training. A more behaviorally oriented treatment approach focuses on the development of self-care skills (e.g., shoe-tying) through direct instruction and reinforcement.

Reports on occupational therapy treatment of young children with other mental health problems are infrequent in the literature. Baron (3), however, presented a case study of a four-year-old boy with oppositional defiant disorder. A structured play experience with the occupational therapist helped this child over a period of many weeks to give up his resentful and argumentative behavior and to develop a more spontaneous and genuine approach to play. Key elements of this treatment included a slow and careful building of trust through brief, frequent, one-on-one play with activities selected by the child from a limited choice given by the therapist; modification of the social play environment so that competition was reduced; and teaching and reinforcement of social skills such as taking turns.

Another serious mental health problem of early childhood is reactive attachment disorder, in which the child stops responding to other people because he has been neglected or ignored; this sometimes leads to failure to thrive, a condition in which the child may stop eating and withdraw totally. In such cases, the most intensive work is with the parents, teaching them how to provide more affection and better care.

Very small children with mental health problems are seldom treated in inpatient settings. Because of the important role of parents and family life in a child's development, the philosophy has been to keep the child with the family wherever possible. Therefore, children may attend day treatment centers, special preschools, or programs at community mental health centers, or may be treated in their homes, often with the involvement of the parents.

Occupational therapy for infants and small children with mental health problems is considered a very demanding and complex area of practice (6). In addition to emotional and social deficits, it seems that children with mental health problems are more likely than children without such problems to experience developmental motor delays (12). The occupational therapist uses special developmental assessments and data collection instruments, such as the Play History (4, 23), to evaluate the child's abilities, interests, and needs. Treatment programs are usually highly individualized, although they may take place in groups. Groups provide an experience of working with others, sharing, waiting, and taking turns, skills that prepare the child to succeed during his school years.

Some of the goals of treatment with this very young population may include developing trust and social interactions, increasing gross and fine motor coordination, improving sensory processing and perceptual skills, and facilitating more spontaneous play. In addition to sensorimotor and sensory integrative methods, play therapy and expressive art activities are sometimes used to help children develop and express their fantasies. Occupational therapy assistants who wish to work in this area will need to develop additional expertise beyond their basic education and should receive extensive supervision from a qualified OTR.

Later Childhood

The grade school years are ones in which the child refines his growing abilities in many areas. The roles of student and contributing family member are gradually adopted. The child develops a more sophisticated awareness of social norms and expectations, and of the needs of others. He learns to delay gratification for increasingly longer periods. In addition, the child becomes more physically coordinated and more intellectually sophisticated. He acquires vast amounts of knowledge and increasingly complex skills through his schoolwork and peer relationships.

The child continues to need the love, support, and encouragement of his parents and family in order to feel secure enough to attempt new challenges. Some mental health professionals believe that the family has such an effect on the mental health of the child that it may be the cause of emotional and behavioral problems. Others believe that the family is a factor, but that other factors such as biological predisposition and experiences at school and elsewhere are also involved.

Fortunately, mental health problems in middle childhood are infrequent, although more common than in early childhood. Among the problems that are seen in children during these years are conduct disorders, in which the child behaves in an antisocial fashion (e.g., stealing, cutting school), and other disorders which show up in physical behaviors (eating problems, stuttering, bedwetting, etc.). Drug and alcohol problems may also appear at this age. Attention deficit disorder often continues into middle childhood, or makes its first appearance at this time. Some children have difficulty learning in school and may be diagnosed with learning disabilities.

Children of school age are treated on an outpatient basis and hospitalized only when they are so out of control that they will harm themselves or someone else. They may be seen in school settings, in day treatment settings, or in afterschool programs.

Typically, the occupational therapy staff work with other professionals such as the special education teacher, the speech therapist, the child life specialist, and the school psychologist. The goals of treatment might include increasing trust and social relatedness, developing cooperation, improving self-esteem and self-awareness, enhancing self-control, developing body awareness and sensorimotor skills, and improving coordination, perceptual skills, and cognitive abilities.

Occupational therapy treatment models vary depending upon the setting and its philosophy, but may involve sensory integrative, behavioral, psychoanalytic, and environmental approaches. Children with attention deficit disorder or learning disabilities may be taught progressive relaxation and stress management techniques. Computer games have been used to evaluate cognitive and perceptual problems, and as rewards or reinforcers for participating in other treatment activities. As with the treatment of small children, occupational therapy intervention in middle childhood is considered a complex specialization, and one in which the COTA will benefit from additional training and supervision.

Adolescence

The most important task of the adolescent is to develop an identity separate from his parents—a social and sexual identity that will enable him to lead an independent life. Occupational choice, previously discussed, is a process that contributes to the development of identity in adolescence. Other important experiences center around the peer group of other adolescents. Through a variety of interactions and relationships with others his own age, the adolescent explores his values and interests and develops social skills. It is not unusual for an adolescent to experience insecurity, mood swings, loneliness, depression, and anxiety in response to the changes in his body and in the expectations of others toward him. These are normal responses to a challenging life adjustment. Sometimes, however, the problems are more severe.

Major psychiatric disorders such as schizophrenia and affective disorders (mania and depression) often make their first appearance in adolescence. Schizophrenia, as discussed in Chapters 3 and 5, is a disorder that is poorly understood, but that manifests itself in extreme personal disorganization. The psychotic symptoms of hallucinations and delusions can usually be controlled only with prolonged use of powerful medications, but even with medication, many schizophrenics have difficulty setting goals or structuring their time; their sense of self-identity is frequently impaired. If it occurs as early as adolescence, schizophrenia interferes with further psychosocial development; in other words, the developmental task of forming a separate identity is extraordinarily difficult, and later development suffers as a consequence.

Affective disorders (mania and depression) may also first appear in adolescence and have a better prognosis or predicted outcome than does schizophrenia. Nonetheless, they are serious disorders, and suicide is a growing risk among adolescents, especially those with affective disorders.

Substance abuse disorders are mental health problems that involve use or excessive use of drugs, alcohol, or other mind-altering substances. Adolescents may fall into substance abuse after experimenting with drugs or alcohol in order to be accepted by their peers. Some adolescents who have other mental health problems use these substances as "self-medication," to deaden their feelings of anxiety or depression.

Although adolescents may be treated in outpatient or community settings, it is not unusual for them to be hospitalized, especially when they are psychotic and in need of medication. Separate wards or adolescent services are provided wherever there are sufficient numbers of adolescent patients to justify the expense. Most adolescent inpatient services use a milieu therapy approach (see Chapter 7). Because the adolescent is trying to develop a separate identity, he will often act out or rebel against authorities (e.g., treatment staff). If the staff is too permissive or inconsistent, the adolescent fails to grasp what the boundaries of reasonable behavior really are; on the other hand, if the staff is too punitive and restrictive, the adolescent may become withdrawn and confused. Staff who work with adolescents are usually trained on the job in how to support the adolescent's independence while setting firm limits on unacceptable behavior.

Occupational therapy for adolescents is a specialized practice area. The registered therapist may use specialized evaluation instruments such as the Adolescent Role Assessment (5) to learn how the adolescent is adjusting to school, family life, and friendship. Goals of treatment may include development of self-esteem and self-identity skills, development of occupational choice, training in daily living skills, development of sensorimotor skills especially in relation to body image, and acquisition of prevocational behaviors.

In selecting activities for adolescents, occupational therapy staff must consider current fashions in activities and technology. Franklin (8), for example, reported that adolescents responded more favorably to a computer-based values clarification program than to a traditional paper and pencil version. Computers for word-processing and graphics design were incorporated by Baron (2) into the tasks available to adolescent members of a newspaper treatment group. In this group, the variety of job tasks and the structure and limitations provided by the leader helped members acquire and develop a sense of internal control and direction.

In working with adolescents who have mental health problems, the occupational therapy assistant may lead self-care and other activities of daily living (ADL) groups, provide sessions on sex education and birth control, or run vocationally oriented programs such as work groups and assembly lines. All of these can be powerful therapeutic experiences for adolescents whose parents are poor role models. Because adolescents are still in school most of the day, occupational therapy and other clinical services are scheduled around their schoolwork.

Early Adulthood

The years from 18 to approximately 40 are filled with challenges and opportunities. The young adult, having completed the process of occupational choice, strives to achieve success in his chosen career. Having attained a sense of his own identity as a separate person, he is able and eager to develop friendships and intimacies with others. The search for a marital or intimate partner is a primary task of this age group. Married couples who choose to have children are faced with the new role responsibilities of parenthood. Thus, early adulthood is a period characterized by a search for intimacy with others, and a desire to achieve and contribute to the future in some way, whether through a career or through raising children (or both).

Many of the patients seen in mental health settings in the 1990s fall into this age range, in part because much of the general population is in this group, the result of the tremendous number of babies born from 1946 to 1961. But in addition, young adulthood is the period during which many of the major psychiatric disorders of adult life are first noted. Also, for those individuals who are insecure in their jobs, or in their personal and sexual and family lives, this can be a period of severe stress and difficult adjustment. High unemployment and uncertain job security are realistic factors that can impede occupational success. The fact that there are more women than men in the population means that some women will not be able to find marriage partners. Also, the rise in infertility problems in this age group means that many will not be able to have their own biological children. Homosexual adults may fear rejection on the job and in social situations because of their sexual preferences (and fears of AIDS). All of these factors are potentially stressful and may lead to mental health problems.

Among the mental health problems and psychiatric disorders often seen in young adults are adjustment reactions, alcohol and drug abuse, schizophrenia, affective disorders, eating disorders, anxiety disorders, and various personality disorders. Adjustment reactions or disorders are maladaptive or ineffective reactions to life stress; instead of dealing with the stress in a positive way (that is, by trying to solve problems and rise above the situation), the individual may feel depressed or anxious, or function poorly at work or in social situations. It is believed that these people do not have an underlying psychological problem, but rather are reacting to stress. Occupational therapy intervention for patients suffering from adjustment disorders focuses on helping them identify and work toward specific goals. A crisis intervention approach (described in Chapter 7) is often used.

Alcohol and drug abuse is probably more prevalent among young adults than among adolescents. Alcoholism is a disease that has many definitions; what all these definitions have in common is excessive or uncontrolled use of alcohol, whether continuously or episodically. Alcoholics typically deny that they have a drinking problem; this attitude prevents them from seeking help or accepting it when it is offered; this is considered part of the disease. Another problem alcoholics have is with their use of time; they spend their leisure hours drinking and often have no other consistent leisure pursuits. As the alcoholic becomes more dependent on alcohol he is likely to have job problems and end up losing his job.

The goals of occupational therapy for alcohol and drug problems usually include development of self-awareness and self-responsibility, identification of personal goals, vocational assessment and work adjustment, and time management and leisure planning skills development. In particular, recovering alcoholics need to learn new activities and routines for their spare time, to replace the empty hours once filled with drinking. Frequently, the occupational therapist and assistant work with a treatment team that may include medical staff, creative arts therapists, and psychologists and alcohol counselors. Programs and occupational therapy approaches to persons with alcoholism and other substance abuse disorders are discussed in more detail in Chapter 9.

Eating disorders include anorexia and bulimia. Anorexia is a disorder in which the person (usually female) literally starves herself, believing that she is fat even though she is really emaciated. Bulimia is a disorder in which the person goes on eating binges, and then makes herself vomit. It is believed that anxiety about self-control versus control by others is one of the factors in both of these conditions. Occupational therapy usually includes assessment and modification of the patient's habits and beliefs related to eating and food, education in nutrition and cooking, sensorimotor and expressive activities for development of a more positive body image, and training in daily living skills. Chapters 5 and 9 contain more information on these disorders and on occupational therapy approaches to their treatment.

Many of the young adult patients seen in occupatonal therapy have diagnoses of either schizophrenia or affective disorder. For some, this is a continuation of a disease first diagnosed in adolescence; these people may have had multiple hospitalizations since then. Others have their first episode during their twenties or thirties. Some cases seem to be able to be controlled with medication, so that the person leads a fairly normal life, free of severe episodes that require hospitalization. However, the majority of cases of schizophrenia and affective disorders become classified as *chronic conditions,* meaning that the disease continues throughout life.

Young adult chronics, as these patients are called in the psychiatric literature, are considered very challenging by mental health professionals. Patients with alcohol and drug disorders and borderline and other personality disorders may also be placed in this category. Although young adult chronics may have limited skills for independent living, they are usually "street smart" and able to survive on their own in a marginal way. Large numbers of the homeless are in this group. Many of these people reject the stigma or label of mental illness, refuse to identify themselves as patients, and move in and out of treatment at whim. It is not unusual for these patients to become involved in criminal activities, and thus they may as easily be imprisoned as hospitalized.

Obviously, not all patients classified as young adult chronics share these characteristics. Sheets, Prevost, and Reihman (21) proposed a classification of three different groups of young adult chronics. Shown in Table 6–1, this classification system is useful for planning treatment and for thinking about the kinds of occupational therapy services that are most useful for patients in the different groups. For example, the low-energy, low-demand patient will need a structured environment and will probably not be difficult to manage, because she accepts herself in the role of patient. The challenge is to motivate this patient to do the best she can, within the limits of her disability. The high-energy, high-demand patient, by contrast, will be very difficult to manage and hard to keep in a program. This patient decides what to do based on what he wants at the moment. Thus, if he wants something, and his therapist will not give it to him right now, he is likely to walk out and not come back until he is in trouble or runs out of other options. The patient's entire life is characterized by impulsivity and an absence of planning. It is this group of patients that are most likely to end up in jail. Because of legal decisions that have awarded mental patients the right to refuse treatment, there is, unfortunately, very little that can be done to force these patients to remain in rehabilitation programs.

The high-functioning patient is more receptive to help, as long as it is provided in a manner that meets her self-esteem needs and aspirations. The patient is likely to be

TABLE 6–1. *Three types of young adult chronic patients*

Low-energy, low-demand group	High-energy, high-demand group	High-functioning group
Well ensconced in role of patient	Able to shop around from agency to agency to get what they want	Generally higher socioeconomic status and better appearance
Do not do well, even in remission	Fluctuating functional abilities and interests	New to mental health system
Concretely attached to programs and program places	"Give me what I want or stay out of my life" attitude toward mental health services	Resist mental health program involvement on the basis of conviction
Probably entered mental health system in early adolescence	Low frustration tolerance, acting out, encounters with the law	Some entered mental health system because of alcohol or drug abuse
Passive, poorly motivated	Frequently evicted, mobile	Want to understand their disorders and ways of preventing relapses
Accepting of mental health services	Expectations of self-reliance	
Appear burned out at an early age	Includes "revolving door" patients and street people	Want to blend into general population without being identified as mental patients

Reprinted with permission of the American Psychiatric Association (© 1982) from Table 2 in Sheets JL, Prevost JA, Reihman J. Young adult chronic patients: three hypothesized subgroups. *Hosp Commun Psychiatry* 1982; 33:197–203.

better educated and to hold very specific career goals. She does not want to be identified as a patient, but will actively participate in a treatment program if it is provided somewhere that is not identified as a hospital or part of the mental health system. It is believed that these patients respond best to a psychoeducational approach; this means that occupational therapy for daily living skills and prevocational skills and the like should be provided in classroom-type settings, with educational objectives and homework assignments. When skills are presented in this format the patient can perceive them as education rather than therapy, thus accommodating her need not to be identified as a patient.

Occupational therapy goals for young adult patients focus on the development of adult life skills and the fulfillment of the patient's personal aspirations. Typical goals include completing one's education, identifying vocational interests and aptitudes, acquiring prevocational and vocational skills, obtaining and maintaining employment, developing daily living skills, improving social skills, identifying and developing leisure interests, and structuring leisure time. The registered therapist performs the evaluations and formulates the treatment goals and plan, working closely with the patient.

The occupational therapy assistant might provide tutoring or academic assistance while the patient works toward a GED (general equivalency diploma) or other educational goal. Other roles for the COTA include running classes or training programs for daily living skills, social skills, leisure skills, and job search skills, and day-to-day supervision of work-oriented programs.

Midlife

Ferol Menks, an occupational therapist, defines midlife as "the point in the life cycle when the individual realizes that time is limited and that he or she cannot accomplish everything hoped and planned for"

(14). The goals that were selected and pursued during the early adult years may have already been reached, or may seem unattainable. Around age 40, the adult begins to reevaluate his life's direction, feeling that this may be his last chance to make major changes.

Erikson conceptualizes the major task of the middle adult years somewhat differently, terming it the crisis of *generativity versus stagnation*. Generativity is a "concern in establishing and guiding the next generation" (7). Unless the adult in the middle years is able to direct this energy successfully, he will feel stagnant or purposeless, cut off from the stream of human achievement that extends into the future.

One obvious avenue for achieving generativity is through one's children, but this path is not open to everyone, and for many does not by itself satisfy this urge. For those who are working, this need may be transformed into a concern with nurturing the careers of younger workers. Some adults may alternatively seek out ways to contribute their expertise and energies through church or community organizations.

The adult at midlife assesses whether his work is satisfying and worthwhile. If the work is found lacking either in opportunities for further achievement or in personal satisfaction, the individual may move into a second career. This may necessitate a return to school, a transition that some find stressful.

Additional developmental stresses center around the process of aging. During this period the adult experiences a decline in physical capacities, a change in sexual energies, and a significant cosmetic deterioration (wrinkles, etc.). Women go through menopause, and men experience a lessening of sexual potency. All of these changes signify that one is no longer young. Different people react differently to this. Some undergo cosmetic surgery, subject themselves to intense exercise programs, seek younger sexual partners, and attempt to stay the forces of time. Others accept these changes gracefully, as a condition of life, and move on to other concerns.

The children of adults in this age group tend to be teenagers. Dealing with the rebellion and turmoil of adolescent children can be a challenge and joy, or a significant stress, depending upon the adult's coping skills. Eventually, these children will mature, leave home, and create lives and families of their own; some adults find this prospect alarming because it means the end of their own roles as parents. In addition, the midlife adult is frequently faced with the needs of his own aging parents, who may be dependent in some way on his care, and whose presence is a reminder of the inescapability of death.

Thus, the stresses on the midlife adult are multiple. Successful negotiation of this stage involves understanding and accepting the aging process, and identifying and pursuing goals in work or family or community life that enable one to contribute to the future in a way that feels significant to the individual.

Psychiatric patients in this age range can be divided into three groups. The first group consists of those who have had mental health problems for many years—problems that have continued (and often worsened) as they aged. The second group comprises persons with various adjustment disorders, those who are unable to master or resolve the crises and stresses of adult life, and who resort to maladaptive behaviors such as drug and alcohol abuse, overeating, or withdrawal. The third group consists of individuals who are in the process of developing presenile dementias such as Alzheimer's disease. Each of these groups has different needs in terms of treatment.

Many of the middle-aged adults who have had mental conditions for many years tend to be somewhat "burned out." This means that they have little energy and seem passive and almost indifferent to what goes on around them. They will go along with treatment programs, but do not seem terribly invested in their own progress; getting through each day seems enough of a challenge. Not every person in this category is burned out, however. Some are "career patients" who have come to identify themselves in the patient role; they use the mental health system to meet their needs for physical safety, food, shelter, and economic assistance. Occupational therapy interventions for adults with chronic disorders of long standing focus on improving and maintaining daily living skills, providing opportunities for productive work in a shetered environment, and facilitating as much independent function as the person can handle.

The second group, those with adjustment reactions to the crises and stresses of adult life, need assistance in identifying and resolving the issues that confront them. As was mentioned earlier, crisis intervention is a widely used approach. Menks (15) has also described a *conflict-resolution model,* in which the occupational therapist guides the patient through five steps, which begin with identifying the problem and end with implementing a plan of action. The problems addressed are varied, ranging from how to use leisure time, to how to compensate for a career that feels demeaning and pointless, to how to cope with divorce or the death of a spouse.

In the third category are people with primary degenerative dementia, a kind of organic brain syndrome that is progressive. Alzheimer's disease, which is in this category, may show its first signs as early as age 40. Memory impairment or forgetfulness is usually the first symptom; the person first has trouble remembering details (dates, names, facts), and the memory loss becomes more profound as the disease progresses. Gradually, so much of the memory is lost that the person is unable to complete simple activities because he does not remember that he started them. There are personality changes as well; though these are not always noticeable in the early stages, they become more bizarre and inappropriate over time. Ultimately, the person loses physical neuromotor control over his body, becomes incontinent and less mobile, and eventually dies.

Because the symptoms of Alzheimer's disease progress slowly at first, the patient in the early stages of the illness can usually continue his customary activities with a few minor adjustments. For example, at work he may have to be supervised more closely, or switch to duties that require less attention to detail. Similarly, family members will have to compensate for his deficits in the home. If, for example, the patient is the cook in the family, he will need supervision to make sure he does not cause a fire. Occupational therapists and assistants work with these early-stage patients and their families in the home wherever possible. The goals of intervention are to assess what areas and activities are causing difficulty for the patient, to evaluate his current strengths and deficits, and to help the family adapt the environment and provide the social support the patient needs.

It is important that Alzheimer's disease patients remain at home or in the accustomed environment for as long as possible, since they are better able to function in familiar environments than in new ones (13). In the later stages of their illness these patients cannot remain in the community because they need either medical care or round-the-clock supervision. They are most frequently placed in nursing homes, although some are hospitalized in large public institutions. Occupational therapists and assistants provide services that help them remain alert and function to the best of their present capacities. These generally include reality orientation (described in Chapter 22), sensory stimulation (e.g., olfactory and tactile stimulation), and physical activities (exercise, ball play, dancing). Memory training is sometimes used with higher functioning (early or middle stage) patients.

Late Adulthood and Aging

The most important psychosocial task of the older adult is believed by many experts to be the development of an understanding and appreciation for what he has accomplished during his life. Erikson (7) has called this the crisis of *ego integrity versus despair.* Erikson believed that in order to feel that his life has been worthwhile, the older adult needs to see himself as only a small part of the human community, which will endure beyond his own death.

In addition to this major developmental task, the older adult often must deal with significant life stress. One's aging body, retirement and the loss of a career role, the deaths of spouses and cherished friends, economic worries, and the loss of one's home are just a few of the stresses that press on the older adult's diminished energies. New hobbies, new friendships, and new roles as volunteer or grandparent may compensate for some of these losses, but many older adults find it difficult to make these adjustments.

Shimp (22) reminds us that many of our cherished "truths" about older people are in fact myths. While many retirees are satisfied and relieved to give up their productive roles, many others happily undertake volunteer and paid jobs into their nineties. Also, the notion that the aged cannot adapt to life stresses needs careful examination in each case. Even a severe stress such as acute care hospitalization can be endured and managed successfully, given sufficient motivation and hope.

Depression is the most common psychiatric diagnosis in the elderly population. A person in a very deep or severe depression can become so withdrawn and self-involved that he appears demented (cognitively impaired); for this reason, the condition is sometimes misdiagnosed as an organic mental disorder. When the depression is finally recognized and properly treated (usually with medication), the person's attention and cognitive functions return to normal. After depression, Alzheimer's disease and other organic mental disorders are the psychiatric conditions most commonly diagnosed in the aged population. Coincidentally and confusingly, depression is often a symptom of organic mental disorder.

Occupational therapy may be provided to the older adult in his home, in a geriatric day center, or in a hospital or nursing home. The purpose of occupational therapy intervention is to help the older adult maintain or achieve a feeling of competence or self-reliance, and to prevent further deterioration in functioning. Environmental adaptations made by the occupational therapist can allow higher functioning individuals to continue living in their own homes; this is very important for maintaining their sense of self-identity and a personal daily routine. In addition, the therapist or assistant may provide leisure counseling, assist in the development of hobbies, and facilitate social involvement.

Occupational therapy interventions for the older adult in a nursing home or geropsychiatric ward are similar to those described earlier for the midlife adult with Alzheimer's disease. The occupational therapy assistant may use reality orientation and remotivation techniques and life review activities (described in Chapters 20, 21 and 22), or instruct nursing staff and volunteers. Other aspects of occupational therapy intervention for this group are described in Chapter 7.

Because not all individuals in a nursing home function at such a low level, the occupational therapist must plan programs that allow people with different capacities to participate and that provide challenges to each person at his own level. The therapist begins by assessing how well each patient functions in terms of his social, physical, and cognitive functioning and his self-care skills. The Parachek Geriatric Rating Scale (16, 17) is sometimes used for this and may be administered by the COTA. The Parachek Scale allows the observer to rate 10 different functions in the three categories of physical capabilities, self-care skills, and social interaction. The scoring system and treatment manual that accompany the scale assist the therapist in assigning patients to different groups, based on functional level as determined by their scores on the rating scale. Parachek recommends that crafts and cognitive activities like games and puzzles be provided for higher functioning patients, simple group activities and self-care for those with scores in the middle range, and sensory stimulation for those with the lowest scores. She recommends physical activities for all three groups, and adapts the activities to compensate for more limited function in the low scoring group.

The occupational therapy assistant who works with the geriatric population must be very receptive to the needs and concerns of the older individual. It is important to respect and accommodate the habits and beliefs that the person has built up over a lifetime. Because they have lost so many of the things that were once important to them, older people often fear the loss of their identity and self-direction, and may feel threatened when a health professional pushes them too far, too fast. Also, because of a generalized slowing of physical capacities, older people may respond less quickly and usually need more time to answer questions and learn new things. Finally, the older individual thinks often and deeply about his past and enjoys telling stories about it; this recounting is an important psychological process for establishing a sense of ego integrity. It is important for the COTA to recognize the value of this reminiscence and encourage it.

SUMMARY AND CONCLUSION

We can think of life as a puzzle or a project that we can work out only by traveling down a path that is not always clear. A turn in the road may bring us face to face with obstacles that must be dealt with before we can proceed. We each have different tools (our native talents and acquired skills) to help us work out the puzzle and to clear the path. Sometimes, though, the obstacle seems unconquerable, and this is when mental health problems arise.

Problems can occur at any age, at any point along the path; some individuals are more vulnerable to these problems than others. The role of the mental health professional is not to solve the problem or clear the path, but to enable the person to tackle and master his own obstacles, so that he can clear his own way and proceed. To do this well, we must know as much as we can about human development, because this forms the underlying structure of each person's path; knowledge of major developmental milestones and tasks helps us predict the person's capabilities at each point in the life span and alerts us to stresses that might affect him.

We must also know as much as possible about occupation and its role in human life, and we must value it highly. Occupation is an essentially human tool for tackling the puzzles of life. It gives us a sense of purpose and competence, channels our energies, and sustains our forward movement on life's path. Without occupation, there is no progress; everything stops. When occupation is disordered, without goals and direction, life becomes chaotic. And when the ability to use occupation is impaired because of disability or disease, the individual is deprived of one of the most valuable tools a human being can possess. The role of occupational therapy is to restore this ability, to enable and support each person's ability to use this powerful tool to solve his life's puzzles, to master stresses and obstacles, and to propel himself on the path to the future.

REFERENCES

1. Angier N. The purpose of playful frolics: training for adulthood. *The New York Times* October 20, 1992; CXLII (49,125):C1–C8.
2. Baron KB. The model of human occupation: a newspaper treatment group for adolescents with a diagnosis of conduct disorder. *Occup Ther Mental Health* 1987; 7(2):89–104.
3. Baron KB. The use of play in child psychiatry: reframing the therapeutic environment. *Occup Ther Mental Health* 1991; 11(2/3):37–56.
4. Behnke CJ, Fetkovich MM. Examining the reliability and validity of the play history. *Am J Occup Ther* 1984; 38:94–100.
5. Black MM. Adolescent role assessment. *Am J Occup Ther* 1976; 30:73–79.
6. Burnell DP. Children with severe emotional or behavioral disorders. In: Clark PN, Allen AS, eds. *Occupational therapy for children*. St Louis: Mosby; 1985.
7. Erikson E. *Childhood and society*. New York: Norton; 1963.
8. Franklin D. A comparison of the effectiveness of values clarification presented as a personal computer program versus a traditional therapy group: a pilot study. *Occup Ther Mental Health* 1986; 6(3):39–52.
9. Ginzburg E. Toward a theory of occupational choice. In: Peters HC, Hansen JC. *Vocational guidance and career development*. New York: Macmillan; 1971.
10. Haskell M. Love and other infectious diseases, 1990. In: Maggio R, compiler. *The Beacon book of quotations by women*. Boston: Beacon Press; 1992:208.
11. Kielhofner G. A model of human occupation. 2: Ontogenesis from the perspective of temporal adaptation. *Am J Occup Ther* 1980; 34:657–663.
12. Kramer LA, Deitz JC, Crowe TK. A comparison of motor performance of preschoolers enrolled in mental health programs and non-mental health programs. *Am J Occup Ther* 1988; 42:520–525.
13. Liu L, Gauthier L, Gauthier S. Spatial disorientation in persons with early senile dementia of the Alzheimer type. *Am J Occup Ther* 1991; 45:67–74.
14. Menks F. Changes and challenges of mid life. 1: A review of the literature. *Occup Ther Mental Health* 1980; 1(3):15–28.
15. Menks F. Challenges of mid life: An occupational therapy conflict resolution model. *Occup Ther Mental Health* 1980; 1(4):23–32.
16. Miller ER, Parachek JR. Validation and standardization of a goal-oriented, quick screening geriatric scale. *J Am Geriatr Soc* 1974; 22:224–237.
17. Parachek JF. *Parachek geriatric rating scale*. 3rd ed. Phoenix, Ariz: Center for Neurodevelopmental Studies; 1986.
18. Peterson TW. Recent studies in autism: a review of the literature. *Occup Ther Mental Health* 1986; 6(4):63–75.
19. Reilly M. *Play as exploratory learning*. Beverly Hills, Calif: Sage Publications; 1974.
20. Robinson AL. Play: the area for acquisition of rules for competent behavior. *Am J Occup Ther* 1977; 31:248–253.
21. Sheets JL, Prevost JA, Reihman J. Young adult chronic patients: three hypothesized subgroups.

In: Hospital and Community Psychiatry Service of the American Psychiatric Association. *The young adult chronic patient: collected articles from H&CP.* Washington, DC: American Psychiatric Association; 1983. (Originally published in *Hosp Commun Psychiatry* 1982; 33:197–203.)

22. Shimp S. Debunking the myths of aging. *Occup Ther Mental Health* 1990; 10(3):101–111.
23. Takata N. The play history. *Am J Occup Ther* 1969; 23:314–318.
24. Vaillant GE, Vaillant CO. Natural history of male psychological health. x: Work as a predictor of positive mental health. *Am J Psychiatry* 1981; 138:1433–1440.

ADDITIONAL REFERENCES AND SUGGESTED READINGS

Agrin AR. Occupational therapy with emotionally disturbed children in a public elementary school. *Occup Ther Mental Health* 1987; 7(2):105–114.

American Psychiatric Association. *Diagnostic and statistical manual of mental disorders.* 3rd ed, revised. Washington, DC: American Psychiatric Association; 1987.

Anonymous. First person account: a father's thoughts. *Schizophrenia Bull* 1983; 9:439–442.

Barris R, Keilhofner G, Watts JH. *Psychosocial occupational therapy: practice in a pluralistic arena.* Laurel, Md: RAMSCO; 1983.

Burnell DP. Children with severe emotional or behavioral disorders. In: Clark PN, Allen AS, eds. *Occupational therapy for children.* St Louis: Mosby; 1985.

Cermak SA, Stein F, Abelson C. Hyperactive children and an activity group therapy model. *Am J Occup Ther* 1973; 26:311–315.

Christiansen CH, Davidson DA. A community health program with low achieving adolescents. *Am J Occup Ther* 1974; 28:346–353.

Erikson E. *Identity: youth and crisis.* New York: Norton; 1968.

Fazio LS. Tell me a story: the therapeutic metaphor in the practice of pediatric occupational therapy. *Am J Occup Ther* 1992; 46:112–119.

Giles GM. Anorexia nervosa and bulimia: an activity-oriented approach. *Am J Occup Ther* 1985; 39:510–517.

Hatfield AB. The family as partner in the treatment of mental illness. *Hosp Commun Psychiatry* 1979; 30:338–340.

Henig RM. *The myth of senility: the truth about the brain and aging.* Washington, DC; American Association of Retired Persons, and Glenview, Ill: Scott Foresman; 1985.

Herman BE. A sensory integrative approach to the psychotic child. *Occup Ther Mental Health* 1980; 1(1):57–68.

Hilowitz EC. Computers as a tool in pediatric private practice. *Occup Ther Newspaper* 1985; 39(10):5.

Hilowitz EC. How to buy software. *Occup Ther Newspaper* 1985; 39(11):7.

Hospital and Community Psychiatry Service of the American Psychiatric Association. *The young adult chronic patient: collected articles from H&CP.* Washington, DC: American Psychiatric Association; 1983.

Kernberg P. Update of borderline disorders in children. *Occup Ther Mental Health* 1983; 3(3):83–91.

Kielhofner G. *A model of human occupation: theory and application.* Baltimore: Williams & Wilkins; 1985.

Kohler ES. The effect of activity/environment on emotionally disturbed children. *Am J Occup Ther* 1980; 34:446–451.

Kwako R. Relaxation as therapy for hyperactive children. *Occup Ther Mental Health* 1980; 1(3):29–45.

Levinson DJ. *The seasons of a man's life.* New York: Ballantine Books; 1978.

Lewis CB. *Aging: the health care challenge: an interdisciplinary approach to assessment and rehabilitative management of the elderly.* Philadelphia: FA Davis; 1985.

Lindsay WP. The role of the occupational therapist in treatment of alcoholism. *Am J Occup Ther* 1983; 37:36–43.

Linn M, Caffey EM, Kiett J, Hogarty GE, Lamb HR. Day treatment and psychotropic drugs in the aftercare of schizophrenic patients. *Arch Gen Psychiatry* 1970; 36:1055–1066.

Mace NL, Rabins PV. *The 36-hour day: a family guide to caring for persons with Alzheimer's disease, related dementing illnesses, and memory loss in later life.* Baltimore: The Johns Hopkins University Press; 1981.

Maiorana R. Early recognition and management of alcohol problems: occupational therapy treatment. *Am Occup Ther Assoc Mental Health Special Interest Section Newsletter* 1984; 7(2):1–2.

Mellencap A. Adolescent depression: a review of the literature, with implications for nursing care. *J Psychosoc Nurs Ment Helath Serv* 1981; 19(9):15–20.

North C, Cadoret R. Diagnostic discrepancy in personal accounts of patients with 'schizophrenia.' *Arch Gen Psychiatry* 1981; 38:133–137.

Palmer F, Barrows C. Vocational activities for adolescents: a program description. *Am Occup Ther Assoc Mental Health Special Interest Section Newsletter* 1985; 8(4):1–2.

Reed KL. *Models of practice in occupational therapy.* Baltimore: Williams & Wilkins; 1984.

Reisberg B. *A guide to Alzheimer's disease for families, spouses and friends.* New York: The Free Press (Collier); 1981.

Scheidlinger S. Group treatment of adolescents: an overview. *Am J Orthopsychiatry* 1985; 55:102–111.

Shannon P. The adolescent experience. *Occup Ther Mental Health* 1983; 3(2):73–81.

Sheehy G. *Passages: predictable crises of adult life.* New York: Bantam Books; 1978.

Sholle-Martin S. Application of the model of human occupation: assessment in child and adolescent psychiatry. *Occup Ther Mental Health* 1987; 7(2): 3–22.

Sholle-Martin S, Alessi NE. Formulating a role for occupational therapy in child psychiatry: a clinical application. *Am J Occup Ther* 1990; 44:871–882.

Smyntek L, Barris R, Kielhofner G. The model of human occupation applied to psychosocially functional and dysfunctional adolescents. *Occup Ther Mental Health* 1985; 5(1):21–39.

Snyder S. Comprehensive inpatient treatment of the young adult chronic patient. *Occup Ther Mental Health* 1985; 5(2):47–52.

Snyder S. Comprehensive inpatient treatment for the young adult patient. *Occup Ther Mental Health* 1985; 5(2):47–58.

Talbot JF. An inpatient adolescent living skills program. *Occup Ther Mental Health* 1983; 3(4): 35–43.

Wasow M. *Coping with schizophrenia.* Palo Alto, Calif: Science and Behavior Books; 1982.

Willson M. *Occupational therapy in long-term psychiatry.* Edinburgh: Churchill-Livingstone; 1983.

PART 2

Context

7

Treatment Settings

I was being admitted to a locked unit of a long-term psychiatric clinic. My belongings were searched, then locked away, and I was stripped and dressed in bed clothes—those horrible green hospital-issued "smock things" that tie in the back with two ill-spaced and sometimes nonexistent ties. Thus clad and dehumanized I was sent to "mingle with the other patients."

IRENE M. TURNER (38)

There are many different environments or treatment settings in which occupational therapists and assistants work with psychiatric patients. Each treatment setting has its own purpose, treatment philosophy, funding pattern, and population that it serves. These factors influence the behavior of patients and staff, and the role of occupational therapy and of the occupational therapy assistant. Daily staff schedules, evaluation and treatment responsibilities, and the kinds of activities and services vary from setting to setting.

This chapter presents an overview of the major types of treatment settings in which occupational therapy services are provided to patients with psychiatric problems. The role and responsibilities of the assistant within each setting will be discussed. Concepts from the model of human occupation about the effect of the environment on occupational behavior will be explored with regard to how particular treatment settings may affect patients' behavior. Since some settings may use theories or practice models other than those described in Chapters 2, 3, and 4, some of these other models will be described briefly.

THE SCOPE OF PATIENTS

As discussed in Chapter 5, mental health problems for which people seek and receive treatment range from transient situational disturbances to severe and progressive illnesses. Among the less severe problems are mild depression and anxiety brought on by life circumstances; many people seek help with these problems from their family physicians, and may be referred to treatment with a psychiatrist, psychologist, or social worker. Mild problems are rarely treated by occupational therapists unless the patient experiences sustained difficulty in carrying out daily life activities; even then, verbal therapy with another mental health professional may be the only treatment provided. Most mild mental health problems resolve themselves more or less satisfactorily as the patient learns to cope with his life situation, or when the situation itself changes. Depending on the funding and programs available in a local area, some occupational therapy services may be available to people with mild mental health problems through community mental health centers, home health services, and prevention programs.

People with more serious mental health problems are often hospitalized or referred to an outpatient mental health center where occupational therapy personnel work with them as part of a team of professionals. Some of the people admitted to these settings, such as battered women and emotionally disturbed children and the frail elderly, are suffering from social and economic problems as well as mental disorders. Drug and alcohol abusers, individuals with personality disorders and eating disorders, and the mildly mentally retarded may also be seen.

Despite the fact that some occupational therapy personnel work with these populations, the majority of occupational therapists and assistants who work in mental health hospital and community settings provide services to more severely disabled psychiatric patients. It has been estimated that there are some 1,700,000 to 2,400,000 persons suffering from chronic mental illness nationwide (37). Serious mental health problems are often first recognized when the patient becomes so symptomatic or disorganized that he needs to be hospitalized or (in the case of substance abuse) admitted for detoxification. Often, but not always, this initial hospitalization is the first of a series. Chronic illnesses (see Chapters 5 and 6) are severe and progressive, leading to decreased ability to function in the community and in some cases to lifelong incarceration. Many patients with severe and chronic problems can learn to function adequately in the community with varying degrees of supervision from mental health professionals, at least in the early years of their illness. The rehabilitation and community reintegration of chronic mental patients, particularly those with schizophrenia, has been demonstrated to be most successful in centers where occupational therapy services are provided (26).

THE SCOPE OF SETTINGS

Treatment settings in which occupational therapists and assistants are employed to work with the mentally ill range from high-security inpatient wards, in which violent or suicidal patients can be adequately supervised, to community settings, in which people who do not need hospitalization are seen. Most inpatient psychiatric settings have some occupational therapy personnel on staff; these settings may be large public institutions, nonprofit voluntary psychiatric hospitals, general hospitals, or proprietary hospitals. The aged and those suffering from Alzheimer's disease and other organic mental disorders may be treated in nursing homes. The criminally insane may be treated on forensic units of large state hospitals, and other criminal offenders may receive services within correctional institutions.

Occupational therapists and assistants may also work with special diagnostic groups who may be treated separately, on their own ward, or in special outpatient programs or live-in facilities in the community. Some of these special populations are described in Chapter 9. Groups that might receive separate treatment include battered women, sex offenders, child abusers, drug and alcohol abusers, persons with dementia, AIDS patients, and persons with eating disorders. It is believed that these groups have special needs that are best met when they are treated with peers who have similar problems. Sometimes separate wards are created for research into the effectiveness of medications or other treatments for persons with a particular diagnosis (e.g., paranoid schizophrenia).

Outpatient settings include aftercare clinics attached to hospitals with inpatient services, various walk-in programs in community mental health centers, and social and community agencies. Children and adolescents may be seen in school settings or in afterschool programs at community centers such as libraries or YWCAs. Those who are very ill may be hospitalized or incarcerated in long-term treatment centers. Home health agencies sometimes provide occupational therapy services in the home to persons suffering from mental disorders, but usually only if there is another (non-psychiatric) diagnosis.

Occupational therapists and assistants are also employed in workshops and vocational rehabilitation centers, which provide patients with psychiatric disabilities the opportunity to perform productive work under noncompetitive conditions. Some of these centers provide prevocational and vocational training, and have programs that enable patients to make the transition to community employment.

INPATIENT SETTINGS

Inpatient settings consist of hospitals and other environments (e.g., skilled nursing facilities) in which nursing care is available around the clock. Patients who need supervision because they are violent or because they are so disorganized that they cannot meet their own needs for food, clothing, and shelter can often be protected only in this type of setting. Inpatient settings are generally divided into two subcategories: acute and chronic. Acute inpatient settings provide services on a short-term basis, generally for patients who have become ill suddenly, or who have a history of psychiatric illness and suffer a sudden recurrence of psychotic symptoms. Some acute settings are locked, so that patients are prevented from escaping and harming themselves or others. Chronic inpatient settings provide supervision and services for patients who have illnesses that cause serious disabilities that impair community living (generally schizophrenia or organic mental disorders). Chronic patients may remain in these settings for many years, even until they die; chronic settings for very disorganized patients are usually locked. Long-term inpatient treatment, in which patients who were not so seriously ill remained for months or years, was the norm only 30 years ago; today this has given way to outpatient treatment, which recognizes that people get better faster in their own communities.

Large State Hospitals and Other Public Institutions

This category includes municipal hospitals, state hospitals, county hospitals, and Veterans Administration and U.S. Public Health Service facilities. Funding for these institutions is provided by city, state, and federal monies. Most such facilities have inpatient and outpatient services, and they may have specialized units for forensic (criminal) cases, addiction and alcoholism, the aged, children, and adolescents. Some are located in urban centers. Most are very large, consisting of several buildings on a sprawling campus, often located in rural areas. Family members may find it difficult to visit patients because of distance.

The deinstitutionalization of psychiatric patients, compelled by the Community Mental Health Act of 1963, resulted in the discharge of many who were previously inmates of large state psychiatric hospitals. At present the population of these centers consists of three main categories: patients who are too violent or suicidal to be released, patients who have intact families or social support systems but who are so severely impaired and disorganized that they cannot live in the community even with this support, and those who lack social support from family or others and who (despite apparently adequate skills) have shown on repeated discharges that they cannot succeed in the community without it. Yet another group of patients, although competent to remain for long periods in the community, may be admitted for brief, occasional hospitalization, often precipitated by stressful life events. Admissions of young adult chronic patients (described in Chapter 6) have increased in recent years. These patients are more difficult to manage and to treat than are their older counterparts.

Patients are admitted to state hospitals on a geographic basis, in which a region is divided into "catchment areas;" the patient is sent to the particular state hospital whose catchment area includes his place of residence. Large public institutions are typically understaffed, not only in occupational therapy and other activity programs, but also in basic medical and nursing services. Sometimes the physicians employed there have no psychiatric training or are recent immigrants whose command of English is so limited that their ability to understand and be understood by patients and other staff is grossly impaired. Funding is erratic and hiring freezes and shortages of supplies are common.

Despite these drawbacks, such facilities provide many opportunities and challenges for occupational therapists and assistants. The variety of diagnoses seen and the possibilities for working with patients of different ages and severity of illness permit therapists to develop a depth and breadth of experience. Also, because patients tend to remain for longer periods, or are frequently readmitted, therapists can develop long-term therapeutic relationships, can observe the progression of the disease process, and can experience the effect of their interventions over time. Also, because of staff shortages, occupational therapists and assistants not infrequently are promoted to administrative or management positions that might not be available to them in other settings.

The types of services provided by occupational therapy in these settings are comprehensive, and because of this difficult to describe completely. Hemphill (17) states that all too often the role of occupational therapy today in most such settings is that of "activity provider." The activities provided—crafts, indoor sports, and games—may divert the patient's attention from her illness but do not help her develop skills she needs to leave the hospital and survive on her own in the community. She recommends that occupational therapy focus instead on rehabilitation with the aim of independent living.

Inpatient wards are generally divided into acute and chronic; on acute wards the emphasis is on medical treatment and control of symptoms through use of medica-

tions. Occupational therapists and assistants may provide general activities aimed at simulating normal patterns of daily living; patients' performance and behavior during activities is monitored to determine the effect of the medical treatment and the patient's readiness for discharge. On chronic wards, depending on the level of disability among the patients, occupational therapy may include sensory integrative treatment, maintenance of or training in daily living skills, current events and discussion groups, and general exercise. There are often fewer staff on chronic wards, and the occupational therapy assistant may be charged with providing services for as many as 50 to 100 patients. The occupational therapy program may be carried out on the ward, in special activity rooms within each hospital building, or in a centralized activities building elsewhere on the hospital campus. Some large state hospitals utilize the off-unit programming approach, in which activities are provided in a centralized location away from the living units. These off-unit sites are ideal for activities like work and school that would be done away from home if one were living in the community. Grooming and other activities of daily living are best taught and practiced in the ward setting, which is closer to the home environment (18).

Because of the emphasis on returning patients to community living wherever possible, occupational therapy on both acute and chronic wards emphasizes evaluation of and training in daily living skills. If and when patients are discharged, they may be assigned to a satellite clinic near the patient's home, at which they can receive whatever aftercare services they need, including occupational therapy; these clinics are staffed and administered by the state hospital system.

Some state psychiatric hospitals have quarterway houses on or near the hospital grounds. These live-in settings allow patients to practice living in the community while still receiving direct supervision from trained staff. Once they have demonstrated an ability to function under these conditions, patients are discharged to independent community living. Transitional services, such as visits by outpatient counselors and telephone counseling, are usually provided.

Acute Care Inpatient Wards

Acute care inpatient wards provide a secure environment in which patients who are seriously ill can be evaluated and treated for a short time; after this they are either discharged (with or without an outpatient treatment plan) or transferred to a long-term unit or other facility such as a state hospital. Acute care wards may be housed in a general hospital, a large private hospital (voluntary or proprietary), or a public institution; they are usually locked for the protection of the patients and the general population. Goals for occupational therapy in the acute care setting include observing and reporting patient performance and response to medication, improving patient performance in preparation for return to the community, assisting in discharge planning, and helping to stabilize behavior (2).

Inpatient stays have gotten shorter as a result of pressures from third-party payers; stays of a week or less are not uncommon. Discharge planning is a primary focus in the acute care setting. Consequently, occupational therapy evaluation is a key element. Areas for evaluation include cognitive level, self-care skills, and independent living skills. Lengthy evaluation is not possible, and any evaluation method used must give quick results that can be used in discharge planning.

The volume of note writing and documentation has increased, since initial and discharge notes must be written on every patient; with 10 to 20 admissions a week this means that 20 to 40 notes are written every week.

Much of the staff's time is spent in meetings, communicating observations and findings about patients, and planning for their discharge; up to half of the occupational therapy staff's time may be given to meetings. Therapists are sometimes frustrated when patients fail to attend occupational therapy groups or must leave in the middle of a group to attend an interview or have a test done; different occupational therapy departments have policies or strategies for dealing with this problem.

Robinson and Avallone (35), for example, developed an *activities health* approach, based on the idea that activity (function) can be healthy even when the person is dealing with a serious mental illness. This approach aims to maintain activities health during hospitalization by providing a normal routine selected by the patient from a typical array of work, rest, and leisure activities. To the extent possible, the program provides opportunities for patients to engage in more specific and individualized tasks similar to those done before hospitalization. Three other objectives of occupational therapy in the activities health approach are to monitor the effects of medication on the patient's ability to function, to work with the patient to assess her activities health and routine, and to recommend services needed to improve everyday functioning after discharge.

Another approach has been to provide activity groups to meet the general needs of patients on the unit; the goals of such groups may be to build self-esteem, increase awareness of self and others, develop group skills, or express feelings (34). Typical activities include games, group sports, and art projects. The purpose is to provide a positive experience that might restore patients' confidence in themselves and increase their interest in and ability to relate to other people.

Peloquin (32) developed the *interview/therapy set* as yet another approach to providing evaluation and treatment for large numbers of acute care patients who stay less than two weeks. Therapy set is the process of orienting patients to the pur-

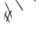

pose, goals, and procedures used in a particular treatment. This approach uses three forms—an open letter, an activity guide, and a checklist of goals—to help patients understand the value of occupational therapy and to encourage their participation. The letter, which describes the purpose of occupational therapy in simple language, is given to all literate patients as soon as they are organized enough to understand it. The activity guide is a self-administered data collection instrument. It is divided into sections consisting of several yes/no questions about problems the patient might be having; each section ends with a brief description of how occupational therapy can help. The checklist of goals, shown in Fig. 7–1, is used to develop a treatment program for each patient, based on objectives identified from the patient's answers on the activity guide. The therapist checks off the goals the patient is to concentrate on and the activities he is to attend to work on them; a copy of the form is given to the patient and another is placed in the chart. The interview/therapy set procedure is an efficient way to provide occupational therapy evaluation and treatment in an acute care setting.

The occupational therapy assistant employed on an acute care inpatient unit is likely to begin his day by attending a morning meeting with other unit staff. This meeting, which lasts less than one hour, might begin around 8:30 A.M., and be led by nursing staff. The purpose is to inform all staff about any new admissions and about the general behavior of patients and events on the ward in the last 24 hours. Following this there may be a general community meeting with the patients; again, the purpose is to introduce new patients, say goodbye to those about to be discharged, and discuss feelings or recent events on the unit. Depending on the program needs identified by the supervising occupational therapist, the assistant may be excused from one or both of these meetings, so that he will have time to prepare supplies or set up for activity groups.

After the community meeting, therapy groups begin, typically running for about 45 minutes to 2 hours; the length of a group depends on its purpose and the attention span of the patients. The assistant may lead a group alone or with another COTA or a student or volunteer, or might assist the registered therapist by providing supplies and tools and instructing and supporting individual patients as directed. Occupational therapy groups may take place on the unit, in the day room, or in a special activities room; in larger hospitals patients may attend activities on other units or in a separate occupational therapy clinic or building. The assistant may be assigned to escort patients to and from off-unit activities; sometimes this responsibility is shared with nursing staff or with the registered therapists. Usually no other therapies are scheduled during the times that occupational therapy groups are running; this does not guarantee, however, that patients will not be called away for lab tests or interviews and evaluations by other staff.

A meeting with other occupational therapy and activity therapy staff may be scheduled during lunch because there is little other time when staff from different units can meet to exchange information. Staff from a particular unit can hear how their patients are performing in other groups, and they can let other staff know about patients from other units whom they are treating in their groups. After lunch there may be another scheduled occupa-

---

FIG. 7–1. Occupational therapy goals toward improved functional performance. From Fig. 2 of Peloquin SM. The development of an occupational therapy interview/therapy set procedure. *Am J Occup Ther* 1983; 37:457–461. Copyright © 1983 by the American Occupational Therapy Association, Inc. Reprinted with permission.

OCCUPATIONAL THERAPY GOALS TOWARD IMPROVED FUNCTIONAL PERFORMANCE

NAME: _____ ROOM: _____ DATE: _____

OCCUPATIONAL THERAPY WILL BE WORKING TO HELP YOU IN THE FOLLOWING AREAS, HOPING THAT YOU WILL EXPERIENCE THE BENEFIT OF ACTIVITY THAT HAS PURPOSE.

With Your Thinking Skills:

_____ improving your concentration by providing crafts, hobbies, and daily exercises that require you to concentrate

_____ reducing your confusion through activities that provide clear directions for you to follow

_____ building your problem-solving skills through activities and puzzles that encourage you to figure out problems

_____ keeping you alert and thinking in order to prepare you to return to your home and community

_____ helping you reduce racing thoughts through organized and calming projects

_____ providing you with opportunities to organize your thinking and behavior through structured tasks

With Your Feelings About Yourself:

_____ boosting your self-esteem through daily successes in activity groups

_____ increasing your self-confidence by having you work independently

_____ increase your feelings of being in control by having you experience the control you have over yourself physically and emotionally

_____ encouraging you to work through hurt or other upsetting feelings through energetic types of activities

_____ maintaining your work and social skills through a full and balanced daily routine

With Your Use of Leisure Time and Available Coping Resources:

_____ teaching you ways to use your free time in a healthier, more satisfying way

_____ encouraging you to look around your community to help you find groups and activities that can help you better satisfy your personal needs

_____ encouraging you to regularly use a part of each day for spontaneous fun and relaxation

With Dealing With Other People:

_____ increasing your comfort level and ability to trust others by involving you in pleasant groups

_____ providing you with the support that comes from belonging to a group

_____ providing you with opportunities to communicate with others

_____ providing you with situations in which you must share, interact, and stay in touch with society's demands

_____ encouraging you to use energetic activities to provide healthy outlets for the strong feelings you are experiencing

With Your Ability to Handle Stress:

_____ reducing your anxiety level through energetic crafts, exercise, and games

_____ teaching you to reduce stress and its symptoms through
    yoga (11:30)
    relaxation techniques (4:15)
    relaxing hobbies

With Your Physical Condition:

_____ improving your general health, strength, and coordination through
    chair exercise
    yoga
    recreational games, sports groups
      requiring physical activity

_____ keeping you in a good physical condition and functioning at your best level

_____ helping you to reduce physical discomforts such as stiffness, shakiness, and pain, through relaxation exercises

_____ helping you to reduce any unpleasant side effects from your medication or treatment through exercises

Other:

In Order to Do the Above, You Should Attend:
___ MORNING CRAFTS ___ MORNING EXERCISES (11:30) ___ RECREATION/WORKSHOPS (1:00)
___ RELAXATION (4:15) ___ RECREATION (6:00)

Suzanne M. Peloquin, OTR/L
Registered Occupational Therapist

Copy given to patient _____

tional therapy period, again lasting 45 minutes to 2 hours; patients may attend the same activities morning and afternoon.

Although occupational therapy groups may be scheduled morning and afternoon five days a week, the individual occupational therapy staff member may be responsible for only five to eight of these sessions, attending treatment team meetings at the other times. There may be two to four treatment teams on a single inpatient unit; each team is assigned patients for which it is primarily responsible in terms of evaluation and treatment and discharge planning. Each team includes the various disciplines of psychiatry, psychology, social work, nursing, and occupational or activities therapy. Weekly or biweekly meetings are necessary to coordinate information and plans for patients.

The final 90 minutes to 2 hours of each day is used for various tasks such as evaluation of individual patients, supervisory meetings, library research, and program planning. However, much of this time is needed for documentation; initial and discharge notes must be written on every patient, as well as progress notes for the few patients who stay for longer periods.

Proprietary Hospitals

Proprietary hospitals are private hospitals run for profit; because of their profit orientation, these hospitals generally accept only paying patients, excluding those who do not have private insurance and adequate funds. Often, only the private patients of doctors on staff are admitted; sometimes these doctors are themselves part owners of the hospital. The treatment team approach, as described in the section on acute care inpatient units, is less often used in proprietary hospitals; instead, the individual physicians write orders on their own patients, which they intend other staff to carry out. Patients may be treated with a combination of psychotropic medication,

electroconvulsive therapy, and psychoanalytically oriented verbal therapy. Physicians' attitudes toward occupational therapy vary from indifferent to enthusiastic. Occupational therapy departments may provide a range of diversional and therapeutic activities, including discussion groups, games, sports, gardening, task groups, and leisure and socialization experiences. Work-oriented and rehabilitative services may be included in settings where the physicians understand and endorse this approach.

OUTPATIENT SETTINGS

Outpatient settings are places where people can go to receive treatment while they live at home. Some outpatient settings, such as satellite clinics and aftercare clinics, are affiliated with hospitals; others are privately administered and get their funding from a combination of private and public sources. All share a philosophical orientation that the patient will get better faster, and stay out of the hospital longer, if she can live independently in her own community.

Community Mental Health Centers

Community mental health centers (CMHCs) are very large agencies that provide a wide range of services within residential communities. Occupational therapists and assistants may be employed by the agencies themselves or by specific programs or services within these agencies, such as vocational rehabilitation, transitional living programs, psychosocial rehabilitation programs, or day treatment centers. One example of the role of occupational therapy in CMHCs is an activity program for psychogeriatric patients (older patients with psychiatric problems) in which the members participate in eating, singing, discussion, movement, and craft activities designed to foster social skills and increase self-esteem (29). Another is the program administered by Hill (an OTR) and Brittell (a COTA) at the Herkimer Outreach Center in New York State, which provides functional skill development, stress management, and socialization experiences (19).

Community mental health centers have traditionally been, and continue to be, very dependent on public funding. Widespread development of CMHCs was spurred by the Community Mental Health Centers Act of 1963 (PL 88–164). CMHCs were intended to be nonprofit agencies, established initially with government funding, whose purpose was to provide for the treatment and rehabilitation of the mentally ill within the community. Under amendments passed between 1965 and 1979, the centers were expected to provide inpatient and outpatient services, partial hospitalization, round-the-clock emergency services, and consultation, as well as children's services, services to the elderly, and alcohol and drug services. During these years federal funding was allotted by service categories, thus ensuring that a variety of services were available and that special groups such as the elderly and children received attention.

The shift to block grants in 1981 with the Omnibus Budget Reconciliation Act (PL 97–35) meant that states and CMHCs were no longer required to provide all of the services previously mandated. A study by Jerrell and Larson (23) documents several programmatic shifts that have occurred as a result of this legislation. One is that the chronically mentally ill and those with severe acute mental illnesses have benefitted from increased funding for program development. Consequently, more comprehensive and coordinated services, including vocational rehabilitation, residential programs, and emergency care, are now available for these patients. However, other groups, including children and adolescents, the elderly, and alcohol and drug abusers, have received less attention. In addition, a two-tier system has emerged, with one level of treatment available to those patients with private insurance and another (with more limited services) for those dependent on public funding.

The implications of these changes for occupational therapy services are not clear. Certainly the emphasis on vocational rehabilitation, psychosocial rehabilitation, and structured day programs for chronic patients will mean a greater need for occupational therapy, at least in the short run. Only the documented success of existing occupational therapy services within the community will help ensure that these services continue to receive funding. Even with evidence of need and success, many of these programs will be underfunded or unfunded unless professionals unite with patients and their families to demand continued and increased public support.

Partial Hospitalization and Day Hospitals

Partial hospitalization began in the Soviet Union in response to an acute shortage of psychiatric hospital beds in 1933 (31, 33). This approach has been applied extensively in Great Britain but has been underutilized in the United States (36). Partial hospitalization provides a less costly alternative to inpatient treatment and serves as a transition to community life. Rather than living day and night in a hospital, the patient lives in the community and visits the partial hospitalization setting to receive treatment services. Day treatment allows patients to receive training in daily living skills and to develop social interaction skills while they remain in the community where they will ultimately need these skills. This approach has been found to be cost-effective, less restrictive for patients, and clinically as therapeutic as inpatient treatment (14, 31).

The term "day hospital" is synonymous with partial hospitalization, and more easily understood by patients. Adult day care, described later in this chapter under settings for the aged, is also a partial hospitalization program. Depending on local practices patients may be referred to day treatment directly from inpatient settings, or by therapists or outpatient centers as an alternative to hospitalization.

The goals of partial hospitalization include management of short-term problems, rehabilitation for independent living, treatment of mental disabilities, and support services (14). The staff is interdisciplinary, but varies tremendously depending on availability of trained personnel. The roles and scope of practice of occupational therapy within a partial hospitalizaton program depend on the mix of professional staff. For example, while a nurse might be better trained to provide information on the uses and effects of medication, the COTA might lead a group on medication education if no nurse is available. Other roles for occupational therapy include provision of rehabilitation groups and individual programming for independent living skills, teaching of problem-solving skills and stress management, and vocational development.

The therapeutic program within a day hospital usually consists of a mix of community meetings, small-group learning sessions, and individual case management. Community meetings encourage patients to take an active voice in deciding program policies and field trips and other special activities, and thus promote leadership and self-assertion among the patients. Small-group sessions facilitate the development of skills such as money management, basic hygiene, work habits, health and safety, nutrition and basic cooking, home management, communication, and self-expression. Patients are scheduled for groups depending on their current needs and whether they possess prerequisite skills. Groups may be run by occupational therapists or assistants, other activity therapists, social workers, or other staff.

Case management is a method of tracking each patient's progress by assigning individual staff members to be responsible for the overall program of a few patients. Thus, every staff member from the psychologist to the mental health therapy aide coordi-nates the treatment of one to five patients; this includes setting treatment goals and methods in collaboration with the patient, as well as various administrative duties such as making sure the patient has enough medication, that she attends medical appointments, and that she applies for and receives any necessary public assistance monies. Occupational therapy assistants may be given case management responsibilities in some settings.

A typical focus for occupational therapy is vocational services. One such program described by Richert and Merryman (33) was organized around Mosey's levels of group interaction skill (see Chapter 3) and Allen's cognitive levels (see Chapter 3). The authors report that approximately 90 percent of the recipients of these services were functioning at cognitive levels 4, 5, or 6. In addition to rehabilitation groups at the various levels of group interaction skill and cognitive level, the program provided for actual work experiences within the hospital setting. Level 4 patients were found to function at the prevocational level, needing structured, concrete, well-supervised experiences. Level 5 patients were in general more capable of independent functioning, with 24 percent engaged in volunteer work. Unpaid volunteer work was used extensively in this program for several reasons. It met the esteem needs of those who had previously worked at more responsible jobs, and it offered a gradual transition to paid employment. Volunteer work also safeguards the patients' benefit programs (which might terminate if paid employment were found).

Another approach, reported by Coviensky and Buckley (9), was the provision of a structured activities program outside of but linked to the partial hospitalization program. The purpose was to provide a structure of work and play for those clients too severely impaired to function in less structured settings. The three components of the program were work, play, and milieu. The work component included volunteer work outside the program (Red Cross, nursing homes, etc.) and tasks and chores within the program setting (meal preparation, gardening, etc.). The recreational component included varied activities typical of normal adults: games, sports, walks, readings, and the arts. The milieu component was provided through daily community meetings at the start of each day, consistent expectations applied by all staff equally, and careful design of the environment to provide for both privacy and interaction.

Community Programs

Various community programs administered by private nonprofit agencies (sometimes with links to CMHCs) have been developed with the aim of helping chronic patients survive and succeed in the community after discharge from the hospital. Fountain House, in New York City, is perhaps the best known of these agencies; its program originated the psychosocial club model (see section on "Additional Treatment Theories and Practice Models" later in this chapter). It provides inexpensive housing, a graded program of job training and employment first within the facility and later in the community, and a myriad of leisure and social activities in an evening and weekend program, as well as psychiatric and social services.

Other community programs administered by independent agencies may be less comprehensive, concentrating on just one aspect of continuing care, such as leisure and recreation, or vocational rehabilitation. Others provide rehabilitative living arrangements, including halfway houses and supervised apartments; patients gradually learn the skills, habits, and attitudes they need to live on their own in the community by practicing them under the supervision and direction of staff.

The specific job functions of occupational therapists and assistants employed by these independent agencies vary. Occupational therapists and even assistants may have supervisory and administrative responsibilities; assistants may be asked to carry out activity programs, or to provide direct patient care, or to act as consultants to other professionals serving the patient and her family.

Prevention Programs

One of the aims of the Community Mental Health Centers Act of 1963 was the prevention of future mental health problems in disadvantaged populations and other groups at risk; despite this stated objective, these programs have not been a consistent priority for federal funding. Ironically, programs sometimes receive funding for start-up costs but are unable to obtain continued funding once they have demonstrated their effectiveness.

Prevention programs described in the occupational therapy literature include several for children. One provided developmental therapy to preschool children in an early intervention program (10). Activities such as mirror play, sand and water play, various art and craft activities, puppetry, singing, and nature walks were designed to enrich the experiences of children with developmental delays. Another program, which met once a week in a local library, provided enriching activities to all of the preschool and kindergarten-age children who attended (not only the developmentally delayed) and included parent participation (7). A third provided recreational and educational opportunities for 350 children ranging from preschoolers to high school seniors (20).

Another study by Grossman (13) examined risk factors for child psychopathology in preschoolers attending a Head Start program. The author suggested a role for occupational therapy in the teaching of parenting skills to mothers experiencing role strain due to limited personal resources (education, money, skills, and social support).

Working in prevention programs requires special skills. Occupational therapists and assistants trained in and accustomed to the medical model, in which they work closely with physicians and other professionals in the health care system, may find the role blurring and diffuse structure of community programs confusing and isolating. Successful workers must be able to create their own programs, sometimes despite community indifference, and provide services flexibly, as needed by the people in the community.

Prevocational and Vocational Rehabilitation

Programs that aim to develop the patient's ability to function in a job or joblike situation fit in this category. A range of programs exists to meet very different needs. For example, those who have never worked usually start in prevocational programs, which help participants acquire work skills by requiring and reinforcing behavior appropriate for a work setting. Once prevocational skills (work habits and attitudes) are developed, the patient can move on to a vocational program, which prepares him for a specific kind of work. Those who, because of the severity of their disabilities, will never be able to enter competitive employment are often placed in a sheltered workshop. Sheltered workshops employ the disabled in productive work; because the disabled work so slowly they are often paid on the basis of how much work (how many pieces) they produce. Tasks one might see in a sheltered workshop include sorting, counting, and bagging plastic tableware; assembling ball-point pens; or counting and packaging envelopes. The use of work activities will be further discussed in Chapters 17 and 19.

Prevocational and vocational programs and sheltered workshops may be found in both inpatient and outpatient settings, and as independent community programs. Occupational therapists and assistants may administer such programs or serve as consultants or group leaders. The ability to analyze, grade, and adapt activities to enable the disabled to perform them is an essential skill.

AGE-SPECIFIC SETTINGS

Children, adolescents, and the aged are often treated in separate facilities or programs designed to meet their particular developmental needs. These include both outpatient and inpatient programs, community-based programs, and special residential programs.

Children's Treatment

Children with psychotic disorders or severe behavior problems are often hospitalized, usually in a children's psychiatric hospital or a children's ward; these facilities have their own staff, which usually includes one or more occupational therapists as well as teachers, child psychologists, speech and language pathologists, and the usual medical staff. Children who have enough control over their behavior to live in the community may reside with their parents or in special residences, yet attend special schools for the emotionally handicapped. Other children, with milder problems, may attend regular public or private schools while receiving treatment in afterschool programs on an outpatient basis.

Working with children requires broad and detailed knowledge of child development and an understanding of the role of activities and play in the child's life. Knowledge of sensory integration theories and methods may also be needed. Mosey's levels of group interaction skill may be applied with children who lack age-appropriate skills for relating to peers in the classroom (1).

Occupational therapy programs for children may focus on consultation to parents or teachers, to help them provide play and self-care experiences that will interest the child and facilitate development of specific skills. Occupational therapy activity programs are usually fit in around the school schedule, or may be carried out in the classroom with the assistance of the teacher.

Adolescent Treatment

Adolescents may need inpatient treatment for schizophrenic or depressive disorders (which often make their first appearance in adolescence), for alcohol or drug abuse problems, for lifelong disturbances originating in childhood psychiatric disorders, or for transient disturbances caused by unpleasant or difficult life events. Adolescents who have psychiatric problems also must deal with the biological and emotional upheaval of puberty and the identity conflicts of the adolescent period. Staff members may act as surrogates for parents or may be viewed as parent-like authorities. Adolescents may need to work through many problems as they attempt to exercise more freedom and take increasing responsibility for their own lives. Milieu therapy models (see other practice models later in this chapter) are often applied in adolescent inpatient and residential settings.

The role of occupational therapy in an adolescent program usually includes provision of a meaningful range of structured therapeutic activities that approximate those enjoyed by adolescents in the community at large. Prevocational and vocational activities and training in social skills and daily living skills are often included; sensory integration and specialized cognitive treatments for learning disabilities may be used with some groups. Leisure and physical education activities are extremely important for this age group. To promote free exchange of feelings and ideas about body image and self-esteem, it is recommended that males and females be seen in separate groups for physical activities like weight training, aerobics, or yoga (28). Education about human sexuality and universal pre-

cautions is essential, and may fall under the scope of occupational therapy in some settings.

Many adolescents benefit tremendously from role modeling and direct training in simple household tasks such as cleaning, cooking, home maintenance, and clothing care. Weissenberg and Giladi (39) reported on a Home Economics Day program provided within an adolescent day hospital. Once a week, for an entire day, the adolescent clients planned, organized, and carried out meal preparation for the center. This provided an opportunity to learn and practice skills and habits in a realistic situation, but with normal time pressures and performance expectations individually tailored to the capacities of the clients.

Working on an adolescent service requires an ability to tolerate and set limits on provocative and rebellious behavior, while supporting reasonable attempts at independence. This is sometimes difficult for younger students and staff, who may identify too closely with issues patients are dealing with.

Settings for the Aged

Aged individuals with mental health problems may be treated in settings ranging from their own homes, to community senior centers, to nursing homes and inpatient settings. Community geriatric centers may provide activity programs, counseling, and meals; participants usually do not have serious psychiatric disorders but often experience periodic or chronic depression or anxiety because of losses associated with aging. The centers may be housed in their own facilities, or more typically within another community agency like a YMCA or church basement.

Some larger settings are able to provide a continuity of services from psychiatric inpatient to community aftercare (15). Such a comprehensive array of services, if well coordinated, maximizes independent functioning and permits patients to be served in the least restrictive environment. This is especially important for this age group, as older people tend to sustain more losses (physical, social, economic) and for this reason experience increased stress. The patient may be admitted first for acute care and at this level would be introduced to ward level groups that address specific needs such as decreasing anxiety, promoting understanding of and adjustment to the hospital environment, and providing information and skills needed for successful community functioning (e.g., obtaining benefits). At the next level, the patient would be encouraged to attend activities at a senior center on the hospital grounds. The third level would be placement as an outpatient in the geriatric day center. Finally, at the fourth level, the patient living in the community would visit the center periodically and receive limited services at home.

Adult day care (2, 3, 16, 31) is a relatively recent treatment model for this age group. A partial hospitalization program, adult day care has been subdivided into two types, with very different funding resources and programming conditions. *Medical/rehabilitative oriented day care programs* are funded through Medicaid and some private insurers, for the purpose of providing physical rehabilitation services similar to those traditionally located in hospitals (3). *Psychosocial/supportive day-care programs,* funded by Title XX of the Social Security Act and Title III of the Older Americans Act, aim to provide a daily program of care for the slightly confused or frail elderly person, and are thus more psychosocial in emphasis (3). Occupational therapy services in the psychosocial/supportive day-care model are similar to those in the partial hospitalization model described earlier in this chapter. Instead of a vocational orientation, these programs focus on avocational skills and social activities. Adaptive equipment and environmental modifications are provided to maximize functioning for clients with physical and mental impairments (3).

Older individuals who have severe psychotic disturbances (e.g., schizophrenia or organic mental disorders) are usually restricted to nursing homes and the geriatric wards of large public institutions. Because the aged tend to have more physical illnesses than younger members of the population, these facilities provide skilled nursing and medical services. Occupational therapy is often provided by assistants, with the registered therapist serving as part-time consultant; services may include orientation to the facility, reality orientation, memory training and assistance, sensory awareness, environmental modification, and training in daily living skills and use of assistive devices. Social and recreational programming, music activities, and exercise and craft programs may be provided by occupational therapy personnel or by recreational therapists or activity leaders.

HOME HEALTH CARE

Home health care is a rapidly developing segment of the health care market; government and private insurance programs have limited inpatient stays, and once discharged, people with chronic or debilitating illnesses prefer to be treated in their homes, rather than have to travel to health care centers. Although most patients in need of occupational therapy home health services have disabilities that are primarily physical, secondary psychiatric disabilities are quite common especially when the first diagnosis is neurological. Sadly, occupational therapists with a medical rehabilitation orientation may fail to document psychosocial services provided in the home (24). Without documentation, such services will not be recognized or reimbursed.

The success of Supportive Care, an independent home health business founded by Susan Maertz, COTA, shows that supportive home care for elderly persons suffering from decreased mental abilities is a viable and desired service (27). The occupational therapy assistant might provide memory aids, training in coping mechanisms and crisis management, and supervision of hygiene, grooming, and nutrition.

Another model program in Portland, Oregon (21), utilizes two occupational therapists on a team with four nurses to provide mental health services in the home. Most of the clients served by this program were found, on evaluation, to be functioning at Allen cognitive level 4. Level 4 patients need assistance to transfer skills from one environment (hospital) to another (home) and to solve routine problems, and thus can benefit from occupational therapy intervention.

Most private insurers today do not reimburse occupational therapy as a home health service unless other services (nursing, physical therapy) are also required. Generally, the first diagnosis must be nonpsychiatric for the patient to qualify for home health care. Home health therapists may circumvent this problem by training family members in management of the physically disabled patient who also has a psychiatric problem. Current efforts by the American Occupational Therapy Association and its membership to change home health policies are directed at educating legislators, insurers, and consumers about how occupational therapy can reduce health care costs and increase the functional independence of disabled people.

COMMUNITY RESIDENCES

Community residences constitute a broad category that includes all the places, other than the family home, where a patient might live in the community. *Group homes* are places where patients live together in the community, with varying levels of supervision from staff. Sometimes each patient has his own room and bathroom; in other facilities patients may have their own bedrooms but share all other living areas.

Some group homes have live-in managers or house parents, and many provide other services through their affiliation with hospitals or CMHCs. *Board and care homes* or *proprietary homes* are a specific kind of group home, operated on a for-profit basis; patients sleep in the facility and eat all their meals there, but other services may not be available. A survey of board and care homes found that the smaller homes provided more activities, more community excursion, and more opportunities for social productivity than did larger homes (30).

Chronic patients in large cities are sometimes housed in *single-room occupancy hotels* (SROs) or in welfare hotels or shelters for the homeless; these settings are typically bleak and often very dangerous. However, with the recent housing shortage and destruction of older housing to make room for new development, many chronic patients are now homeless.

Some community residences are designed to expose the patient to a more natural living experience, and to provide opportunities to acquire and practice independent living skills. A halfway house is a transitional residence, not a permanent home. It is designed for people with disabilities who are not yet ready to live in the community but who do not need to be confined to an institution. Halfway houses are often associated with hospitals, and some are on hospital grounds, but many others are free-standing or associated with community mental health agencies. The overall program in a halfway house aims to promote independence in the residents. Two very different approaches to this are the "nurturing" and the "high expectation" approach (11). The nurturing approach sees the halfway house as an intermediate location for someone who is still quite ill and therefore incapable of much responsibility; in this approach the staff takes charge of running the house. In the high expectations approach residents are expected to manage the house and to deal with pressures and responsibilities.

Freidlob, Janis, and Deets-Aron (11) described a halfway house in California for veterans with neuropsychiatric disorders, staffed by two occupational therapists. The program design provided three segments of treatment. The first focused on nutrition and interpersonal and housekeeping skills. The second aimed to promote independence and the focus shifted to vocational skills and community resources. The third segment provided for ongoing supervision of residents as they semi-independently pursued their individual daily routines, which might include school, work, and community recreation. Graduates of the program were invited back once a month to share experiences and get support from fellow graduates and staff. Halfway houses and supervised apartments are also described under the psychosocial rehabilitation practice model later in this chapter.

Occupational therapists and assistants working in community residences may provide services ranging from recreational, leisure, and socialization activities to training in independent daily living skills, and case management.

ENVIRONMENTAL CONCEPTS OF HUMAN OCCUPATION

The model of human occupation and other occupational therapy theories acknowledge that all human activity arises from the human being's basic urge to explore and master his environment. Treatment settings are different from the natural and man-made environments in which most people spend their time, and thus have different effects on the activity behaviors of patients. Before we explore what these effects might be, it is important to review some of the basic concepts of person-environment interaction from the model of human occupation.

All occupational behavior depends on environmental interaction. The person must be able to have an effect on his environment. In general, the more complexity and novelty in the environment, the greater the person's urge to explore it. However, if there are too many new and different and complicated things in the environment, the person may feel overwhelmed and become unable to act purposefully. Dunning (10) identified three features of the environment that have an effect on social and occupational behavior: space, people, and tasks. *Space* includes the size and kind of space, the objects within it, and how they are arranged. *People* includes not only the number of persons but also the roles they fill and the expectations they have of each other. *Tasks* are defined by objects in the environment that compel certain task behaviors (e.g., a workbench versus a card table), and by social pressures. Through these three features, environments communicate expectations for occupational behavior.[1]

In general, we can safely assert that inpatient treatment settings have deficits or at least differences in all these areas, as compared to typical home, work, and leisure settings. The space typically has fewer interesting objects in it; because of safety precautions inpatient settings may seem bare. Curtains, carpets, and stuffed furniture may be absent, thus creating an atmosphere more like an airport lounge in an underdeveloped nation than any room in an American home. Patients may be prohibited from placing decorations on the walls. The lighting is likely to come from fluorescent ceiling fixtures rather than incandescent floor and table lamps. Overall the space may feel barren, sterile, and somewhat depressing (even to staff members).

Although there are usually a lot of people around, many of these are staff. It is clear

---

[1] Other authors have recently reconceptualized the features of the environment that affect occupational behavior in the model of human occupation. They identify four environmental layers: objects, tasks, social groups and organizations, and culture. Interested readers can pursue this further in Barris et al. (6).

to everyone that the staff are in charge; they are seen by themselves and the patients as more competent than the patients. Therefore, they tend to perform almost all of the necessary tasks in the setting, including preparing and serving meals, caring for laundry and housekeeping, and preparing and cleaning up after activities. Patients may be involved in any or all of these tasks, but usually under the supervision of staff.

Even this superficial examination of the environmental characteristics of inpatient treatment settings shows that they communicate an expectation that patients need to do very little, and that they probably will not be able to do even that very well. This is less true of many outpatient settings, but even these settings do not often communicate an expectation that the patient perform at anything like a normal level.

To help the patient develop and maintain the skills and behaviors he will ultimately need to function on his own, the occupational therapy assistant may need to alter some features of the treatment environment. Space can be altered by rearranging furniture, placing folding screens to eliminate distractions, and painting walls or adding wall coverings to the extent permitted; patients should be involved in making these decisions and doing the work where practical. The assistant can control the effect of people in the environment by looking at his own role as group leader and the roles of volunteers and students in occupational therapy groups; the less the staff does, the more patients will feel they need to do themselves. Making tasks available to patients will often require working with the administrators of the setting to change policies; there is no reason why patients should not be allowed (or required) to do their own laundry, but administrators may feel that this would be inconvenient, inefficient, or interfere with ward routine.

Treating patients in their homes presents different opportunities to apply environmental concepts. A patient's home, or any environment (e.g., his office) that he creates for himself, communicates his interests and his habits to the careful observer. The objects with which he surrounds himself, the care given to different rooms or parts of rooms, the age of the furnishings and the amount of use they seem to have received, all indicate their relative importance to the patient. For example, Levine (25) describes a home in which the furniture in all the rooms but the kitchen was 40 years old and quite worn, but the kitchen was freshly painted and had new appliances; she inferred that the kitchen was the center of the family's activities.

Usually the patient has more control of the environment in his home than in the hospital; this increases his sense of personal causation. The therapist is the guest, and relinquishes control naturally to the patient, thus supporting the patient's motivation to control and master his environment.

Another situation that may call for a different application of environmental concepts occurs when the patient travels with the assistant out into the community. Observing how the patient reacts to the different stimulation presented by shops, bus stops, and public agencies may reveal hitherto unsuspected skills, and may help the assistant identify what kinds of environmental changes will facilitate more independent behaviors.

In summary, demands from the opportunities present in the environment have a profound effect on human occupational behavior. Almost all treatment settings, but especially inpatient units, convey only limited expectations for patients to participate in and be competent at daily life tasks and occupational roles; occupational therapy personnel may increase expectations for patients to perform by selectively altering features of the environment. Working with patients in their homes or in various community environments may provide information about which environmental features best facilitate independent functioning for a particular person.

ADDITIONAL TREATMENT THEORIES AND PRACTICE MODELS

Different treatment settings base their therapeutic efforts on different theories. Although the major theories used in psychiatric treatment in the United States today were described in Chapter 2, and the currently most popular practice models for psychiatric occupational therapy in Chapters 3 and 4, there exist many other treatment theories and practice models that the occupational therapy assistant might encounter on the job; this section will briefly describe five of these.

Milieu Therapy

Milieu therapy, and a related practice model called the therapeutic community, are based on the assumption that the treatment ward or day treatment center is a social system. Like other social systems it has rules, hierarchies, and roles that must be filled if the system is to function. Milieu therapy is an approach that attempts to give patients as much responsibility as they can possibly handle, and to enable them to take charge of their own decisions and day-to-day environment. Because milieu therapy shifts responsibility for decision-making to patients, staff who are used to having more authority will need to adjust their expectations and behavior (5).

Community meetings and patient government are methods used in milieu therapy. *Community meetings* are scheduled gatherings of all staff and patients; they may occur once a week or more frequently. Recent events affecting the patients or staff and plans for the future are typical topics for discussion; disagreements between patients or between patients and staff are often aired, and sometimes resolved, at these meetings. *Patient government* is a method for enabling patients to have more control over conditions that affect them in the

treatment facility; officers or an executive committee of patients are elected by the patients themselves. The officers or committee then set or implement policies desired by the patients. Realistically, however, some policy changes sought by patients cannot be implemented, particularly in inpatient settings, since rules about locked doors, scheduled mealtimes, and the like are set by hospital administration; therefore, patient government has limited power. *Resident council* is a similar patient government system sometimes used in nursing homes and large community residences. Ironically, these various methods of patient government are frequently included on inpatient units whose overall approach is clearly medical and authoritarian and therefore incompatible with self-determination by patients; this is the very opposite of milieu therapy and is probably confusing for everyone concerned.

The underlying philosophy of milieu therapy holds that each individual in the community is capable of contributing in some way to general community life. Therefore, patients are assigned housekeeping and other tasks wherever possible; again, because of bureaucratic and legal restrictions on "unpaid labor" it is not possible to enforce a consistent milieu in inpatient settings. The psychosocial rehabilitation approach described in the next section, which is based on milieu therapy concepts, demonstrates that these concepts are workable in community settings.

Psychosocial Rehabilitation (The Psychosocial Club)

Psychosocial rehabilitation is an environmental approach designed to improve the ability of chronic mental patients to maintain themselves in the community by providing support, training, and activities that reinforce and enable independent functioning. It is a multidisciplinary approach, involving the professional disciplines of social work, vocational rehabilitation, occupational therapy, therapeutic recreation, and others, as well as paraprofessionals trained on the job, and volunteers. The fundamental premise is that, by providing supports and reinforcement within the environment where the patient spends most of his time, the patient can be encouraged to attempt, practice, and succeed at the skills he needs to get along in day-to-day life.

Psychosocial rehabilitation focuses on the social, rather than the medical, aspects of mental illness. Thus, although psychotropic medication and consultation with the psychiatrist may be available, these are seen as adjunctive rather than essential services. Comprehensive psychosocial rehabilitation centers, such as Fountain House in New York City, typically provide five basic categories of service: socialization programs, daily living skills counseling and training, vocational rehabilitation and transitional employment, transitional living arrangements, and case management. In keeping with the philosophy that people with chronic mental illness can maintain themselves in the community if they receive appropriate support, the persons who attend psychosocial rehabilitation programs are referred to as "members" rather than patients.

Socialization programs are at the heart of the psychosocial rehabilitation approach. By participating in organized activities and casual "lounge programs," members acquire social and leisure skills and meet others with similar needs and interests. Informal activities such as playing pool or cards, watching television, reading, and chatting are typical of lounge programs. Organized activities might include cooking, sewing, home repair, crafts, and theater trips. Depending upon facilities and funding, other activities such as swimming, skiing, camping, and hiking may be available. Programs that provide only socialization opportunities and not the other elements of psychosocial rehabilitation described below are sometimes called *psychosocial clubs* or *clubhouse programs*. Membership is seen as voluntary.

Daily living skills programs may include opportunities for self-assessment, counseling with particular problems, and training in desired skills. After many years of illness, usually including several hospitalizations, the person with chronic mental illness may be quite unaccustomed to performing chores and tasks the rest of us take for granted. By providing information, advice, and opportunities to learn and practice new skills, the daily living skills counselor enables members to acquire such skills as using public transportation, caring for an apartment, shopping for and caring for clothing, and shopping for and cooking food. This is a role for which the occupational therapy assistant is particularly well prepared.

Prevocational rehabilitation and transitional employment are services aimed at helping members acquire job-related skills and obtain jobs in the community. Prevocational rehabilitation helps members become acculturated to basic work habits and the social rules typical of community work settings. Members attend work groups where they perform jobs needed by the center, or contracted for by the center with businesses in the community. They are expected to behave in a businesslike, productive, work-oriented manner, and are counseled about behaviors they need to change. Clerical groups, janitorial and maintenance groups, thrift shops, and simple assembly line work are typical activities. After a period of successful performance in a prevocational program members are placed, through the transitional employment program, into entry-level jobs in the community. These jobs may be unpaid or pay only minimum wage, but they give members a chance to be productive in a real-life setting; work experiences are not usually meant to become full-time jobs, but are seen rather as stepping-stones to other, permanent positions.

Transitional living arrangements encompass a range of supervised residential opportunities. The halfway house or supervised community residence is usually the first step; here members can receive room and board and round-the-clock supervision from trained staff (often paraprofessional *house parents* or *residential counselors*). Usually members are expected to be out of the house during the day, either working or looking for work, or attending a day treatment program. During the evening and on weekends they may be supervised as they help prepare their own meals; do the shopping, laundry, housecleaning, and other chores; and organize and carry out their own leisure and social activities. Supervised apartments are the next step; the apartments are usually leased (or, less commonly, owned) by the psychosocial rehabilitation program, which then sublets them to members. Several members live together in one apartment, sharing housework and other responsibilities. Staff visit periodically to provide counseling and support and to oversee cleanliness and other basic issues.

Occupational therapists and assistants may be disturbed by the role blurring that occurs among staff in psychosocial rehabilitation settings, and may fear that their unique occupational therapy identity will become lost as they take on responsibilities (such as case management) that are typically part of other disciplines, and as members of other disciplines become leaders of activity groups. To work successfully in these settings, occupational therapists and assistants need to be comfortable taking on management roles (22).

It is important to recognize that psychosocial rehabilitation embodies concepts from *moral treatment* (see Chapter 1) that guided the early development of occupational therapy; although other professionals and nonprofessionals may run activity groups that meet the interests of the members, it is not reasonable to jump to the conclusion that they are "practicing occupational therapy" any more than is the swim instructor at the YWCA or the crafts instructor in an adult education center.

Family Therapy

Family therapy approaches are based on the belief that the patient's illness may be caused by, and at the very least is intimately connected with, his family relationships. The patient's behavior is seen as an expression of demands and opportunities controlled by the family. According to family therapy theories, any approach that attempts to treat the patient's illness without treating the family is misguided.

Different theories give various explanations of the relationship between the patient's illness and the family system. At one extreme, some theories hold that the patient's illness is not his own, but rather the symptom of a sick family; the family uses the patient as a safety valve to express its unconscious conflicts and psychopathology. Other theories take the view that, regardless of its etiology, the patient's illness creates such a strain on other family members that they need support and guidance to learn how to maintain their own self-esteem and integrity while responding effectively to the patient. All family therapy approaches view the patient and his family as an interactive social system; what happens to one family member reverberates and affects all the others. The family and the patient are treated together, sometimes by two therapists.

Few occupational therapists practicing in mental health use family therapy approaches as their major practice model, yet most acknowledge and support family therapy concepts. For example, when helping a chronic schizophrenic acquire independent daily living skills, the therapist may talk with the family about what the patient is able to do on his own; otherwise the family may continue to do things for him that he can do himself. Similarly, families overcome with grief, guilt, and frustration about the disabilities of the patient may benefit from objective advice and information provided by knowledgeable mental health professionals.

When occupational therapists practice in a treatment setting where family therapy is the prevailing practice model, they may find that certain occupational therapy methods are viewed by the administrators as incompatible with the overall philosophy of the setting. Sensory integration approaches may be considered too "medical" to be used, for example.

Stress Management

Defined medically, stress is a condition experienced by humans and other biological organisms when equilibrium is disrupted by outside forces. These outside forces are called *stressors*. A *psychosocial stressor* is an event or situation that the patient or client experiences as emotionally or psychologically stressful; an example is learning that one's electricity is about to be turned off for nonpayment of bills. Open systems theories, of which the model of human occupation is one example, assume that biological organisms require a certain amount of stimulation from stressors in order to develop and function. When the demands from stressors are too great, however, the organism can become overwhelmed by stress and unable to function.

Stress management is an educational approach that teaches people about stressors and the effects of stress, and trains them in techniques for controlling psychological and emotional stress. Usually a stress management program begins with an assessment of recent psychosocial stressors and reactions to them; positive events (for example, getting married or getting a promotion) as well as negative ones can be stressors. Participants are asked how they react

to each stressor; specific behaviors such as overeating or sleeping too much are identified. Depending upon the participant's needs, as identified through evaluation, he is then instructed in skills and coping techniques. Some of these include meditation, relaxation exercises, yoga, exercise, assertiveness training, relaxation, and time management. Participants may attend groups where they learn to explore and share feelings about stressful life events. The specific value of occupational therapy in stress management programs is its unique ability to assess dysfunctional patterns of occupational behavior and restore more natural and adaptive patterns through the use of purposeful activities.

Some stress management programs similar to that described above are administered by occupational therapists, or codirected by them with professionals from other disciplines. One model provides for continuity between the hospital and the community, to ensure transfer of skills (8). Often, occupational therapists and assistants use stress management techniques in combination with other treatment methods; for example, training in independent daily living skills can be enhanced when participants are taught how to be reasonably assertive with shopkeepers and how to use relaxation techniques to reduce stress when frustrating things happen.

Crisis Intervention

Crisis intervention is a practice model, related to stress management, that aims to help people deal with problems when they are in the middle of them. The patient (usually referred to as the "client," since often the person is suffering only from an immediate psychosocial stressor) can walk in, during the hours the clinic is open, and receive advice, support, and resources to solve her immediate problem.

People in crisis tend to be overwhelmed by their feelings and then sometimes become confused, passive, and unable to act. They may abandon their usual activities and develop maladaptive behaviors such as denying reality, complaining rather than acting, or giving up entirely. Rosenfeld developed an approach using nuclear tasks to help people in crisis; his model includes the steps shown in Table 7–1. This model seeks to restore normal occupational behavior patterns by engaging the client in nuclear tasks. A *nuclear task* is a purposeful activity that requires the person in crisis to marshal his resources and get on with his life. Rosenfeld has identified three types of nuclear task: remotivating tasks, skills and coping tasks, and symbolic tasks. Remotivating tasks help the person in crisis get started doing something; by doing something the person shows himself that he is not helpless. An example is a woman cleaning out a closet even though she is preoccupied about having lost her job. Skills and coping tasks help the person acquire the skills needed to resolve or work on the crisis; for instance, the woman may need to practice interviewing skills before looking for another job, or she may need to work on her wardrobe and personal presentation. Symbolic tasks are activities, usually chosen by the person himself, that show resolution of the crisis; for example, a couple whose infant died suddenly might, after some time, decide to have a party and include friends who have young children.

Whereas the nuclear task approach is an occupational therapy practice model, other crisis intervention methods are used by other mental health professionals in psychiatric emergency rooms, in hospitals and CMHCs, in satellite and aftercare clinics, and in some home health programs and community agencies. A crisis hotline is one example that may be familiar.

SUMMARY

Occupational therapists and assistants may be employed in many different kinds of settings to provide services to persons with mental health problems. Each setting has its own philosophy, and several alternative practice models that might be used in these settings have been presented. Each setting presents opportunities and demands that affect both staff and patients, and that shape the role of occupational therapy. Recognizing that no treatment setting is ideal, and

---

TABLE 7–1. *The nuclear task approach to crisis intervention*

To Identify Nuclear Tasks Through Evaluation:
- Use expressive activities when indicated to promote expression of affect.
- Seek evidence of task failures and functional deficits that contribute to the crisis.
- Identify uncompleted tasks that disturb and/or motivate the client. Assess the symbolic and realistic value of these tasks for resolving the crisis.
- Assess the client's functional resources. Identify patterns of attribution and activity that tend to promote or diminish effective coping responses.

To Promote Performance of Nuclear Tasks in Treatment:
- Help the client see and accept the challenge inherent in the crisis.
- Promote reasonable attributions to counteract the client's negative, harsh, and hopeless self-estimates.
- Undertake graded remotivating activities designed to yield rapid success in affecting uncompleted task elements of the crisis.
- Teach new functional skills and coping behaviors necessary to surmounting the crisis.
- Discuss and implement activities that test or signify progress toward recovery.
- Plan daily activity routines that promote a sense of orderliness, control, and certainty, thereby creating islands of comfort and enjoyment in the client's sea of troubles.

Reprinted from Table 2 of Rosenfeld MS. Crisis intervention: the nuclear task approach. *Am J Occup Ther* 1984; 38:382–385. Copyright © 1984 by the American Occupational Therapy Association, Inc. Reprinted with permission.

that some are worse than others, occupational therapists and assistants can make their treatment settings more effective by applying concepts from the model of human occupation. These concepts about how humans interact with their environments can be used to understand the effects of each type of setting on patients and staff. By manipulating some of the variables known to affect human performance (such as environmental demands and availability of interesting objects), occupational therapy personnel can facilitate more exploratory behavior and competence in their patients, thus compensating for the negative effects of unstimulating and stressful treatment environments.

REFERENCES

1. Agrin AR. Occupational therapy with emotionally disturbed children in a public elementary school. *Occup Ther Mental Health* 1987; 7(2): 105–114.
2. American Occupational Therapy Association. Facts about occupational therapy in acute psychiatric admissions. *Fact Sheet—AOTA*. Rockville, Md: 1992.
3. American Occupational Therapy Association. Occupational therapy in adult day-care (position paper). *Am J Occup Ther* 1986; 40:814–816.
4. American Occupational Therapy Association. Roles and functions of occupational therapy in adult day-care. *Am J Occup Ther* 1986; 40:817–821.
5. Appelbaum AH, Munich RL. Reinventing moral treatment: the effects upon patients and staff members of a program of psychosocial rehabilitation. *Occup Ther Mental Health* 1989; 9(3): 69–86.
6. Barris R, Kielhofner G, Levine RE, Neville AM. Occupation as interaction with the environment. In: Kielhofner G, ed. *A model of human occupation: theory and application.* Baltimore: Williams & Wilkins; 1985.
7. Benzing P, Strickland R. Occupational therapy in a community-based prevention program. *Occup Ther Mental Health* 1983; 3(1):15–30.
8. Courtney C, Escobedo B. A stress management program: inpatient-to-outpatient continuity. *Am J Occup Ther* 1990; 44:306–310.
9. Coviensky M, Buckley VC. Day activities programming: serving the severely impaired chronic client. *Occup Ther Mental Health* 1986; 6(2): 21–30.
10. Dunning H. Environmental occupational therapy. *Occup Ther* 1972; 26:292–298.
11. Friedlob SA, Janis GA, Deets-Aron C. A hospital-connected halfway house program for individuals with long-term neuropsychiatric disabilities. *Am J Occup Ther* 1986; 40:271–277.
12. George NM, Braun BA, Walker JM. A prevention and early intervention mental health program for disadvantaged pre-school children. *Am J Occup Ther* 1982; 36:99–106.
13. Grossman J. A prevention model for occupational therapy. *Am J Occup Ther* 1991; 45: 33–41.
14. Gusich RL, Silverman AL. Basava day clinic: the model of human occupation as applied to psychiatric day hospitalization. *Occup Ther Mental Health* 1991; 11(2/3):113–127.
15. Harwood KJ, Wenzl D. Admissions to discharge: a psychogeriatric transitional program. *Occup Ther Mental Health* 1990; 10(3):79–100.
16. Hasselkus BR. The meaning of activity: day care for persons with Alzheimer's disease. *Am J Occup Ther* 1992; 46:199–206.
17. Hemphill BJ, Werner PC. Deinstitutionalization: a role for occupational therapy in the state hospital. *Occup Ther Mental Health* 1990; 10(2): 85–99.
18. Hibbard T, Campitelli J, Lieberman HJ. Off-unit activities programming for long-stay psychiatric inpatients: clinical and administrative effects. *Occup Ther Mental Health* 1989; 9(1):49–61.
19. Hill L, Brittell T. The role competence model. (Draft of unpublished paper). Herkimer, NY: Herkimer Outreach Center; 1985.
20. Jaffe E. The role of the occupational therapist as a community consultant: primary prevention in mental health programming. *Occup Ther Mental Health* 1980; 1(2):47–62.
21. Javernick JA. Focus: home care—delivering psych services in the home: do OTs have a role? *OT Week* September 3, 1992; 6(35):14–15.
22. Javernick JA. Focus: mental health—OTs expand their horizons at Way Station. *OT Week* October 15, 1992; 6(41):14–15.
23. Jerrell JM, Larson JK. Community mental health services in transition: who is benefiting? *Am J Orthopsychiatry* 1986; 56(1):78–88.
24. Kunstaetter D. Occupational therapy treatment in home health care. *Am J Occup Ther* 1988; 42:513–519.
25. Levine R. The cultural aspects of home delivery. *Am J Occup Ther* 1984; 38:734–735.
26. Linn MW, Caffey EM, Klett J, Hogarty GE, Land HR. Day treatment and psychotropic drugs in the aftercare of schizophrenic patient. *Arch Gen Psychiatry* 1979; 36:1055–1066.
27. Maertz S. COTA share. *Occup Ther Newspaper* 1984; 38(4):7.
28. Melia MA, Weikert K. Evaluation and treatment of adolescents on a short-term unit. *Occup Ther Mental Health* 1987; 7(2):51–66.
29. Menks F, Sittler S, Weaver D, Yanow B. A psychogeriatric group in a rural community. *Am J Occup Ther* 1977; 31:376–384.
30. Nagy MP, Fisher GA, Tessler RC. Effects of facility characteristics on the social adjustment of mentally ill residents of board-and-care homes.

Hosp Comm Psychiatry 1988; 39:1281–1285.

31. Norman AN, Crosby PM. Meeting the challenge: role of occupational therapy in a geriatric day hospital. *Occup Ther Mental Health* 1990; 10(3):65–78.

32. Peloquin SM. The development of an occupational therapy interview/therapy set procedure. *Am J Occup Ther* 1983; 37:457–461.

33. Richert GZ, Merryman MB. The vocational continuum: a model for providing vocational services in a partial hospitalization program. *Occup Ther Mental Health* 1987; 7(3):1–20.

34. Rider BB, Gramblin JT. An activities approach to occupational therapy in a short-term acute mental health unit. *Am Occup Ther Assoc Mental Health Specialty Section Newsletter* 1980; 3(4):1–3.

35. Robinson AM, Avallone J. Occupational therapy in acute inpatient psychiatry: an activities health approach. *Am J Occup Ther* 1990; 44:809–814.

36. Rosie JS. Partial hospitalization: a review of recent literature. *Hosp Comm Psychiatry* 1987; 38:1291–1298.

37. Talbott J. Chronic and episodic illness: possibility of future funding. Presented at the annual meeting of the American Orthopsychiatric Association, New York, April 20–24, 1985.

38. Turner IM. The healing power of respect—a personal journey. *Occup Ther Mental Health* 1989; 9(1):17–32.

39. Weissenberg R, Giladi N. Home economics day: a program for disturbed adolescents to promote acquisition of habits and skills. *Occup Ther Mental Health* 1989; 9(2):89–103.

ADDITIONAL REFERENCES AND SUGGESTED READINGS

Aronson R. The role of an occupational therapist in a geriatric day hospital setting—Maimonides Day Hospital. *Am J Occup Ther* 1976; 30:290–292.

Barris R. Environmental interactions: an extension of the model of human occupation. *Am J Occup Ther* 1982; 36:637–644.

Barris R, Kielhofner G, Watts JH. *Psychosocial occupational therapy: practice in a pluralistic arena.* Laurel, Md: RAMSCO; 1983.

Becker RE, Page MS. Psychotherapeutically oriented rehabilitation in chronic mental illness. *Am J Occup Ther* 1973; 27:34–38.

Bocks T, Gordon H, Brozost B. Individualized psychosocial assessment of chronic psychiatric patients in a day treatment setting. *Am Occup Ther Assoc Mental Health Special Interest Section Newsletter* 1981; 4(3):3–4.

Brodkin AM. Family therapy: the making of a mental health movement. *Am J Orthopsychiatry* 1980; 50(1):4–17.

Erikson JM. *Activity, recovery and growth.* New York: WW Norton; 1976.

Gabriel J. Day treatment. *Am Occup Ther Assoc Mental Health Special Interest Section Newsletter* 1981; 4(4):1–2.

Grossman J. Nationally speaking . . . preventive health care and community programming. *Am J Occup Ther* 1977; 31:351–354.

Groth B, Toppson J. COTA share: improving the COTA professional image in therapeutic activity programming. *Occup Ther Newspaper* 1983; 37 (4):7.

Hatfield AB. The family as partner in the treatment of mental illness. *Hosp Commun Psychiatry* 1979; 30:338–340.

Howe MC, Weaver CT, Dulay J. The development of a work-oriented day center program. *Am J Occup Ther* 1981; 35:711–718.

Jerrell JM, Larson JK. Community mental health services in transition: who is benefiting? *Am J Orthopsychiatry* 1986; 56(1):78–88.

Kannegieter RB. Environmental interactions in psychiatric occupational therapy—some inferences. *Am J Occup Ther* 1980; 34:715–726.

Kiernat JM. Geriatric day hospitals: a golden opportunity for therapists. *Am J Occup Ther* 1976; 30:285–289.

Mann WC. A quarterway house for adult psychiatric patients. *Am J Occup Ther* 1976; 30:646–647.

Mosey AC. *Activities therapy.* New York: Raven Press; 1973.

Mueller S, Suto M. Starting a stress management programme. *Am Occup Ther Assoc Mental Health Special Interest Section Newsletter* 1983; 6(2): 1–3.

Penner DA. Correctional institutions: an overview. *Am J Occup Ther* 1978; 32:517–524.

Reed KL. *Models of practice in occupational therapy.* Baltimore: Williams & Wilkins; 1984.

Reed KL, Sanderson SR. *Concepts of occupational therapy.* 2nd ed. Baltimore: Williams & Wilkins; 1983.

Rogers JC. Roles and functions of occupational therapy in long-term care: occupational therapy and activity programs (AOTA position paper). *Am J Occup Ther* 1983; 37:807–810.

Rosenfeld MS. Crisis intervention: the nuclear task approach. *Am J Occup Ther* 1984; 38:382–385.

Rosenfeld MS. A model for activity intervention in disaster-stricken communities. *Am J Occup Ther* 1982; 36:228–235.

Schechter L. Occupational therapy in a psychiatric day hospital. *Am J Occup Ther* 1974; 28:151–153.

Sheehan S. *Is there no place on earth for me?* Boston: Houghton Mifflin; 1982.

Short JE. Changing role expectations of psychiatric occupational therapists. *Occup Ther Mental Health* 1984; 4(3):19–27.

Talbott JA. Toward a public policy on the chronic mentally ill patient. *Am J Orthopsychiatry* 1980; 50(1):43–53.

Tiffany EG. Psychiatry and mental health. In: Hopkins HL, Smith HD, eds. *Willard and Spackman's occupational therapy.* 6th ed. Philadelphia: JB Lippincott; 1983.

Webb LJ. The therapeutic social club. *Am J Occup Ther* 1973; 27:81–83.

Whitmer GE. From hospitals to jails: the fate of California's deinstitutionalized mentally ill. *Am J Orthopsychiatry* 1980; 50(1):65–75.

Williams DH, Bellis EC, Wellington SW. Deinstitutionalization and social policy. *Am J Orthopsychiatry* 1980; 50(1):54–64.

Williams R, Benese N. The day hospital at the Burke Rehabilitation Center. *Am J Occup Ther* 1976; 30:293.

Willson M. *Occupational therapy in long-term psychiatry.* Edinburgh: Churchill Livingstone; 1983.

8

Psychotropic Medications and Somatic Treatments

Some griefs are med'cinable.

WILLIAM SHAKESPEARE (3)

The introduction in the 1950s of drugs that could control hallucinations and other psychotic symptoms ushered in a new era in psychiatric rehabilitation. Suddenly, patients who had been unapproachable, out of control, and out of touch with reality were calm and could engage in occupational therapy and other rehabilitative treatments. In the succeeding decades many more types of psychotropic, or mind-changing, drugs have been discovered and introduced. These drugs are effective in reducing symptoms and returning people to their premorbid level of functioning.[1] This chapter will present information on the major types or classes of drugs used in psychiatric practice today, their therapeutic uses, and side effects. It will also describe specific occupational therapy interventions to help patients understand how medications influence their ability to function in purposeful activities. The use of electroconvulsive therapy (ECT) and other somatic (body-oriented) treatments will also be discussed. The reader is reminded that the effectiveness of drug therapy and somatic treatments is

attributed to neuroscience concepts, described in Chapter 2.

PSYCHOTROPIC MEDICATIONS

Psychotropic means "mind changing." Thus, psychotropic medications are drugs that alter or change the way the mind works. Many drugs have psychotropic qualities. These include medications prescribed for mental disorders, medications that are prescribed for physical disorders but that produce mind-altering side effects, and other mind-changing but illegal drugs (for example, PCP and LSD).

This chapter will consider only the first of these three groups: the psychotropic medications that physicians prescribe to treat the symptoms of mental illness. It is essential for the COTA to know about these different drugs. Although he cannot prescribe drugs (only the physician can do so), the COTA *is* in a position to observe the effects of the medication on the patient's symptoms and performance of everyday activities. He can see firsthand whether the patient is able to function better today than yesterday, or whether side effects such as tremors are interfering with his ability to perform routine tasks. The physician relies

---

[1]For a more detailed (and highly readable) discussion of these medications and treatments, the books by Lickey and Gordon (1, 2) are recommended.

on occupational therapy and nursing staff and patient self-reports to help him monitor how well a medication is working, whether it needs to be changed, or whether the dosage should be increased or reduced. In addition, the physician relies on staff to support his medical decisions and help the patient understand that some side effects are temporary. For these reasons it is important for the COTA to know the different classes of drugs, the problems for which they are prescribed, and the more common side effects.

Table 8–1 lists six major categories of drugs: antipsychotic drugs, antiparkinsonian drugs, antimanic drugs, antidepressant drugs, antianxiety drugs, and psychostimulants. Within each category the brand names of individual drugs are listed. Because there are several different classes (or chemical groups) of antidepressants, drugs in this category are grouped by class. Several different type styles are used to indicate the severity and frequency of the various side effects (see the key accompanying the table). In particular, the reader should note that side effects shown in boldfaced type are serious, either life-threatening or indicators of possible permanent damage. These side effects *must* be reported to the nurse or doctor immediately, *and* the assistant must also record (in the chart) the symptom and the person to whom it was reported.

Antipsychotic drugs, also known as *neuroleptics,* are prescribed most often for patients with schizophrenia and other psychotic disorders. These drugs control psychotic symptoms, such as hallucinations and delusions, and generally bring the patient into better contact with reality. The neuroleptics are also used to reduce violent or potentially dangerous behaviors in manic episodes and with drug abusers. Unfortunately, these drugs have no effect on the so-called "negative" symptoms of schizophrenia (apathy, disinterest in other people and one's environment, self-absorption,

and lack of motivation). Therefore, patients receiving these drugs are very much in need of occupational therapy and other rehabilitative services that help them function better in daily life.

Among the many side effects of neuroleptics are movement disorders (extrapyramidal syndrome), a tendency to sunburn very easily (photosensitivity), dry mouth, and blurred vision. Postural hypotension is another frequent side effect; the patient's blood pressure drops when he rises from lying to sitting, or from sitting to standing, causing him to black out or feel faint. Many patients on these drugs also suffer from a decrease in sexual interest, and may experience milk secretions from the breast (lactation). Side effects are most unpleasant during the first 10 days of treatment. After this time the movement disorders tend to diminish, although the cholinergic effects (dry mouth and blurred vision) may remain.

Tardive dyskinesia is potentially the most serious of the side effects of neuroleptics. It is a movement disorder that may become permanent unless the patient is removed from medication. The initial signs include facial movements, writhing motions of the tongue, and small writhing motions of the fingers. Any suspected signs of tardive dyskinesia should be reported to the physician immediately. Some unfortunate individuals may develop permanent tardive dyskinesia if their medication is not discontinued soon enough. This movement disorder can be very disfiguring and embarrassing to some patients, causing social rejection, impairments at work, depression, and suicidal acts (5). But other patients may be quite unconcerned. If you notice a patient who is receiving neuroleptics displaying any behaviors that seem similar to those described here, you should contact the doctor or nurse immediately and document this in the chart.

Because extrapyramidal syndrome is a frequent but unwelcome effect of neuroleptic medication, *antiparkinsonian drugs*

TABLE 8–1. *Therapeutic and adverse effects of psychotropic drugs*

Drug class/individual drugs	Therapeutic effects	Side effects
ANTIPSYCHOTIC DRUGS (NEUROLEPTICS) Compazine, Haldol, Loxitane, Mellaril, Moban, Navane, Permitil, Prolixin,[a] Serentil, Sparine, Stelazine, Taractan, Thorazine, Trilafon, Vesprin	Sedation Decrease in delusions Decrease in hallucinations Decrease in psychomotor agitation Control of other psychotic symptoms	Extrapyramidal syndrome Parkinsonism Akathisia Dystonia Akinesia Photosensitivity **Increase in psychosis** **Excessive sedation** **Postural hypotension** **Tardive dyskinesia** DRY MOUTH BLURRED VISION ALLERGIC SKIN REACTION
(CLOZAPINE) Clozaril	Relief from both positive (agitation, delusions, hallucinations) and negative (apathy, withdrawal) symptoms of schizophrenia	**Agranulocytosis** (potentially fatal blood condition) Seizures
ANTIPARKINSON DRUGS Akineton, Artane, Cogentin, Kemadrin, Parlodel, Parsidol, Symmetrel	Control of extrapyramidal side effects caused by use of antipsychotic medications (above).	Dry mouth Blurred vision Dizziness Nausea
BETA BLOCKERS Inderal	Currently under investigation for treatment of tardive dyskinesia and panic disorder	Insomnia Dizziness Fatigue Weakness Hypotension Cold hands and feet Tingling hands and feet **Various cardiac syndromes** Nausea Diarrhea Depression
ANTIMANIC DRUGS (Lithium compounds) Cibalith-S, Eskalith, Lithane, Lithium Carbonate, Lithobid, Lithonate, Lithotabs	Decrease in activity level Reduction in mood swing Normalization of sleep Decrease in speech production Increased attention span Improved judgment	DIARRHEA DROWSINESS **Slurred speech** **Loss of balance** **Confusion** VOMITING Fine hand tremor NAUSEA Thirst WEAKNESS/ INCOORDINATION BLURRED VISION Ataxia
ANTIDEPRESSANT DRUGS (TRICYCLICS) Adapin, Amitid, Amitril, Asendin, Aventyl, Elavil, Endep, Etrafon, Janamine, Limbitrol, Norpramin, Pamelor, Pertofrane, Sinequan, SK-Pramine Surmontil, Tipramine, Tofranil, Triavil, Vivactil	Relief from depression Reduction in suicidal risk and ideation Increased activity level Normalization of sleep Decreased weight loss	DROWSINESS **Constipation** **Urinary retention** **Seizures** **Postural hypotension** Weight gain Anxiety/agitation NAUSEA Dry mouth BLURRED VISION Tremors

TABLE 8–1. (*Continued*)

Drug class/individual drugs	Therapeutic effects	Side effects
Anafranil	This tricyclic antidepressant is under investigation for treatment of obsessive-compulsive disorders	Drowsiness Dizziness Fatigue Blurred vision Tremors Seizures **Various cardiac syndromes** Hypotension Dry mouth Constipation
(MAO INHIBITORS)[b] Marplan, Nardil, Parnate	Relief from depression and symptoms of depression as listed under tricylics	Dizziness Constipation Dry mouth **Postural hypotension** **Hypertensive crisis** **Headache** **Nausea** **Vomiting** **Drowsiness** **Weakness/fatigue** Tremors/twitching
(TETRACYCLICS) Ludiomil, Norval	Relief from depression and symptoms of depression as listed under tricyclics	**Hypotension** Palpitations Tremor **Constipation** Visual disturbances **Seizures**
(FLUOXETINE) Prozac	Relief from depression and symptoms of depression as listed under tricyclics	Headache Nervousness Insomnia Drowsiness Anxiety Tremors Dizziness Fatigue Rash Nausea Diarrhea Dry mouth Anorexia Weight loss Excessive sweating
(TRAZODONE) Desyrel	Relief from depression and symptoms of depression as listed under tricyclics	**Priapism** Nervousness Drowsiness Dizziness Fatigue Nausea Dry mouth Hypotension
(BUPROPION) Wellbutrin	Relief from depression and symptoms of depression as listed under tricyclics	Agitation Headache Blurred vision Insomnia Drowsiness Tremors Seizures Dizziness Nausea Constipation Dry mouth Anorexia Weight loss

TABLE 8–1. (*Continued*)

Drug class/individual drugs	Therapeutic effects	Side effects
ANTIANXIETY DRUGS (BENZODIAZEPINES) Ativan, Centrax, Libritabs, Librium, Lipoxide, Paxipam, Reposans-10, Serax, Tranxene, Valium, Xanax	Reduction of anxiety and tension Reduction of symptoms of alcohol withdrawal Relief of muscle spasm	Fatigue/drowsiness Ataxia Confusion Depression Hypotension Nausea Slurred speech Tremors Vertigo/dizziness Blurred vision
(MEPROBAMATE) Equanil, Meprospan, Meribam, Miltown, Neuramate, Sedabamate, Tranmep	Reduction of anxiety and tension	Physical dependence Drowsiness Slowed reaction time Slurred speech Vertigo/weakness Visual disturbance
(HYDROXYZINE) Anxanil, Atarax, Durrax, E-Vista, Hy-Pam, HYzine-50, Quiess, Vistacon, Vistaril, Vistazine	Reduction of anxiety and tension Control of symptoms in acute alcohol withdrawal	Drowsiness Dry mouth
(OTHERS) BuSpar, Trancopal	Reduction of anxiety and tension	Drowsiness Dizziness Headache Nervousness Nausea Rash Dry mouth
PSYCHOSTIMULANTS (USED FOR CHILDREN WITH ATTENTION-DEFICIT DISORDERS) Cylert, Desoxyn, Ritalin	Reduction of hyperactivity Increased attention Control of impulsivity Reduction of mood swings	Impaired growth Tics Insomnia Anorexia Hallucinations
(USED FOR OLDER PATIENTS WITH COGNITIVE DEFICITS) Cenalene, Menic, Metrazol, Nico-Metrazol, Vita-Metrazol	Improved mental functions Increased activity level	Insomnia Anorexia Nausea/vomiting Diarrhea Headache

More common effects (both therapeutic and adverse) are printed in ordinary type. Not all effects are seen to the same extent in all drugs of a given class. Very serious side effects that should be reported to medical staff and documented in the chart are shown in bold type. Side effects that are usually short-term or temporary are shown in capital letters.

[a]Prolixin in injectable form of Prolixin Deconoate is effective for two weeks between injections.

[b]Patients taking MAO inhibitors should not eat the following foods: aged cheeses, wine, beer, pickled herring, beans, yogurt, liver, and yeast. They must also avoid alcohol and the use of over-the-counter preparations for hay fever and allergies. Use of these substances with MAO inhibitors can precipitate a hypertensive crisis which may lead to death. Headache, chest pain, and sore neck are possible signs of hypertensive crisis and should be reported immediately to physician or nurse *and* documented in the chart.

are often prescribed simultaneously. These drugs reduce the extrapyramidal symptoms, thus enabling the patient to engage more easily in activities in which physical coordination is a factor. Unfortunately, these drugs may exacerbate the dry mouth, blurred vision, dizziness, and nausea the patient is already experiencing.

Antimanic drugs control the symptoms of mania and are prescribed for affective disorders in which manic symptoms are present. All of the drugs in this group contain lithium carbonate, a common metal salt. Lithium is toxic, and because of this frequent blood tests are performed to ascertain the level of lithium in the blood. During the first two or three weeks of receiving lithium, many people experience uncomfortable side effects such as diarrhea, dry mouth, frequent urination, drowsiness, and fatigue. These side effects usually diminish with time, and patients need to be encouraged to stick it out until this happens. The only lasting side effect seems to be a fine hand tremor, which is sometimes controlled by having the patient take another drug, propranolol, simultaneously. Gross bilateral hand tremors and ataxia, jaundice or yellowing of the skin or eyes, diarrhea, and vomiting are signs of possible overdose and should be reported to the physician immediately and documented.

The major therapeutic value of *antidepressant drugs* is relief from depression and the suicidal risk and social withdrawal associated with it. There are three major classes of antidepressant drugs, and several new drugs that fit in none of these classes. Each class will be discussed separately. Often, the physician will need to prescribe brief trials of different drugs before the one that produces the desired effect for a particular patient is identified.

Tricylic antidepressants derive their name from their chemical composition, which consists of three rings. These drugs are very commonly prescribed for depressive disorders, but do not begin to take effect until seven to ten days after they are first prescribed, and reach full effectiveness only after three weeks. As the drug begins to take effect the COTA will notice a gradual increase in the depressed person's ability to function. Common side effects of tricyclics include dry mouth, blurred vision, and constipation (and these can be relieved with lemon drops, magnifying glasses, and bran). Epileptic seizures may also be precipitated in susceptible patients.

Monoamine oxidase (MAO) inhibitors produce an antidepressant effect by interfering with the breakdown of certain brain chemicals. These drugs are usually prescribed to patients who have shown a poor response to tricyclics. MAO inhibitors also take up to three weeks to reach their full effect, and can be used only in patients who are willing to follow a strict dietary regimen. The amino acid tyramine interacts with MAO inhibitors to cause a hypertensive crisis (sudden increase in blood pressure), which may lead to cerebral hemorrhage and death. Tyramine is found in aged cheese, wine, beer, yogurt, tea, coffee, avocados, bananas, soy sauce, pickled herring, and other foods, and patients on MAO inhibitors must avoid them. COTAs who work with patients in food preparation should avoid foods that contain tyramine when patients on MAOs are involved.

Tetracyclic antidepressants have only recently been introduced in the United States. Their name comes from their chemical composition (four rings). It is believed that these drugs operate in a way similar to the tricyclics, but their side effects seem to be less severe.

Other antidepressants include fluoxetine (Prozac) and trazadone (Desyrel). Each is believed to produce fewer side effects than the tricyclics or MAO inhibitors. Desyrel, in some male patients, produces priapism (persistent erection). Patients experiencing this side effect must discontinue the medication immediately and notify their physician to avoid long-term problems.

Antianxiety drugs are used to control anxiety in disorders that are *not* psychotic (neu-

TABLE 8–2. *Drug side effects and recommended occupational therapy adaptations and interventions*

Side effect	Adaptations and interventions
Extrapyramidal syndrome	In general, report all extrapyramidal symptoms to physician or nurse when first observed and then report changes as they occur.
Parkinsonism—Muscular rigidity, tremors, drooling, shuffling gait, mask-like face.	1. Use gross motor activities that involve rotation of the head and trunk. 2. Avoid activities that require patient to work against resistance.
Akathisia—Restlessness, muscular tension (often worse in the legs than the arms).	1. Help patient select activities that allow for movement, getting up and down, etc. 2. Avoid activities that require prolonged periods of sitting or standing still. 3. Put patient at a separate table if persistent movement is disruptive to others.
Dystonia—Painful, sudden muscle spasms, often localized to the neck, jaw, eyes, or back. Patient may arch back, roll eyes, etc.	1. Help patient engage in activities that do not require fine coordination or attention to detail. 2. Avoid use of power tools, sharps, etc.
Akinesia—Muscular weakness and fatigue, reduction of movement.	1. Permit breaks in activity. 2. Avoid activities where patient must work against resistance, or for a long time.
Tardive dyskinesia—A movement disorder thought to be caused by prolonged use of neuroleptics. Movement patterns may be either choreiform (jerky, twitching) or athetoid (writhing) and often include facial distortions such as tongue thrust, lip smacking, tics, and chewing. Early signs include facial tics, slight but definitely abnormal eye or lip movements, rocking, and swaying.	1. *If new, notify physician at once.* Side effects can be reversed if caught early, but if neglected may become permanent. 2. *If chronic,* and if patient is aware and concerned, provide support and encouragement. Allow patient to verbalize his embarrassment and discomfort.
Postural hypotension—Patient feels faint or blacks out when he rises from lying to sitting or from sitting to standing. This is due to the effect of gravity.	1. Notify physician. 2. Teach patient to sit up slowly, stand up slowly. Stand close to patient and be prepared to support him at the waist. Do not try to support the patient by grabbing his arm. 3. Encourage patient to use furniture and other supports to maintain balance. 4. Avoid activities that involve sudden postural changes. 5. Avoid gross motor activities to reduce sudden movements.
Dry mouth—Patient feels thirsty.	1. Allow patient to get water whenever he needs to do so. 2. Have hard (sucking) candies available. Lemon drops are best. Some people prefer sugar-free breath mints. 3. Educate patient about the dehydrating effect of caffeinated drinks and alcohol.
Blurred vision—Vision may be blurry, or in some cases patient may experience double vision.	1. Help patient select activities that do not involve fine visual attention. 2. In gross motor activities, use mats and soft equipment to avoid injury. 3. In crafts, use large pieces that are easily seen (e.g., one inch mosaic tiles). 4. Provide magnified reading glasses (several levels of magnification) to be used in the occupational therapy clinic.
Hand tremors—Rhythmic involuntary hand movements (see also ataxia below).	1. If patient is on a new trial of a lithium-based antimanic medication, and tremor is gross, notify physician. Gross bilateral hand tremor may be a sign of drug toxicity. 2. If patient has been on lithium for one month or more, fine hand tremors are frequent. Help patient learn to compensate by stabilizing elbow or arm to prevent tremor.

TABLE 8–2. (*Continued*)

Side effect	Adaptations and interventions
	3. If patient is on neuroleptics and tremor has a writhing or worm-like appearance, notify physician. These movements may indicate tardive dyskinesia.
Ataxia—Failure of muscle coordination, manifested as clumsiness when a motor action is attempted (e.g., walking or doing a craft).	1. If patient is on a new trial of lithium-based antimanic medication, notify physician immediately, as this may be a sign of drug toxicity. 2. Prepare to provide support when patient gets up out of a chair or turns corners while walking. 3. Help patient select and engage in activities in which incoordination will not interfere with success.
Nausea	1. Have soda crackers, graham crackers, and bread available. 2. Over-the-counter antacids are sometimes recommended by the physician. Because these preparations may interfere with the action of some antipsychotic and other medications, physicians' approval is required.
Photosensitivity—Patient is extremely sensitive to effects of the sun, and will sunburn after brief exposure. This is most commonly seen in patients who are taking certain neuroleptics	1. Educate patient about photosensitizing effect of medications. 2. Have patient wear sunscreen, long sleeves, hat, and sunglasses. Be sure patient applies sunscreen to tops of feet, backs of hands, ear lobes, top of head (bald men). 3. Keep time in the sun as brief as possible. 4. Observe patient closely for signs of sunburn.

roses, personality disorders, etc.). These drugs are sometimes called the *minor tranquilizers,* to differentiate them from the *major tranquilizers,* or neuroleptics. There are two chemical classes of antianxiety drugs: the benzodiazepines and the meprobamates. It is not especially important for the occupational therapy assistant to know the difference. Both classes have similar therapeutic effects and adverse side effects.

Psychostimulants are drugs that stimulate and increase mental and physical activity. Oddly, and paradoxically, they have the opposite effect in children, and are sometimes prescribed for control of hyperactivity in children with attention deficit disorder. Side effects, which include impaired growth, tics, and insomnia, must be carefully monitored. Another group of psychostimulants is sometimes prescribed for older patients who have memory deficits and other cognitive problems.

Patients with mental health problems are often prescribed more than one type of medication. For example, a neuroleptic may be used with lithium to reduce acute psychotic symptoms of mania. Not only are different psychotropic drugs used in combination with each other, but patients who have medical conditions are generally taking other medications as well. Because drugs interact with each other, the physician is especially careful to prescribe only those medications that are compatible with ones the patient is already taking. Use by patients of drugs that are not prescribed or that are not documented in the medical record (e.g., those prescribed by the family physician for a medical problem) should be reported to the psychiatrist in charge of the case.

Although the occupational therapy assistant cannot prescribe medications or reduce their undesirable side effects, he can help patients adapt to the way their bodies respond to these side effects. Table 8–2 (see pages 142–143) provides information about selected side effects and provides strategies the occupational therapy assistant can employ to help patients deal with them and function better. Occupational therapy staff can also assist by monitoring patient compliance with prescribed drug regimens, and by observing and reporting to the physician any undocumented drugs that the patient may be taking.

SOMATIC TREATMENTS

Somatic treatments are those which act upon the body to produce an effect on the mind. These include electroconvulsive therapy and psychosurgery, among others. *Electroconvulsive therapy* (ECT) is sometimes incorrectly called "shock therapy." The patient is given a muscle relaxant, after which a brief electrical current is applied to his temples, causing a convulsion. No one is certain why this treatment is effective, but it does relieve severe depression and reduce the life-threatening risk of suicide in 80 to 90 percent of depressed patients who fail to respond to drug therapies. Usually 8 to 12 ECT treatments are given over several weeks. The only side effects are occasional headache immediately after a treatment, and short-term memory loss (lasting a few weeks). The patient usually does not remember the treatment at all, and the only permanent memory loss may be of events in the few days before the treatment. Patients receiving ECT are often confused and may not remember (for example) who the occupational therapy assistant is, or that they were working on a particular project in occupational therapy. Guidelines for responding to this type of confusion and memory loss are described in Chapter 11.

Psychosurgery was a common treatment in previous decades,[2] when it was erroneously believed that surgically cutting the connections between the prefrontal cortex and the hypothalamic area of the brain would relieve mental symptoms. This procedure, called a lobotomy, often left the patient with impaired judgment and a complete lack of motivation. Psychosurgical techniques are only rarely practiced today, for relief of intractable depression or violence, and it is unlikely that the occupational therapy assistant will encounter patients who have received this treatment.

SUMMARY

Psychotropic medications are drugs that affect the way the mind works. Physicians frequently prescribe these drugs and other somatic treatments such as ECT for patients with mental health problems. Although psychotropic medications have great value in reducing or controlling the symptoms of mental illness, unpleasant side effects may also occur. For many patients, the choice is between a side effect and symptoms of a mental disorder, either of which will interfere with their ability to carry out everyday activities. The occupational therapy assistant working with psychiatric patients needs to be aware of the different kinds of medication and their effects, both therapeutic and adverse. By observing the patient closely day after day, the COTA can notice the effects of medication on the patient's functional level; this information, when communicated to the physician, aids in the proper adjustment of dosage level. In addition, the COTA can adapt activities to enable the patient to succeed despite drug side effects, and can educate the patient to the effects of the drugs he is taking and teach him strategies he can use to deal with these effects.

REFERENCES

1. Lickey ME, Gordon B. *Drugs for mental illness: a revolution in psychiatry.* New York: WH Freeman; 1983.

---

[2]For a detailed and sobering discussion of the history of psychosurgery, see Valenstein (4).

2. Lickey ME, Gordon B. *Medicine and mental illness—the use of drugs*. New York: WH Freeman; 1991.
3. Shakespeare W (1610). *Cymbeline* III, ii, 33. In: Barlett J, ed. *Familiar quotations*. 15th ed. Boston: Little, Brown; 1980:243.
4. Valenstein ES. *Great and desperate cures*. New York: Basic Books; 1986.
5. Yassa R, Jones BD. Complications of tardive dyskinesia. *Psychosomatics* 1985; 26:305–313.

ADDITIONAL REFERENCES AND SUGGESTED READINGS

Allen CK. *Occupational therapy for psychiatric diseases: measurement and management of cognitive disabilities*. Boston: Little, Brown; 1985.
Bailey DS, Cooper SO, Bailey DR. *Therapeutic approaches to the mentally ill*. 2nd ed. Philadelphia: FA Davis; 1984.
Baker CA, publisher. *Physician's desk reference*. 46th ed. Oradell, NJ: Medical Economics Company; 1992.
Crawford AL, Kilander VC. *Psychiatric and mental health nursing*. 6th ed. Philadelphia: FA Davis; 1985.
Frances A, Weiden P. Promoting compliance with outpatient drug treatment. *Hosp Comm Psychiatry* 1987; 38:1158–1160.
Hemphill BJ, Smith DA. Did you know . . . there are at least eight scales for identifying and measuring tardive dyskinesia? *Am Occup Ther Assoc Mental Health Specialty Section Newsletter* 1982; 5(1):4.
Hemphill BJ, Smith DA. Did you know . . . that many of your patients . . . *Am Occup Ther Assoc Mental Health Specialty Section Newsletter* 1982; 5(2):2.
Klawans HL, Goetz CG, Tanner CM. *Textbook of clinical neuropharmacology and therapeutics*. 2nd ed. New York: Raven Press; 1992.
Opler LA, Katz I, Kobayashi J, Ruiz P. Tardive dyskinesia and institutional practice: current issues and guidelines. *Hosp Commun Psychiatry* 1980; 31:239–245.
Saffir JS. The theoretical implications of chlorpromazine as a variable in therapy based on sensory integrative theory. *Am J Occup Ther* 1978; 32:460–466.
Smith DA. Effects of psychotropic drugs on the occupational therapy process. *Am Occup Ther Assoc Mental Health Specialty Section Newsletter* 1981; 4(1):1–3.
Swonger AK, Constantine LL. *Drugs and therapy: a handbook of psychotropic drugs*. Boston: Little, Brown; 1983.
Tiffany EG. Psychiatry and mental health. In: Hopkins HL, Smith HD, eds. *Willard and Spackman's occupational therapy*. 6th ed. Philadelphia: JB Lippincott; 1983.
Townsend MC. *Drug guide for psychiatric nursing*. Philadelphia: FA Davis; 1992.
Tyrer PJ. *Drugs in psychiatric practice*. London: Butterworths; 1982.
Van Schroeder C, Chung R. Occupational therapy impacts the care of patients at risk for tardive dyskinesia. *Am Occup Ther Assoc Mental Health Specialty Section Newsletter* 1985; 8(2):1, 3–4.
Werner A, Campbell RJ, Frazier SH, Stone EM, Edgerton J, eds. *A psychiatric glossary*. 5th ed. Washington, DC: American Psychiatric Association; 1980.

9

Special Populations

*No people are uninteresting. Their fate is like
the chronicle of planets.*

Yevgeny Yevtushenko (28)

The purpose of this chapter is to present some special diagnoses and conditions that the occupational therapy assistant might encounter in a psychiatric setting. Some of these conditions have a medical and a psychiatric component (substance abuse, eating disorders, AIDS). Homelessness, the last topic in this chapter, is more social in origin. This chapter is intended to supplement Chapters 5 and 7, to give greater detail on some conditions that might require additional understanding of the treatment context. By treatment context we mean not only the physical and social environment, but also the clinical team environment. To work successfully with the groups of patients discussed in this chapter the occupational therapy assistant will need to understand background information on the etiology and treatment, and will need to appreciate the special concerns of other persons involved in the patient's recovery.

ALCOHOL AND SUBSTANCE ABUSE

We are considering alcohol and drug abuse patients a special population for several reasons. First, particular behavioral patterns are characteristic of this group. These behavioral patterns are often rein-

forced or enabled by those with whom the abuser associates (family, employer). Second, successful recovery by this group of patients usually requires involvement with and commitment to a 12-step program such as Alcoholics Anonymous. Third, alcohol and drug problems are often compounded by associated medical and psychiatric conditions. The occupational therapy assistant will certainly encounter alcohol and substance abusers frequently as patients, in settings as diverse as burn units, general medical services, trauma units, physical rehabilitation centers, and mental health settings. Fourth, staff who work with this population often choose to pursue certification or credentialling as alcohol and drug abuse counselors. Such certification supplements their basic professional education and enhances their status and credibility in the eyes of other certified counselors. Finally, occupational therapy intervention has a specific focus with this group, and the occupational therapy assistant can take a significant role.

In this section we will describe the various abused substances and their effects, the mental and social characteristics of substance abuse, and occupational therapy interventions. We will also discuss the various 12-step groups and will briefly consider the dual-diagnosis patient.

Abused Substances and Their Effects

Alcohol consumption is a fact of life in American society and in most other cultures worldwide. Alcohol abuse is epidemic, but socially sanctioned. According to the American Psychiatric Association alcohol and drug abuse is "by far the predominant cause of premature and preventable illness, disability, and death in our society" (3). It is estimated that one in ten adult Americans is alcoholic and that each of these significantly affects at least four other individuals, impairing the quality of their lives (5). A 1984 report puts the annual cost of alcoholism at $89.5 billion for treatment and social/economic losses in worker productivity, property damage, and early death and disability from alcohol-related accidents (automobile, fire, falls, violence) (3).

In small quantities, alcohol has been promoted as beneficial by the medical profession. A glass of wine a day is believed to confer some protection against premature cardiac and vascular disease. As explained in Chapter 5, there are varying degrees of *unhealthy* involvement with alcohol. Generally, alcoholics begin drinking in their teens or twenties, and the disease becomes progressive, leading to abuse and ultimately to dependence. More males than females are heavy drinkers. There is a familial pattern of alcoholism, which may have a genetic component. However, one cannot discount the effect of observing, as a young child, the drinking behavior of family members.

Three patterns of alcohol abuse are recognized: regular daily drinking, heavy weekend drinking, and periodic or episodic binge drinking. A person who abuses alcohol but who is not yet dependent on it will be able to go for days and weeks and even months of abstinence without suffering withdrawal symptoms. Once the disease has reached the dependence stage, however, the individual will experience withdrawal when alcohol is withheld. Symptoms may include delirium tremens, or the DTs (characterized by fever, tremors, ataxia, and even hallucinations). Sweating and high blood pressure are other symptoms of withdrawal.

Chronic excessive alcohol use may lead to lasting neurological damage and dementia. Medical conditions caused by alcohol include liver damage; gastric damage; premature aging; impotence and infertility; and increased risk of heart disease, respiratory disease, and neurological disorders. Depression is associated with alcohol abuse and may be either a contributing factor or result of alcoholism. Many alcoholics have been prescribed psychotropic medications (antidepressants such as Prozac, or antianxiety drugs such as Xanax) by physicians who were not aware of their alcohol abuse. Children born to alcoholic mothers may suffer fetal alcohol syndrome, characterized by facial abnormalities, mental retardation, and pervasive developmental defects.

Marijuana is the most widely available illegal drug in America. It is often used in combination with alcohol or other drugs. Marijuana impairs a variety of cognitive and perceptual-motor functions including concentration, judgment, short-term memory, perception, and motor skills. Marijuana may adversely affect reproduction and may exacerbate pre-existing heart conditions. Because it is smoked and because it contains many known carcinogens, it may be more damaging to the lungs than tobacco. It has been linked to depression and is suspected as the primary cause of "amotivational syndrome" in adolescents. This syndrome is characterized by loss of interest and initiative, difficulty concentrating, and diminished functional performance at school and work (3).

Cocaine derives from the leaves of the South American coca plant. As a white powder, it can be snorted through the nose or dissolved and injected. Crack is a smokable form of cocaine, and produces a rapid "high." Crack is more addicting than other forms of cocaine because the "low" that follows rapidly from the "high" increases the desire for the drug. As with alcohol abuse, cocaine abuse may follow either an episodic or a chronic daily pattern. Cocaine abuse may lead to serious medical problems including frequent and tenacious upper respiratory infections, heart failure, reproductive problems including miscarriage, stroke, seizures, and personality changes and violent psychosis. Newborns exposed to cocaine *in utero* may share the same physical problems as the abusing mother and may suffer serious birth defects and deformities. Further, they may be irritable and have difficulty bonding to the mother or accepting nourishment (3).

Opiate narcotics, which may be either natural or synthetic in origin, include heroin, morphine, and meperidine (Demerol). Use of these drugs leads to addiction in about 50 percent of cases. Associated medical conditions include heart problems and the risk of acquiring acquired immune deficiency syndrome (AIDS) or other infections from contaminated needles. Children born to opiate-addicted mothers will suffer withdrawal sysmptoms and may die as a result (3).

Other frequently abused drugs include phencyclidine (PCP or angel dust), lysergic acid dyethylamine (LSD), amphetamines, amyl nitrite and other inhalants, and various prescription drugs.

Psychological Characteristics and Social Factors

Alcohol and substance abuse problems are believed to originate in learned patterns from childhood that predispose to substance abuse. Children of substance abusing parents are likely to become substance abusers themselves because they did not experience a normal nurturing and growth-producing environment. In some cases the child is rejected and/or sexually abused by the drinking parent and ignored or smothered by the nondrinking parent. In other cases, the child reverses roles with the parent, providing care for the parents and siblings and taking on cooking and other household chores. Another pattern leading to adult alcohol abuse is having been overprotected in childhood, which restricts risk-taking (a major source of self-esteem) and limits the development of necessary social skills (16). While these predisposing patterns are not shared by all alcoholics, they are common to many.

Substance abusers as a group tend to employ a characteristic set of defense mechanisms. Moyers (16) summarized the literature on the *preferred defensive structure* (PDS) of alcoholics. The PDS is a group of strategies for achieving one's goals. Moyers reminds us that the alcoholic may have acquired these strategies in childhood to avoid experiencing painful feelings. *Denial* is the first line of defense, as it permits the substance abuser to ignore the disease and to escape accountability for its consequences. Further, even in sobriety, this defense is used to avoid painful confrontation with the consequences of one's actions. *Projection,* or the transfer onto others of one's own feelings, is also used to disguise one's unacceptable negative feelings. For example, the alcoholic who is himself quite angry (but can't face this) believes a neighbor is angry with him and this "makes" him drink. *Rationalization,* or giving reasons for drinking behavior, helps the alcoholic distance himself from his own compulsion to drink by blaming it on, for example, his wife or his employer. Chapters 10 and 11 give more detail on appropriate and helpful responses to these elements of the PDS.

Another characteristic defense is a preference for *dichotomous thinking.* This either-or, black-and-white, reasoning has been attributed to unpredictable experiences in childhood. Dichotomous thinking leads to wild variability in behavior. For example, extreme perfectionism and attention to detail may alternate with sloppy indifference. Another example is swinging from overdependence on staff to withdrawal and aloof independence. Moyers recommends that the patient be involved in carefully designed experiences that permit her to recognize and explore a middle ground between the two extremes. For example, the patient who is alternately overdependent and too independent needs to recognize differences in situations that call for more or less dependence on others.

Social factors that must be understood for effective work with the alcohol or substance abuser include codependency, enabling behaviors of others, and social/leisure deficits. *Codependency* refers to the unhealthy involvement of a non-substance abuser in controlling a substance abuser. Codependent behavior is most common in spouses and immediate family members, but may occur in others with whom the alcoholic associates. *Enabling* is a codependent behavior characterized by making it easier for the substance abuser to continue to drink and/or drug. Examples of enabling include picking up the slack by taking care of the user's responsibilities (calling in sick for him) and providing money and other forms of material support.

While the alcoholic may risk losing his job due to his alcoholic behavior, in some cases the employer may actually be an enabler. Some occupations provide many job-related drinking occasions, and excessive consumption is condoned—for example, hangovers are accepted as normal or tardiness is overlooked. Richert (20) reported an association between evening or night shifts and alcohol consumption.

After years of spending most leisure hours in drinking-related pursuits, the typical alcoholic has a network of drinking companions, a set of familiar drinking locations, and sometimes a repertoire of drinking-related activities (watching sporting events, gambling, or playing cards, etc.). These habits related to the use of leisure time are a major problem for the recovering alcoholic, who must relearn how to enjoy leisure in a sober way.

Alcoholics Anonymous

No discussion of substance abuse would be complete without mention of Alcoholics Anonymous (AA), a self-help group whose purpose is to help its members achieve and maintain sobriety. Founded in 1935, AA is entirely funded by member contributions. Membership in AA is based on AA's third tradition, that "the only requirement for membership is a desire to stop drinking" (1). AA is commonly accepted as the most successful program for maintaining sobriety, and professionals who work with alcoholics actively encourage involvement with AA.

The foundation of the AA program is the 12 steps.[1] The first 3 steps engage the alcoholic in admitting his powerlessness over his disease and promote willingness to seek help from AA and from other sources. The remaining 9 steps provide a structure for understanding the consequences of one's actions, for mending impaired social relations, for maintaining a sober life-style, and for carrying the message of hope and strength to other alcoholics. Every day, all over the world, countless AA groups meet (usually for about one hour) in church basements, hospitals, detention centers, detox units, schools, and other public places. The atmosphere in a typical AA group is warm and accepting, welcoming of all regardless of social status, and nurturing especially to those members who have "had a slip."

In the decades since the founding of AA, other 12-step groups have sprung up on this model. These include Narcotics Anonymous (NA), Cocaine Anonymous (CA), Debtors Anonymous (DA), Overeaters Anonymous

---

[1]Text of the 12 steps can be found in any AA publication (Reference 1, and others listed in recommended additional readings at the end of the chapter), and a list of local meetings open to professionals and interested others may be obtained from any local chapter of AA.

(OA), and Al-Anon and Al-A-Teen for families affected by an alcoholic member.

Credentialling and Certification in Alcohol and Substance Abuse Counseling

Alcoholism and substance abuse counselors provide assessment and therapy services to recovering substance abusers, usually through agencies designed for this population. Many occupational therapy personnel working with substance abusers have found it desirable to obtain certification or credentialling as substance abuse counselors. Such credentialling confers a degree of credibility among the substance abuse mental health professional community; uncredentialled therapists are sometimes viewed with distrust. Requirements for credentialling vary among the 50 states. In most cases, the counselor must have some college credits, must take some courses related to alcohol and substance abuse, and must work for a specified number of supervised hours doing substance abuse counseling before sitting for a state-administered examination. To maintain credentialling, counselors are required to demonstrate completion of a certain number of continuing education units per year. Occupational therapy assistants interested in pursuing such credentialling should contact the offices of alcoholism and substance abuse services in their state capital.

Occupational Therapy Interventions

Occupational therapy for the substance abuse patient is directed to improving functioning and providing skill development in specific areas. Evaluation focuses on use of time (especially leisure time), cognitive and perceptual skills, social skills and self-expression, daily living skills, and role acquisition. Viik et al. (26) tested the Assessment of Occupational Functioning (AOF), a screening tool based on the model of human occupation, with an alcoholic population.

They found that clear differences in occupational functioning exist between newly sober inpatient alcoholics and those with one or more years of sobriety. Newly sober alcoholics had a preference for activities associated with alcohol, whereas alcoholics with longer recovery preferred activities associated with sobriety. The *Barth Time Construction* (see Chapter 14) has also been used to obtain information about the alcoholic's use of time generally and of leisure time specifically. Mann and Talty (12) designed a *Leisure Activity Profile* (LAP) to distinguish between alcoholic and nonalcoholic use of leisure time. The assumption is that alcoholics tend to choose activities that are related to alcohol. One role of occupational therapy can be to introduce and promote participation in other activities, and to model and facilitate a spontaneous and "fun" attitude toward leisure. The LAP contains a list of 38 activities, half of which are associated with alcohol consumption. Preliminary data (12) suggest that the LAP differentiates well between alcoholics and nonalcoholics, but the LAP needs further research study and development before it will be considered reliable and valid for clinical use.

Once sober, the alcoholic has few resources for spending the large amounts of leisure time now available. Recovering alcoholics are instructed to avoid "people, places, and things" that lead to drinking. Some newly sober alcoholics use their leisure time attending several AA meetings per day. Others may band together with other alcoholics to attempt leisure activities (such as an AA softball team or tennis league). Occupational therapy can help by assessment through the Interest Checklist or similar inventory (see Chapter 14) and by intervention through providing opportunities to plan and experience sober leisure activities. Voorhies[2] describes a continuum of

---

[2]Personal communication from Susan Voorhies, COTA/CAODAC, of HCA Regional Hospital Rediscovery Unit, Jackson, Tenn. Activities developed in consultation with Anne Brown, OTR, MS.

occupational therapy activities for leisure development. These include a Leisure Education Group, in which members explore their own leisure habits, learn about alternative activities, and investigate interests. A Gym/Recreation Group helps members to develop physical and social skills and promotes release of energy through physical activity and competition. A Community Resource Group provides for planned trips into the local community to demonstrate the range of oppportunities available and to present alternatives to being socially isolated. A Family Recreation Night (see below) helps the recovering patient reintegrate into the role of family member and recreator. Voorhies notes that the more active and spontaneous the groups, the better the response. Since patients no longer have the option to create feelings of well-being through chemicals, they respond positively to altering their feelings through activity.

Voorhies also describes a successful alumni volunteer program, in which recovered alcoholics return to the treatment center on a regular basis to help others. They go with patients to AA and NA meetings, hold AA Big Book[3] studies groups, or spend leisure time with them. In addition to helping the newcomer, the alumni volunteer is strengthening his own recovery by following AA's 12th step of reaching out to the "still-suffering alcoholic."

Perceptual and cognitive functions may be impaired by alcohol and substance abuse, and are sometimes evaluated by occupational therapy. Van Deusen (25) examined the treatment of perceptual-motor dysfunction in alcohol abusers, noting that tactile perception, figure-ground discrimination, and visual-spatial relations may be impaired in this group. The etiology or causes of perceptual-motor dysfunction in alcoholics are not clearly established. In many cases, the deficits disappear or diminish after a period of recovery and abstinence. It is not clear whether rehabilitation has an effect; the evidence suggests that younger persons (with shorter time in active alcoholism) fare better than older alcoholics in recovering a more normal level of perceptual-motor skill. Van Deusen further noted that treatment of such deficits by occupational therapy staff is appropriate only where the deficit can be shown to impair the person's ability to perform activities of daily living. Van Deusen recommends that occupational therapy staff working with this population collect data on the types and degree of impairment they observe in this group.

In the area of social skills and self-expression, substance abusers benefit from learning new ways to cope with feelings (rather than resorting to use of the drug of choice). Expressive activities (art, clay, poetry, drama) are sometimes used to assist the recovering alcoholic to recognize and convey emotions that she has been used to blocking out by drinking and/or by defense mechanisms such as denial and projection. Since there is a risk to the patient of overexposure and becoming overwhelmed by feelings that seem raw and new, expressive activities must be used with delicacy and judgment. Use of expressive activities for this purpose is not generally the role of the entry-level occupational therapy assistant, and requires direction and supervision from someone more experienced with this technique.

Assertiveness training is often provided to assist the recovering substance abuser to acquire more appropriate skills and more successful strategies for interacting with others. This enlarges the repertoire of social behaviors available to help the newly sober patient achieve his goals in his interpersonal relationships. Stress management and relaxation skills training can also be used to develop an understanding of what the individual finds stressful, and to teach a number of activities that can be used to promote relaxation.

[3]The Big Book refers to the basic text, *Alcoholics Anonymous,* which gives the history and method of the 12-step program and includes 40 autobiographical sketches.

In the area of daily living skills, many patients in recovery benefit from money management activities. Often, a large portion of their disposable income went to purchasing their drug of choice, and the recovering patient may have limited ideas about how to budget money and control spending (19). Time management, parenting skills, nutrition and meal planning, food preparation, housekeeping, and use of community resources are other areas of daily living skills that may need attention with this group of patients.

In the area of work, different areas can be targeted for intervention, depending on the functional level of the patient. Some higher-functioning substance abusers have experienced much success in their careers; despite their alcohol or drug use, they were reliable and in many cases ambitious and conscientious workers. This group may need information and assistance in planning leisure time activities, in developing a social network, and in managing work time so that it does not become obsessive. Another group of recovering patients may at some point in the past have had successful work experiences, but they have been fired from their jobs because of alcohol or drug-related behaviors. This group needs help in redeveloping work habits and skills so that they can reenter the worker role. Résumé writing and job search skills are also appropriate interventions for this group. Yet another group, of much lower functioning patients, has little or no experience of success in the role of worker. This group may require a full range of vocational and prevocational assessment and training. Occupational therapy can address the basic task skills and work-related social behaviors through work groups and volunteer positions. In some cities, alcoholics with several months of sobriety can obtain vocational testing and training from the Employment Program for Recovering Alcoholics (EPRA), which is associated with AA.

Recovering alcoholics and substance abusers need also to rebuild their relationships with their families. Moyers (17) outlined an approach to working with families to break down destructive and enabling patterns and to establish healthier ones. Voorhies[4] described a Family Recreation Night group, which meets one evening per month. Up to nine patients, each with an average of three adult family members and the patient's children, meet to play games and do nonthreatening group activities (i.e., Taboo, Pictionary, Outburst, etc.). The games are adapted for all ages to promote cohesiveness and participation of everyone. This group provides opportunities for a family experience of leisure activities, helps build social skills and insight into the appropriate tasks of a family member, and prepares the patient for leisure with the family after discharge.

Dual Diagnosis Conditions

Dual diagnosis refers to the patient with two diagnoses—substance abuse and another Axis I or II psychiatric disorder. Many substance abusers have personality disorders, coded on Axis II. Of more concern, however, are the dual diagnosis patients with Axis I diagnoses of schizophrenia or affective disorders. In general, dual diagnosis substance abusers have fewer skills and correspondingly more functional impairments than patients who have only the diagnosis of substance abuse. They are more prone to relapse and require more structure. Occupational therapy interventions for these patients need to be more training-oriented, teaching daily living skills and task skills, and reinforcing appropriate behavior.

EATING DISORDERS

As stated in Chapter 5, *eating disorders* include several different conditions revolv-

----

[4]Personal communication from Susan Voorhies, COTA/CAODAC, of HCA Regional Hospital Rediscovery Unit, Jackson, Tenn. Activities developed in consultation with Anne Brown, OTR, MS.

ing around abnormal behavior in the consumption and retention of food. *Anorexia nervosa* is characterized by abnormally low body weight with refusal to gain weight and a disturbed body image. *Bulimia nervosa* is characterized by binge eating followed by self-induced vomiting or other drastic measures to reduce body size (fasting, use of laxatives). Some clinicians also include *obesity* (excessive body weight) in the category of eating disorders.

Anorexia has been recognized as a clinical condition for over 300 years (27). Many different approaches have been attempted, including behavioral (14) and psychoanalytic (22). Current understanding suggests that many eating disorder patients have suffered childhood trauma, including in many cases sexual abuse. Roth (23) describes these patients as needing to control themselves and others through their food intake. The typical eating disorder patient was controlled in childhood by an overprotective and intrusive parent who did not permit her to acquire the normal experiences that lead to self-assessment and the development of healthy reality-based self-esteem. Instead, the young girl adopts a false ideal of low weight, behind which she hides her chronic feelings of emptiness and low self-esteem.

As with alcohol abuse, to a significant degree our society promotes the development of eating disorders. The popular press and broadcast media represent the ideal female as muscular, underweight, and unrealistically thin. Dieting, powdered and canned food substitutes, and aggressive exercise are all marketed as desirable for reducing weight to keep up with the popular ideals, themselves highly unrealistic. To illustrate, in sizing of children's clothes, not even three-year-olds are expected to have a waist as small as 18 inches. Yet, we have been enculturated to believe that women should strive to this ideal popularized in the figure of Scarlett O'Hara.

Focuses for occupational therapy intervention with anorexic patients include the development of behaviors that support role performance as an adult female (cooking and menu planning, reasonable exercise routines, and acquiring and caring for a wardrobe). In addition, occupational therapy must address underlying problems related to distorted body image, deficient self-esteem, and limited assertiveness. In a review of the literature, Rockwell (22) found that the following types of activities were preferred by occupational therapists working with eating disorders patients: art therapy, cooking/menu planning, crafts, stress management training, and group discussion/activities.

Art therapy facilitates the identification and expression of feelings and beliefs about the self. This can help the patient with low self-esteem explore the reasons for feeling so inadequate. Body image issues can also be expressed and examined. McColl et al. (13) suggest, however, that such an activity should not be forced on the patient. Because the feelings of ineffectiveness run so deep, the activities that work best are those that the patient selects.

Cooking and menu planning are important activities for this group. Bailey (4) notes that the eating disorder patient typically has extensive knowledge of the calorie content of foods but little knowledge of other aspects of food content such as vitamins and nutritive value. In addition, a cooking group supports the experience of preparing and consuming normal-sized portions of food. For bulimic patients, cooking groups provide an opportunity to experience in a more normal way foods that might previously have led to bingeing (9). The patient can bake a cake and share it with the group, having only one portion herself.

Meyers (15) reported on a case study of one 27-year-old mother of two with a diagnosis of anorexia and bulimia. This patient felt that crafts gave her a positive experience of control. She could use her hands for something more productive and useful than putting them down her throat to force vomiting of food. She saw the craft experience as a "microcosm of real life with many different people working side by side." The patient found the body image group a struggle, and had difficulty letting go of her ideal of a smaller size. As she gained weight, she found it painful to accept the change in body shape and the need for larger new clothes.

In the therapeutic relationship with an eating disorder patient, Meyers (15) indicates that unconditional caring must be accompanied by the expectation for change. In other words, while accepting the patient for where she is and valuing her for who she is, all staff must convey the attitude that they expect the patient to work toward a normal weight and to cease self-destructive eating behaviors.

Eating disorder patients present a clinical challenge. Good supervision is a must. Because of the risk of death and physical illness from poor nutrition, these patients must be monitored by medical staff.

MULTIPLE PERSONALITY DISORDER

Multiple personality disorder is a rarely diagnosed condition in which there exist within the same person at least 2 different personality states. The number of personalities may be as high as 200 in some cases (2). These personality states are often manifested by observable differences in behavior, dress, grooming, voice, and other outward characteristics. Commonly, the different personalities are unaware of the existence of the others. This means that when one personality "takes over," the individual might not remember the previous personality's behavior or experiences. Multiple personality disorder is diagnosed far more frequently in females than in males. It is associated with childhood abuse, most often sexual in nature. Substance abuse and self-mutilating behavior may also be present.

The usual approach of the primary therapist to treating someone with multiple personality disorder involves befriending or making an alliance with the various personalities and helping the individual become aware of them and integrate them with each other. Treatment of multiple personality disorder requires extensive clinical training. Integration of the various personalities with each other can occur only when the patient works over a long period with a highly trained therapist (usually a psychiatrist, social worker, or psychologist). Treatment of this condition is therefore beyond the scope of the occupational therapy assistant's expertise. While it is possible that one might encounter such a patient in practice, this is unlikely due to the rarity of the condition. The occupational therapy assistant should expect to receive explicit direction and intensive supervision for any work with such a patient.

The focus of occupational therapy for this condition has only recently been discussed in the occupational therapy literature. However, occupational therapy is the rehabilitation service most frequently recommended (21). Because the disorder begins in childhood, many of the personalities are childlike and some are preverbal (without language). Therefore, nonverbal media such as arts and crafts may be the best way to reach these personalities and encourage them to express themselves (11). Richert and Bergland (21) in a review of the literature stated that task-oriented groups seemed better suited for lower-functioning patients and verbal groups such as assertiveness training for higher-functioning patients.

The occupational therapist or assistant must be alert to which personality is currently present. The therapist's response will have to change when a different personality comes forward, as for example when the "normal adult" host personality gives way to a frightened child alter personality (8). Dawson (6) suggests that one approach to integrating different personalities is to get them to work together on a long-term task. Many other fascinating approaches have been considered and applied to the treatment of this rare condition. The assistant who encounters the multiple personality disorder patient in clinical practice is advised to obtain supervision and to consult the references listed at the end of this chapter.

ACQUIRED IMMUNE DEFICIENCY SYNDROME

Acquired immune deficiency syndrome (AIDS) is a complex medical condition involving the progressive destruction of the body's immune system and a consequent vulnerability to other diseases such as pneumonia and Kaposi's sarcoma, a form of cancer. The human immunodeficiency virus (HIV) that causes AIDS is transmitted through infected blood and bodily fluids, primarily through unprotected sexual contact and intravenously by infected needles. The material in this chapter will address the psychosocial aspects of AIDS. The physical aspects of AIDS are addressed in most OT textbooks on physical disabilities, and in several of the references listed at the end of this chapter. Information on universal precautions and infection control can be found in Chapter 9.

Patients with AIDS constitute a special population for several reasons. First, the risks of disease transmission to the immune-compromised and vulnerable patient, and of HIV infection to others, require scrupulous attention to infection control measures. Second, persons with AIDS or HIV infection must make an adjustment to the reality of the disease. For some this includes an admission to self of how their own actions (unsafe sex, IV drug use) exposed them to infection. For many, especially in the gay community, ongoing grief over the deaths of many friends and acquaintances compounds this. For all, it means adjusting to the prospect of diminishing function and the loss of valued roles, to physical deterioration, and to early death. Finally, many persons with AIDS suffer from dementia. AIDS-related dementia is similar to other dementias, often starting with mild signs such as forgetfulness and social withdrawal, and leading in time to physical withdrawal, motor paralysis, and total indifference and inability to communicate with others. Approaches to cognitive problems, including dementia, are covered in Chapters 11 and 22.

While the psychiatric symptoms of AIDS (depression and dementia) respond to the standard treatments (drugs, psychotherapy, environmental and activity modification) for these conditions, these patients require additional attention to the stress and disruption associated with the illness. Viewed from the model of human occupation, AIDS disrupts at all levels. Belief in self often diminishes, valued roles are lost over time, performance skills deteriorate, the sphere of interests shrinks, and the patient's world becomes much smaller. The social reaction of others who fear infection or who are repulsed by the patient's behavior accelerates this process. Persons infected with AIDS may lose their jobs or be denied health benefits. While legal remedies are available, the patient who faces the prospect of premature death has little reason to believe that the problem can be resolved in his lifetime.

Denton (6) proposed roles for occupational therapy intervention at three phases in the illness. At *Phase I* or *pre-AIDS,* intervention focuses on psychosocial support and education about disease transmission. The patient who is recently diagnosed as HIV-positive benefits from a supportive relationship that allows him to express his grief and anxiety and to develop coping strategies. Stress management and training in problem-solving skills is most effective at this point. Education in safe sex procedures and values clarification about responsibility to keep others safe from infection is crucial. The focus should be on helping the patient to maintain as normal a life as possible and to develop coping skills.

At *Phase 2* or *early to mid-stage disease,* the patient (who is now physically ill) requires environmental modifications, adaptive equipment, and other rehabilitation measures. Activities that promote a feeling of self-worth and of contributing to the social network may be valued by the patient at this time, according to Denton. Schindler (24) discusses the importance of helping the AIDS patient to continue to participate in valued roles, and to continue to present himself or herself as a useful and involved member of society. For example, a young woman who was physically wasted and also depressed needed assistance to purchase new clothing and to care for her appearance.

Another role for occupational therapy with patients at Phases 1 and 2 is the provision of health promotion activities. Gutterman (10) describes strong patient interest in topics such as skin care, nutrition, yoga, therapeutic touch, massage, and alternative holistic health modalities.

At *Phase 3* or *end-stage treatment,* the patient (who is approaching death) benefits from efforts to keep him involved in activities of interest to him. Expressive media may be helpful in engaging the patient to release and explore feelings. Piemme and Bolle (18) recommend that staff working with patients at this stage of illness prevent professional burnout by strategies such as weekly support groups, multidisciplinary meetings, and other activities that allow health care providers to discharge feelings with each other.

HOMELESS PERSONS

Homelessness is not a psychiatric condition. It is a social problem. We are considering the plight of homeless persons within this chapter because a large number of them are mentally ill. Many of those who are homeless would have been institutionalized 40 years ago. As discussed in Chapter 1, deinstitutionalization has achieved the goal of releasing psychiatric patients

from the inappropriately restrictive environment of the state mental hospital but without providing appropriate community supports. Immediately after deinstitutionalization, released mental patients moved into the least desirable community housing. With the real-estate boom and speculation of the 1970s and 1980s, much of this housing was destroyed to be replaced by more profitable, more expensive homes. Lacking both financial resources and cognitive skills, displaced patients were not able to find affordable housing. Thus, though "free," many patients are materially worse off in the community, where they lack shelter and structure.

Working with the homeless mentally ill patient presents many challenges. The fact that the patient has no stable, nurturing environment is a challenge that cannot be ignored or wished away. In addition, many of the homeless mentally ill are dual diagnosis patients, having both psychiatric and substance abuse diagnoses. In New York City, it is not unusual to encounter the homeless mentally ill Vietnam veteran who has diagnoses of personality disorder, post-traumatic stress disorder, HIV infection, and multiple substance abuse. Compounding the multiple diagnoses and the homelessness of these patients is the fact that many have serious physical conditions. Also, many are resistant to treatment, preferring life on the streets to unpredictable interventions by mental health providers. From the patient's point of view, he understands and has adjusted to street life. Getting involved with the mental health system may rob him of the niche he has carved out in the homeless community without providing him with anything better.

Pritchett[5] described her work as associate director of Project Reachout, a program for the mentally ill homeless on New York

---

[5]From an address by Judy Pritchett, OTR, for the Mental Health Special Interest Group of the Metropolitan New York Occupational Therapy Association, December 9, 1992. Ms. Pritchett may be contacted at Project Reachout, 593 Columbus Avenue, New York, NY 10024 (212-595-3066).

City's Upper West Side. Case managers in vans roam through Central Park, looking for likely candidates for the program. As these patients are notoriously difficult to engage, staff members approach in a manner that allows the patient to keep his distance. Through repeated contacts, and offers of sandwiches and other tangibles, the targeted individual is usually induced to speak with the staff. Once engaged, the patient is invited to the offices of Project Reachout. To get into a van with strangers, regardless of what they promise, requires a considerable leap of faith on the part of the patient, who may have previous experience of forced hospitalization. The staff member who made the original contact becomes the case manager for the patient, and provides food, coffee, clothing, showers, and aid in obtaining entitlements. Working on a personal contract with the patient, once trust has been established, the worker then introduces the need to take medication. The client must agree to this and follow through before the worker will make a referral to permanent shelter. Once a person has been placed in a shelter, a letter certifying ongoing participation in the Project is given each day as a condition of continuing to stay in the shelter.

As soon as the patient is brought to Project Reachout, interventions to help him change his lifestyle from homelessness to community living begin. Pritchett remarks that the change from homelessness to a home is "as disorienting as suffering a CVA, in terms of its effects on lifestyle." Patients are given clean clothing and are encouraged to save their dirty clothes and launder them weekly. A mock SRO (single room occupancy hotel) room in the center is used to demonstrate how a room in a shelter might be set up and used. A cooking group using communal facilities such as those found in SROs orients the patient to kitchen skills, and also teaches survival skills (that food left around will be stolen). Patients are taken on short shopping trips for food, clothing, and small appliances. Activity groups and training sessions around

grooming (haircuts, nail care, etc.) and safety (sex education, STD transmission, use of condoms) are provided.

Various structured leisure and expressive activities are included in the day program. In the early stages, more psychotic clients may remain outside the groups, using the offices of the project as a safe harbor and coffee shop. Pritchett believes that the success of outreach projects depends on tapping into the values of the clients, many of whom would like to work, to have a home, and to be a "regular person" with a social life and a family. Viewed from the model of human occupation, many of the mentally ill homeless have developed a work identity as entrepreneurs with a focus of panhandling, collecting and redeeming bottles, and other marginal but materially productive activities. To attract such clients, the outreach program must offer something that meets the same esteem needs. A work program in a church basement and a variety of "real world" jobs with stipends have been developed by Project Reachout. Even so, some patients find their prior homeless occupations more attractive than the substitute occupations offered by the Project.

As occupational therapists and assistants, our goal is to help the patient achieve and maintain the highest level of occupational functioning possible in his situation. Thus, we must be creative and compassionate and flexible in our understanding of the customs and culture of the homeless, and we must adapt our interventions so that the patient learns something that will actually be useful to him. A major role for occupational therapy with the homeless mentally ill is in helping them recognize and resolve problems of everyday living, such as obtaining and taking prescription medications, finding and caring for clothing, and managing money. In every case, the skills taught must be targeted to the situation experienced by the patient.

For example, problem-solving skills in how to obtain food and supervised activities on a day-by-day basis might be really important, whereas learning involved cooking techniques (that assume a well-equipped kitchen) would be irrelevant and might be seen as insensitive. Barth[6] described her work with a group of homeless substance abusers in a men's shelter in New York City. One activity especially valued by the group was the preparation (in the shelter kitchen) of simple food for an Alcoholics Anonymous meeting. The AA group, in which they previously felt inadequate, welcomed this contribution, and the result for the homeless men was an instant increase in status and recognition.

SUMMARY

This chapter has presented an introduction to some special populations that might be encountered by the certified occupational therapy assistant. We have considered substance abuse, eating disorders, multiple personality disorders, AIDS, and the homeless mentally ill. Effective intervention with each of these populations requires additional knowledge that can be found in the references listed. We recommend additional training and supervision by experienced professionals for those COTAs who wish to work intensively with these special populations.

REFERENCES

1. Alcoholics Anonymous World Services, Inc. *Twelve steps and twelve traditions*. 3rd ed. New York: Alcoholics Anonymous World Services, Inc; 1953.
2. American Psychiatric Association. *Diagnostic and statistical manual of mental disorders*. 3rd ed, revised. Washington, DC: American Psychiatric Association; 1987.
3. American Psychiatric Association. *Let's talk facts about substance abuse* (pamphlet). Washington, DC: American Psychiatric Association; 1988.
4. Bailey MK. Occupational therapy for patients with eating disorders. *Occup Ther Mental Health* 1986; 6(1):89–116.
5. Cassidy CL. Occupational therapy intervention in the treatment of alcoholics. *Occup Ther Mental Health* 1988; 8(2):17–26.
6. Dawson PL. Understanding and cooperation among alter and host personalities. *Am J Occup Ther* 1990; 44:994–997.
7. Denton R. AIDS: guidelines for occupational therapy intervention. *Am J Occup Ther* 1987; 41:427–432.
8. Fike ML. Considerations and techniques in the treatment of persons with multiple personality disorder. *Am J Occup Ther* 1990; 44:999–1007.
9. Gills GM, Allen ME. Occupational therapy in the rehabilitation of the patient with anorexia nervosa. *Occup Ther Mental Health* 1986; 6(1):47–66.
10. Gutterman L. A day treatment program for persons with AIDS. *Am J Occup Ther* 1990; 44:234–237.
11. Higdon JF. Expressive therapy in conjunction with psychotherapy in the treatment of persons with multiple personality disorder. *Am J Occup Ther* 1990; 44:991–993.
12. Mann WC, Talty P. Leisure activity profile measuring use of leisure time by persons with alcoholism. *Occup Ther Mental Health* 1990; 10(4):31–41.
13. McColl MA, Friedland J, Kerr A. When doing is not enough: the relationship between activity and effectiveness in anorexia nervosa. *Occup Ther Mental Health* 1986; 6(1):137–150.
14. McGee KT, McGee JP. Behavioral treatment of eating disorders. *Occup Ther Mental Health* 1986; 6(1):15–25.
15. Meyers SK. Occupational therapy treatment of an adult with an eating disorder: one woman's experience. *Occup Ther Mental Health* 1989; 9(1):33–47.
16. Moyers PA. An organizational framework for occupational therapy in the treatment of alcoholism. *Occup Ther Mental Health* 1988; 8(2):27–46.
17. Moyers PA. Treating the alcoholic's family. *Am Occup Ther Assoc Mental Health Special Interest Section Newsletter* 1990; 13(3):2–4.
18. Piemme JA, Bolle JL. Coping with grief in response to caring for persons with AIDS. *Am J Occup Ther* 1990; 44:266–269.
19. Raymond M. Life skills and substance abuse. *Am Occup Ther Assoc Mental Health Special Interest Newsletter* 1990; 13(3):1–2.
20. Richert GZ. Vocational transition in acute care psychiatry. *Occup Ther Mental Health* 1990; 10(4):43–61.
21. Richert GZ, Bergland C. Treatment choices: rehabilitation services used by patients with multiple personality disorders. *Am J Occup Ther* 1992; 46:634–638.
22. Rockwell LE. Frames of reference and modalities used by occupational therapists in the treatment of patients with eating disorders. *Occup Ther Mental Health* 1990; 10(2):47–63.
23. Roth D. Treatment of the hospitalized eating disorder patient. *Occup Ther Mental Health* 1986; 6(1):67–87.

---

[6]Personal communication by Tina Barth, OTR, of Health Related Consulting Services, New York.

24. Schindler VJ. Psychosocial occupational therapy intervention with AIDS patients. *Am J Occup Ther* 1988; 42:507–512.
25. Van Deusen J. Alcohol abuse and perceptual-motor dysfunction: the occupational therapist's role. *Am J Occup Ther* 1989; 43:384–390.
26. Viik MK, Watts JH, Madigan MJ, Bauer D. Preliminary validation of the assessment of occupational functioning with an alcoholic population. *Occup Ther Mental Health* 1990; 10(2):19–33.
27. Waltos DL. Historical perspectives and diagnostic considerations. *Occup Ther Mental Health* 1986; 6(1):1–13.
28. Yevtushenko Y. *People: selected poems*. Baltimore, Md: Penguin; 1962: 85.

ADDITIONAL REFERENCES AND SUGGESTED READINGS

General

American Psychiatric Association, Task Force on DSM-IV. *DSM-IV options book: work in progress.* Washington, DC: American Psychiatric Association; 1991.
Bonder BR. *Psychopathology and function.* Thorofare, NJ: SLACK; 1991.
Pacquette M, Neal MC, Rodemich C. *Psychiatric nursing diagnosis care plans for DSM-III-R.* Boston: Jones and Bartlett; 1991.
Perry S, Frances A, Clarkin J. *A DSM-III-R casebook of treatment selection.* New York: Brunner Mazel; 1990.
Spitzer RL, Gibbon M, Skodol AE, et al. *DSM-III-R case book.* Washington, DC: American Psychiatric Association; 1989.

Substance Abuse and Codependency

Adair J. The role of occupational therapy in the treatment of co-dependency. *OT Forum* June 21, 1991; VI(24):9–10.
Alcoholics Anonymous World Services, Inc. *Alcoholics anonymous.* 3rd ed. New York: Alcoholics Anonymous World Services, Inc; 1976.
Alcoholics Anonymous World Services, Inc. *Living sober.* 3rd ed. New York: Alcoholics Anonymous World Services, Inc; 1975.
American Occupational Therapy Association. *AOTA resource guide on substance abuse.* Rockville, Md: American Occupational Therapy Association; 1992.
Bean-Bayog M. Alcoholism as a cause of psychopathology. *Hosp Comm Psychiatry* 1988; 39:352–354.
Galantir M. Taking issue—treating substance abusers: why therapists fail. *Hosp Commun Psychiatry* 1986; 37:769.
Gangl ML. The effectiveness of an occupational therapy program for chemically dependent adolescents. *Occup Ther Mental Health* 1987; 7(2):67–88.
Henisse PA. The addicted patient—are we treating the problem or the symptom? *OT Forum* June 21, 1991; VI(24):12.
Herrington RE, Jacobson GR, Benzer DG, eds. *Alcohol and drug abuse handbook.* St Louis, Mo: Warren H Green; 1987.
Kasl CD. *Many roads, one journey: moving beyond the 12 steps.* New York: Harper; 1992.
Katz SJ, Liu AE. *The codependency conspiracy: how to break the recovery habit and take charge of your life.* New York: Warner Books; 1991.
Klein JM. Abstinence-oriented inpatient treatment of the substance abuser. *Occup Ther Mental Health* 1988; 8(2):47–59.
Klein JM, Miller SI. Three approaches to the treatment of drug addiction. *Hosp Comm Psychiatry* 1986; 37:1083–1085.
Lange BK. Ethnographic interview: an occupational therapy needs assessment tool for American Indian and Alaska Native alcoholics. *Occup Ther Mental Health* 1988; 8(2):61–80.
Scarth PP. Services for chemically dependent adolescents. *Am Occup Ther Assoc Mental Health Special Interest Section Newsletter* 1990; 13(3):7–8.
Schroff JT. The role of an OTR consultant in a medical detoxification unit. *OT Forum* March 20, 1992; VII(7):4–11.
Stensrud MK, Lushbough RS. The implementation of an occupational therapy program in an alcohol and drug dependency treatment center. *Occup Ther Mental Health* 1988; 8(2):1–15.

Eating Disorders

Alexander N. Characteristics and treatment of families with anorectic offspring. *Occup Ther Mental Health* 1986; 6(1):117–135.
Barris R. Occupational dysfunction and eating disorders: theory and approach to treatment. *Occup Ther Mental Health* 1986; 6(1):27–45.
Schlundt DG, Johnson WG. *Eating disorders: assessment and treatment.* Boston: Allyn and Bacon; 1990.

Multiple Personality Disorder

Angel SL. Toward becoming one self. *Am J Occup Ther* 1990; 44:1024–1027.
Baldwin LC. Child abuse as an antecedent of multiple personality disorder. *Am J Occup Ther* 1990; 44:978–983.
Braun BG. Multiple personality disorder: an overview. *Am J Occup Ther* 1990; 44:971–976.
Dawson PL. Understanding skepticism toward multiple personality disorder. *Am J Occup Ther* 1990; 44:1048–1049.
Fike ML. Clinical manifestations in persons with

multiple personality disorder. *Am J Occup Ther* 1990; 44:984–990.

Fike ML. Childhood sexual abuse and multiple personality disorder: emotional sequelae of caretakers. *Am J Occup Ther* 1990; 44:967–969.

Frye B. Art and multiple personality disorder: an expressive framework for occupational therapy. *Am J Occup Ther* 1990; 44:1013–1021.

Sachs RG. The sand tray technique in the treatment of patients with dissociative disorders: recommendations for occupational therapists. *Am J Occup Ther* 1990; 44:1045–1047.

Sepiol JM, Froelich J. Use of the role checklist with the patient with multiple personality disorder. *Am J Occup Ther* 1990; 44:1008–1012.

Skinner ST. Occupational therapy with patients with multiple personality disorder: personal reflections. *Am J Occup Ther* 1990; 44:1024–1027.

Skinner ST. Multiple personality disorder: occupational therapy intervention in acute care psychiatry. *Occup Ther Mental Health* 1987; 7(3):93–108.

Acquired Immune Deficiency Syndrome

American Occupational Therapy Association. Position paper: human immunodeficiency virus. *Am J Occup Ther* 1989; 43:803–804.

Anderson J, Hinojosa J, Bedell G, Kaplan MT. Occupational therapy for children with perinatal HIV infection. *Am J Occup Ther* 1990; 44:249–255.

Atchison BJ, Beard BJ, Lester LB. Occupational therapy personnel and AIDS: attitudes, knowledge, and fears. *Am J Occup Ther* 1990; 44:212–217.

Cornblatt MS, Ayres MJ, Kolodner EL. A legal perspective on AIDS. *Am J Occup Ther* 1990; 44:244–246.

Hansen RA. The ethics of caring for patients with HIV or AIDS. *Am J Occup Ther* 1990; 44:239–242.

Johnson JA, Pizzi M, eds. *Productive living strategies for people with AIDS.* Binghamton, NY: Haworth Press; 1990.

Marcil WM, Tigges KN. *The person with AIDS—a personal and professional perspective.* Thorofare, NJ: SLACK; 1992.

O'Rourke GC. Case report—the HIV-positive intravenous drug abuser. *Am J Occup Ther* 1990; 44:280–283.

Peloquin SM. AIDS: toward a compassionate response. *Am J Occup Ther* 1990; 44:271–278.

Perry SW, Markowitz J. Psychiatric interventions for AIDS-spectrum disorders. *Hosp Commun Psychiatry* 1986; 37:1001–1006.

Pizzi M. Challenge of treating AIDS patients includes helping them lead functional lives. *OT Week* August 18, 1988; 2(32):6–31.

Pizzi M. The model of human occupation and adults with HIV infection and AIDS. *Am J Occup Ther* 1990; 44:257–264.

Pizzi M. Nationally speaking—the transformation of HIV infection and AIDS in occupational therapy: beginning the conversation. *Am J Occup Ther* 1990; 44:199–203.

Pizzi M. Women, HIV infection and AIDS: tapestries of life, death, and empowerment. *Am J Occup Ther* 1992; 46:1021–1027.

Siwolop S, Ticer S, Rhein R, et al. The AIDS epidemic and business. *Business Week* March 23, 1987:122–132.

Sladyk K. Teaching safe sex practices to psychiatric patients. *Am J Occup Ther* 1990; 44:284–286.

Vincent TA, Schkade JK. Knowledge and attitudes of occupational therapy students regarding AIDS. *Am J Occup Ther* 1990; 44:205–210.

Weinstein BD. Assessing the impact of HIV disease. *Am J Occup Ther* 1990; 44:220–226.

Weinstein BD, De Neffe LS. Hemophilia, AIDS, and occupational therapy. *Am J Occup Ther* 1990; 44:228–232.

Homeless Persons

Cohen NL, ed. *Psychiatry takes to the streets.* New York: Guilford Press; 1990.

Lamb HR, Bachrach LL, Kass FI, eds. *Treating the homeless mentally ill.* Washington, DC: American Psychiatric Association; 1992.

RECOMMENDED RESOURCES

Alcoholics Anonymous General Services Office
475 Riverside Drive
New York, NY 10115

Cocaine Anonymous
1-800-347-8998

Hazelden Educational Materials
(for alcohol and drug abuse treatment and recovery)
Pleasant Valley Road
P.O. Box 176
Center City, MN 55012-0176
1-800-328-9000

Narcotics Anonymous
Greater New York Office
5790 Broadway
Bronx, NY 10463
1-212-601-6856

National Institute on Alcoholism
5600 Fishers Lane, Rm 10-05
Rockville, MD 20857
1-800-662-HELP

National Institute on Drug Abuse
5600 Fishers Lane, Rm 16-105
Rockville, MD 20857
1-800-662-HELP

PART 3

Interacting with Patients

10

Therapeutic Use of Self

Without the caring elements that ground the therapist-patient relationship and the dialogue that grounds collaborative treatment planning, occupational therapy would be reduced to a sterile science of occupation.

SUZANNE M. PELOQUIN (7)

Wanting to help other people is one reason why students choose to enter a field like occupational therapy. Although occupational therapists and assistants help people primarily by using activities, they also help them by the way they relate to them, by encouraging them to become more aware of their own abilities and more confident about using them. Relating to people is a skill used by all health professionals, and by lawyers, clergymen, and others whose work involves dealing with people. In all these fields, the ability to listen and to communicate is essential. Relating to patients requires even greater skill than relating to nonpatients. Psychiatric patients may not have had good experiences in the past relating to other people. They may be fearful and have trouble expressing themselves. The way we relate to patients, what we say and what we do not say, in words or in actions, affects them deeply, whether or not we are aware of it.

 Being aware of oneself and of the patient and being able to control what one communicates is called *therapeutic use of self.* It is different from other ways of relating to people, because the purpose of the relationship is different. The relationship between the patient and the health care worker is not an equal one. The patient expects that the health care worker, in this case the occupational therapy assistant, will be able to help him with his problems, to make him feel better; the assistant, on the other hand, expects to be able to help the patient. The purpose of their relationship is to help the patient identify problems he is having, to help him set reasonable goals, and to help him work toward their accomplishment.

To understand the special nature of the therapeutic relationship it is helpful to consider two important differences between that relationship and a relationship one might have with a friend. The first is that in a friendship each person expects something from the other. By contrast, in the therapeutic relationship, the patient expects to receive help and the therapist or assistant expects to give it, but neither expects the help to be returned. The second is that in a friendship both people are responsible for making sure the relationship is rewarding and mutually satisfying. In a therapeutic relationship, the therapist is responsible for developing and maintaining a good relationship with the patient.

Relating to patients effectively, like other skills, comes more easily to some people than to others. Fortunately, it *is* a skill, which like any other skill can be developed through effort and practice. Reading about it is only the beginning, for like riding a bicycle it can be mastered only with experience. Still, before attempting to relate to patients it is helpful to know something about what is expected. In this chapter we will examine the role that occupational therapy staff typically take toward patients, we will explore some of the qualities that patients find helpful in therapists, and we will discuss some techniques the occupational therapy assistant can use to relate to the patient effectively. We will also look at some of the reactions both the patient and the assistant may have to each other. Finally, we will consider some of the legal and moral aspects of the therapeutic relationship and discuss how to end a therapeutic relationship with a patient.

ROLES OF THE OCCUPATIONAL THERAPY ASSISTANT IN THE THERAPEUTIC RELATIONSHIP

Unlike other health professionals who help patients primarily by talking with them, occupational therapists and assistants help patients most often by doing things with them, and helping them do things by themselves. The occupational therapy assistant must take on a variety of special roles while at the same time involving patients in activities. These roles include those of instructor, coach, supervisor, role model, problem solver, environmental manager, and group member (1, 3, 8).

When teaching a patient to do an activity, the assistant is in the role of instructor. She analyzes what the patient needs to learn, what he already knows, his ability to learn, and how he learns best (demonstration, oral direction, etc.). She creates activities and materials that will help the patient experience what he needs to learn. She presents the instructions so that he can understand

them, she encourages him to practice, and she corrects errors as he makes them.

As coach she coaxes the patient, supports his efforts, and urges him to do even better. As supervisor she oversees his efforts, checks the quality of his work, monitors his progress, and supplies him with new tasks and new challenges.

We have already seen that people learn by imitating other people. Watching another person is a natural way to learn something new or difficult. Since patients do not always have the skill to serve as role models for each other, the occupational therapy assistant frequently takes on this responsibility. When serving as a role model, the assistant must not only identify what is to be learned but also be able to explain why. She must be able to make the patient believe that this new skill is important. Finally, she must demonstrate the appropriate skill or behavior and help the patient imitate it.

Occasionally, the occupational therapy assistant may be asked to model behaviors he does not already know and feel comfortable with. For example, an assistant who has little experience with or interest in group sports may be asked to run a volleyball game. If this happens, it might be better if she arranged with her supervisor for someone more experienced to lead the game and for her to learn by assisting the leader. In so doing she can also serve as a role model who is not afraid to try something new.

The assistant steps into the role of problem solver when she helps the patient identify problems and set goals for treatment. In this role she helps the patient understand the results of his evaluation. She helps him choose what he would like to work on first. She also explains why she is recommending a particular activity or method of doing an activity; this sets an example for problem solving that the patient can later imitate. She tries to involve the patient in the process of solving his own problems. This may require that she ask questions rather than state everything she knows; she may have already identified a solution to the problem but deliberately encourages the patient to solve the problem himself by withholding her solution until he has done so. The same approach can be used whenever problems arise during the course of an activity.

Whenever the assistant changes the nature of the task, the tools and materials involved, or the social or physical context in which the activity occurs, she is acting as environmental manager. She recognizes that the patient's ability to participate in and succeed at the activity is a function of the environment, and she observes the environment carefully to see what changes will help the patient perform better. In this role she also tries to instruct the patient about how the environment affects him, and how he might change it for himself. For example, the assistant may observe that the rock music playing in the background seems to distract the patient from what he is doing; she might select instead instrumental music with a slower tempo and softer sounds (e.g., classical guitar or electronic music). She would then urge the patient to consider how he feels and how he performs the activity with the two types of music.

Finally, when the assistant is running a group, she often must take on a variety of roles within the group; this is because patients do not always have the skills necessary to perform these roles themselves. For example, she may need to settle disputes between two group members if neither they nor the other members are able to do so. When she does this she is also modeling the appropriate behavior for this role, and should follow the guidelines for serving as a role model. Group roles and the role of the assistant as leader of a group will be discussed in detail in Chapter 17.

In summary, the occupational therapy assistant is required to assume many different roles when helping patients with activities, individually or in a group. Her success in treating patients will depend very much on her ability to recognize and step into whatever role is required for each situation. Regardless of the particular role, she, like other health professionals, should try to embody the therapeutic qualities that have been identified over the years as helpful to patients. As you read about these qualities, try to recall a wonderful relationship from your past, and try to identify specific events that illustrate them. A relative, family friend, counselor, or teacher who listened to you carefully and made you feel special probably demonstrated most of these qualities in your relationship.

THERAPEUTIC QUALITIES

Empathy

Empathy is the ability to understand how the other person feels. The occupational therapy assistant should not only try to see the world from the patient's point of view, but should also get this across to the patient. Listening to what the patient says and encouraging him to say more about it helps the assistant understand how the patient feels. When the patient believes that the therapist truly understands his point of view, he is likely to communicate more and work harder in therapy.

Sensitivity

In the therapeutic relationship, sensitivity is an alertness to the patient's needs and an awareness of your effect on him. The effective therapist is acutely attuned to the patient's behavior, especially his nonverbal behavior. A patient's body language and other nonverbal behaviors often give a more accurate picture of her true feelings than do the words she uses. For example, the occupational therapy assistant might suspect that the patient who says she is looking forward to being discharged really feels otherwise if she bites her lip and looks at the floor. These behaviors convey anxiety and depression. By recognizing this, the assistant can give the patient the opportunity to discuss her true feelings. If she had taken the patient at her word, this might not have happened.

Respect

The patient needs to be recognized as a unique individual, with interests and values of his own, which may be quite different from those of the occupational therapy assistant. A male patient may not, for example, think it particularly important to learn how to cook. Perhaps in his culture cooking is seen as "woman's work," or maybe his wife or mother does this for him and he has no interest in it or desire to do it for himself. The assistant should help this patient select a more meaningful activity unless he really needs to learn to cook in order to, for example, live on his own.

Different cultures have different expectations for what should happen between a patient and a mental health worker. To illustrate, an Asian patient who has not really been assimilated into American culture may be very confused at being asked to participate in planning his own treatment. Because his culture emphasizes authority, he will expect the health professional to have the answers (6). Similarly, some older Hispanic women may not understand the health professional's recommendation that they assert themselves and ask their husbands to take on more responsibility, since in their culture the woman's role is to support and nurture the man, regardless of how little he does in return (4). To engage patients from different cultures, the assistant will need to understand and appreciate the values and traditions to which the patient is accustomed. This means that every time she encounters a patient from a different culture, the assistant has to educate herself in what that culture expects.

Warmth

Warmth is the sense of friendliness, interest, and enthusiasm the therapist conveys. It is shown by smiling, eye contact, leaning forward, touching, and other nonverbal behaviors. All of these should be used selectively, depending upon the situation and the patient's ability to tolerate the therapist's warmth. Some patients are very uncomfortable about being touched, and the therapist must be sensitive to this. The way the therapist displays warmth must vary with the situation; smiling is appropriate when praising a patient's efforts, but not when listening to a tearful recitation of his problems, or when confronting him when he breaks the rules of the group. In the latter two situations, the therapist's warmth is conveyed through eye contact, body position, and tone of voice.

Genuineness

Genuineness is the ability to openly be oneself in a situation. To do this the therapist must first be aware of himself and be comfortable with who he is. The therapist who has mastered this is able to say and do what he really means; his verbal and nonverbal messages say the same thing. He is not afraid of making mistakes or not knowing the answer to every question and is willing to admit it. He does not need to distance himself from patients with an artificially professional role; he finds it easy to be in the role of therapist without being phony or defensive.

Self-Disclosure

Self-disclosure is the practice of revealing things about oneself. In a therapeutic relationship the patient is asked to unveil many private facts and feelings. Indeed, he may be required to reveal so much that he at times feels like a specimen under a microscope. By letting the patient know some facts about herself the occupational therapy assistant evens the score a little, and makes the relationship seem more equal. It is important, however, that the assistant reveal only as much as is needed to make the patient more comfortable. Timing is very important; self-disclosure is most helpful when the patient has asked for it (verbally or nonverbally) and very detrimental when it interrupts the patient in the midst of expressing himself. Also, patients from some cultures may see therapist self-disclosure as unprofessional and offensive.

In addition, it is important to know what *not* to disclose to a patient. These include details about one's personal life such as one's address and phone number. Unfortunately some patients may want to seek out staff after they are discharged, and this can be difficult and sometimes dangerous for the staff member and her family. Finally, whatever is disclosed should be for the patient's benefit; the assistant should never burden the patient with her own problems.

Specificity

Specificity is the art of stating things simply, directly, and concretely, focusing only on what is relevant. The effective therapist points out what is happening without labeling it or turning it into an abstract principle or a value judgment. For example, she says, "When you walk away while I am talking to you I get the feeling you don't want to hear what I have to say," rather than "You're being hostile." When giving directions, she states them in language simple enough to be understood. For instance, she tells the patient to find the center of the block of wood by "drawing lines across from corner to corner," rather than by "finding where the hypotenuses of the right angles meet."

Similarly, when helping a patient understand what is happening during an activity, the therapist should identify relevant details and help the patient see them. For example, when the patient makes a mistake and becomes upset and wants to quit the activity, the therapist should help him see exactly what he needs to do to correct his error.

Immediacy

Immediacy is the practice of giving feedback right after the event to which it relates. Patients benefit from learning about their successes and their mistakes while they are happening, rather than later when they or the therapist may have forgotten important details. Immediacy also includes the idea of focusing the patient's attention on the here and now. Patients sometimes become preoccupied with things over which they have no control, like what they will do if they win the lottery, or what Dr. Jones said to one of the nurses. The more someone is allowed to do this, the less able he will be to make real-life decisions and carry them out. These patients need to become involved in something that is really happening.

To sum up, the occupational therapy assistant should try to cultivate the therapeutic qualities discussed above. This is a lifelong project; these qualities cannot be developed overnight. Once developed, they need constant nurturing, evaluation, and refinement. Research studies have documented that, regardless of the health professional's training or theoretical orientation, patients get better sooner, and with more lasting results, when they are treated by health professionals who possess these traits.

TECHNIQUES FOR RELATING TO PATIENTS

1. *When trying to develop a relationship with a new patient, try to make the first*

contacts brief. Introduce yourself, explain your purpose for getting to know the patient, briefly describe what the patient might gain from occupational therapy, and set a time for your next meeting. If you place yourself for a moment in the patient's position, you will understand why she might feel overwhelmed by meeting so many new people at one time, all of them eager to ask her questions. Instead, promote trust by orienting the patient to occupational therapy and providing her with a schedule for the first few days.

2. *Use language that conveys what you mean and that will accomplish your purpose.* When attempting to get a patient to explore his feelings or to give general information about himself, open questions should be used. Remember that an open question asks for an answer longer than a few words. For example, "What have you been doing today?" is likely to produce a lengthier reply than "Did you go to the exercise group?" On the other hand, a closed question, of which the latter is an example, is more useful when you really want to know something specific, like whether the patient has finally gone to the exercise group that she has been avoiding.

Similarly, avoid suggesting that a choice exists when there really is none. If occupational therapy is a required activity for all patients, asking "Would you like to come to occupational therapy now?" risks angering the patient once he learns he has to come after all. Instead, say "It's time for occupational therapy. We will be meeting in the day room." This gives the patient time to collect his thoughts and get ready for the group, but also makes clear that he is expected to attend.

3. *Be comfortable with occasional silences, your own and the patient's.* Everyone needs time to collect his thoughts, and patients may need more time because their thinking is slowed by the disease process or the drugs they are receiving. While you are waiting for the patient to answer, observe his nonverbal behavior to determine whether he is confused by the question, has not heard it, or is merely trying to compose his answer. In any case, avoid showing that you are impatient or in a hurry by tapping your feet or looking at your watch or the door.

4. *Use minimal responses such as "Go on" or "Uh-huh" to show that you have been listening and to encourage the patient to keep talking.* At times patients may find it hard to express themselves, or to believe that you are really interested, and encouragement is essential. Remember that minimal responses can also be nonverbal, such as leaning forward or making eye contact.

5. *Actively listen to what the patient is communicating.* Pay attention to nonverbal clues as well as to the words used. Verbalize what you see. If the patient is twirling her hair and tapping her nails on the tabletop, state this: "I notice you're tapping your nails and twirling your hair." This allows the patient to say that she "always does that when I'm nervous," and thus helps her interpret and understand her own behavior. Saying to the patient, "You seem nervous," makes the therapist seem the authority and the patient a laboratory specimen.

6. *Try to get the patient to focus on one thing at a time.* Patients may have trouble concentrating and may skip from topic to topic or gloss over something painful to avoid dealing with it. By saying, "I'd like to go back to what you said about banks making you angry because I think it might have something to do with the problem you said you have sticking to a budget," the therapist opens an important topic for a more thorough discussion. Some patients may resist this at first or be too anxious to stay on the topic; if so, the therapist should drop the subject and try to bring it up at another time.

7. *Ask for clarification when you do not understand something the patient has said or done.* Since your purpose is to get the patient to explain further, your request should be phrased so as not to put the

patient on the defensive. For example, "Would you repeat that? I didn't hear it" is much easier for the patient to take than "You really have to talk louder if you expect me to answer you." Likewise, when commenting on something a patient has done in an activity, it is better to say, "You've glued the pictures so that they face in different directions. I'm not sure that I see why. Can you tell me about it?" than "Why did you do that?"

8. *Promise only what you can deliver.* Patients will take any staff member at his word when he promises something, and will be hurt if the promise is not kept. Occupational therapy assistants, like other staff, are often so busy that they forget or run out of time to do things they meant to do. The artful therapist will leave herself a way out by saying, for example, "I'll try to bring you some purple yarn this afternoon, if I get out of the meeting in time." If she finds that she is unable to do something she has promised, the therapist should go to the patient and briefly explain why, indicating if and when she *will* be able to do it: for example, "I can't find the purple yarn but I'll ask my supervisor about it tomorrow morning and let you know."

ISSUES THAT ARISE IN THERAPEUTIC RELATIONSHIPS

In certain respects, relationships between patients and staff are no different from other human relationships. Human beings bring to their associations with each other an array of past experiences, emotions, and predispositions. To pretend otherwise is silly. By familiarizing himself with the most common emotional issues, the occupational therapy assistant will be more prepared to deal with them when they arise.

Transference and Countertransference

Transference occurs whenever one person (usually the patient) unconsciously relates to the other (usually the therapist) as if that person were someone else. Usually the "someone else" is an important person in the patient's life. For example, the patient may begin to act as though the therapist were her older brother, who always took care of her and mediated her conflicts with her friends.

Countertransference occurs when the other person (usually the therapist) unconsciously falls into the role the first person has transferred onto him. In the example discussed, if the therapist began to do special favors for the patient and step into her quarrels with her peers, this would be countertransference. It would be easy for the therapist to fall into this role unconsciously if he had a younger relative or friend for whom he had played this role in the past.

It is crucial to recognize that transference and countertransference occur on an unconscious level; this makes them very difficult to deal with. If patient and therapist continue to act out the roles prescribed by the transference, the patient will not learn that there are other ways of relating to people who remind her of her brother. The relationship with this therapist will not benefit the patient. If, on the other hand, the therapist can recognize what is going on he can observe the patient's transference to find out more about how the patient expects other people to act. Once he learns, for example, that one of the things she expects from males is to defend her in conflicts with others, he can bring this up for discussion. He can also, by refraining from entering into conflicts between the patient and her peers, help her to explore other ways of relating to people, and help her learn to solve problems and conflicts by herself.

There are two ways to identify when a transference is happening. The first is to observe your own behavior and study how you relate to patients, especially noting if you relate differently to different patients. The second is to learn from your supervisor and other staff, who have more objectivity because they are not involved in the immediate situation. Students, beginning therapists and assistants, and even experienced staff are sometimes amazed to learn that they have gotten involved in the countertransferential relationship with a patient. Certainly there is no reason to be surprised, and even less reason to be ashamed, to find out that you have become enmeshed in a patient's transference. The patterns and feelings we have developed over many years of dealing with our families and others close to us are so much a part of us that it is natural for them to be set in motion by patients who remind us of important people from our pasts.

Dependence

It is quite common for patients to depend on staff members, whom they perceive as having more knowledge, skill, and power than they do themselves. The degree to which patients are allowed or encouraged to depend on staff needs to be carefully monitored if the patient is ever to learn to depend on himself. Purtilo (5) differentiates three types of dependence, only two of which belong in the therapeutic relationship.

Detrimental dependence is excessive dependence by the patient on the health professional. In other words, the patient is capable of doing more on his own and for himself, but he and the therapist have become entangled in a relationship in which she does these things for him. Detrimental dependence undermines the therapeutic relationship, the purpose of which is to help the patient identify and work on his problems.

Constructive dependence is a more productive kind of dependence, in which the patient relies on the health professional to provide something that the patient cannot provide for himself. For example, a patient with poor daily living skills may need the therapist to tell him whether or not his clothing is appropriate for a given occasion, such as a party or a job interview.

Self-dependence is the person's ability to depend on himself, to identify and solve his own problems. It is synonymous with independence. Some patients will have trouble seeing their own abilities and strengths, and may believe they need more assistance from the therapist than perhaps they really do. Other patients may have an exaggerated view of their own capacities or may be afraid of depending on another person, and for this reason may not ask for help or may decline assistance when it is offered. The occupational therapy assistant should help patients become aware of the extent of their abilities and encourage them to rely on their own resources whenever they can and to ask for help when they cannot.

Helplessness, Anger, and Depression

Students entering fields such as occupational therapy may fantasize that they will "save the world" by making a big difference in the lives of their patients. However, when they finally begin to work with them they not infrequently learn that some patients served by occupational therapy are so severely disabled that no amount of intervention will really improve their ability to function. Instead, such patients need large amounts of time and attention from staff merely to maintain the few skills they already possess. In addition, patients may have unrealistic hopes and expectations that occupational therapy will help them accomplish things that are simply beyond their capacity.

Both patients and therapists occasionally feel helpless, frustrated, and angry about this. The patient may feel that the occupational therapy assistant is not doing enough for him. The assistant may feel that she is doing all she can, but that what she does is not good enough. If these feelings are allowed to fester they become open sores that drain the very life out of the treatment relationship. Rather than getting angry at the patient or feeling bad about herself, the assistant should take some positive steps to understand and change the situation. One way is to share her feelings with other staff; more experienced staff are likely to have a perspective that the student or new therapist does not; on the other hand, a fellow student or junior staff member may be in the midst of a similar crisis and have lots to share herself. Another way is to get involved with a support group in the local occupational therapy association.

A third way is to enter therapy or counseling. This is the traditional way for new therapists to learn more about themselves, release and deal with the troublesome feelings patients can arouse, and learn about the therapeutic relationship first hand, from the patient's point of view.

Sexual Feelings

It is quite common for patients to develop sexual feelings toward staff. They may confuse the closeness and warmth of a therapeutic relationship with the intimacy of a sexual one. Dealing with the patient's subtle or not-so-subtle expressions of his sexual needs can be very difficult for students and beginning therapists. The therapist may need to explain firmly but warmly that it is not appropriate for her to become sexually involved with a patient. She can explain that she cannot help him work on his problems if she becomes sexually or emotionally involved. If the patient resists this reasoning, she can always fall back on the excuse that "it's hospital policy."

Dating patients is never a good idea, even after they are discharged. Consider a situation in which a student from a distant state became sexually involved with a patient with a spinal cord injury during a physical disabilities internship. The patient fell into a deep depression, refused to attend occupational or physical therapy, and developed a lingering respiratory infection when the student ended her field work and returned home.

There are several lessons to be learned from this example. One is that therapists need to be aware of their own needs when they are working with patients. In studies of therapists who became sexually involved with patients, about 90 percent admitted to feeling vulnerable, needy, or lonely at the time (2). It can be tempting to get involved with a patient who seems attractive, especially when one's current social life is not particularly satisfying or is perhaps nonexistent. Being away from home, friends, and family may have made the student more vulnerable to becoming involved.

The second lesson is that sexual relationships with patients can result in very unpleasant consequences for the student or therapist. In this situation, the student was abruptly terminated from her fieldwork. A working therapist would probably have been fired or severely disciplined. There are sound reasons for being extra cautious with psychiatric patients; every year there are accounts (although rare) of mental health workers being murdered or harmed by patients they have become too closely involved with.

The third and most important lesson is that no matter how much fun the relationship was at the time, in the end the patient suffered. Causing unnecessary pain to a patient violates his rights, betrays the occupational therapy code of ethics, and places the student and the facility at risk for a malpractice lawsuit.

Fear and Revulsion

Contact with some psychiatric patients can bring up extremely difficult feelings of fear and revulsion or contempt. One fear arises from the risk of contagion, from patients who have potentially communicable diseases such as HIV infection and tuberculosis. Any fear of catching a disease from a patient should be discussed with one's supervisor. Application of universal precautions against infection (see Chapter 12) is necessary to protect both patients and staff. However, the fear may still remain. The best way to become more comfortable is to learn all there is to know about the routes of transmission of the disease in question.

Another kind of fear is the fear of the unknown, the unfamiliar, and the different. Again, education and information about differences, be they in cultural practices or sexual preference, can bring the therapist or assistant closer to understanding the patient's view of the world.

One may naturally feel repulsed by a patient who has committed an act of violence against another person. Sometimes, one may feel distanced even from the patient who has experienced a violent act. When patients confront us with scary experiences, it is natural to want to avoid the feelings they evoke. An honest talk with a supervisor or with another professional who works closely with the patient will help the beginning therapist understand these feelings and develop strategies to keep them from contaminating the therapeutic relationship.

ETHICS

A code of ethics is a set of moral principles that guide the practice of a profession. It consists of rules and guidelines about what is considered proper conduct for the professional in his relationship with the general public and with the person receiving his services. In occupational therapy the patient is the person to whom the professional has the greatest obligation, one which is based on the trust implied by the patient's willingness to be placed under the occupational therapist or assistant's care. The specific obligations of occupational therapy staff toward the patients in their care include:

1. *Placing the patient's interests above one's own.* The patient always comes first.

In a fire or other emergency the patients should be helped to leave the building before staff see to their own welfare. Likewise, in less dramatic situations, the occupational therapy assistant should attend to the patient's needs even if this means she must defer her own. For example, helping a patient to the bathroom is more important than talking to another staff member or to a friend on the phone.

2. *Directing one's energies toward the accomplishment of the treatment goals.* Every encounter with a patient should be related to that patient's problems and goals. An evaluation should be performed and a treatment plan developed and documented as soon as possible, so that the patient can be made aware of the purpose and direction of his treatment.

3. *Respecting the patient's rights, including his right to refuse treatment.* The right to refuse treatment is based on the individual's right to determine what is best for his own welfare as written in the U.S. Constitution. A patient can be forced to accept treatment against his will only if he has been involuntarily admitted to the hospital or declared legally incompetent. Treatment in each of these situations requires a special court order which must be renewed periodically. Patients also have a right to receive treatment regardless of their race, creed, or origin, or the personal likes or dislikes of the occupational therapy assistant.

4. *Respecting the confidentiality of the therapeutic relationship.* The patient has the right to expect that information about his condition, his personal life, and his treatment will be given only to those directly concerned with his care. It is *never* appropriate to share this information with anyone outside the treatment facility. In practical terms, this means that any notes or copies of hospital records should have the patient's name and address (and those of his family and friends) removed completely before they are shared with teachers or classmates. Similarly, one should refrain from talking about patients, even to another

professional, in public places like the bus or the cafeteria.

Students and beginning therapists often wonder whether they should share secrets a patient has told them with other staff. Usually they should. Some exceptions are obvious—for example, if the patient is planning a party or a treat for a staff member. In general, however, the entire treatment team is charged with caring for the patient. By withholding information from other staff, the therapist is impairing the staff's ability to provide the patient with the best possible care. Reporting a patient's confidences is absolutely necessary when the patient threatens to harm himself or someone else; such threats should never be taken lightly.

5. *Safeguarding the patient's welfare while under your care.* Although this principle applies equally to all patients, special precautions are necessary when working with psychiatric patients, because they are more likely to harm themselves or others due to confusion, incoordination, impaired thinking, or inability to control their impulses. The occupational therapy assistant needs to be consistently alert to where her patients are and what they are doing. She must take care to account for tools, sharp objects, and other materials that could be used in a suicide attempt or an assault. She must make sure that confused patients do not become lost or hurt themselves accidentally. Safety procedures will be covered in detail in Chapter 12.

6. *Maintaining one's own competence to provide occupational therapy treatment.* The patient has every right to expect that the occupational therapy assistant will provide skillful treatment based on current knowledge in occupational therapy. Consequently, the occupational therapy assistant has an obligation to keep up to date on advances in his area of practice. In some states occupational therapy personnel must show evidence of continuing education courses to renew their state licenses or certificates.

7. *Safeguarding the patient from negligence, abuse, and substandard care.* Most malpractice suits involve situations in which the patient was harmed because a health professional failed to attend to his needs or caused him injury directly or indirectly. For example, the occupational therapy assistant could be sued if he was responsible for leading or co-leading an activity from which a patient escaped and later killed himself. Similarly, if a patient who was confused as a side effect of receiving electroconvulsive therapy cut himself on a power tool in the workshop, the staff member in charge would be held accountable.

A patient has the right to a reasonable standard of care. This does not necessarily mean the absolute latest in experimental medical technology, but rather the kind of care that is usual and considered adequate by most professionals in the field. The patient also has a right to receive treatment only from those who are qualified to give it. The occupational therapy assistant should know and follow her own job description, and should refuse to perform tasks for which she is not qualified or trained. Even when she is following orders the occupational therapy assistant is still legally responsible for her own actions.

TERMINATING THE THERAPEUTIC RELATIONSHIP

Saying goodbye is hard, especially when we have been close to someone. This is no less true of the therapeutic relationship; new therapists are often surprised not only by the strength of their patients' feelings, but by their own as well. Many different circumstances can bring an end to the relationship between patient and therapist—the patient's discharge, the patient's successful accomplishment of his treatment goals, a change of job or living situation for patient or therapist, or a recognition that the patient cannot benefit from further treatment. Ending a relationship can be uncomfortable and difficult, but ending it well can resolve unfinished issues and strengthen the patient's confidence to deal with the real demands and opportunities that his life holds.

The occupational therapy assistant can help the patient learn and grow during the termination process by using some simple techniques. One technique is to ask the patient to take some time to think about what he has gained from the treatment, and to have him talk about it. Another is to ask the patient how he is feeling about leaving, or about the therapist's leaving. If the patient is leaving a group, or the group itself is breaking up, the members should each be given time and encouragement to talk about their feelings, to express what they have gotten out of the group, and to say goodbye to each other.

Sometimes new therapists are concerned that saying goodbye takes too much valuable time away from other treatment activities or from the main business of a group. They need to recognize instead that terminating a treatment relationship deserves as much attention as beginning one. Termination is a potent opportunity to reinforce whatever gains have been made in treatment. In addition, it can help prepare the patient to deal with the natural losses and terminations that await him in the future.

To sum up, the relationship between the occupational therapy assistant and the patient strongly influences the way the patient sees himself and his abilities. At its best, the therapeutic relationship increases the patient's confidence and strengthens his will to try new things and become more fully himself. By being conscious of her feelings and the way she acts toward patients, and by taking the risk to learn and accept more about herself, the assistant can begin to understand and learn to master this complex and powerful treatment tool.

REFERENCES

1. Barris R, Kielhofner G, Watts JH. *Psychosocial occupational therapy—practice in a pluralistic arena.* Laurel, Md: RAMSCO; 1983.
2. Bouhoutos JC. Therapist-client sexual involvement: a challenge for mental health professionals and educators. *Am J Orthopsychiatry* 1985; 55:177–189.
3. Mosey AC. *Activities therapy.* New York: Raven Press; 1973.
4. Olarte SW, Massnik R. Benefits of long-term group therapy for disadvantaged Hispanic outpatients. *Hosp Commun Psychiatry* 1985; 36:1093–1097.
5. Purtilo R. *Health professional/patient interaction.* 3rd ed. Philadelphia: WB Saunders; 1984.
6. Taui P, Schultz GL. Failure of rapport: why psychotherapeutic engagement fails in the treatment of Asian clients. *Am J Orthopsychiatry* 1985; 55:561–569.
7. Peloquin SM. Sustaining the art of practice in occupational therapy. *Am J Occup Ther* 1989; 43:219–226.
8. Willson M. *Occupational therapy in long-term psychiatry.* Edinburgh: Churchill Livingstone; 1983.

ADDITIONAL REFERENCES AND SUGGESTED READINGS

American Occupational Therapy Association. Principles of occupational therapy ethics. *Am J Occup Ther* 1988; 42:795–796.
Bailey DS, Cooper SO, Bailey DR. *Therapeutic approaches to the mentally ill.* 2nd ed. Philadelphia: FA Davis; 1984.
Bruce MA, Christiansen CH. Advocacy in word as well as deed. *Am J Occup Ther* 1988; 42:189–191.
Burnett-Beaulieu S. Occupational therapy profession dropouts: escape from the grief process. *Occup Ther Mental Health* 1982; 2(2):45–55.
Cassidy JA. Access to health care: a clinician's opinion about an ethical issue. *Am J Occup Ther* 1988; 42:295–299.
Dillard M, et al. Culturally competent occupational therapy in a diversely populated mental health setting. *Am J Occup Ther* 1992; 46:721–726.
Fidler G, Fidler J. *Occupational therapy: a communication process in psychiatry.* New York: Macmillan; 1963.
Hays JS, Larson K. *Interacting with patients.* New York: Macmillan; 1963.
Herzberg SR. Client or patient: which term is more appropriate for use in occupational therapy? *Am J Occup Ther* 1990; 44:561–564.
King M, Novik L, Citrenbaum C. *Irresistible communication: creative skills for the health professional.* Philadelphia: WB Saunders; 1983.
Kyler-Hutchison P. Ethical reasoning and informed

consent in occupational therapy. *Am J Occup Ther* 1988; 42:283–287.

Maholick L, Turner D. Termination: that difficult farewell. In: Briggs AK, Agrin AR, eds. *Crossroads: a reader for psychosocial occupational therapy*. Rockville, Md: American Occupational Therapy Association; 1981. (Originally published in *Am J Psychother* 1979; 33.)

Neuhaus BE. Ethical considerations in clinical reasoning: the impact of technology and cost containment. *Am J Occup Ther* 1988; 42:288–294.

Peloquin SM. The patient-therapist relationship in occupational therapy: understanding visions and images. *Am J Occup Ther* 1990; 44:13–21.

Sabol PS. The contagion factor in depression. *Am Occup Ther Assoc Mental Health Special Interest Section Newsletter* 1985; 8(1):2–3.

Schindler VJ. Psychosocial occupational therapy intervention with AIDS patients. *Am J Occup Ther* 1988; 42:507–512.

Steich TJ. Malpractice and occupational therapy personnel. *Occup Ther News* 1985; 39(6):8.

Wolf S. Counseling: for better or for worse. In: Briggs AK, Agrin AR, eds. *Crossroads: a reader for psychosocial occupational therapy*. Bethesda, Md: American Occupational Therapy Association; 1981.

11

Responding to Symptoms and Behaviors

The staff members were very patient with me. I resented their intrusions and their restrictions, but, at the same time, I dimly recognized their actions as evidence of caring and support. Someone sat with me when I could concentrate on a project, such as an embroidery sampler, which I enjoyed although I was not allowed to keep the needle or scissors. I began to feel less like a prisoner because I was given some freedom and because the staff seemed to respect me and care about my getting well.

IRENE M. TURNER (22)

Imagine that you are entering a locked psychiatric ward to start your first occupational therapy fieldwork in psychosocial dysfunction.[1] A patient approaches you and asks you one question after another: "Who are you? What's your name? Are you the new patient? Are you a volunteer? Did you see the football game last night? Do you like football? I've got season tickets. Wanna go with me tonight?" At the same time, you can see two or three other patients standing and sitting around the halls, heads hanging, eyes downcast. Another is pacing the hall, touching and trying every doorknob. Meanwhile, your supervisor is right behind you, and while you are grateful for the support, you are also worried that you will say or do the wrong thing to the patients.

Do you feel that you could handle yourself in this situation? If you are like most

people when they first begin working with psychiatric patients, you would probably feel anxious and uncomfortable. At times it seems not only that you don't know what to do, but also you haven't the vaguest idea how to prepare yourself for this experience. You don't even know what questions to ask your supervisor. The purpose of this chapter is to give you a way of thinking about how patients act and about how best to respond to them. We will first examine why patients act the way they do, because this helps us understand how to approach them. Then we will discuss some responses you can make to them.

A FRAMEWORK OF CONCEPTS ABOUT SYMPTOMS

When patients say and do bizarre things, our first reaction may be to label them as "crazy." All we have accomplished by this is to protect ourselves, by saying that patients are somehow different from us, that the way they act is not the way normal peo-

---

[1]Much of the material in this chapter derives from Early MB. *T.A.R. introductory course workbook: occupational therapy—psychosocial dysfunction.* Long Island City, NY: La Guardia Community College.

ple act, that their actions make no sense, and that there is no way to understand them. However, if we step back from this reaction and examine the reasons behind it, we may see that we already know a great deal about why patients act as they do.

In most important ways patients are exactly like other people. All people have emotional needs, such as the need to belong and to be accepted by other people, the need to be loved and approved of by those around them, and the need to explore and master their environments. With most people we encounter it is usually pretty easy to understand what they want from us, and how to make them comfortable with us and with themselves. Patients with psychiatric problems are usually not so easy to understand, however. They still have basic needs to be loved and accepted, but the way they express these needs may cause other people to reject them. Other people cannot understand what they want; of course, they themselves do not always know. Consider the following dialogue:

> COTA (observing that patient is applying the modeling clay to the front, rather than the back of the copper tooling): Wait. It goes on the other side, like this . . . (demonstrates on sample she is holding).
> Patient (shouting): You don't know what you're doing. This is ridiculous. How can someone as incompetent as you help anyone get better? You're so out of it yourself that it's pathetic. Where's a supervisor? You ought to be fired. Out of my way! (storms off to a corner of the room and lights a cigarette).

What went wrong here? Why is the patient reacting this way? What is he feeling? What should the COTA do about it?

One possible interpretation of this patient's behavior is that he felt ashamed at not recognizing that he was doing the project incorrectly. After all, it looked like a simple project to him. He interpreted the COTA's comment as a criticism not just of his error but of his entire being. He had wanted to feel competent; that is why he chose such a simple project. He felt as

though he was falling apart, that there was nothing he could do right, not even a very simple thing like copper tooling. Indeed, it seemed to him that he was completely worthless, that he would never be able to leave the hospital and return to his family and his job. So he displaced all of his frustration with himself onto the COTA. He blamed her for his failure, because it was too painful for him to face. And all of this happened unconsciously; the patient's unconscious protected him from learning the awful truth—that he had made the mistake himself.

Do you see that in some ways his reaction seems perfectly natural? Yes, it might be "immature" or "hostile," but it is a reaction we can understand. We all use defense mechanisms to keep from facing facts that we find threatening. Perhaps you interpreted this patient's behavior differently. Many interpretations are possible. The point is that if we take the time and make the effort to grapple with what patients are really feeling and why, we can often see that their reactions make sense, that their behavior does not just come from nowhere, and that in many ways they are no different from us. This may be a scary idea to face. It raises questions about how sane we are and how safe we are from becoming "crazy."

Whereas some patients may become verbally abusive as this patient did, others may withdraw, and still others may become suspicious. Some may burst into tears and apologize for ruining the project. Such reactions, while understandable, are nonetheless extreme or peculiar. Behaviors like these are termed *symptoms,* because they show that some disease or abnormal state is present that is causing the patient to act this way. Symptoms are visible behaviors that show underlying problems.

To understand the role of symptoms in psychiatric disorders, it may be helpful to recall the concepts of object relations theory (Chapter 2). According to object relations theory, the ego mediates the conflicts between the id (needs and primitive drives), the superego (moral principles), and external reality (real life demands and obstacles). When the ego is not able to solve these conflicts, anxiety results. Anxiety is the most common symptom in psychiatric disorders and occurs in a wide range of diagnoses. Anxiety is a state of tension and uneasiness caused by conflicts that the ego is unable to resolve.

Other common symptoms, such as depression, withdrawal, and hostility are sometimes just the way the person deals with anxiety. It may be helpful to think of these symptoms as "maladaptive ego defenses" (see Table 2–1). In other words, the individual (consciously perhaps, but most often unconsciously) uses the symptom to reduce the anxiety she is experiencing. For example, a woman who is angry at her husband may develop migraine headaches; this lets her get back at him by making him take care of her without her having to express her anger directly.

Although symptoms are sometimes effective strategies for avoiding anxiety, they create other problems and may actually increase anxiety. A teenage girl who feels depressed and insecure about her social skills and appearance may withdraw from her peers, thus eliminating a potential source of anxiety. As she continues to withdraw, however, her peers may consider her less and less socially acceptable, thus making it harder for her to approach them, and thus increasing her anxiety.

Whatever symptom the patient displays, it can help us identify what the patient needs, and what she is compensating for by acting this way. For example, a patient who identifies with a staff member (copying her clothing and hair style or mannerisms) may be compensating for a feeling that she herself is really inadequate or inferior. Or a patient who makes excuses for (rationalizes) her own behavior may be having trouble accepting herself and her own responsibilities. And a patient who denies feelings or facts that are unpleasant may be protecting himself from these painful thoughts.

It must be remembered that the symptoms are not the disease. They are only the behavioral evidence of the disease. Most of the symptoms we will consider in this chapter occur in many different psychiatric disorders. The psychiatric disorder, or diagnosis, is a name given to a group of symptoms that commonly occur together. This is similar to the way a physical diagnosis is made. For example, the patient who has a fever, a cough, and red spots on his chest is diagnosed as having measles, because of the symptoms occurring together. Any one of these symptoms by itself, or combined with other symptoms, might have led to a different diagnosis.

When a psychiatrist evaluates a patient and assigns a diagnosis, she considers the person's history and his presenting symptoms. Although this is similar to the way a doctor might diagnose measles, there is an important difference. Our understanding of psychiatric disorders is not as advanced as that of physical disorders. Although a psychiatrist is able to describe how a patient is behaving, and can recognize important clues in his history, she is not always able to reach a diagnosis that another psychiatrist would agree with. Indeed, on the next admission, the psychiatrist may reevaluate her own diagnosis and assign a different one. It is not uncommon for a patient to have had different diagnoses on different admissions, especially to different hospitals. You may be wondering whether psychiatric diagnoses are of any use at all. Psychiatrists use diagnoses to select what drugs or other treatment they will use to help the patient.

For your purposes, as an occupational therapy assistant, you may find that the patient's diagnosis is *not* particularly helpful. Instead, you might find that the patient's symptoms give you more of a handle on the situation, because they give you clues about what the patient needs. Also, because symptoms impair functioning in predictable ways, they give you clues about where the patient might be having difficulty. After all, the purpose of occupational therapy is to help the patient be able to meet his needs and carry on his life's activities. By identifying the symptom and deciphering the underlying need, we take the first step toward helping the patient satisfy it.

Often, the particular symptoms displayed are more characteristic of the individual's personality than of the psychiatric diagnosis she has been given. To illustrate, a patient with a diagnosis of schizophrenia may show obsessive-compulsive behavior such as bizarre rituals (touching doorknobs) and obsessive tidiness. Those behaviors originate in the way she was brought up, and what her parents were like, and are not by themselves evidence of schizophrenia. Another person, also diagnosed with schizophrenia, might show a different symptom. For example, she might repeatedly assault others. Although everyone observing the patient can identify the symptom or behavior that is maladaptive, psychiatrists often have difficulty agreeing on *why* the patient has that particular symptom, and what the underlying process really is.

It is important to remember also that the patient is much more than the sum total of her presenting symptoms. Although much of her behavior may appear to be unreasonable or bizarre, she usually has some behaviors or qualities that are fairly healthy, which we can call assets. The patient may have the ability to do crossword puzzles or play basketball well, or may spontaneously help other patients when they have difficulty. A patient's assets are just as important as her symptoms. In fact, they are probably more important, since they can help the patient control and master her symptoms. For example, when a depressed, withdrawn patient helps another patient do a needlework stitch, she feels that she has done something useful. She may be able to stop thinking about her problems for a little while. If she is able to continue doing something at which she feels competent, she will feel more in control, more able to cope with her problems.

As you continue in your reading of this chapter, it is important to remember the concepts we have covered so far:

1. Symptoms are the behavioral evidence of underlying psychological or physiological problems.
2. Symptoms may be seen as an expression of unmet needs (e.g., for love and belongingness) or of unresolved conflicts.
3. Identifying the symptom and deciphering the underlying need can help in planning treatment to meet the need.
4. Symptoms are not diagnoses. The same symptom may occur in a variety of diagnoses.
5. Symptoms are sometimes more related to a patient's upbringing and underlying personality than to a particular diagnosis.
6. Activities selected for patients with symptoms should reflect the patient's assets, interests, occupational role, and present level of functioning.

RESPONSE VARIABLES

The occupational therapy assistant, faced with a patient who is behaving oddly and who seems very uncomfortable, has three tools at her disposal to help her manage the patient. We will call these tools *response variables,* because we can change them depending on the patient's needs. The three response variables are self, environment, and activity.

Self refers to the assistant's own personality, the way she talks and acts toward the patient. It is synonymous with therapeutic use of self. The way the assistant adapts her personality to meet the patient's needs will have a significant effect on how the patient perceives himself, occupational therapy, and the activity process. As specific symptoms are discussed, guidelines will be given for how to approach (modify your personality for) patients with those symptoms. These guidelines are merely suggestions; they should not be thought of as rules or demands for you to change your entire personality. In general, your relationships with all patients will depend on a warm, interested, and open-minded approach to them and to their needs. You must be comfortable with yourself and with your own behavior if you wish to reach out effectively to patients. Any modifications that you make in your own behavior must be ones that feel right to you.

To feel comfortable in a therapeutic role it is important not to make unrealistic demands on yourself. No one is perfect or perfectly in control of his responses at all times. You will put yourself in the best frame of mind for helping your patients by trying to do the best you can, and accepting the likelihood that you (like everyone else) will make mistakes.

The *environment* is the context in which your interaction with the patient takes place. It includes, for example, the presence or absence of other people, the general noise level, the amount of visual stimulation, the quality of the lighting, the arrangement of the furniture, the ventilation and temperature, and many other factors. Whereas some features of the environment may be beyond your control (e.g., central air conditioning, absence of windows), others may be changed to meet the needs of the patient. Sometimes the patient needs more stimulation, sometimes less. Sometimes the level of stimulation is good, but the type of stimulation needs changing. *Activity* is the thing that you and the patient are doing together. It can range from copper tooling, to writing a résumé, to organizing materials to prepare a meal, to looking at newspaper advertisements for apartments. The list is endless. In selecting activities it is important to consider the patient's interests, occupational roles, previous skills, and present level of functioning. At times familiar activities may offer security, in that they give the patient an opportunity to demonstrate that he can do something well. At other times, for example, when a patient is confused and disorganized, such activities can make her feel

worse, if she is unable to perform them or finds that she cannot do them as well as she had in the past. Finally, and most importantly, regardless of the patient's symptoms, the most effective activities are those that the patient has chosen himself, that mean something to him, and that support his occupational roles. The assistant should encourage patients to choose their own activities, even if the choice is only among two or three alternatives.

RESPONSE STRATEGIES

The rest of this chapter presents information to help you respond effectively to patients showing particular symptoms. For each symptom you will find the following information:

1. The definition of the symptom and a discussion of what it may mean for different patients (that is, what unmet needs it may be disguising).
2. The diagnosis (or diagnoses) in which the symptom commonly occurs.
3. A description of how to use the self therapeutically to help the patient feel more comfortable and function better.
4. A description of how the environment might be modified to meet the patient's needs.
5. The characteristics of suitable activities and recommended modifications in activities.
6. Examples of specific activities.

The ideas expressed here are culled from many sources throughout the history of occupational therapy; they will not work with every patient, and they should not be used mechanically. A word of caution: Do not think of these strategies as a "cookbook." We cannot approach every depressed patient in the same way, no matter what the guidelines say. Every patient is different and brings his own unique ingredients. Just as when preparing a meal it is wise to look in the refrigerator before looking in the cookbook, when working with patients it is important to see what they are bringing to the situation.

Anxiety

Definition

Anxiety is a state of tension and uneasiness caused by conflicts that the ego is unable to resolve.

Discussion

Anxiety is one of the most common symptoms seen in persons with psychiatric illness. It is normal for every person to experience some anxiety, particularly when faced with frightening, challenging, or unpredictable situations. The healthy person controls his anxiety through the unconscious operation of the various defense mechanisms (Table 2–1), the purpose of which is to prevent the person from experiencing consciously any unpleasant conflicts and the anxiety associated with them. To a certain degree, we can think of anxiety as a positive force. It motivates us to attempt new things; for example, your anxiety on first encountering a psychiatric patient may prod you to approach him and try to talk to him.

Although anxiety is experienced to some extent by all persons, normal and abnormal, it becomes pathological (causing illness) only when it is so extreme and so long-lasting that it interferes with effective functioning in daily life situations. Anxiety may occur alone, as the primary symptom, or other symptoms may accompany it. Sometimes it causes other symptoms, just as a fever causes other symptoms (malaise, chills, aches) in the body. For example, in the case of the patient discussed earlier in this chapter, we may conclude that he became angry and hostile because he was anxious about his perceived failure in copper tooling.

We can recognize when a patient is anxious by observing his body language and listening to what he says. Some patients worry aloud; they talk incessantly about things that may never happen. Others fidget: They tap their feet, pull their hair, tug at their faces, drum the tabletop, and pace the halls. Others may express fears about certain places or objects. They may be afraid to go outside or to use the toilet. Regardless of the behaviors through which the patient expresses his anxiety, the therapeutic objective is generally the same: to reduce the anxiety he is experiencing so that he can function.

Diagnoses in Which Anxiety Is a Common Symptom

As a symptom, anxiety may be found in almost every diagnostic category. The only recognized exception is in cases of social deviancy (antisocial personality). It was once believed that criminals, psychopaths, and other deviant individuals experience no anxiety at all. Current understanding, based on reports from such patients that they feel tense, is that they do feel uncomfortable because they know they are different from other people (2).

Strategy for Therapeutic Use of Self

Encourage the patient to talk about what is bothering her and to express how she feels. Answer the patient's questions, if you can, but avoid being drawn into extended discussions of physical symptoms and their possible causes. It helps to first focus on what the patient is concerned about, listen to her fears, and then gradually turn her attention to a neutral topic or something more constructive. For patients who express their anxiety through rituals, phobias, or constantly demanding attention, different responses are needed.

TABLE 11–1. *Flexible responses to anxious behaviors*

Behavior	Recommended Response
Ritualistic, compulsive: The patient carries out unnecessary and apparently meaningless actions, such as checking for dust on doorsills before crossing them.	Never criticize the patient's behavior. Instead, recognize that no matter how ridiculous the ritual may appear, it is one the patient uses to cope with anxiety. You can make the patient more comfortable if you can convince him that you accept him no matter what he does.
Phobic, fearful: The patient is afraid of things that other people do not find frightening (e.g., going shopping, riding in cars).	Encourage the patient to talk about her fears; help her focus on exactly what makes her afraid. This is especially important when the fear prevents her from accomplishing tasks needed in her occupational role (e.g., a homemaker needs to shop for food).
Intrusive-demanding: The patient constantly demands attention, or interrupts when you are working with others.	Reassure the patient that you will be available to help him. Give him a definite time and stick to it. Ignore subsequent interruptions but *do not* become angry with the patient.

Strategy for Modifying the Environment

In general, the environment should be calm, comfortable, and familiar. Anxious patients often become more anxious when overstimulated by too much noise or too many people. Because the treatment setting is different from what the patient is used to, he might be frightened or overly cautious. Giving him a brief tour of the occupational therapy area and a schedule for activities will help him feel more secure and in control.

Strategy for Selecting Activities

Choose activities that produce a successful result without excessive attention to detail. A project that the patient can work on for a while, then get up and move about, and come back to later is ideal. Some anxious patients respond well to activities involving a single motor sequence that is repeated (e.g., quick-point); they seem to use the regular pace of the activity to control and calm their own pace. Gross motor activities, involving either aerobic exercise or stretching/relaxation, can help to reduce the uncomfortable physical symptoms that go with anxiety (tense muscles, neck and back aches, racing pulse, etc.). Meditation, relaxation tapes, or biofeedback can also be used. Stress management techniques such as progressive relaxation, time management, and leisure skills may be helpful.

Examples of Appropriate Activities

Small woodworking kits; those with a small number of pieces (three) are best until you are certain the patient can handle more. An exception is the lobster basket,[2] in which many pieces are identical and assembly is obvious if a finished model is provided.

Simple cooking tasks; for example mak-

[2] Available from S&S Arts and Crafts, Colchester, Conn., and other vendors.

ing chocolate-chip cookies. There are lots of opportunities for the patient to move around while cleaning up or waiting for a batch to be done.

Yoga; this will need physician approval and should be taught by someone who knows the correct body dynamics and techniques. Alternatively, the patient can be helped to relax by taking a walk, raking leaves, or doing housework.

Depression

Definition

Depression is a feeling of intense sadness, despair, and hopelessness.

Discussion

Like anxiety, depression is something most people experience occasionally. Sadness is an appropriate response to painful losses, such as the death of a loved one, being fired from a job, or being rebuffed by a friend. Most people recover from these sad feelings and are able to carry on with their lives. Depression becomes pathological when it lasts longer than most people would consider reasonable and when it interferes with ordinary activities.

The depressed patient typically shows a cluster of symptoms, all related to the depression. The most striking is the depressed mood, often accompanied by crying or irritability. The depressed patient also tends to have a bleak view of himself and of the world in general, and to see the future as hopeless. He feels helpless and hopeless and may feel worthless and guilty. He usually loses interest in people and activities that previously brought him pleasure. The patient's statements in occupational therapy often betray his low opinion of himself: "I'm stupid," "Don't bother with me—the other patients need you more," "I can't even do this right." He is easily frustrated and tends to blame himself for whatever goes wrong.

Other associated symptoms, termed *vegetative signs,* include changes in activity level and biological functioning. Sleeping too much or not being able to sleep, losing one's appetite or overeating, neglect of personal hygiene and grooming, and diminished energy are common. The patient's movements and speech may be slowed down (psychomotor retardation) or speeded up (psychomotor agitation). His mental functions may be dulled; he may have trouble concentrating or making decisions and may be slow to respond to questions. He may be easily distracted and unable to attend long enough to complete simple grooming tasks.

Many theories have attempted to explain the causes of depression. Some neuroscientists believe that there is a genetic or biochemical element; for example, lowered levels of serotonin, a neurotransmitter (brain chemical) have been found in suicidal patients (10). Others believe that the loss of a parent (or similar serious loss) in early childhood may predispose certain individuals to depression in adulthood. Another theory is that the depressed person has a less developed sense of himself than other people do, and because of this he reacts strongly to even mild criticism and setbacks.

The cognitive therapists Ellis (6) and Beck (3) argue that people become depressed because they think illogical thoughts. For example, a woman who forgets to pick up her husband's shirts from the laundry may think this is just another example of her inadequacy as a wife, and may believe that her husband will divorce her or at least criticize her. Cognitive therapy attempts to help the patient identify her irrational negative beliefs and to substitute more logical and positive ideas.

Yet another theory argues that depression operates like the defense mechanisms, to protect the patient from feelings that he fears are even more painful. For example, the "anger turned inward" argument is that instead of becoming angry at the cause of the loss (the person who left, died, or rejected him) the patient turns the anger against himself. Because he unconsciously feels it is bad to be angry he punishes himself by being depressed. Nonetheless he may still feel guilty about being angry, and this contributes to his self-hatred and sense of worthlessness.

In still another theory, Seligman (19) suggests that depressed patients may have learned to feel helpless as a result of repeated failures in which nothing they did seemed to affect what happened. The depressed patient has learned that she cannot control her own life, and has decided to give up trying. She attempts to withdraw from other people, seeking to physically isolate herself by sitting alone, wandering off, or staying in bed all day. In this way she can retreat from a reality that she perceives as threatening, hostile, and unmanageable. The passive and negative behavior of the unemployed, the homeless, and the economically disadvantaged becomes quite understandable when viewed from this perspective.

Seligman concludes that activities in which the patient can experience success and self-control will relieve depression. Neville (18) notes that the volition subsystem is impaired in the depressed patient, as evidenced by a belief that one's life is not in one's control and that the future is hopeless. She, like Seligman, recommends that the depressed patient be exposed to experiences that reinforce his sense of responsibility and self-control.

Diagnoses in Which Depression Is a Common Symptom

Depression occurs in a wide range of disorders. It is the primary symptom in the affective disorders (affective means mood). Depression is common in organic mental disorders. It is frequently seen in schizophrenia, in almost all the personality disorders, and in patients with substance abuse.

As previously discussed, it is a normal response to personal loss, and so is often a symptom of the various adjustment reactions.

Strategy for Therapeutic Use of Self

It is extremely important to allow the patient to talk about what is bothering him; discussion should focus on exactly how he feels and why. The more awareness he develops about the causes of his depression, the more likely he will be able to do something about it. The assistant should listen and reflect back what she hears the patient saying, but should never agree that the situation seems hopeless. Instead, she should help the patient select realistic short-term goals and activities that he can realistically accomplish. She should reinforce good hygiene and grooming and not permit the patient to neglect his personal appearance.

The patient who is silent and withdrawn presents a special challenge. Often, this patient tries to discourage staff contact by becoming more withdrawn or becoming hostile and then fleeing. The assistant should not be tricked by these maneuvers into neglecting the patient. By approaching the patient many different times, each time for only a brief period, the assistant shows she accepts the patient's feelings. As the patient becomes more comfortable with her, he will eventually respond. For example, the assistant may visit the patient in his room and sit with him quietly, perhaps commenting occasionally about events from the news or things that have happened on the unit. After several visits, the patient may be willing to attempt a simple activity on a one-on-one basis. Later, group activities can be attempted while the one-on-one activity is continued.

In general, the therapist should match her tempo to that of the patient, whether the patient is slow-moving or agitated. The therapist should be quite clear in any directions she gives the patient, and avoid giving the patient more choices than he can handle. For example, it is better to present only two activity choices at first. The therapist should avoid praising what the patient accomplishes, and should rather acknowledge his efforts with a simple comment like, "It looks like you've finished that. Is there anything more you'd like to do with it?" The patient is usually quite aware of the difference between his present level of functioning and his past abilities, and excessive praise will make him feel that he must be in very bad shape. The assistant should accept whatever the patient is able to do at the moment, and not pressure him into doing more. It is not unusual for a depressed patient not to want to keep projects that he has made. Not infrequently the project is poorly executed and evidences the patient's low energy level and limited attention to detail. The occupational therapy assistant should accept the patient's decision to reject the project, and should refrain from commenting on it further.

Under no circumstances should the assistant change the subject when the patient talks about his bad feelings, or try to cheer him up. These approaches deny the importance of the patient's feelings and give him the message that the assistant does not accept him or want to deal with his real concerns.

Depressed patients who are receiving medication may be expected to show a decrease in depressive symptoms (symptom remission) within the first three weeks of treatment. At this time the patient may have more energy but still feel depressed, and there is a real risk of suicide; the risk is greater for patients who have previously attempted suicide. Some of the signs that a patient may be thinking of suicide include obvious ones like talking about it or wondering aloud what it would be like to be dead. Others that are less obvious are the appearance of feeling much better for no clear reason, and giving away personal possessions. For example, the patient might present the assistant with her camera or a piece of her own jewelry. Without rebuffing the patient, the assistant should try to get her to talk about why she is doing this. The assistant *must* notify medical staff (nurse, doctor, or primary therapist) if she suspects a patient is contemplating suicide. Otherwise she may hear in the Monday morning staff meeting that the patient threw herself off a roof during her weekend pass. If the patient is being seen on an outpatient basis, the assistant should contact the patient's primary therapist and her own supervisor so that a psychiatrist can evaluate whether the patient needs to be hospitalized.

Strategy for Modifying the Environment

The environment should be subdued. The more severe the depression, the less stimulation should be present. It may be necessary to reduce the lighting and the noise level, and work one-on-one in order to get the patient to focus on an activity. Too much stimulation may cause the patient to retreat further. This is particularly true for withdrawn patients who may not be able to tolerate the presence of others in a group. As the patient becomes more comfortable, the amount of stimulation should be increased gradually; having more materials, supplies, and sample projects visible will increase opportunities for decision making.

The atmosphere on an inpatient ward often restricts opportunities for patients to make choices about even simple things. For example, meals consist of whatever is served, at the time that the staff says is mealtime. Patients who are suicidal may not be permitted to wear their own clothing (so that staff will know not to let them on the elevator). Showering and shaving may be scheduled at the staff's convenience. This atmosphere can further damage the depressed patient's fragile sense of self-control. Therefore, choices should be presented whenever possible. Merely deciding to rearrange the furniture or hang up a picture can increase the patient's sense of responsibility.

Strategy for Selecting Activities

Start with simple, structured, short-term, familiar activities. Unstructured activities should be avoided because the patient will not be able to deal with the decision making needed. The activities must be short-term ones because the patient lacks the attention span for a longer activity and will be able to work only slowly and intermittently. For the same reason, activities that require rapid responses at particular moments (e.g., copper enameling, slip casting) should be avoided, unless a staff member or volunteer is available to assist the patient. Repetitive activities allow the patient to succeed with minimal new learning, since the motions are learned only once and then repeated. Although familiar activities are generally more comfortable, there is a risk that the patient will compare his present to his past performance, further damaging his self-esteem. Therefore, simple, unfamiliar activities are sometimes preferred, at least initially.

The first activities used should be ones at which the patient is guaranteed to succeed. Even a simple task like making a phone call or brushing one's hair can be a first step. Activities are then graded to include more complexity and require more effort as the patient becomes more confident and energetic.

In the beginning the activities should be ones that can be done alone, without the need to interact or share tools or materials with others. Thereafter, opportunities for minimal socialization should be presented as soon as the patient seems comfortable.

Patients who are agitated will benefit from activities in which they use their hands; this substitutes productive actions for nonproductive ones like handwringing and fidgeting.

People who are depressed may avoid crafts, games, and exercise because they seem too pleasurable or too demanding. The patient may be more able to accept an activity that is useful to other people rather than to himself. Staff should try to accept offers of help from depressed patients, in order to reinforce the patient's active choice. Some patients respond well to activities that are tedious, menial, and repetitive (peeling potatoes, mopping the floor); the patient may be using these activities to work off his feelings of guilt. Although the patient should be permitted to do these activities when he chooses, other activities should be introduced gradually.

Gross motor activities can help the patient release tension and promote the intake of oxygen and increased blood flow to the brain. There is ample evidence that this can relieve depression, but the real problem is motivating the patient to attempt it. The patient's low energy level is a serious obstacle, but can sometimes be overcome by simply telling the patient that it's time for the activity (e.g., "We are going to the gym now").

Precautions against suicide or self-abuse should be observed at all times. Although the depressed patient may feel more in control if he can use a sharp tool without harming himself, the assistant must stay alert to this possibility. Even seemingly innocuous objects can be used in a suicide attempt; for example, a depressed patient might use a leather belt or macramé project in an attempt at hanging. Tools and supplies should be accounted for at the beginning and end of every session involving depressed patients and before any patient leaves the room (even to go to the bathroom). Similarly, when working with patients outdoors or in open or unfamiliar settings, the assistant must keep track of where they are; depressed patients may elope and then harm themselves. These precautions apply to inpatient settings only, and would be modified in community settings.

For patients who are chronically depressed, activities that teach them how to manage stress and advocate for themselves are important. This would include leisure skills, assertiveness training, and role-oriented treatment focusing on the roles important to them. These experiences help patients to unlearn helplessness.

Examples of Appropriate Activities

Some simple, structured, short-term, familiar activities include housework, folding laundry, simple cooking, sanding, clerical tasks, and sewing. Obviously, the patient's previous interests and occupational roles will guide the assistant in selecting the particular activity.

Craft activities that may be less familiar but are still highly structured include mosaics, copper tooling, leatherwork, and woodworking. These must be graded down to a fairly simple, short-term level at first. Kits are useful, but the assistant should first attempt the kit herself, as many have one or two steps that are not obvious or that require dexterity or timing.

Gross motor activities include aerobic exercise, dance therapy, running, swimming, ball games, and walking (especially outdoors).

Mania

Definition

Mania is a disturbance of mood characterized by excessive happiness (euphoria), generosity (expansiveness), irritability, distractibility, and increased activity level.

Discussion

The manic individual appears to be operating at 78 rpm in a 33-rpm world. Everything is speeded up. The patient may be hyperactive or agitated. He may speak very rapidly (pressured speech) and skip from topic to topic (flight of ideas). He finds it hard to concentrate on any one thing, instead flitting from one to another; he is often involved in many different activities simultaneously. He may express an unrealistic view of his own abilities, believing that he can accomplish almost anything (grandiosity). He may get involved in very risky enterprises and endanger himself or his family by spending money frivolously, taking expensive trips, extorting money from others, and so on. He seems unaware of or indifferent to the consequences of such actions.

The manic patient typically has very poor judgment, which reveals itself in almost everything he attempts. His style of dress may be eccentric or downright bizarre. He may wear several hats or belts simultaneously or cover his clothing with emblems, buttons, or other decorations. The female manic often wears so much makeup that she looks like a tropical fish.

One of the most disturbing qualities of the manic individual is his attitude toward and effect on other people. He has a lot of energy and often flatters others and gives them gifts. Because of this an unsuspecting staff member can be drawn into a relationship in which he comes to need the manic patient to gratify his own self-esteem.

The manic is also very sensitive to others' vulnerabilities; for example, he may say that he cannot be helped by a certain staff member because that person just got out of school and does not have enough experience. If the staff member really feels insecure about this, the patient may be able to drive him away and to manipulate the self-esteem of other staff who feel superior because they have more experience. By relying on such maneuvers the patient may be able to get the staff fighting with each other, which then takes the pressure off him.

Another tactic used by manic patients is "upping the ante." The patient starts by making what seems like a reasonable request (e.g., to go out in the hall to smoke a cigarette). Once granted the request, the patient asks for something else, and then something else, until he finally makes a request that is completely unreasonable (e.g., to have everyone stop working and take a break). When the therapist refuses to grant the final request, the patient becomes angry and abusive, arguing that the therapist is uptight and rigid.

What purpose do these tactics serve? Why is the manic patient so ready to manipulate others? Some (15) argue that the manic patient is very ambivalent about his need to be taken care of. He needs other people but is simultaneously frightened of depending on them. So he arranges to control and manipulate them. When he finally exhausts their patience and they take control over his behavior, he has the satisfaction of being taken care of without having to ask for it.

Diagnosis in Which Mania Is a Common Symptom

Mania is the primary symptom of a manic episode in an affective disorder, but it can occur in other disorders as well. These include organic conditions caused by substance abuse, paranoid schizophrenia, and some personality disorders.

Strategy for Therapeutic Use of Self

The manic patient's ambivalence about relying on other people raises specific issues for the therapeutic relationship. It is easy to be manipulated by someone who makes you feel special, and the assistant should beware of flattery. Similarly, criticisms by the patient of other staff are often the opening gambit in a game of "You're the only one who can help me."

Manic patients may demand almost constant attention, praise, and approval from staff members. At the same time, their behavior (for which they are seeking approval) is often bizarre and so self-centered that others avoid them. The assistant should be cautious in giving any praise or approval to the manic patient, and should instead firmly and gently focus on how to make the behavior more appropriate. However, it is also essential to avoid criticizing the patient, who is very vulnerable and easily feels rejected. Some psychologists argue that mania is the "flip side" of depression. In other words, the low self-esteem and feelings of despair and hopelessness that characterize depression are often just under the surface of the manic's behavior.

It is important to be firm and consistent with the manic patient. Setting limits on what the patient can do, and enforcing them, shows the patient that *someone* is in control, even if he is not. The patient may also interpret limit setting as a message that the staff cares enough about him to stop him from hurting himself.

As the patient's medication begins to take effect and his symptoms diminish, he may become frightened when he remembers the bizarre and impulsive things he did when he was ill. Reassuring the patient that these behaviors were caused by his illness can make him feel more comfortable. It is important to recognize, though, that the patient may face legal or financial problems as a result of his actions during the manic phase.

Getting the manic patient to focus on just one activity is a challenge. She typically makes grandiose or unrealistic statements (e.g., "I'm very creative. I know weaving and beading and fashion design. I'm going to weave my own fabric and make a beaded evening gown.") The occupational therapy assistant should not go along with these schemes and should suggest other, more realistic activities. The assistant must set firm limits on the use of supplies and materials and not permit the patient to overrun the clinic.

The patient is likely to resist rules and expectations for performance, saying in effect, "My way is much more creative. Don't be a drag." It is important not to get emotionally involved in discussing why a project should be done a certain way; instead, firmly and briefly explain what needs to be done, and show the patient a sample. If the patient insists on doing it differently, there is no point in fighting about it as long as no one is endangered.

Because they are so distractible and have such poor judgment, manic patients should be carefully watched around electrical equipment and other objects that might accidentally cause injury.

Strategy for Modifying the Environment

Controlling the environment to help the manic patient function is based on a single principle: The manic patient will respond to every bit of stimulation present. Therefore, the assistant should eliminate or reduce distractions in the environment to the greatest possible extent. For example, an occupational therapy shop decorated with many finished projects and interesting materials will provoke intense interest in doing everything at once. To avoid this, the assistant should strip the environment of everything but what is essential to the activity. Tools and supplies needed for later steps in a project should be kept out of sight until such time as they are needed.

Remember that *anything* can distract the manic patient. Music, other people, the telephone, the view from the window can all invite the most intense curiosity and involvement. Distractions should be minimized. If possible, have the patient work alone, facing a blank wall.

Strategy for Selecting Activities

Because of the patient's high energy level, activities that permit her to get up and move around are ideal. Short-term activities provide immediate gratification to the patient with poor frustration tolerance

and inability to wait for results. Allen (1) recommends that craft activities be portable, since the patient is likely to carry projects around with her.

Activities should be structured and have three or fewer steps. Activities that are unfocused or creative or that require decisions (e.g., oil painting) should be avoided. Similarly, activities should not require fine coordination or attention to detail. Materials should be controllable, not floppy or unpredictable (e.g., leather or wood rather than clay).

Since the manic patient usually needs to develop a longer attention span, try to provide activities that involve carryover of skills from one day to the next. For example, whipstitch can be done on leather, and later as an embroidery stitch (fabric is floppier and therefore less controllable than leather).

Manic patients may benefit from gross motor exercise because it allows them to move around and use up excess energy. However, it is difficult for the assistant (or anyone) to deal with more than three or four patients in an exercise group if one is acutely manic; for larger groups more staff are needed.

Examples of Appropriate Activities

As with any other patient, it is best to let the manic patient choose his own activity, although the assistant should present only two or at most three choices. Ideas about what activities might be appropriate can be obtained from the patient's history or the evaluation.

Some crafts that might be used are copper tooling, stringing beads, and sanding and finishing prefabricated wooden projects. Some patients respond well to small leather projects (e.g., wristbands, coin purses with hardware already attached). The assistant may need to perform one or more of the steps for the patient, especially if they involve fine coordination (e.g., ending the lacing, applying a snap). Projects in which the patient's name can be part of the decoration appeal to some manic patients.

Some semistructured activities can be used with caution. For example, magazine picture collage will invite chaos unless it is structured; by providing only a few magazines and a pair of scissors at first, then supplying the backing paper after the pictures have been selected and cut out, and the glue only after the pictures have been arranged, the assistant will help the patient stay in control of what she is doing and obtain a better result.

As discussed, gross motor activities such as dance, exercise, and volleyball can help the manic patient work off energy and use his hyperactivity productively. Sometimes it is easier to work one-on-one in an exercise activity with the manic than in a group.

Hallucinations

Definition

A hallucination is a false sensory experience, one that has no basis in external reality. A person experiencing hallucinations may see, hear, feel, smell, or taste things that are not there. Some common hallucinations include hearing voices, seeing animals or people or lights, and feeling burning or crawling sensations on one's skin.

Discussion

It is commonly believed that hallucinations arise from a defect in the way the brain functions. It is as though a connection is loose or a circuit is overloaded. There is a malfunction in the part of the brain that interprets external sensation and that differentiates between what is really happening and what is imagined. Changes in several brain structures and imbalances in several brain chemicals have been suggested as the causes of hallucinations (17).

Auditory (sound) hallucinations occur most often. The patient may hear voices telling him to do things (command hallucinations) or criticizing him, or he may hear music or strange sounds or someone calling his name. He may perceive a sound as much louder or softer than it really is. Visual hallucinations are also common and may involve the patient's seeing walls move, or his face looking strange in the mirror, or people looking transparent or flat. Gustatory (taste) and olfactory (smell) hallucinations are less common, but are seen in patients with temporal lobe epilepsy; usually the hallucinated taste or smell is very unpleasant. Tactile hallucinations may be of itching or burning or a feeling that insects are crawling on or biting one's skin.

The patient usually finds the hallucinations troubling, frightening, and uncomfortable. It is not hard to understand the patient's reaction to voices saying awful, threatening things or spiders crawling over his clothes. However, if the hallucinations are of voices that praise the patient or tell him he has special powers, he may enjoy them. Similarly, hallucinations that enhance reality are usually perceived as very pleasant. For example, the patient may become transfixed by the glittering crystal patterns he sees in an ordinary city sidewalk or by the varied textures and colors on a brick wall. It has been suggested that some patients rely on their "voices" as a substitute for human relationships; this seems more likely when the voices tell the patient reassuring or flattering things.

Diagnosis in Which Hallucinations Are a Common Symptom

Hallucinations can occur in a wide range of psychiatric disorders and may be also present in any physical disorder with a high fever. Some of the psychiatric disorders include schizophrenia (see discussion of perceptual distortions in Chapter 3), manic and depressive psychoses, organic mental disorders, and substance abuse disorders.

In each of these conditions the type of hallucination may differ. For example, auditory hallucinations are common in schizophrenia; these hallucinations are frequently voices that comment on the patient's behavior, usually in an insulting way. In manic and depressive disorders auditory hallucinations may also be present, but they are *mood-congruent*. This means that the voices say things that are consistent with the patient's mood (e.g., telling the depressed patient that he is bad, to kill himself, etc.). In schizophrenia the hallucinations seem unrelated to the patient's mood.

Strategy for Therapeutic Use of Self

The assistant should try to reassure the patient and help her understand what is happening to her, saying for example, "I know that you see rats in the corners, but they are not really there. It's your disease that makes you see them."

Talking in a calm, rhythmic, soothing manner may comfort the patient. The assistant should point out any real sensory stimulus that the patient seems to misinterpret ("That sound was the central air conditioning coming on."). She should avoid sarcastic comments, no matter how tempting. For example, when the patient says he has visitors from another planet, the assistant should not say, "Oh, which one?"

At the same time, however, the assistant should refrain from arguing with the patient about whether or not the hallucinations are real. Instead, she should try to divert attention to some neutral topic or activity and try to draw the patient back to reality. She can acknowledge how the hallucination makes the patient feel without agreeing that it is real. Since it is impossible to know a patient's emotional reaction to a hallucination, the assistant should not assume that the patient feels any particular way about

it. However, patients who are hallucinating often react aversively to being touched by other people; therefore the patient should be given lots of room.

One report indicates that having the patient repeat a word or phrase that is comforting and positive may help reduce the length, frequency, and intrusiveness of hallucinations (17). For example, the patient might say to himself, "I am safe here," or "I have done the best I can and it is good enough."

Strategy for Modifying the Environment

Many patients who hallucinate do so when they are under stress, especially in environments that are too stimulating for them. Sometimes just moving the patient to a quieter, less overwhelming area will make the hallucinations diminish or go away altogether. Therefore, in general, the environment should be calm, quiet, and nondistracting.

However, such patients should not be permitted to isolate themselves from other people entirely, since hallucinations may increase in the absence of any other stimulation. In fact, associating with other people, and especially conversing them them, tends to block auditory hallucinations and focus the patient on reality. MacRae (17) reported that a patient successfully limited his hallucinations by going on a planned walk as soon as the voices began.

Strategy for Selecting Activities

Simple, highly structured activities that encourage involvement and interaction with a few other people are recommended. The structure prevents the patient from drifting away into his private world, and the presence of other people tends to focus him on reality. If possible, the activity should require some minimal interaction with others, if only to ask for a tool. The patient should not be permitted to work alone, apart from the group. Activities should not demand attention to detail or fine coordination since the patient may still be distracted occasionally by the hallucinations.

Some therapists advocate activities that strongly stimulate the senses. They argue that flooding the patient's auditory channels with music or a sing-along may block auditory hallucinations. Allen[3] has observed that hallucinating patients prefer to work with bright colors, and she believes these somehow interfere with the hallucinations. However, it is also apparent that *some* patients' hallucinations seem to get worse when other stimulation is increased, as if the hallucination is trying to compete for the patient's attention. The most accurate information about how a given activity affects a particular patient is obtained from the patient himself. By watching how the patient reacts and listening to what he says, the assistant can usually learn enough about the effects of the activity to determine whether it is working or how it needs to be changed.

Examples of Appropriate Activities

Simple, structured, short-term activities might include coloring "stained glass" (nonreligious) pictures, discussing specific current events, preparing lunch, and assembling wood kits. Familiar, necessary life tasks like doing laundry or housework can also be used where relevant to the patient's interests and occupational roles.

Activities with strong sensory stimulation include those involving music or dance, watching films or television, and cooking and eating. Falk-Kessler and Froschauer (7) described a group activity in which the patients watched and discussed soap operas with the staff. Since psychiat-

ric patients tend to watch many hours of television daily anyway, this seemed a way to control hallucinations and create a bridge from their imaginary worlds to reality.

Delusions

Definition

A delusion is a false belief, one that is contrary to reality as experienced by others in one's cultural group.

Discussion

A true delusion is a belief not based on reality. The patient may believe, for example, that television shows and newspaper stories have special messages for him, or that automobile license plates contain a secret code that he must decipher in order to save the world. These beliefs are called *ideas of reference*. Or a woman may believe that the FBI is taking thoughts out of her brain (*thought withdrawal*) or putting strange ones in (*thought insertion*). She may feel that she is being followed (*delusions of persecution*) or that she has special powers (*delusions of grandeur*).

A delusion is a false belief that is peculiar to the individual. It is different, then, from a cultural belief, which although odd may be embraced by an entire nation or ethnic group. For example, people in some Caribbean countries believe that pulling on an infant's limbs when he is bathed will make him taller, stronger, and more coordinated when he grows up. As another example, Australian aborigines believe that the "real" world that we experience while awake is less powerful and in a sense less real than the "dream world" of sleep and drugged states.

Students often find it hard to remember the difference between a delusion and a hallucination. A delusion is an inaccurate thought or idea. By contrast, a hallucination is a false perception, sensory experi-

---

[3]Allen CK. "Cognitive Disabilities: Part One—Measurement and Management." Workshop given by Advanced Rehabilitation Institutes, New York, 1985.

ence, or feeling. A patient does not have to hear or see something that is not there in order to have a delusional idea; he can base his delusion on events that are really happening. It is just that his interpretation of these events is odd. For example, he may think that the newscaster on television who looks him right in the eye while summarizing a story knows all about him and is giving him a special message. What he actually sees and hears is no different from what any viewer would see; it is his interpretation that is different.

The content and quality of a patient's delusions can give clues about his needs. For example, delusions in which one is special are thought to be a defense against feelings of inferiority and inadequacy. Being a target of persecution also conveys a specialness that may mask poor self-esteem, but because other people are viewed as dangerous, it also allows the person to distance himself from them, thereby not risking their rejecting him first.

Diagnoses in Which Delusions Are a Common Symptom

Delusions may be present in any of the psychotic disorders: schizophrenia, manic and depressive psychoses, and organic mental disorders. Less frequently, they may occur in certain personality disorders (schizotypal personality, paranoid personality) and in eating disorders (anorexia nervosa, bulimia).

Strategy for Therapeutic Use of Self

As a rule, it is better not to discuss the patient's delusions with him, since this tends to reinforce them. Simply change the subject and divert his attention to an activity or something else that is really going on. It is pointless to try to convince the patient that his delusion is not true; doing so will only alienate and anger him.

Developing and organizing delusions that, although odd, make a certain bizarre sense requires a fair degree of intelligence and cognitive skill. Avoid being patronizing. Instead, relate to the patient as an intelligent adult.

Strategy for Modifying the Environment

The environment should be relatively stimulating and provide opportunities for the patient to get involved in real-life activities.

Strategy for Selecting Activities

All activities should be suited to the patient's intellectual level. Since delusional patients tend to have better verbal and cognitive skills, activities that use these skills are recommended. Of course, the activities should be appropriate to the patient's occupational roles and reflect his interests, and the patient should be encouraged to select his own activity.

Activities that are in any way related to the patient's delusions should be avoided. For example, making wire jewelry is a poor choice for a patient who believes that part of her brain was replaced by a complicated electrical device during a recent hysterectomy.

Examples of Appropriate Activities

Some intellectually challenging verbal activities include board games, current events discussion, crossword puzzles, and word games. Chess and computer games might also be used. Aspects of the patient's usual occupation should be incorporated wherever possible; for example, a real estate agent can organize files and develop presentation materials, or a secretary can use a word-processing program.

Paranoia

Definition

Paranoia is a type of thinking in which persecutory and grandiose ideas predominate. General suspiciousness is usually called *paranoid ideation,* whereas very extreme and unbelievable ideas (such as that the attorney general and the police are out to get you) are termed *paranoid delusions.*

Discussion

The paranoid patient feels suspicious of those around him; he is constantly alert and concerned about whether others are harassing him, persecuting him, taking advantage of him, or treating him unfairly. He keeps himself aloof and distant from others, often subjecting family and would-be friends to repeated "tests" of loyalty.

One way to think about paranoia is as a defense against rejection. By believing that others are out to get him, the patient avoids having to risk being rejected when he tries to get close. This keeps him from developing relationships where he fears he might get hurt.

Similarly, he avoids experiencing his low self-esteem by instead thinking that he is special in some way. Paranoid patients seem to need to believe that they are better, more moral, more self-sufficient than other ordinary people. They are afraid to lose their independence and have to rely on another person.

Diagnoses in Which Paranoia Is a Common Symptom

Paranoia is the predominant symptom in paranoid schizophrenia and in a rare condition called "true" paranoia. It is also seen in some psychotic depressions and in paranoid personality disorder. To some extent the suspiciousness shown by patients with borderline and narcissistic personality disorders can be considered a kind of paranoia.

Strategy for Therapeutic Use of Self

The occupational therapy assistant will understand how to approach the paranoid patient if she tries to look at the world from his point of view. In his way of looking at things, everything is potentially dangerous; anyone or anything can threaten his uncertain sense of himself. The assistant should avoid approaching him suddenly, from behind, or in a manner that can be perceived as threatening. It is important not to whisper in the patient's presence, since he will believe you are talking about him.

Similarly, any directions or statements made by the assistant should be clear, consistent, directive, and unambiguous. Paranoid patients are usually very intelligent, often more intelligent than many of the staff, and therefore should be approached as intellectual equals. Arguing with them is pointless; they will always win. They often possess extraordinary memories; therefore it is wise to be truthful and not make promises unless you are certain you can keep them.

Frequently, a paranoid patient in an activity group will isolate himself from other patients and try to strike up a special relationship with whatever staff member is present. Some therapists believe that allowing and encouraging this special relationship helps the patient adjust faster to the group. The patient can be given a special role (passing out supplies, taking attendance) that makes him feel important. The paranoid patient will be threatened by competition, so competitive games or situations in which one person is compared to another should be avoided. The patient should be given the message that he is important and that he should focus on himself and not worry about what other people are doing.

The question of who is in control of a situation is a real concern for the paranoid patient. The assistant must be careful to stay in charge of the situation and not let the patient run away with the show. For example, the patient may want people to sit in assigned seats (usually away from him); by refusing this request outright the assistant may alienate the patient, but by giving in to it she gives him the idea that he has a great deal of power. In such a case the artful assistant will work out a compromise that gratifies the paranoid patient's need to be alone, yet simultaneously affirms her own control of the situation; for example, she may seat the patient at a separate table, but then let other patients sit wherever they wish.

Strategy for Modifying the Environment

The paranoid patient is easily threatened by changes in the environment; therefore, the environment should be kept as stable and reliable as possible. When changes are anticipated (e.g., a new paint job, a need to rearrange the furniture for a special event) the patient should be prepared in advance.

Frequently, the paranoid patient will deliberately isolate himself from other people. This is a self-protective measure, which the assistant should tolerate and support until the patient feels more comfortable. Social contact should never be forced on the patient. After an initial period of isolation he should be encouraged to join others in a group; usually he will first take on the role of watchful observer or that of "special assistant" described above. Gradually, after repeated exposure to the same people, the paranoid patient may begin to relate more spontaneously.

Because the paranoid patient is easily threatened and frightened, there is some potential for violence. Staff should follow the safety guidelines recommended for the hostile and aggressive patient.

Strategy for Selecting Activities

Activities must be ones the patient can control. Structured activities involving controllable materials (e.g., leatherwork) are recommended. Before presenting any activity to the patient, the assistant should make sure that it is appropriate for the patient's intellectual level and complex enough to engage and maintain his interest. In the beginning, activities should be individual, done independently, without need for help or instructions. The paranoid patient usually has the ability to follow diagrams and written directions. Unless there is reason to suspect that the patient is suicidal or assaultive, it is best to give him his tools at the beginning of the session rather than requiring him to come and ask for each one individually.

Examples of Appropriate Activities

Making a wood, leather, or metal project from written instructions is sufficiently complex to challenge this type of patient. Other possibilities include high-level clerical tasks (organizing files, using computerized data bases), design tasks, jewelry making, and puzzles.

Hostility and Aggression

Definition

Hostility is an unfriendly attitude directed toward other people. Aggression is an attack on a person or object; aggression can be verbal, physical, or both.

Discussion

Before discussing some of the reasons why patients may at times be hostile or aggressive, it is important first to distinguish aggression from assertiveness, with which it is frequently confused. Assertiveness is the direct expression of feelings and desires; it has come to be synonymous with "sticking up for oneself." There are situations in which, in order to assert himself, a person must also be aggressive. For example, in New York City parking spaces are at such a premium that it is quite common for two drivers to want the same space. What should the driver who arrived first do? To secure the space for himself he may need to get out of his car and argue about it. Most New York City car owners would consider his "aggression" appropriate.

Another important consideration is that some cultural groups condone aggressiveness by males (especiallly when avenging real or fancied insults to females). Although the degree of aggressiveness displayed may seem extreme (or silly) to someone from a different social class or cultural background, it is accepted and even expected in some cultures.

When working with patients who are verbally or physically aggressive it is important to distinguish between ordinary (or culturally endorsed) self-assertiveness and inappropriate aggression. Although almost everyone feels hostile at times, sometimes with good reason, most people are able to control their feelings and avoid acting them out. When a person is unable to express his feelings in words he may resort to violence; this is especially true if the person has a history of being abused as a child or being violent as an adult.

Patients who become verbally abusive or physically violent may be expressing a variety of unmet needs. The patient may feel threatened or hemmed in, physically or psychologically. Psychiatric centers are often crowded, and the patient may find the physical press of other people and the lack of privacy overwhelming; similarly, the patient may feel confined and frustrated by the rules and restrictions. Some patients use physical or verbal violence as a way of venting frustration, of letting off steam;

often such patients find it difficult to express themselves in words and have not developed any constructive channels for their aggression (e.g., sports activities, hobbies). Other patients use hostility and aggression self-protectively; by keeping others at a distance they make rejection impossible.

Diagnoses in Which Hostility or Aggression Is a Common Symptom

Patients with psychotic disorders (paranoid schizophrenia, manic-depressive psychosis, psychotic depression, organic mental disorders) sometimes become hostile. Usually something has happened to provoke this response, but it is often hard to figure out exactly what. Substance abusers and persons with antisocial personality disorders may also show hostility.

Strategy for Therapeutic Use of Self

Staff should be alert to signs that a patient is feeling tense, threatened, or suspicious. A patient's body language gives clues about his mental state. For example, stiffness or rigidity in the set of the mouth or the shoulders usually signifies anger or anxiety. Threatening gestures or the destruction of objects (no matter how small or insignificant) are other signs. The sooner the possibility of aggressiveness is recognized, the sooner it can be dealt with.

The general approach is to get the patient to talk about what is bothering him, and to help the patient use words to express his feelings rather than just acting them out. It is important not to respond in kind, no matter how insulting or provocative the patient's words are. Try to speak to the patient privately, thus avoiding a public display that may make him feel more threatened. Encourage him to discuss his feelings. Tell him exactly what needs to be corrected about how he is handling the situation, explain that his behavior is affecting you and the other patients, and give him some alternatives for handling it. Avoid punishing or criticizing him; both of these approaches are humiliating and will tend to escalate aggressiveness.

It is important to be direct and clear about what is expected. Follow through by enforcing any limits you set. To illustrate, if you have told Mr. Jones that he will have to leave the group if he touches another patient again, then you had better make sure you have other staff available who can remove him if this happens. Otherwise Mr. Jones may continue to test your limits, since you obviously cannot be taken at your word.

Be especially cautious with patients who say that you (or another staff member or patient) remind them of someone they do not like. This should be considered a warning that the patient may attack when psychotic and out of control. Violent acts are more likely in patients who have a self-reported history of violence than in those without such a history (4).

Strategy for Modifying the Environment

Because of the potential for violence, the hostile patient should be isolated from others who may irritate her. While speaking to the hostile or potentially violent patient the assistant should stand four or five feet away, and to the side, not facing the patient directly. This position gives the patient room and is not confrontational. It is not a good idea to be alone with a patient who may become violent. Similarly, in any room the door should be left open, and the staff member should be positioned closer than the patient to the door. Do not touch the patient. Even what you intend as a comforting touch can be perceived as an attack. Remove all potential weapons from the area. Even brooms and mops have been used to beat people to death, so *think*.

Strategy for Selecting Activities

Unfortunately, there is no handy formula for choosing activities for hostile and aggressive patients. Therapists who follow object relations theory believe activities that encourage sublimation of hostile and aggressive feelings are best. These need not be openly aggressive activities. For example, symbolic activities like art and dance may permit the patient to express her feelings in a more socially acceptable way; this seems especially appropriate for patients with poor verbal skills. Activities that require large, forceful motions (e.g., wedging clay) can also be used to express aggressiveness, but in some patients these may increase aggressiveness (21). Avoid activities that require frustration tolerance and attention to detail. For obvious reasons, do not use activities that involve sharp tools or small, heavy, and throwable objects. Activities that require repetitive motions may help some people organize and control their feelings.

Examples of Appropriate Activities

Active sports and other gross motor activities such as dance are useful for releasing tension. Sanding a large wood project involves repetitive gross motor movements and is mildly destructive; it is an example of an activity that might help reduce tension. Peeling potatoes is another activity that can serve the same purpose; the tool should be a potato peeler with a rounded point (not a knife). Activities that involve sharp or potentially dangerous tools (e.g., woodworking, metal hammering) should be used only when both therapist and patient feel comfortable that the patient can control himself.

Patients who have problems managing, controlling and expressing anger may benefit from anger management (11, 12, 13, 21) and conflict resolution (9) training. Such training gives the patient the skills of preplanning a response to angry feelings, identifying anger when it occurs, problem-solving to handle anger, and empathizing with and forgiving the other party (12).

Seductive Behavior and Sexual Acting-Out

Definition

Seductive behavior is any behavior that would normally be seen as explicitly (openly) sexual or as provoking a sexual response from others. Examples are highly varied. They might be as subtle as touching someone's shoulder or loosening a tie or collar or as blatant as making sexual remarks or asking a staff member for a date. Sexual acting-out is openly sexual behavior in response to unconscious feelings. This includes engaging in sexual acts with other patients. Sometimes the phrase "sexual acting-out" is used to describe extreme behaviors of patients who have lost contact with reality. Such patients may, for example, masturbate openly, disrobe in public, tuck their shirts in their panties and dance around, or fondle other patients.

Discussion

Sexual needs do not just disappear when a person becomes mentally ill; psychiatric patients have the same needs as everyone else, but they have much more difficulty gratifying their sexual needs. Inpatients who may have been used to daily sexual activity before hospitalization find that they can see their sexual partners only on weekend passes. To add to their frustration, the lack of privacy may make masturbation difficult or impossible. Even in outpatient settings, some patients will not have developed enough social skills to be able to form close relationships in which sexual needs can be gratified. So, it should not be surprising that some patients seem preoccupied with sex.

Sometimes what looks like seductive behavior is really a bid to get attention, or to see how a staff member will react. If the patient can make the staff member sufficiently uncomfortable, he can make sure that that person will never confront him about his real problems. Similarly, the patient who feels unattractive or insecure may set up a sexual confrontation so that a staff member will reject him, thus confirming his worst fears.

Additionally, patients who are hallucinating may attempt to remove their clothes because they feel insects crawling on them or because they hear voices commanding them to do so. King (16) points out that sexual promiscuity may have its roots in "skin hunger" or a need for warmth and tactile input. So, it is important to pinpoint the motivation behind the patient's behavior before deciding what to do about it.

Diagnoses in Which Sexual Acting-Out or Seductiveness Is a Common Symptom

The most extreme forms of sexual acting-out (disrobing, open masturbation) usually occur only in psychotic patients or those with psychosexual disorders (exhibitionism, sexual masochism). The other behaviors mentioned may be seen in any patient (or indeed in anyone anywhere).

Strategy for Therapeutic Use of Self

Patients who are behaving inappropriately should be told so. This should be done in a calm, nonjudgmental manner. The patient should be stopped from doing things that will later embarrass her. For example, if she will not stop her lewd dancing, she should be excused from the dance activity for the day. The rules of the particular setting should be strictly enforced (e.g., most inpatient settings forbid physical contact between patients).

Patients who try to involve staff in sexual relationships may be expressing needs that are other than sexual. For example, an adolescent male who fears he is homosexual may behave seductively to a female therapist to test out his own sexual identity. Some patients may confuse the closeness of the therapeutic relationship with the intimacy of a sexual one (discussed in Chapter 10). When a patient behaves seductively toward a staff member, the staff member should carefully explain the nature of the therapeutic relationship and should discourage further overtures gently but firmly. She should avoid *any* physical contact, and should not allow the patient to talk about the possibility of a sexual relationship with her. As a last resort, if the patient is not able to stop, she should arrange for another staff member to work with the patient.

Notify staff and document all sexually preoccupied behavior and remarks, to prevent incidents that may happen at night or when fewer staff are around. Encouarge patients to "tell on" others who abuse them sexually.

Strategy for Modifying the Environment

Crowded situations, in which physical contact is almost unavoidable, are not a good idea. The patient should have room to move.

Strategy for Selecting Activities

No one would dispute that sex is the best activity for gratifying sexual needs. If the patient's religious beliefs permit, and the assistant feels comfortable, masturbation can be suggested as an alternative.

It is possible to release a great deal of sexual tension through forceful gross motor activities. Activities that involve other people, especially with physical contact, should be used cautiously, depending on the patient's tolerance and self-control.

Social skills training and other activities that teach or reinforce appropriate social behavior are also recommended.

Examples of Appropriate Activities

Forceful gross motor activities that can be done alone or without physical contact include, for example, exercise, running, wedging clay, and woodworking. Some examples of activities involving others in physical contact are sports like volleyball, basketball, and touch football, and dance. Activities with limited or no physical contact that still permit physical release include swimming, cycling, weight training and aerobics, and yoga.

Cognitive Deficits: Confusion and Impaired Memory

Definition

A cognitive deficit is an impairment or defect in one or more of the mental functions needed for thinking. Some of these processes are orientation, alertness, concentration, attention span, memory, comprehension, judgment, and problem solving.

Orientation is knowledge of where one is, what time it is (hour, day, date, season), and who one is with. This is sometimes referred to as "orientation to time, place, and person" and abbreviated as "orientation ×3" (meaning orientation in three spheres of information). Problems in this area are described as *disorientation* or *confusion*. Generally, disorientation to time alone is the least severe form; disorientation to place and time is more severe; and disorientation to person, place, and time the most severe.

Alertness refers to awareness of the immediate environment. Problems in alertness may be described generally as *clouding of consciousness,* meaning literally that the patient seems to be in a fog, or by the specific aspect of alertness that is impaired. Concentration and attention span are aspects of alertness.

Concentration is the ability to focus one's mental energies on the immediate task at hand. The intensity of focus is the primary concern. *Attention span* is the length of time that concentration can be maintained. Impairment in attention span is usually referred to as *distractibility* (meaning a tendency to lose focus because another stimulus catches one's interest) or *inattention* (usually meaning the inability to pay attention even though no competing external stimulus is present). Responses to these symptoms will be discussed in the next section.

Memory is the ability to recall past events and knowledge. Health professionals commonly distinguish between short-term memory and long-term memory, to indicate the difference between memory of events from months or years ago (*long-term memory*) and memory of more recent events (*short-term memory*). Thus a patient's ability to remember his date of birth or the names of his children reflects his long-term memory, and his ability to remember whether he had lunch or where he put his eyeglasses reflects his short-term memory. Experimental psychologists sometimes use the term "short-term memory" to refer to memory of events that occurred within the past few seconds, rather than hours or days (23). Since this can cause confusion among treatment staff, make sure that you understand which kind of short-term memory is being described. Problems in remembering important information are referred to as *memory impairment*.

Comprehension is the ability to understand. Comprehension is composed of many separate skills, including the ability to recognize words, to identify objects, to place things in order by time or size or some other quality, and to classify or sort or group objects in a logical fashion.

Comprehension depends upon the development of concepts. We can think of concepts as containers for experiences; for example, our concept of dog includes many different varieties and sizes of dog; when we see a four-legged animal we compare it to other items in the concept "dog" to see if it belongs in this container. A person's ability to comprehend depends on the number of concepts he has available and the way they are organized. To illustrate, an unsophisticated concept of "muscle" might refer just to physical strength ("He's got muscles"). A student of physical medicine or anatomy will have a more sophisticated concept, in fact a highly organized group of concepts, including for example "striated muscles," "voluntary muscle," "antagonist," and "deep hip flexor."

It is important to recognize that trouble in comprehending may have other than psychological causes. Language skills, prior education, and life experience all affect comprehension. Physiological changes from brain damage or chemicals in the body can also impair comprehension. Problems in comprehension are usually described as *inability to comprehend*.

Judgment is the ability to recognize and comply with established social norms and standard procedures. Like comprehension, judgment reflects background and social class. Using foul language probably indicates bad judgment in an otherwise conservative businessman, but may be the social norm for a dock worker. Problems in judgment are usually referred to as *impaired judgment;* some examples are urinating on the street, making sexual innuendos to coworkers, and sitting down on a bench marked with a sign that says "wet paint."

Problem solving is the ability to recognize, analyze, and ultimately figure out solutions for problems that arise in the course of everyday activity. Some examples of problems that most people need to solve are budgeting money and getting from place to place. Everyone but the very wealthy has to figure out how to pay for things like repair of the hot water heater or a new car. When the car breaks down or the subway is delayed, an alternate way of transporting oneself has to be found. Living on one's own in the community depends on the ability to solve problems such as these.

Because cognitive impairments have such a profound effect on a person's ability to succeed on his own, they will be discussed several times in this text. The reader is encouraged to refer to Chapters 6, 22, and 23 for more information.

Discussion

A person who realizes that his thinking is not as clear as it once was, or that he has forgotten and left a pot burning on the stove (for the fourth time) is usually very frightened and anxious. He may begin to check things many times over, or to engage in ritualistic actions. Or he may become anxious and agitated, or even belligerent. Commonly, the patient's long-term memory and recall of events from many years ago are excellent. His problems in short-term memory are deeply disturbing, and he may make up stories to cover them up. This is called *confabulation*.

Often the cognitively impaired patient is also depressed; it is not always clear whether the depression is the cause of the cognitive problems or the result. Most people believe that the depression and the cognitive problems interact with each other in a negative way; the more the person experiences problems in thinking and remembering, the more depressed he will become. Likewise, the more depressed he is, the more likely he is to forget things and have trouble concentrating. Thus the depression and the cognitive problems fuel each other, and the person may become more depressed and more impaired as time goes by.

Some patients with cognitive problems have very *labile* emotions. This means that they rapidly shift from being calm and comfortable to crying or laughing uncontrollably. An elderly nursing home resident might, for example, suddenly burst into tears when she remembers the death of a childhood pet.

Patients who are disoriented frequently become lost, especially in strange new environments (like hospitals and nursing homes). They need help finding their rooms and their way to the bathroom.

Patients with poor judgment usually do not recognize that their judgment is off, that they are doing something inappropriate (like washing their hair in the water fountain) or offensive (like fondling the assistant's derrière). They may try to laugh it off, or to prevent further criticism by becoming hostile. Both of these behaviors can be considered defenses against the anxiety and pain that would result if they really understood what they had done.

Problems in carrying out motor actions are often associated with cognitive deficits. These may be more or less severe and can be analyzed according to Allen's cognitive levels (see Chapters 3, 14, and 23). *Dressing apraxia* is a severe form in which the person has trouble carrying out the proper sequence of actions to get dressed, and may for example put her socks on over her shoes, or wear two skirts.

To summarize, cognitive deficits can seriously impair a person's ability to function. The person with cognitive deficits may have a wide range of emotional reactions in response to decreasing function. When working with the cognitively impaired patient it is important to consider his emotional response and whatever cognitive skills are still intact.

Diagnoses in Which Cognitive Deficits Are Common

Cognitive deficits occur to varying degrees in many different psychiatric disorders. They are always found in organic mental disorders; in these disorders (which include Alzheimer's disease) the impairment is usually severe and progressive (meaning that it gets worse over time).

Cognitive deficits can also occur as a result of physical disease. Any disease that impairs circulation will have an effect on the brain because less blood and therefore less oxygen reaches it. Brain infections and trauma to the head can result in cognitive problems that may be permanent or transient.

Drugs and alcohol affect brain chemistry and therefore can cause cognitive deficits. Phencyclidine (PCP) abuse often results in impaired alertness, concentration, and attention span. Prolonged or extensive alcohol abuse is associated with an organic mental disorder characterized by permanent impairment of intellectual abilities. Some prescription medications, including several used for treatment of psychiatric disorders, can cause temporary cognitive deficits, which disappear when the medication is discontinued.

Finally, patients receiving electroconvulsive therapy (ECT) usually experience disorientation and short-term memory loss for several days after receiving treatments. With time, these mental functions usually recover, although the patient may never be able to remember events from around the time of the treatments.

Strategy for Therapeutic Use of Self

General rules for approaching the patient with cognitive deficits are difficult to prescribe. Patients function at many different levels; some may forget only an occasional fact or today's date; others may be so disoriented that they think Nixon is president or that they are in a factory rather than a nursing home. It is important to approach each patient as an individual, and to pitch your comments and directions to the patient's present level of functioning. By doing this you will help the lower functioning patient feel more secure and will avoid insulting the higher functioning patient. Keeping this important precaution in mind, the following guidelines should be used.

Since being disoriented can be very frightening, be sure to remind the patient of where he is and who you are. For the patient with severe memory impairment (and this includes some patients receiving ECT) it may be necessary to repeat this information each time you see the person. Wearing a name tag with your name and title in large print can help. Keep in mind that the person may have trouble finding the bathroom; orient him to this and any other important aspects of the environment. Other information that a patient might need to know includes the time of day, what is happening now, and what will be happening next.

Although the patient with cognitive impairment may do very inappropriate things because of his poor judgment, the assistant should consistently show a warm and accepting attitude. Patients should not be punished or threatened no matter how inconvenient or unpleasant their behavior has been. Instead, the assistant should gently explain what is expected and then help the patient behave appropriately. It is important to intervene immediately when the patient does something wrong, and to help him correct it then and there. Otherwise he may not know what you are talking about when you mention it to him later.

Whenever the patient is given directions, whether on how to do an activity or how to get to the cafeteria, the directions should reflect the five C's: *calm, clear, concise, concrete,* and *consistent.* Speak in a calm tone of voice, articulating the words clearly. You may need to speak more slowly than you do usually, but your tone of voice should be respectful (not patronizing or impatient). Whatever you have to say, make it brief; the patient's attention span is short. Use common everyday language, not abstract or difficult words that the patient may not comprehend. Finally, use the same words every time you give the directions. Incorporating the patient's own words can be helpful. To illustrate, if the patient asks where you put his "specs," use this word rather than "glasses" or "eyeglasses" when you tell him where to find them. If you expect the patient to remember the directions and use them later, have him repeat them back to you. Better yet, write them down or make sure that he writes them down.

Finally, match your tempo to what the patient seems able to handle. Cognitively impaired patients may take a while to respond; it just takes them longer to process ideas and information.

Strategy for Modifying the Environment

Cognitively impaired patients, more than any other group of patients, need a consistent and well-designed environment. Good lighting will help the patient orient himself. Even at night, lighting should be kept fairly bright. Colored lines (whether tiled, taped, or painted) on the floor leading to the bathroom and other frequently used areas are also good orientation aids. Reflector tape is recommended.

Locations should be clearly marked with signs. Large print should be used. Pictographs or pictorial symbols may be more easily recognized than words; an example is a picture of a cup and saucer on the door of the cafeteria. A sign or symbol on the door of the patient's room may help him find it (making the sign can be a good project). The patient may need to label, mark, or color-code objects in his room to help him find them.

External memory aids such as a clock (large), calendar (large), and radio are valuable. These help orient the patient to time and to current events. For the patient who needs to remember to do things at a certain time, *cueing devices* (14) such as programmable alarm watches and timers can be used. Many different electronic devices are available that store specific kinds of information; an example is one that stores telephone numbers and dials them automatically when the proper code is entered. Sometimes such devices are difficult for the patient to learn to use, in which case their value is questionable. Harris (14) and Skil-

beck (20) describe some of these devices and how they can be used.

Because cognitively impaired patients rely so much on structure and routine in the external environment to help them stay organized, they are very sensitive to any changes. Therefore, the environment should be kept the same from day to day; this is true of the occupational therapy shop as well as the patient's living area.

The question of how much stimulation should be available in the environment is fascinating and much debated. Research has shown that environments with low amounts of stimulation can cause cognitive impairments because they deprive the senses of necessary information. However, it seems equally true that too much stimulation can also cause cognitive impairments, because the person cannot process so much information at one time. Clinicians agree, however, that any stimulation presented should be clear and unambiguous. For example, when music is used, records should be played on a good stereo system rather than a cheap turntable with a worn-out needle.

Another factor to be considered in designing an environment for a patient with cognitive impairments is its similarity or dissimilarity to the patient's home environment. When the patient enters the hospital or nursing home, not only is he often seriously ill and in psychological distress, but his distress is further exacerbated by the strangeness of this new environment. The patient's discomfort can be lessened somewhat if he is allowed to keep mementos of home in his room. He should also be allowed to set up his belongings in whatever way makes sense for him, as this will encourage carryover of dressing and hygiene/grooming routines. Finally, if the patient is planning to return home, or is to be discharged to another facility, his future environment must be considered. Teaching of new skills or reinforcement of old skills should take place in an environment similar to this future one.

Strategy for Selecting Activities

The patient's prognosis must be considered when selecting activities. Some cognitive impairments are transitory and the patient is expected to regain full function (e.g., post-ECT memory impairment). These patients should be given simple, structured, short-term activities to help them maintain their abilities and confidence until they recover. Activities that can be finished in one day are preferred, because the patient may refuse to work on a project two days in a row because he does not remember that it is his. Once the cognitive functions begin to return to normal the patient should be quickly reintroduced to whatever activities and skills she needs in her occupational roles.

Other conditions (e.g., dementia associated with alcoholism) are permanent but stable; the patient will not get better, nor will he get worse. For these patients, the specific cognitive deficits need to be identified and then analyzed in relation to his previous occupational roles. Then the patient can be taught ways to adapt to his disability within these roles or to find new occupational roles more appropriate to his present condition. The general approach is to simplify known activities rather than introduce new ones. Dubovsky (5) gives the example of an electronics engineer who suffered from a mild organic mental disorder, which prevented him from functioning adequately in his job; despite his cognitive deficits he continued to use his skills by teaching basic electronics.

A third group of conditions, unfortunately, are permanent and progressive; the patient will become less and less able to function and will eventually die. These patients need help to maintain whatever skills remain, for as long as possible. The patient should be encouraged to be as independent as he can while he can. Activities for this type of patient should be restricted to those that are familiar, relevant, and necessary. Participation in his own self-care is impor-

tant to help the patient retain a sense of dignity and self-esteem. These patients usually do not have the ability to learn anything new.

Some general guidelines apply to all three groups of patients. The first is that unfamiliar and complex activities should be avoided since they will add to the patient's confusion. Activities that require independent decision making may overwhelm the patient's limited judgment; activities that involve simple choices (e.g., between two colors or two food items) can build the patient's confidence, however. The occupational therapy assistant should help the patient carry out activities that the patient believes are important.

Depending on individual need, the patient may benefit from reality orientation. This approach, which aims to keep the patient aware of what is going on around him, will be described further in Chapter 22. Touring around the halls and practicing travel within the treatment facility is appropriate for severely disoriented patients.

Many patients suffering confusion or impaired memory find it helpful to write things down. These patients should be encouraged to carry a notebook with them at all times; designing and organizing the notebook can be an ongoing activity. Taking an excursion to town to select an appointment book at the stationery or office supply stores can be a way to assess simultaneously the patient's travel and orientation skills.

Examples of Appropriate Activities

Activities that can be used to help orient the patient to reality include current events discussion, patient government or resident council, and reality orientation classes.

Familiar, relevant, and necessary life tasks should emphasize self-care and whatever other tasks may be needed for a particular individual (e.g., cooking, housework, laundry, shopping). Familiar crafts and hobbies can help bolster self-confidence when the ability to do more complex tasks has been lost. Short walks or shopping excursions are also helpful and provide variety, exercise, and a sense of added purpose.

Attentional Deficits and Disorganization

Definition

Attentional deficits are problems in directing attention to a task or in sustaining attention for a reasonable length of time. Disorganization is a lack of planning and order that interferes with successful completion of activities.

Discussion

Attentional deficits and disorganization are often associated with the other cognitive deficits described above. However, since the general management of these symptoms is different, they are discussed separately.

A patient may have trouble concentrating on a task or paying attention to it over time for several reasons. He may be distracted by hallucinations or memories or other internally generated stimuli, or by things around him in the external environment. It is thought that some schizophrenic patients process information more slowly than other people; by the time they figure out what is happening, something else is going on, and they have trouble keeping up (8).

Someone who has trouble paying attention is likely to have trouble with organization as well. However, another possible cause of disorganization is overstimulation; the person has difficulty focusing on one thing at a time because there is so much that catches his attention (this is common in mania). Still another is poor judgment, evidenced by trying to do too many things at one time. Also, a person may appear disorganized simply because he lacks the skills or knowledge to perform the activity. To il-lustrate, someone who has done little cooking will have trouble assembling the necessary ingredients and implements and carrying out the steps efficiently.

Diagnoses in Which Attentional Deficits and Disorganization Are Common

Both of these symptoms occur in organic mental disorders, in PCP and alcohol abuse, and in schizophrenia and affective psychoses. Persons with learning disabilities often have these problems. Normal individuals are likely to have impaired attention and to be disorganized when they are under stress or otherwise preoccupied.

Strategy for Therapeutic Use of Self

It may be difficult to get the patient's attention. If so, say his name, *loudly*. If necessary, shout; although this may feel uncomfortable to you at first, it is the only way to get the attention of severely regressed patients. Patients who do not respond to what you say to them may respond to being touched, firmly but gently on the arm or shoulder.

The patient who is disorganized or who is having trouble paying attention to a task may simply not be capable of doing that particular task at this time; if so, his attention should be directed to another, more simple activity. The new activity should be introduced matter-of-factly, so as to avoid making the patient feel incompetent (e.g., "I think that we should save this for another day; I need to work out some of the details. I'd like you to try this instead.") The goal is to help the patient feel comfortable and competent within the limits of his present abilities.

Strategy for Modifying the Environment

Distractions can be reduced by having the patient work alone, facing a blank wall.

If the patient is being distracted by internally generated stimuli (hallucinations, etc.), vigorous stimulation may be necessary to get his attention.

Strategy for Selecting Activities

Simple, well-delineated activities that have a definite sequence consisting of very few steps are recommended. The assistant may need to do the more difficult steps for the patient. Activities that are creative or that have flexible standards or goals should be avoided; they will only increase disorganization.

Examples of Appropriate Activities

Mosaic tile projects, leather coin purses, plastic-dip flowers, and copper tooling can all be used, although some steps may have to be modified. For instance, oxidizing the copper might be skipped altogether or done by the assistant or a volunteer.

Generally, the most important activities are self-care and the life tasks needed in the patient's occupational role. Helping a housewife organize her kitchen or do the laundry more efficiently will probably be more important to her than learning copper tooling.

SUMMARY

Symptoms are the behavioral evidence of underlying psychological and physiological problems. They give us clues about what the patient is experiencing, what he is having trouble with, and what we might do to make him more comfortable. This chapter has presented some ideas about how to respond to patients who exhibit different symptoms and behaviors. The occupational therapy assistant's response to the patient is composed of three variables: therapeutic use of self, modification of the environment, and selection of activities.

The information presented in this chapter is intended as a general guide and not as a rigid system of rules. It cannot substitute for a proper treatment plan, but can be useful for refining the treatment plan once the general goals and methods have been identified. Each patient is unique and will need an individualized approach. Occupational therapists and assistants cannot treat the patient's symptoms, because symptoms are caused by an underlying disease process. However, the occupational therapy assistant can help the patient function better by modifying the environment so that he can manage it and by selecting activities that utilize his remaining capabilities.

REFERENCES

1. Allen CK. *Occupational therapy for psychiatric diseases: measurement and management of cognitive disabilities.* Boston: Little, Brown; 1985.
2. American Psychiatric Association. *DSM-IIIR: diagnostic and statistical manual of mental disorders.* Washington, DC: American Psychiatric Association; 1987.
3. Beck AT. *Cognitive therapy and the emotional disorders.* New York: International Universities Press; 1976.
4. Convit A, et al. Predicting assaultiveness in psychiatric inpatients: a pilot study. *Hosp Comm Psychiatry* 1988; 39:429–438.
5. Dubovsky SL, Weissberg MP. *Clinical psychiatry in primary care.* Baltimore: Williams & Wilkins; 1978.
6. Ellis A. *Humanistic psychology: the rational-emotive approach.* New York: McGraw-Hill; 1974.
7. Falk-Kessler J, Froschauer KH. The soap opera: a dynamic group approach for psychiatric patients. *Am J Occup Ther* 1978; 32:317–321.
8. George L, Neufeld RWJ. Cognition and symptomatology in schizophrenia. *Schizophrenia Bull* 1985; 11(2):264–285.
9. Gibson D. Theory and strategies for resolving conflict. *Occup Ther Mental Health* 1986; 5(4): 47–62.
10. Goleman D. Clues to suicide: a brain chemical is implicated. *The New York Times,* October 8, 1985; C1–C6.
11. Grogan G. Anger management. 1: a perspective for occupational therapy. *Occup Ther Mental Health* 1991; 11(2/3):135–148.
12. Grogan G. Anger management. 2: clinical applications for occupational therapy. *Occup Ther Mental Health* 1991; 11(2/3):149–171.

13. Harborview Anger Management Program, Harborview Community Mental Health Center, Seattle. Helping angry and violent people manage their emotions. *Hosp Comm Psychiatry* 1987; 38:1207–1210.

14. Harris J. Methods of improving memory. In: Wilson BA, Moffat N. *Clinical management of memory problems.* Rockville, Md: Aspen Systems; 1984.

15. Janowsky DS, Leff M, Epstein RS. Playing the manic game: interpersonal maneuvers of the acutely manic patient. *Arch Gen Psychiatry* 1970; 22:252–261.

16. King LJ. *Sensory integration as a broad spectrum treatment approach.* Philadelphia: Continuing Education Programs of America; 1978.

17. MacRae A. An overview of theory and research on hallucinations: implications for occupational therapy intervention. *Occup Ther Mental Health* 1991; 11(4):41–60.

18. Neville A. The model of human occupation and depression. *Am Occup Ther Assoc Mental Health Special Interest Section Newsletter* 1985; 8(1):1–4.

19. Seligman ME. *Helplessness: on depression, development and death.* San Francisco: WH Freeman; 1975.

20. Skilbeck C. Computer assistance in the management of memory and cognitive impairment. In: Wilson BA, Moffat N. *Clinical management of memory problems.* Rockville Md: Aspen Systems; 1984.

21. Taylor E. Anger intervention. *Am J Occup Ther* 1988; 42:147–155.

22. Turner IM. The healing power of respect—a personal journey. *Occup Ther Mental Health* 1989; 9(1):17–32.

23. Wilson BA, Moffat N, eds. *Clinical management of memory problems.* Rockville, Md: Aspen Systems; 1984.

ADDITIONAL REFERENCES AND SUGGESTED READINGS

Allen CK. *Occupational therapy for psychiatric diseases: measurement and management of cognitive disabilities.* Boston: Little, Brown; 1985.

American Occupational Therapy Association. *Objectives and functions of occupational therapy for psychiatric conditions.* Dubuque, Iowa: Wm C Brown; 1958.

Bailey DS, Cooper SO, Bailey DR. *Therapeutic approaches to the mentally ill.* 2nd ed. Philadelphia: FA Davis; 1984.

Ben-Shlomo LS, Short MA. The effects of physical conditioning on selected dimensions of self-concept in sedentary females. *Occup Ther Mental Health* 1985; 5(4):27–46.

Berger MM. *Working with people called patients.* New York: Brunner/Mazel; 1977.

Corry S, Sebastian V, Mosey AC. Acute short-term treatment in psychiatry. *Am J Occup Ther* 1974; 28:401–406.

Crawford AL, Kilander VC. *Psychiatric and mental health nursing.* 6th ed. Philadelphia: FA Davis; 1985.

Custer VL, Wassink KE. Occupational therapy intervention for an adult with depression and suicidal tendencies. *Am J Occup Ther* 1991; 45:845–848.

Devereaux E, Carlson M. The role of occupational therapy in the management of depression. *Am J Occup Ther* 1992; 46:175–180.

Fidler G, Fidler J. *Occupational therapy: a communication process in psychiatry.* New York: Macmillan; 1963.

Hasselkus BR. The meaning of activity: day care for persons with Alzheimer disease. *Am J Occup Ther* 1992; 46:199–206.

Hays JS, Larson K. *Interacting with patients.* New York: Macmillan; 1963.

Mace NL, Rabins PV. *The 36-hour day: a family guide to caring for persons with Alzheimer's disease, related dementing illness, and memory loss in later life.* Baltimore: The Johns Hopkins University Press; 1981.

Reisberg B. *A guide to Alzheimer's disease for families, spouses, and friends.* New York: Macmillan; 1981.

Sabol PS. The contagion factor in depression. *Am Occup Ther Assoc Mental Health Special Interest Section Newsletter* 1985; 8(1):2–3.

Seligman MEP. *Learned optimism.* New York: Alfred E Knopf; 1991.

Simon E. *A manual for self-instruction in psychiatric occupational therapy OT-203 the recognition of hostility.* Buffalo, NY: Erie Community College; 1974.

Solomon K. Learned helplessness in the elderly: theoretic and clinical considerations. *Occup Ther Mental Health* 1990; 10(3):31–51.

Watson LJ. Psychiatric consultation–liaison in the acute physical disabilities setting. *Am J Occup Ther* 1986; 40:338–342.

Willson M. *Occupational therapy in long-term psychiatry.* Edinburgh: Churchill Livingstone; 1983.

12

Safety Techniques

The cautious seldom err.
CONFUCIUS (2)

Psychiatric hospitals and outpatient treatment settings are usually pretty safe places; they have to be, because psychiatric patients are probably more likely than other people to harm themselves, either by accident or on purpose. Some patients are suicidal, others have histories of violence, and others are just confused or careless and likely to get lost or get into accidents. When these patients are treated in the hospital they are usually placed on locked units. Such units restrict the use of sharps and other objects that can be used violently or self-destructively, and some provide padded seclusion rooms for separating violent or out-of-control patients from others.

When patients leave a locked unit to come to occupational therapy, or when occupational therapy is conducted on the unit, special precautions need to be taken so that they do not harm themselves. Steich (9) advises that occupational therapy personnel are legally liable for negligence if a patient injures himself because staff failed to follow proper procedures. No matter what the setting or type of patient, it makes sense to follow standard general safety, public health, and fire code regulations and to teach patients about them so that they can follow them at home.

This chapter will present guidelines for general safety in the occupational therapy department, and will review some basic first aid measures. Universal precautions

(for the prevention of disease transmission) will be addressed first. This chapter is not meant to substitute for training in up-to-date disease prevention methods or basic first aid. The reader is encouraged to seek the most recent information on disease prevention and to enroll periodically in a hands-on first aid course.

The chapter will also introduce special safety precautions for working with patients who are at risk for elopement, suicide, or assault, and will discuss the value of teaching patients about safety.

UNIVERSAL PRECAUTIONS

"Universal precautions" refers to the set of procedures recommended by various governmental and health agencies for the purpose of preventing the spread of infection. The precautions particularly target infections that are caused by disease agents that may be found in blood and other bodily fluids. The HIV virus, responsible for acquired immune deficiency syndrome (AIDS) and the hepatitis B virus are two examples. The reader is reminded to obtain and follow the most recent guidelines available; these change as more research and information becomes available.[1]

---

[1] The guidelines contained herein were released effective March 6, 1992.

Health care students and workers worry about the risk of contracting AIDS from patients. For occupational therapists and assistants the risk is much smaller than for some other professions in which contact with bodily fluids is more likely. Even for these professions, the risk of catching AIDS is insignificant compared to the risk of catching more infectious diseases such as tuberculosis. Many different disease-causing agents can be transmitted from person to person. Remember that the patient can contract a disease from the health care worker as well. For these reasons it is important that health care workers observe basic infection control procedures and universal precautions with *all* other persons in the work environment.

Employers (hospitals, etc.) are required to have an exposure control plan and to provide adequate hand-washing facilities (including single-use towels or hot air blowers) and protective barriers such as gloves for the use of employees who may contact blood or other bodily fluids (11). Small community-based programs might not reliably provide these controls and supplies, and so the obligation falls on the occupational therapy assistant to learn and follow the current federal guidelines.

Hand Washing

The first and most effective method of disease prevention is regular and thorough hand washing. Marcil (6) lists the following times at which occupational therapy personnel should wash their hands:

1. Before starting work
2. Before and after treating individual patients
3. Before and after removing gloves
4. During performance of normal duties
5. Before and after the handling of food
6. After personal use of the toilet or toileting of a patient
7. After sneezing, coughing, or contact with oral and nasal areas
8. Before eating or preparing food
9. Prior to leaving the rooms of patients on isolation or precautions
10. On completion of duty

While this list was generated in relation to work with AIDS patients, it should be applied in all clinical settings, including mental health.

Hand-washing Procedure

The key points of any hand-washing sequence are to clean all hand surfaces and crevices, to use soap and reasonably hot water, to avoid recontamination from sink or faucets or other surfaces, and to use clean disposable towels or hot air to dry the hands. The following steps are basic:

1. If they are kept in another location, bring at least three paper towels to sink.
2. Remove hand jewelry including watch.
3. Turn on water to good stream of tolerable but hot water.
4. Using soap, make a good lather.
5. Using one hand, wash the other up to and including the wrist, taking care to clean between fingers and under fingernails.
6. Repeat procedure for other hand.
7. Dry hands, using one towel and a patting motion. Follow with a second and if needed a third towel.
8. Use last towel to turn off faucets.
9. Use last towel to turn doorknob or open door of sink area.
10. Discard towels in trash container.
11. Apply hand lotion to prevent cracking of skin (a route for infection to enter).

Protective Barriers

Because a few psychiatric patients do not have control over their bodily functions, because some patients may have poor habits of personal hygiene, and because medications may cause vomiting, the occupational therapy worker may encounter a patient's bodily fluids. For this reason, protective barriers (primarily gloves) must be worn when cleaning areas that have been or *may* have been contaminated. Band-Aids should be used to cover tiny cuts and even hangnails at all times, and should be changed whenever hands are washed.

Infection Control of Common Areas

The occupational therapy clinic for psychiatry appears less "medical" than the clinic for physical disabilities. The home-like appearance and the informal atmosphere should not be taken as an excuse for avoiding proper infection control. Tables, counters, and other surfaces should be washed and disinfected daily (and any time contamination is suspected). Adequate supplies of cleaning materials such as hand soap, paper towels, a pail and mop, sponges, detergents, and disinfectants should be maintained. Disposable gloves, utility gloves, Band-Aids, and a first aid kit should be kept in each occupational therapy area.

Linens used in homemaking groups should be replaced or laundered after each use. Cosmetics and personal hygiene items (combs, toothbrushes) should never be shared. For personal hygiene sessions, patients should bring their own supplies, or the therapy assistant should provide brand new items for each patient. Cosmetic companies will often provide samples on request for this purpose.

By federal regulations, eating, drinking, smoking, applying cosmetics or lip balm, and handling contact lenses are prohibited where there is a likelihood of occupational exposure to blood or bodily fluids (11).

Universal Means Universal

It is natural to feel that certain patients, especially those similar to oneself or one's family and friends, could not possibly be a source of infection. With this feeling comes the temptation to "relax" and to omit or tone down the infection control procedures. It is not possible to tell whether someone is infected just by looking at them. Using universal precautions *universally,* with all patients, limits the spread of infection from person to person. And if the precautions are *always* used, mental energy is not wasted on figuring out whether or not to use them. Consistent, universal application of the procedures is the only responsible and ethical course of action for the health care worker.

CONTROLLING THE ENVIRONMENT

Patients often say that they enjoy coming to occupational therapy because the clinic has so many interesting things in it. Unfortunately, some of these "interesting things" are not very safe unless handled properly. The safety of the patients and the staff can largely be protected by organizing the OT clinic properly and by having all staff follow certain procedures.

1. *Keep track of your keys.* In some settings occupational therapy staff attach their keys to their clothing with a metal or plastic clip, a leather thong, or a spiral cord. Do not set your keys down and turn around to do something else.

2. *Make sure restricted items are not taken onto inpatient wards.* Depending on the setting, patients may not be permitted to have certain objects on the ward. Some examples include razors, belts, anything in a glass container, hair lifts, hair picks or rat-tail combs, plastic bags that are head size or larger, wire hangers, or anything breakable (1). In practical terms this means that the patient may not be able to bring some finished projects and some supplies back to his room. Examples include ceramic pieces, leather lace, yarn and cord and macramé, and cosmetics in glass containers. Any questionable items should be

discussed with nursing staff *before* they are brought onto the unit.

3. *Have everything ready before the patients arrive in the clinic or treatment area.* If the assistant has to run around finding supplies and tools and getting people started, she cannot at the same time pay attention to where all the patients are and what they are doing. For the same reason, any tools or supplies that might be needed in the course of the group should be available in the same room, in neat and accessible storage. If staff is busy rummaging through the supply cabinet, patients have ample opportunity to get in trouble. *Never leave patients from a locked ward alone and unattended.*

4. *Use shatterproof mirrors.* This solves the problem of patients hurting themselves or another person with pieces of a broken mirror, but this precaution may not be needed in every setting, depending on the patient population.

5. *Use good judgment about who is allowed to come to occupational therapy.* Patients on suicidal or elopement observation may not, in some settings, be permitted to leave the unit. Even if they are allowed to come to occupational therapy, the assistant or therapist running the activity should carefully consider the risks before permitting the patient to attend the group. Is this patient going to take so much energy and attention that the other patients will be neglected? Is this a safe activity for this particular patient? Will other staff be available close by in case there is a problem?

6. *Organize tool and supply cabinets to permit a fast, accurate count of all potentially dangerous items.* There are several ways to achieve this. Many clinics use a shadow board, in which every tool has a shadow or outline marking its place. Any tool that is missing can be identified immediately. The shadows can be cut out from brightly colored contact paper or painted on. Having patients return tools to the rack at the end of the session helps them develop good work habits and feel more responsible

and in control (4). Allen[2] recommends using transparent plastic containers for small items; these containers are available as flat, compartmented boxes, or as small standing chests of drawers. Knives and other sharp objects must be kept in locked storage.

7. *Alert patients to potential dangers in activities.* You should inform them about any materials that may cause injury, and teach them how to prevent it. For example, paper, foil, and ceramic glaze may cause cuts. A reed, dowel, or wire can cause eye injuries. Wood has splinters.

8. *Follow safety precautions for toxins.* Many of the substances used in activities can be harmful or fatal if ingested; others have been classified as carcinogens. The occupational therapy assistant should read the label of every spray can and jar in the clinic and follow the precautions indicated. It is very harmful, for example, to breathe even small amounts of the mist from hair spray, silicone spray used on tiles, and spray paint or lacquer. The fumes from magic markers and plastic dipping films and resins can cause dizziness. Most leather dyes are toxic, as are most wood finishes. Exposure to wood dust can cause allergic reactions, and prolonged or repeated exposure is associated with increased incidence of nasal cancer.[3] Some glues and their vapors are toxic. Ceramic glazes that contain lead should not be used in occupational therapy, nor should any paint containing lead (e.g., flake white oil color) or cadmium (cadmium red, etc.). Anything that might irritate the eyes or lungs (e.g., grout) should be used cautiously. Provide adequate ventilation whenever solvents or aerosol sprays are used.

Do not transfer dangerous materials to unmarked containers. Keep them in their original containers wherever possible. If a

---

[2]Allen CK. "Cognitive Disabilities. 1: Measurement and Management." Workshop given by Advanced Rehabilitation Institutes, New York, 1985.

[3]A summary of the health effects of common wood finishes and solvents is presented in Mustoe (7).

small amount is poured out for patients to use, it should be put in an appropriate container (not paper or plastic or styrofoam) and discarded after the session. Place jars and containers of all liquids toward the center of the table where they are less likely to be knocked over.

Because of the danger from accidental ingestion of toxins or carcinogens, eating, drinking, and smoking should be prohibited in areas where these supplies are used.

9. *Know and use proper safety equipment.*[4] Safety goggles, appropriate clothing, and sometimes dust masks should be worn by patients and staff using any power tool. Neoprene gloves should be worn when handling alcohols and solvents. Vapor masks should be worn when solvents are used in large quantities or for a long time (as in furniture stripping and refinishing). Eyewash kits should be available. Staff who are in a hurry may be tempted to do without safety equipment "just this once." Just this once may be one time too many; we all pick up lots of carcinogens in other ways, and it is the cumulative effect that matters; every little bit just adds to it.

Remember that some individuals may have allergies to different foods, fibers (e.g., wool), and animals. The dust from plaster and clay can be very irritating to the lungs, skin, and eyes.

10. *Observe local fire code regulations.* Flammables should be kept in a separate cabinet designed for that purpose. Fire extinguishers and fire blankets should be mounted in logical places, wherever fire or flammables are used. The occupational therapy assistant should know how to use them. Warning signs for "no smoking" and "no eating and drinking" and signs indicating the location of safety equipment should be clearly visible.[5] Doorways and fire exists should never be obstructed.

Patients should not be permitted near the ceramic kiln when it is operating. The door to the kiln should be padlocked so that no one will open it while it is on.

11. *Pay attention to the condition of the floor.* Clean up spills immediately. Highly waxed floors are often slippery and dangerous for shop and kitchen areas. It makes sense to sweep up sawdust and debris in the workshop fairly frequently; this means every half hour or so depending on the level of use.

12. *Eliminate electrical hazards.* Be sure that the current is sufficient for the demand; do not overload a circuit or use multiple-outlet plugs. Appliances with a three-prong plug need to be grounded; if there is no three-prong outlet available, do not use the appliance unless the green grounding wire is screwed into the switchplate. Make sure that electricity and water cannot come into contact with each other in the clinic. Have electrical outlets near sinks or other water sources disconnected, if necessary. Arrange for damaged cords and plugs to be repaired or replaced immediately. Be sure that electrical equipment is unplugged or switched off when leaving the clinic. This is especially important for devices that have a heating element (irons and curling irons, copper enameling kilns, and coffee makers). It is often a good idea to have a central power cutoff installed for shop areas or kitchens.

13. *Observe food safety guidelines and fire safety precautions in the kitchen.* Since the occupational therapy kitchen is used by so many staff and patients, things can get out of hand fairly quickly unless all staff take responsibility for keeping it clean and safe. Generally one person is designated to have final responsibility, and this is often the occupational therapy assistant. The refrigerator and freezer should be kept at the proper temperature. Leftover quantities of food packed in cans should be transferred to other containers and clearly marked, including the date. The refrigerator should be cleaned out once a week to discard items that have spoiled or are about to.

---

[4]Safety equipment appropriate for shops where solvents, carcinogens, and flammables are used can be obtained from Lab Safety Supply, Janesville, WI 53567-1368.

[5]These fire safety items are also available from Lab Safety Supply.

The OT kitchen should be equipped with good, thick, potholders and mitts. The oven should be well insulated to prevent accidental burns. Patients and staff should roll up their sleeves and wear aprons while working at the stove. Handles of pots should be turned in, so that they do not stick out past the edge of the stove. Patients need to be observed closely; it is not at all unusual for a patient to try to pick up something hot with a bare hand or reach into boiling water. Because patients may have poor coordination, have them set containers on a firm surface before liquids are poured into them. This is most important when the liquids are hot.

14. *Apply techniques for proper positioning, energy conservation, and work simplification, and teach these to patients.* Occupational therapy assistants generally learn these techniques in relation to persons with physical disabilities, but they are needed for *all* patients. Observe and correct the patient's body and hand position to prevent repetitive strain injuries. Provide for rest breaks. Teach patients how to be organized in their approach to a task. Refer to physical disabilities texts for particulars if you are unfamiliar with these ideas.

15. *Provide increased structure for patients at lower cognitive levels.* Be alert to the changing functional level of patients, especially those undergoing changes in medications. A patient may approach a famiiliar task with confidence and yet be a danger to himself due to cognitive impairment. Trace and Howell (10) analyze the preparation of a cup of instant coffee, citing numerous risks for unsafe behavior.

MEDICAL EMERGENCIES AND FIRST AID

Occupational therapy assistants need to know how to respond to medical emergencies whether they work in inpatient or outpatient settings. Fainting and seizures and minor cuts, burns, and contusions are the most common medical emergencies. Serious burns and wounds, fractures, poisoning, heart attacks, and strokes are less common, but still occur. The outcome of these serious conditions depends heavily upon the ability of the person nearest the scene to respond quickly and correctly.

The general rules for responding to a medical emergency are to:

1. Summon help. In inpatient settings medical staff is usually close by. In outpatient settings you may have to telephone the emergency number or the local police or hospital.
2. Remove the person from further danger. This can be done while help is being summoned.
3. Apply recommended first aid procedures. The specific procedures depend on the nature of the problem. If you do not know the proper procedures, find someone who does and wait until help arrives.

In moving the patient and applying first aid, remember and follow all universal precautions to avoid contact with bodily fluids.

Seizures

Some of the medications used to treat psychiatric disorders are associated with an increased likelihood of seizures. The occupational therapy assistant should know what a seizure looks like, and what to do if a patient has one.

The usual pattern in a seizure is for the person to become rigid and statue-like for a few seconds, and then begin to move with an all-over jerking motion. The person may void urine or feces or stop breathing, and will probably turn somewhat blue. When you notice that a patient is about to have a seizure you should:

1. Get the patient away from anything that might accidentally injure him during the seizure. Help position the patient lying down with something under his head. Remove eyeglasses. Loosen restrictive clothing.

2. *If the person's mouth is open,* place a soft object between his teeth. The purpose of this is to prevent the person from accidentally biting his tongue. A good object to use is a tongue depressor covered with several layers of gauze and then wrapped well with adhesive tape. A rolled handkerchief or other sturdy cloth object can be substituted. Do not try to force the patient's mouth open if it is shut.
3. After the jerking stops, turn the person's head to the side to allow fluids to drain from the mouth. Give artificial respiration *only if needed.*
4. Keep the person lying down. Do not give the person anything to eat or drink.
5. Get medical help.

Bleeding

Bleeding can range from relatively minor to quite serious and potentially fatal. Because sharp objects and power tools are used in occupational therapy, it is important for all staff to know how to respond to a bleeding emergency. The first goal is to stop the bleeding; it may be necessary to send someone else for help, and sometimes the only person available will be another patient. Be sure the person summoning help knows whom to contact and what to say to them. To stop the bleeding, do the following:

1. Don gloves and then apply direct pressure over the wound. Use a gauze pad or clean cloth, but if none is available use your gloved hand. Apply steady, even, firm pressure.
2. Elevate the injured part above the level of the person's heart. This slows down the flow of blood because of the force of gravity.
3. If the bleeding still does not stop, apply pressure on the artery supplying blood to that part. The pressure point for the brachial artery is on the inside of the upper arm about halfway between the el-

bow and the armpit. The pressure point for the femoral artery is in the crease of the hip joint, just to the side of the pubic bone. Use the flat part of your fingers, not the fingertips. Pressure should be applied to the artery only if direct pressure and elevation have failed to stop the bleeding.
4. *Do not* apply a tourniquet unless you have been trained to do so.

Burns

Most of the burns that occur in occupational therapy are relatively minor first-degree burns and can be treated with basic first aid procedures. Second- and third-degree burns require immediate medical attention. Because second- and third-degree burns are treated differently, and it can be difficult to tell which is which unless you have seen them before, the occupational therapy assistant should summon help when the burn has any blistering or when skin is missing or charred. For first-degree burns, where the skin is reddened but not blistered, the following should be done:

1. Rinse or soak the burned area in cold (not iced) water.
2. Cover with a Band-Aid or gauze pad.
3. *Do not* use butter or ointment.

Scalding with boiling water is a potential danger in the kitchen. If boiling water is poured on the person's clothes the first step is to remove the clothing.

Sunburn

Photosensitivity, or increased sensitivity to the sun's rays, is a side effect of some medications used to treat psychiatric disorders, and of some other common prescription medications (e.g., tetracycline). Because some occupational therapy activities may be conducted out of doors, the occupational therapy assistant needs to be aware of the medications patients are receiving. Sunburn can be prevented by having the patient wear an effective sunblock, a hat, and (if necessary) clothing with long pants and sleeves. Be sure the patient applies sunblock everywhere, especially to the shoulders, the top of the head (bald men), and the tops of the feet and backs of the hands if these are bare. Sunglasses are recommended, since the eyes are also affected by the medications.

Strains, Sprains, Bruises, and Contusions

All of these common injuries cause soft-tissue damage; blood vessels under the skin are broken and bleed into surrounding areas, but there is no external bleeding. Pain, discoloration, and swelling will result if these injuries are not treated promptly. The procedure is:

1. Apply ice. This decreases the bleeding, thus limiting the swelling, discoloration, and pain.
2. Rest the injured part. This prevents further injury.
3. Apply pressure. Wrap an elastic bandage around the injured part. The bandage should give support, yet not cut off the blood flow. A purple-blue color and numbness are signs that the bandage is too tight.
4. Elevate the injured part above the level of the heart. The force of gravity will reduce the blood flow.

PSYCHIATRIC EMERGENCIES

Elopement

The psychiatric meaning of "elopement" is much less romantic than its everyday meaning. Elopement means running away from the treatment facility without being discharged in the normal way. Patients may elope because they just don't want to be there, or because they don't want to receive treatment, or because they have something specific they want to do, like kill themselves or hurt someone else.

Preventing elopement starts with securing doors and windows. Doors should be locked except when in use. Windows should be kept closed, or if opened should have gates or window guards. Some circular lock fittings on screens or windows can be opened by using the lids of some magic markers; occupational therapy staff should be alert to this possibility when ordering supplies.

When escorting patients to and from a locked unit, the COTA should be especially careful; it is easy to "lose" a patient if your back is turned. Similarly, patients who want to escape from a locked unit may lurk by the door, waiting for an unsuspecting staff member to unlock it. Sometimes these patients are disoriented and confused and won't know where to go once they do escape; others may have a definite plan. Always look behind you to see who is nearby when you are opening a locked door. And be sure to notify nursing staff when you take patients off the ward.

Trips into the communiy present special concerns. Sometimes it is hard to determine in advance just who is likely to try to run away during a trip. Two staff members should always accompany patients from a locked unit if there are four or more patients in the group; it is best to have two staff members even with smaller groups, since one can stay with the group if the other needs to go after someone who is running away. If you are alone with a group and a patient elopes, return the other patients to the ward or to the care of a responsible staff member before going after the one who ran away.

Suicide

Some of the basic precautions for dealing with the suicidal patient have already been covered in the section on depressed patients in Chapter 11. In addition, the occupatinal therapy assistant must be alert to the possibility that the patient will try to elope from the treatment facility, and that the patient may try to remove objects from the occupatinal therapy clinic in order to use them in a later suicide attempt.

Suicidal patients who succeed in eloping from a locked inpatient unit may try to commit suicide immediately, by the first means possible (throwing themselves in front of a moving car or train, or off the roof or out of a high window). Therefore, the occupational therapy assistant should take precautions to prevent the patient from eloping. The patient must be escorted from the unit to occupational therapy alone or in a small group; no staff member can be expected to keep track of more than four patients when any of them are on suicidal observation. Depending upon the setting, and the complexity of the physical layout, it may be safe to escort only two or three patients at a time. Similarly, such patients should be excluded from community field trips. Occasionally staff from other disciplines (e.g., psychiatrists) may put pressure on the occupational therapy staff to take suicidal patients on trips; this is even more common when the patient appears to be getting better. The occupational therapist or assistant should refuse to do this if she suspects at all that the patient may be suicidal.

The occupational therapy assistant needs to be especially alert to ways in which tools and supplies can be used in a suicide attempt. The list of possible dangers is extensive: toxins (e.g., leather dyes), flammables (e.g., turpentine), sharps (needles, pins, scissors, leather knives), matches, objects that can be used in hanging (belts, yarn, leather lace) and so forth. The patient who is intent on suicide will use anything at hand; she may break a mirror or a light bulb, stick a fork in an electrical socket, or try to drown herself in the toilet. The fact that suicidal patients can use apparently harmless objects to injure themselves poses

a real problem in occupational therapy. Patients who are grossly suicidal should not be permitted off the unit or in the occupational therapy clinic. But since some patients may be more impulsive and suicidal than they appear, every precaution should be taken with patients who have any history of suicidal ideation or actual suicide attempts.

All supplies and tools should be kept under lock and key; tools (and needles, pins, matches, flammables and toxins, and items in glass containers) should be counted before patients enter the clinic, and before any of them leave. When patients have to leave the room to go to the bathroom or get a drink of water a staff member must accompany them; likewise, any sharps should be accounted for since it only takes a few minutes to bleed to death if the wound is in the right location.

Assault

Patients who are assaultive should not be seen in occupational therapy until they are properly sedated with medications; there is simply no reason to risk the safety of the other patients and the staff. However, occasionally a patient may become assaultive while in occupational therapy. Often this is an escalation of hostility; sometimes the assaultiveness could have been contained if staff had noticed the situation and responded to it more quickly (see the section on hostility in Chapter 11). At other times the assault occurs without warning, seemingly unprovoked, and frequently the patient has no memory of the incident after it occurs; patients who have abused PCP are especially prone to this.[6]

If, by any chance, the situation does get out of control and the patient strikes out at the assistant or any of the patients or ap-

---

[6] Allen CK. "Cognitive Disabilities. 1: Measurement and Management." A workshop given by Advanced Rehabilitation Institutes, New York, 1985.

pears ready to do so, the assistant should take the following steps, in order:

1. Call for more staff.
2. Remove other patients from the area.
3. Attempt to calm the patient.

If you need more staff, express this clearly. In other words, yell or scream if you must. Don't hesitate to ask a higher functioning patient to telephone or go for help. Similarly, a more competent patient can escort the others to a safe area.

Talking to the disturbed patient in a calm, soothing tone may help her calm down; if you can get the patient to talk about what's bothering her she will usually be more manageable. More staff will be needed to calm and subdue the patient if she should actually get out of control. Under no circumstances should the assistant attempt to overpower the patient. Someone experiencing psychotic rage is extremely powerful; all of her energy is directed at striking out. As many as six adult males may be required to restrain a single patient. There are two exceptions to this general rule: The assistant may be able to restrain a small child (10 years old or younger); and the assistant may feel compelled to step in if the safety of other patients is in danger. In either case the assistant should first call for more staff.

The use of restraint and force should be considered a last resort; every attempt to calm the patient by other means should be exhausted first. Because the correct use of restraint is more easily learned by demonstration and practice than by reading about it, it will not be covered in this text. Students should expect to learn restraint techniques during their fieldwork, if such techniques are needed in the setting.

If a violent incident should occur, the assistant should follow the treatment setting's procedure for reporting such incidents. Once the incident is over and the patient is calmed or removed from the scene, she should encourage other patients who may have been present to express their feelings about what has happened.

An additional set of rules applies to patients who become violent or assaultive in an outpatient setting. One of the professional staff will probably contact the police or ambulance service. Assaultive patients should not be allowed to remain in the community because they are likely to commit further violent acts.

TEACHING PATIENTS ABOUT SAFETY

Independent living in the community requires a basic knowledge and application of household and personal safety precautions, basic first aid, and emergency procedures. Helping patients master these skills is a service the occupational therapy assistant can provide. Ogren (8) suggests that health and safety skills for community living should include knowledge of emergency phone numbers, simple first aid, household safety hazards, and how and where to obtain medical care. Kartin and Van Schroeder (3) advocade, in addition, instructcion in personal safety (use of locks, how to deal with strangers) and earthquake procedures. They list sample activities for safety instruction, including making photographs or cartoons of common safety hazards, having guest speakers from fire or police departments or from the hospital or the Red Cross, and having patients list emergency numbers on an index card to keep by the telephone. Because many patients lack knowledge and judgment, education about safe sex techniques is also important. Reproducible activity sheets for reinforcing safety precautions can be found in Korb, Azok, and Leutenberg (5).

We cannot anticipate every emergency or bizarre situation that a patient may encounter and have to respond to in the community. Rote learning of specific safety procedures is not sufficient preparation for safe living in the community (12). Safety instruction must also incorporate activities that require the patient to identify problems and generate alternative responses. The occupational therapy assistant should develop the habit of clipping newspaper articles and collecting stories and anecdotes about health and safety situations a patient might run into. These can be turned into a file of paper-and-pencil activities or discussion topics.

SUMMARY

All occupational therapy staff have a legal and professional obligation to ensure the health and safety of their patients, their coworkers, and themselves. Since life is not always predictable, the occupational therapy assistant needs to acquire a habitual attitude of alertness, attention, and common sense. The goal of occupational therapy is to help patients enjoy and master the activities and skills they need to function in their lives. We need to teach patients that pleasure, comfort, and satisfaction in performing many everyday activities rely on reducing the potential for injury and infection by using appropriate safety measures.

REFERENCES

 1. Bailey DS, Cooper SO, Bailey DR. *Therapeutic approaches to the care of the mentally ill*. 2nd ed. Philadelphia: FA Davis; 1984.
 2. Confucius. The Confucian analects, bk. 4:23. In: Bartlett J, ed. *Familiar quotations*. 15th ed. Boston: Little, Brown; 1980; 463.
 3. Kartin NJ, Van Schroeder C. *Adult psychiatric living skills manual*. Kailua, Hawaii: Schroeder Publishing and Consulting; 1982.
 4. Kidner TB. The hospital pre-industrial shop. *Occup Ther Mental Health* 1982; 2(4):63–69. (Originally published in *Occup Ther Rehab* 1925; 4(3):187–194.)
 5. Korb KL, Azok AD, Leutenberg EA. *Life management skills II—reproducible activity handouts created for facilitators*. Beachwood, Ohio: Wellness Reproductions; 1991.
 6. Marcil WM. AIDS facts and implications for occupational therapy. In: Marcil WM, Tigges KN. *The person with AIDS: a personal and professional perspective*. Thorofare, NJ: SLACK; 1992.
 7. Mustoe G. Respiratory hazards—choosing the right protection. *Fine Woodworking* 1983; 41: 36–39.
 8. Ogren K. A living skills program in an acute psychiatric setting. *Am Occup Ther Assoc Mental Health Special Interest Section Newsletter* 1983; 6(4):1–2.
 9. Steich TJ. Malpractice and occupational therapy personnel. *Occup Ther News* 1985; 39(6):8.
10. Trace S, Howell T. Occupational therapy in geriatric mental health. *Am J Occup Ther* 1991; 45:833–837.
11. US Department of Labor *Universal precautions: department of labor final rule on bloodborne pathogens*. US Department of Labor; 1992.
12. Willson M. *Occupatinal therapy in long-term psychiatry*. Edinburgh: Churchill Livingstone; 1983.

ADDITIONAL REFERENCES AND SUGGESTED READINGS

American Red Cross, Handel KA. *The American Red Cross first aid and safety handbook*. Boston: Little Brown; 1992.
Bertorelli P. Keeping ten fingers—injury survey pinpoints hazards in the shop. *Fine Woodworking* 1983; 42:76–78.
McCann M. *Health hazards manual for artists*. New York: Foundation for the Community of Artists; 1978.
Southmayd W, Hoffman M. *Sports health—the complete book of athletic injuries*. New York: Quick Fox; 1981.

Occupational Therapy Process

13
Overview of the Treatment Process

Possibly, if the therapist's primary task is to help the person function in the future, then the visualization of future possibilities is an important aspect of occupational therapists' clinical reasoning.

MAUREEN HAYES FLEMING (6)

The whole idea behind occupational therapy is to help the patient develop and use the skills he needs to function as best he can within the limits of his disability. The entire treatment process is directed toward this final purpose. From the moment the occupational therapy department is first notified that the patient needs service, every action should be directed toward this end. Throughout the treatment process the patient needs to know what is being done, and why; occupational therapy staff should involve the patient and his family in making decisions about the treatment, as this is the best way to ensure that the patient will follow through with it and that it will have a lasting effect on his life.

This chapter will provide a brief overview of the treatment process, beginning with a listing and discussion of the eight stages in the process. We will describe each of these stages, explain how they are related to each other, and highlight the role of the occupational therapy assistant in each stage. We will also consider clinical reasoning, a complex cognitive and affective process by which the therapist analyzes the patient's situation and generates ideas for intervention. Although the registered therapist is responsible for controlling and

documenting the treatment process, the assistant may be delegated some of this responsibility. In addition, because the assistant has a different (often more extensive) contact with the patient, the contributions of the assistant are invaluable in determining treatment goals and direction.

EIGHT STAGES IN THE TREATMENT PROCESS

The occupational therapy treatment process begins with the referral and ends with the patient's termination from treatment. These are the first and last of the eight stages of the treatment process. The eight are referral, screening, data collection and evaluation, treatment planning, treatment implementation, reevaluation, discharge planning, and termination from treatment. The eight stages are summarized in Table 13–1, are described briefly below, and are discussed in more detail in later chapters.

The treatment process begins with the referral, which is a request for service. In most states occupational therapy services can be reimbursed only if they are initiated by an order or referral signed by a physician (4). In other words, federal and state

TABLE 13–1. *Eight stages in the treatment process*

1. REFERRAL. Occupational therapy service is requested orally or in writing. In most cases a physician's order or written referral is needed for reimbursement. The occupational therapy assistant relays the referral to the supervising OTR.

2. SCREENING. Occupational therapy staff observe the patient and/or collect information from interviews and from his medical record in order to determine whether he needs further occupational therapy evaluation and treatment. The COTA reports to the OTR and may collaborate in making recommendations.

3. DATA COLLECTION AND EVALUATION. More information about the patient is collected once it has been decided that he needs occupational therapy services. The registered therapist determines what information is needed and how to obtain it and assigns the assistant to data collection and evaluation tasks. The occupational therapy assistant may follow a structured set of questions to interview the patient or his family, and may be assigned to gather information from the patient's medical record. The assistant may carry out structured evaluation procedures.

4. TREATMENT PLANNING. Information gathered from interviews, medical records, and evaluations is analyzed to determine what the patient's problems are and how to solve them. Working with the patient, the therapist or assistant (depending on the focus of treatment) determines short- and long-term goals based on the identified problems. The occupational therapist or assistant selects the methods and specific treatment activities to be used to work toward these goals.

5. TREATMENT IMPLEMENTATION. The treatment plan is carried out. The occupational therapy assistant is often responsible for this aspect of the treatment process, involving the patient in purposeful activities designed to achieve the goals stated in the treatment plan.

6. REEVALUATION. The occupational therapist or assistant evaluates the patient again, after some of the treatment has been carried out. The purpose of reevaluation is to see whether the treatment plan is working and whether it needs to be changed.

7. DISCHARGE PLANNING. The occupational therapist works with the patient and the rest of the treatment team to make sure that the patient will be able to function to the best of his ability after he leaves the treatment setting. Discharge plans should include living arrangements, employment and leisure, and/or continuing treatment, depending on the patient's need. The occupational therapy assistant may collaborate with the therapist on the discharge plan.

8. TERMINATION OF TREATMENT. The patient is discharged from the program. His achievements in the program and his future plans are discussed. A final note is written, documenting the goals and outcome of the occupational therapy program.

medical care programs and private insurance companies will pay for occupational therapy services only if a physician has requested the service in writing. This applies to outpatient as well as inpatient settings.

An example of a referral form for an inpatient setting is shown in Fig. 13–1. The physician completes the form, indicating a problem or problems he wishes occupational therapy to address. Mayer (10) points out that occupational therapy staff sometimes need to educate physicians in how to write referral problems so that they are related to the patient's functioning. For example, "patient needs to divert mind from hypochondriacal concerns" shows the relationship between the patient's inactivity and his symptoms, whereas "patient needs

arts and crafts" does not. Some physicians prefer that the occupational therapist write the referral and submit it to the physician for his signature.

Sometimes referrals are made orally; the physician may just say that he would like the patient seen by occupational therapy. Whether the request is oral or written, the occupational therapy assistant should promptly notify his supervisor of the referral. The supervisor will then decide what role the assistant will take in the patient's evaluation and treatment. Some patients who have problems with daily living skills may not have been referred to occupational therapy; in such cases the occupational therapy assistant should initiate the referral by speaking with the doctor about the patient's need for treatment. Regardless of

Sample Referral Form

BUTLER HOSPITAL
PROVIDENCE, RI
REQUEST FOR
OCCUPATIONAL THERAPY

EVALUATION/CONSULTATION

Date of Request _____

Name _____Unit_____ ___Age_____

Physical handicaps/physical precautions _____

_____

Referral problem (s)_____ ___ _____

_____ ___ _____

Assessment Question _____

_____

Evaluation requested

_____ Bay Area Functional Performance Evaluation (BaFPE)
_____ Activities of Daily Living Evaluation (ADL)
_____ Vocation Evaluation
_____ Assessment for Occupational Therapy program
_____ Other

Requested by _____MD

_____

_____

Recommendation and action (DAP format):

FIG. 13–1. From Mayer MA. The medical referral: a tool for professional dialogue and treatment planning. *Am Occup Ther Assoc Mental Health Special Interest Section Newsletter* 1984; 7(1):2. Copyright © 1984 by the American Occupational Therapy Association, Inc. Reprinted with permission.

who initiates the referral, it must always be documented in the patient's chart.

Screening is used to determine whether or not the patient needs occupational therapy evaluation or treatment. If you have ever been to a hospital emergency room you were probably screened by the emergency room nurse. This process is sometimes called *triage;* the nurse decides how serious your problem is and either sends you home with a clinic appointment for another day, or tells you to take a seat and wait, or admits you immediately if your condition is serious. Screening in occupational therapy is similar to this. You can think of screening as a filter through which the patient must pass before he is admitted to the occupational therapy program. Not every patient needs occupational therapy, and some of those who need it may be too ill to attend until after the medication begins working.

The purpose of screening is to answer the following questions: Does this patient have any problems functioning in his daily life activities and his occupational roles? Are these problems treatable by occupational therapy? Is the patient enough in control of himself to attend occupational therapy and benefit from it? If not, should he be evaluated by occupational therapy after he receives some medication and it begins to take effect?

Screening is usually done by interview or observation of the patient, and sometimes by review of the patient's history and medical record. The occupational therapist decides what information is needed and may direct the occupational therapy assistant to collect some of it by interviewing the patient or his family, reviewing his medical record, or observing his performance in an activity and recording his behavior on a structured form such as a checklist or rating sheet. The assistant then organizes the information and reports it to the registered therapist, who makes the final decision about admitting the patient to occupational therapy.

Sometimes screening is done before the referral has been received; this is more common in short-term settings with a high turnover rate or where there are large numbers of patients but not enough occupational therapy staff to serve all of them. The supervising occupational therapist must decide who can benefit most, or who needs the service most, and then must obtain a documented referral.

In some psychiatric settings all patients are routinely referred to occupational therapy, and screening is not done. In acute inpatient settings the patients are often too symptomatic and out of control to attend occupational therapy, but the occupational therapist must still see these patients and document that they cannot be evaluated further until their symptoms subside.

Data collection and evaluation begin once it has been determined, with or without a formal screening, that the patient needs occupational therapy services. The registered therapist is responsible for this process; she decides what data are needed and may direct the assistant to interview the patient, observe the patient in activities, or administer structured evaluations and tests. Information is gathered from wherever it can be obtained—the medical record, the patient himself, his family or employer, other treatment settings, or mental health professionals who have worked with the patient in the past. Evaluations and tests are selected based upon what the patient appears to need to be able to do to function in his life.

The purpose of collecting data about the patient is to identify the specific skills and supports he needs to function effectively in his daily life activities. The purpose of evaluation is to assess the patient's current level of functioning and to identify skills and talents and interests that, if developed more, might help him function better. All evaluation procedures must be related to these

goals or they may not be reimbursable. Results of the evaluations are recorded in the patient's chart. The patient's current level of functioning is sometimes called the *baseline*. Treatment effectiveness is measured by comparing the patient's level of functioning after treatment to this baseline level. Because data collection and evaluation are covered in detail in Chapter 14 they will not be discussed further here.

Treatment planning involves identifying the patient's problems and selecting goals that are reasonable to achieve and methods to achieve them. The purpose of treatment depends upon the patient's prognosis, or the degree to which we can predict he will recover from his disability and be able to resume a normal life. We can judge whether a specific patient is likely to achieve a specific treatment goal only when we know his prognosis.

Some higher functioning patients with good prognoses will be able to develop new skills, or improve their present ones, and return to a reasonably independent life in the community. Other patients may be able to succeed in the community only if their environment and responsibilities are modified to compensate for their disabilities, and if they have family or treatment personnel to whom they can turn for support. Some patients will actually function less and less well as time goes by, but will be able to maintain their abilities longer if occupational therapy is provided.

The patient's problems are identified by analyzing the information gathered from interviews, medical records, and evaluations. The occupational therapist tries to assess the patient's potential to benefit from treatment, on the basis of his prognosis and history. This assessment is the basis for determining the general direction of intervention and for setting treatment goals. Intervention may be focused on prevention of predicted future disability; an example would be to educate a potential child abuser in other methods of controlling her child. A second possible focus is rehabilitation, or the development of necessary life skills and the underlying functions (such as cognitive skills) that support them. The patient's development of self-care or work skills is an example of rehabilitation. The third major focus is maintenance, or helping the patient keep on functioning as best he can despite his disability, even though his functioning is likely to remain the same or deteriorate because of his disease.

Once the focus of intervention has been determined, the specific goals are selected, preferably in collaboration with the patient and/or his family. At the same time that she is defining the goals, the therapist is usually thinking about the methods she will recommend be used to reach them. She knows what treatment groups, activities, and other resources are available in the treatment setting and the surrounding community and should have some ideas about how to work on the goals. She can then make recommendations and suggest alternative plans to the patient and his family.

The therapist must estimate how long it will take the patient to achieve a treatment goal. Those that will take a long time are termed long-term goals, and the therapist breaks these down into smaller steps, or short-term goals, so that the patient will see that he is accomplishing something even though his final target may be far off. Some goals do not need to be divided into steps because they are inherently short term.

The occupational therapy assistant who has been involved in the patient's evaluation will often also assist the registered therapist in developing the treatment goals. Because the assistant has considerable expertise in independent daily living skills and therapeutic activities, he is often called upon to collaborate in selecting and adapting the treatment methods. He may be assigned to explain the treatment plan to other staff, and to the patient and his family. Careful treatment planning is crucial to the ultimate outcome of treatment and will be covered in greater detail in Chapter 15.

Treatment implementation is the actual performance of the methods and activities outlined in the treatment plan. The occupational therapy assistant is often responsible for much of the actual treatment, which may be done individually or in groups, and which may use a wide variety of therapeutic media and other resources. Pelland (12) notes that students or novice therapists may occasionally fail to use the documented plan and may more often have difficulty determining which of the documented plans should be pursued first. Lack of experience with timing and with the clinical environment may also cause confusion and poor implementation. Supervision is essential at this stage.

Regardless of the specific activity or approach employed, treatment should be executed thoughtfully, with careful attention to the patient's interest in and understanding of the treatment. The occupational therapy assistant must be certain that the patient is aware of the purpose of the treatment and must help him understand why it is important to him and his life. Peloquin (13) gives suggestions as to how to assist the patient to link the activities used with their purposes. The first is to explain the purpose of the group or activity. The second is to encourage the patient to think about the purpose, and to ask him to share his view. The third is to discuss the skills used and link them to the activities or tasks performed. Finally, she recommends that the therapist summarize what has transpired. This four-step process ensures that the therapist has verbalized the purposes to the patient and has engaged the patient in understanding the purpose of the occupational therapy treatment.

Several chapters in this text are devoted to describing specific treatment activities, so only the most general aspects of treatment implementation have been discussed here. The reader is directed to Chapters 17 through 23 for more specific information.

Reevaluation is any evaluation performed after the initial evaluation. Reevaluation is usually done after some of the treatment has been performed, although it is sometimes necessary to reevaluate a patient who has not yet received any treatment; two different examples are the patient whose functioning has deteriorated since the first evaluation, and the patient who could not be properly evaluated at first because he was too symptomatic.

At first it might appear that reevaluation after successful treatment is unnecessary, a cumbersome afterthought that takes staff time away from other (treatment) activities. However, occupational therapists can prove how effective their treatment has been (and thus justify reimbursement and continued funding) only by comparing the results of the initial evaluation with those of the reevaluation. The occupational therapy assistant follows the direction of the registered therapist in carrying out reevaluation, which in all respects except timing is identical to the initial evaluation.

Discharge planning is a vital aspect of the treatment process, but one that unfortunately is often performed in a slipshod fashion because of time pressures and limitations on how long the mentally ill are allowed to remain in inpatient settings. Inadequacy of community resources to meet the needs, and underfunding of mental health services in general, make discharge planning difficult at best.

Ideally, planning for discharge should begin at admission. The questions to be addressed include: Where will the patient live, and with whom, when he is discharged? What activities will structure his day—work, leisure, self-care, organized day treatment, or a combination of these? Will the patient need additional services to carry out his daily life activities? If so, what are they? What is the best place for this patient to receive continuing treatment—an aftercare service of the hospital, a community mental health center, a home health agency? Although only the very wealthy or well-insured patient receives so extensive a discharge plan today, perhaps within

our lifetimes we will yet witness a mental health care system comprehensive enough to make this kind of discharge planning customary for every patient.

Accurate assessment of the patient's ability to function, and identification of the conditions under which he is likely to function best, are the foundation on which good discharge planning is built. The occupational therapist and assistant may be the only members of the treatment staff in a position to observe regularly how the patient performs routine tasks and how he deals with problems that arise. This information is crucial for predicting whether the patient will be able to function in the community and for identifying the degree and kind of support he will need.

Because the social worker often has final responsibility for discharge planning in many inpatient settings, occupational therapy staff may need to communicate their observations and recommendations to the social worker. The occupational therapy assistant, who is likely to have firsthand knowledge of the patient's abilities, interests, and preferences, should share this knowledge with the registered therapist and others responsible for discharge planning and may collaborate with the team on the discharge plan.

Termination of treatment is the final step in the treatment process. As discussed in Chapter 10, termination is an opportunity for the patient and the occupational therapist and assistant to review what has transpired over the course of the treatment. The patient should be helped to identify and assess his accomplishments, and to formulate goals for himself to work on in the future. Occupational therapy staff should double-check any arrangements for continuing treatment to make sure that the patient will be able to follow through on them. Finally, a discharge note must be written in the patient's chart, documenting the evaluation findings, treatment goals, and outcome of treatment, including recommendations for continuing treatment elsewhere.

Depending on the setting, some stages in the treatment process may be eliminated or deferred. Restrictions on the length of inpatient hospitalization may effectively collapse the stages of the treatment process. For example, if the patient will not be allowed to stay in the hospital for more than 14 days, it is not really possible to do anything but evaluate him and work out a good discharge plan, leaving the treatment planning and implementation to the staff of the outpatient treatment facility. Chapter 7 describes different kinds of treatment settings and the types of services the occupational therapist and assistant might provide in each of them.

The eight stages in the treatment process form a unified whole. Although they are discussed separately here, in the mind of the experienced clinical therapist they often merge together. From the moment she receives the referral information, the therapist begins to sort and analyze her knowledge of and ideas about the patient, and to weigh alternative plans for his treatment and discharge arrangements. Students and new therapists and assistants may wish to consider each stage separately at first, while they are trying to learn what happens and what to do at each stage, but they should always try to see the connections between them. For the therapist will be able to convince the patient of the importance of each stage only when he himself understands the continuity of the entire process.

CLINICAL REASONING

Faced with the task of developing a treatment plan for a psychiatric patient that the patient will find meaningful and empowering for her life, the therapist needs a logical approach to gathering information about the patient and using it to generate treatment goals and methods. Although many different approaches to organizing data and planning treatment have been presented over the years in the occupational therapy literature, until recently little has been written about how experienced and skillful clinicians approach the problem of planning treatment for patients. How does the therapist know which practice model to select, which evaluations to administer, which problems to target, and which approaches to use?

At the beginning of this chapter, we described clinical reasoning as a complex cognitive and affective process. By this we mean that clinical reasoning requires both thinking and feeling. The therapist, educated in many theories and practice models, and trained in various techniques, must consider and logically analyze which theories and methods best apply to the situation of this patient. At the same time, she must feel for the patient in his situation—she must step back from her role as therapist and step into the patient's "story." She must come to understand how his life looks to him. In her Eleanor Clarke Slagle Lecture in 1983, Rogers identified three crucial questions on which the therapist should focus. As listed and elaborated in Fig. 13–2, these questions form the core concerns of the clinical reasoning process.

The first question—What is the patient's status?—is an assessment question. Before the therapist begins to think about treatment goals and methods she must develop an understanding of who the patient is, what his problems are, what his strengths are, and how motivated he is for treatment. The therapist manages and coordinates data gathering and evaluation to obtain information to answer these questions. This is not a random process: The therapist selects from among the many evaluations available the ones she feels are most likely to yield useful results. She bases her selection in part upon facts about the patient's age, sex, diagnosis, history, and current and past occupational roles. She knows instantly, for example, that a successful 33-year-old lawyer admitted with a diagnosis of manic episode is not going to need an ac-

---

First question: What is the patient's status?
  What is the patient's occupational role status?
  What problems does he have?
  What strengths does he possess?
  What is he motivated to try?

Second question: What are the available options?
  What approaches are available?
  What outcomes are predicted for each of these? What results can we expect?
  How much time is needed to reach the objectives using each of these approaches?

Third question: What ought to be done?
  Which options are consistent with this patient's values?
  Has the patient been informed of the consequences of different treatment options and been allowed to
    choose among them?

FIG. 13–2. The focus of clinical inquiry. Adapted from Rogers JC. Eleanor Clarke Slagle lectureship 1983—Clinical reasoning: the ethics, science, and art. *Am J Occup Ther* 1983; 37:601–616.

tivities of daily living evaluation, but that a 33-year-old homeless man with a 15-year history of schizophrenia probably will. The more coherent and organized the therapist's knowledge of occupational therapy theory and methods, and the more experience she has with psychiatric patients in general and with this type of patient in particular, the more efficient and focused her assessment is likely to be.

To arrive at an answer to the second question—What are the available options?—the therapist must search her memory for knowledge and past experience that relates in any way to the patient's problem. This would include thoughts about occupational therapy theory and techniques acquired through basic or continuing education or in clinical practice, or through reading journal articles or talking with or observing other professionals. The therapist thinks about previous patients who were similar to this one, considers the outcome of the treatment they received, and tries to imagine how that treatment might work with this patient. Ultimately, the therapist generates a mental list of all possible treatments that might address this patient's problems.

The third question—What ought to be done?—focuses on the ethical aspects of treatment. As Rogers states, "Simply because a goal appears technically feasible for the patient does not mean that it should be set as a goal" (14). The patient has a right to self-determination; she has a right to design her own life as she deems best. The notion that through human occupation each person becomes what she does, and by doing shapes her own identity has always been at the core of occupational therapy (3). In other words, the patient should select her own treatment goals, and these may conflict with those the therapist would choose. Ultimately, the patient has a right to refuse treatment. Professional ethics oblige the therapist to try to persuade the patient to accept a treatment that she knows or suspects will improve the patient's condition, or without which her condition will deteriorate. This does not mean that she will accept the plan, or that she can be made to do so. Whatever we may feel about society's obligation to the mentally ill, legal and constitutional protections guarantee them the right to refuse treatment when they are not an immediate danger to themselves or others.

More recently, the AOTA and the AOTF

(American Occupational Therapy Foundation) have sponsored a Clinical Reasoning Study, seeking to specify and examine in detail the reasoning processes of experienced occupational therapists (1, 2, 5, 6, 7, 8, 9, 15, 16). Fleming (5) suggests that experienced therapists shift easily among three reasoning tracks. *Procedural reasoning* applies to the disability and the treatment options. For example, thoughts about the patient's diagnosis of schizophrenia, its long-term implications of diminished functioning, and the possible treatment interventions (sensory integration, psychosocial club approach, etc.) are considered procedural. *Interactive reasoning* applies to understanding and relating to the patient as an individual. This reasoning track focuses on the relationship with the patient, with communicating receptivity and acceptance for his needs and concerns. *Conditional reasoning* includes the larger context, the "what if" brainstorming of events that might change the current conditions, and the need for the patient to participate. This involves the use of imagination to create mental scenarios of what might happen if a given approach were tried, to create a picture of what the patient's life might have been like before the onset of illness, to see a future vision of what is possible for him.

The cultivation of hope is a critical element in the treatment process. Mattingly (7) describes the use of the narrative method, which involves telling a story that will capture interest and spark confidence in the patient. This may require the creation of a context in which boring and repetitive tasks can be seen as a kind of game, for example. Another way to nurture optimism and motivation is to specifically and concretely link the present task to a future vision of the patient's life.

The process of clinical reasoning described above is a continuous one; ideas about what needs to be assessed, and how, and what treatment methods are possible and which ones to choose are constantly being generated in the therapist's mind, from the moment the patient is first referred until she is finally discharged. The occupational therapy assistant collaborates with the registered therapist in this process of clinical inquiry by helping to gather data, to generate treatment alternatives, and to recommend treatment choices based on knowledge of the patient's needs and values. Although not finally responsible for the treatment plan, the assistant attempts, like the therapist, to observe the patient carefully and objectively, to formulate questions and hypotheses about her, and to develop treatment options.

The role of the occupational therapy assistant in the clinical reasoning process has not been addressed in the literature. This is unfortunate, as the assistant is positioned close to the patient in the treatment situation and for this reason often has access to information not shared with staff who spend less time with the patient. The assistant is most likely to have a more complete version of the patient's "story," based on numerous meetings and much time spent together. Often, the assistant is viewed by the patient as less threatening, and more on an equal level, in contrast to the authoritative position accorded other staff. This perceived equalization of status may engage the patient to share information he might withhold (intentionally or not) from the registered therapist or from the doctor or social worker. For the same reason, suggestions made by the assistant are taken a little differently by the patient, and may be more easily accepted and enacted. Occupational therapy assistants need to recognize, cultivate, and tap their power to clarify and contribute to the clinical reasoning process.

SUMMARY

In this chapter, the treatment process has been presented as a sequential one, with eight discrete stages. In practice, these stages blur together at times, as the therapist and assistant explore different options for understanding and helping the patient. Using clinical reasoning, we try to understand the patient's problems from his point of view. We try to learn how he sees things, and to envision the world he would like for himself, even if he is not ready to see it clearly. We mentally review the various possibilities for treatment approaches and try to imagine how the patient might react. This requires a back-and-forth process of gathering new data even while we are proceeding with treatments planned on the basis of data previously collected. In this sense, treatment is not so much like a path with a clear-cut beginning and ending, but more like an expanding network of possibilities that we explore together with the patient.

REFERENCES

1. Cohn ES. Clinical reasoning: explicating complexity. *Am J Occup Ther* 1991; 45:969–971.
2. Crepeau EB. Achieving intersubjective understanding: examples from an occupational therapy treatment session. *Am J Occup Ther* 1991; 45:1016–1025.
3. Fidler GS, Fidler JW. Doing and becoming: purposeful action and self-actualization. *Am J Occup Ther* 1978; 32:305–310.
4. Fine SB. *Occupational therapy: the role of rehabilitation and purposeful activity in mental health practice.* Rockville, MD: American Occupational Therapy Association; 1983.
5. Fleming MH. The therapist with the three-track mind. *Am J Occup Ther* 1991; 45:1007–1014.
6. Fleming MH. Clinical reasoning in medicine compared with clinical reasoning in occupational therapy. *Am J Occup Ther* 1991; 45:988–996.
7. Mattingly C. The narrative nature of clinical reasoning. *Am J Occup Ther* 1991; 45:998–1005.
8. Mattingly C. What is clinical reasoning? *Am J Occup Ther* 1991; 45:979–986.
9. Mattingly C, Gillette N. Anthropology, occupational therapy, and action research. *Am J Occup Ther* 1991; 45:972–978.
10. Mayer MA. The medical referral: a tool for professional dialogue and treatment planning. *Am Occup Ther Assoc Mental Health Special Interest Section Newsletter* 1984; 7(1):1–2.
11. Neistadt ME. The classroom as clinic: applications for a method of teaching clinical reasoning. *Am J Occup Ther* 1992; 46:814–819.
12. Pelland MJ. A conceptual model for the instruction and supervision of treatment planning. *Am J Occup Ther* 1987; 41:351–359.
13. Peloquin SM. Linking purpose to procedure during interactions with patients. *Am J Occup Ther* 1988; 42:775–781.
14. Rogers JC. Eleanor Clarke Slagle lectureship 1983—Clinical reasoning: the ethics, science, and art. *Am J Occup Ther* 1983; 37:601–616.
15. Rogers JC, Holm MB. Occupational therapy diagnostic reasoning: a component of clinical reasoning. *Am J Occup Ther* 1991; 45:1045–1053.
16. Schwartz KB. Clinical reasoning and new ideas on intelligence: implications for teaching and learning. *Am J Occup Ther* 1991; 45:1033–1037.

14

Data Gathering and Evaluation

It is not only by the questions we have answered that progress may be measured, but also by those we are still asking. The passionate controversies of one era are viewed as sterile preoccupations by another, for knowledge alters what we seek as well as what we find.

FRIEDA ADLER (1)

Any plan for treatment is only as good as the information on which it is based. We have to learn how the patient is functioning now and how he has functioned in the past if we are to help him function better in the future. Only when this information is accurate and reasonably complete will we be able to see what problems the patient is faced with, and what strengths and talents he possesses to cope with them. Only then can we begin to consider how to help him improve or maintain his ability to deal with his problems and get on with his life.

This chapter will describe the kinds of information occupational therapists and assistants usually collect about patients with mental health problems. It will discuss the purpose of evaluation and explore some of the concepts used to organize information once it is gathered. It will contrast the roles of the registered occupational therapist and the occupational therapy assistant and explain how to gather data by looking at medical records, observing the patient, administering evaluations, and interviewing the patient and others who know him.

Methods for recording and reporting information will also be discussed. Selected occupational therapy interviews and evaluations will be described in detail, including

the purpose of each evaluation and how to administer it. Some standardized tests and other less commonly used evaluations a COTA might be asked to administer to patients will also be described.

THE PURPOSE OF EVALUATION

Evaluation is the planned process of collecting and interpreting information gathered by observation, interview, review of medical records, and testing (4). The word "assessment" is used instead of "evaluation" in official documents of the American Occupational Therapy Association. While the meanings of the two terms are slightly different, for the purposes of this chapter we will use them interchangeably.

The main purpose of evaluation in psychiatric occupational therapy is to find out what things the patient needs or wants to be able to do, and whether or not he can do them. If he cannot do the things he needs and wants to do, the occupational therapist wants to know why not, and whether he might be able to do them if some changes were made. Although procedures vary depending on the setting, the type of patients, and other factors, in general evaluation seeks to answer the following questions:

What activities and occupational roles is the patient expected or required to perform?

What skills and habits are needed to carry out these activities and roles?

Which of these skills does the patient have already?

Which ones has he had in the past, but stopped using for one reason or another?

Which ones has he never developed?

What are this patient's interests? What values and goals does he want to pursue? What else motivates him?

To what extent is it possible for him to develop skills he has never had or redevelop ones he has stopped using?

What aspects of the environment facilitate or interfere with his ability to use his skills? What environmental modifications can help him function better?

What has been the effect of the patient's illness on his functioning, as he experienced it? What is the prognosis?

We could go on listing questions for several more pages, but these summarize the main points. It may help to return to this list later when you actually participate in evaluating a patient.

ASSETS AND DEFICITS

The purpose of all data collection and evaluation, as stated previously, is to find out how the patient has functioned in the past and how he is functioning now. We want to know what kinds of things he needs to be able to do in order to manage his daily activities and to carry out his occupational roles. Only when we know what the patient needs and wants to be able to do does our evaluation of what he can and cannot do have any meaning.

To appreciate this point, look at the following descriptions of behavior. Try to figure out whether each is an asset (strength) or a deficit (problem). An *asset* is a useful, adaptive behavior, one that helps the patient get what he needs and carry out his daily life activities. A *deficit* is a behavior that interferes with him meeting his needs and doing the things he needs and wants to do:

1. He didn't listen to the directions. He just went ahead on his own.
2. She stared out the window during the lecture.
3. She always wears tailored suits to work.
4. He praised each child who finished the block design puzzles.

How did you classify these behaviors, as assets or as deficits? Most people would say that the first two are deficits and the second two are assets. But is this always true? In the first example, the man may have already known the directions; in that case, didn't it show initiative for him to proceed on his own? In the second example, isn't it possible that the woman already knew the information in the lecture, or that she was thinking over a point the lecturer had made?

A woman who wears tailored suits would be appropriately dressed for many jobs. If she were a lawyer, banker, or sales executive, that is the way she would be expected to dress. However, if she were a special education teacher or an occupational therapist working with children with multiple handicaps, dressing this way would make it difficult for her to do her job. Similarly, praising a child who has done something well encourages him to keep trying and to do new things, and is a desirable behavior in a teacher or therapist. On the other hand, when a psychologist is testing a child's intelligence he is supposed to follow the test instructions exactly, and is not supposed to add to them or alter them. Praising the child may change the results of the test.

As all of these examples illustrate, a given behavior may be an asset or a deficit, depending upon a person's life situation and occupational and social roles. Of course, some behaviors are almost always deficits, regardless of context. Very poor hygiene and grooming can only interfere with getting along with other people socially or on the job. There are other behaviors that are almost always assets: for example, cooperating with others. In general, however, we need additional information about the patient before we decide which of his behaviors are deficits and which are assets.

Some of the basic information that can clarify whether a behavior is an asset or a deficit are the patient's age, sex, family situation, education, occupation, work history, leisure habits and history, self-care habits, social relationships, and cultural background. Information about the patient's interests, goals, and values may further define what he feels is important. His diagnosis, prognosis, and prescribed medications must also be known because they may affect what he is able to do in the future.

CONCEPTS CENTRAL TO THE EVALUATION PROCESS

All of the information we have listed so far consists of many small and interrelated facts, which are sometimes better understood and organized by using the concepts of life space, social support, life-style, and expected environment.

Life space is the interaction among the individual's cultural group membership, interests and value orientation, and physical and psychological environment. It is important to know the patient's cultural group because each group has its own values and heritage of "normal" behavior. For example, a 28-year-old mother of two may be expected to behave differently depending on whether her background is Cuban, Jamaican, Italian, Norwegian, Jewish, or Hindu. Her cultural group membership may dictate whether it is acceptable for her to have a career outside the home, to wear pants, or to go shopping on Saturdays (or Sundays).

An individual's interests and values may be a reflection of his cultural group or may be in conflict with it. Sometimes the person's family or cultural group pressures him into abandoning his natural interests and values. We saw an example of this in the case of David (Chapter 2), whose childhood interest in sports and games was discouraged by his parents.

The remaining aspect of life space is the person's physical and psychological environment. This includes *all* of the environments he passes through or is exposed to in his daily life activities. Does he live in the city or the country, alone or with other people, in a house or an apartment? On a psychological level, is his neighborhood clean, safe, and pleasant, or dirty, dangerous, and frightening? Are there parks and recreation facilities nearby? Does he live near friends and family, or is he relatively isolated? How much of his neighborhood does he know and use? If he works, what is his work environment like? What kinds of environments does he pass through on his way to and from work?

The interrelationships between a person's cultural group membership, interests and value orientation, and environment are often complex. One way to experience this interrelatedness of life space is to think about how your life would be different if you moved your home to a different location. How would you travel to school? What would you do in your spare time, and with whom, and where? How far would you have to walk to the grocery store, dry cleaner, handball court, swimming pool, park, or church? Would you be able to keep in touch with your old friends? Where and how would you meet new ones?

Life space influences what you are able to do and what you *have* to do. For example, some people who live in cities prefer not to own automobiles because they believe they waste energy and pollute the environment. However, if one of these people were forced to move to the country he would probably have to buy a car, just to get around. If the nearest supermarket is eight miles away and there is no public transportation, there really is not much choice. Valuing the environment so much that you refuse to drive a car would be a deficit. Many times, behaviors that are assets in one life space are deficits in another, and vice versa.

People who have immigrated to the United States from other parts of the world may find that their traditions and cultural values seem out of place. They are faced with difficult conflicts and choices about how much they will become involved with American culture, and how strongly they will cling to their own cultural traditions. To a lesser extent this is also true of second- and third-generation Americans.

Watanabe (38) points out that occupational therapists must study not only what the patient's life space is like, but also how much of the available life space he uses. For example, the person who stays indoors, watching television and reading most of the time and venturing out only to do routine and predictable chores, is using very little of the life space accessible to him. He is ignoring social and recreational opportunities nearby. He has restricted his world to a small corner of the real world that is out there.

Occupational therapists are concerned also with the *social support* available to the patient in his environment. Social support is the way in which and the extent to which relationships with other people facilitate the patient's meeting his needs and carrying out his daily activities. For example, the chronic schizophrenic who lives with his parents in a ranch house in a middle-class suburb has a very different social support system from a chronic schizophrenic who lives in a single-room occupancy hotel in a big city and has no contact with his family.

Along with the patient's life space and social support, we also need to know about her *life-style*. Life-style refers to the way the person allocates her time and energy in activities of self-care, work, rest, and lei-

sure. How does she budget her time among these various activities? How much does she sleep or watch television? Does she schedule time for leisure and play activities? How much time does she spend on self-care and homemaking?

Research has shown that life-style has a measurable effect on health. For example, competitive and hardworking people tend to develop heart disease more frequently than other people. However, this may not be true for every individual, and occupational therapists and assistants should be cautious about imposing their own values about the balance of work and leisure on their patients.[1]

The way time is allocated among activities is only one aspect of life-style; how and why the person pursues each activity is equally important, as the following example illustrates:

> Ms. F., an architect, is at the top of her field. Her designs have won top honors in major competitions. Ms. F.'s major leisure interest is tennis. She is an excellent player and frequently wins local tournaments. She follows a daily exercise program to train and develop her muscles for tennis. She says that she wishes she could see more of her friends and family but feels her schedule won't permit it.

Ms. F. seems to work as hard in her "leisure" as she does in her job. Both are highly competitive and stressful. She seems to thrive on this, and Ms. F.'s drive and discipline are assets to her in both areas. There isn't much variety in her activities, however. Everything seems to revolve around work and tennis. Ms. F. would probably feel a failure in either area very deeply, because she has nothing to balance them. Consider, for example, how Ms. F. might react to an automobile injury that left her dominant side partially paralyzed.

In addition to general background information about the patient, his occupational

---

[1] Allen CK. "Cognitive Disabilities. 1: Measurement and Management." Workshop given by Advanced Rehabilitation Institutes, New York, 1985.

roles, his life space, and his life-style, it helps to know what kind of environment the patient will be going to after he is discharged. This is sometimes called the *expected environment* (32). Some few patients will be transferred to another inpatient facility. Others will go to halfway houses, board and care homes, single-room occupancy hotels, community residences, or supervised apartments. A few will find new apartments on their own, and some will return to their homes. When the expected environment is different from the previous environment, the patient's life space changes, and sometimes he needs to develop new skills or to change the way he does everyday activities. Someone who will be living on his own for the first time (even in a supervised apartment) will need to be able to care for his own clothes, budget his money, and manage other self-care tasks.

To summarize, the main purpose of evaluation is to assess to what extent the patient is able to carry out his daily life activities and occupational roles with a sense of purpose, pleasure, and competence. Which of his present behaviors are assets and which deficits can only be determined when the patient's life space, social support, life-style, and expected environment are considered.

ROLES OF THE REGISTERED OCCUPATIONAL THERAPIST AND THE OCCUPATIONAL THERAPY ASSISTANT

It is important to understand the interrelated roles of the OTR and the COTA during the evaluation of the patient. The registered therapist has final responsibility for obtaining and interpreting the information needed to plan treatment. She decides what information is needed, and how to get it (3).

The registered therapist identifies the areas that need to be evaluated. For a patient with mental health problems the relevant areas might include activities of daily living, psychosocial and cognitive skills, work skills (including homemaking and child care), play and leisure skills, academic skills, sensory integrative skills, and skills needed to relate to others alone or in a group (3, 4). Other areas may be assessed, depending upon the theory that the therapist is following. For example, in the model of human occupation, over 60 different evaluations are available to examine factors as diverse as the patient's locus of control (sense of self-control versus control by others or by fate) and environmental press (degree and kind of stimulation and demands from the patient's environment). Patients who have, or who are suspected to have, physical limitations need to be evaluated in these areas too.

The occupational therapist chooses the methods she will use to obtain the information she needs, and she explains her evaluation plan to the patient, to his family (where relevant), and to other health professionals involved with the patient. She may carry out all of the evaluation herself or assign parts of it to the occupational therapy assistant.

Before assigning any part of the evaluation to the certified occupational therapy assistant, the registered therapist must feel confident that the COTA would obtain the same or very similar results to what the OTR would obtain, using the same evaluation instrument. This is known as *establishing service competency* (3). Service competency can be established by using standardized or criterion-referenced tests and comparing the results obtained by the COTA with those obtained by the OTR. (A criterion-referenced test provides clear descriptions for performance for each rating.) Another way to establish service competency is to have raters view and rate the same videotaped performance. The OTR is responsible for the evaluation and for assisting the COTA to develop service competency in areas that will be delegated. The COTA is responsible for making sure

that she has established service competency in a given instrument before undertaking independent use of the instrument.
The COTA should also indicate areas in
which she feels she could easily develop
service competency, given sufficient training.

When the evaluation is completed, the
therapist organizes, analyzes, and interprets the information. She summarizes the
patient's assets (strengths) and deficits
(problems), and reports this in an initial
evaluation note, which becomes part of the
patient's medical record. She bases her plan
of treatment on the initial evaluation and
uses it to make recommendations about
other services that might benefit the patient. Because the evaluation is the foundation of the rest of the treatment process,
it is extremely important that it be as accurate and complete as possible. Often, because of an extremely short hospital stay,
the evaluation is less complete than the
therapist would like; more thorough evaluation is possible in outpatient settings
where patients may be seen over a longer
period.

The role of the COTA in evaluation is to
collect data as directed by the OTR (3, 27).
The OTR decides what methods and procedures the COTA should use. Experienced
COTAs may be given more responsibility
for selecting evaluation methods in some
areas, such as daily living skills. All evaluation methods performed by the COTA are
structured; each has a definite procedure
and is performed the same way each time it
is administered. The COTA gathers the information, performs the evaluations, and
records her observations. She then organizes the information she has collected and
reports it to the OTR. The report may be
oral or written, depending upon the requirements of the setting. Finally, the COTA
may be assigned to record this information
in the patient's medical chart or report it to
other professionals working with the patient.

THE COTA'S METHODS AND AREAS OF DATA COLLECTION

Once she has established service competency on the particular interview protocol (outline), the COTA may be asked to interview the patient, a family member, or
someone else who knows the patient well.
An interview is a conversation between the
evaluator and someone else, the purpose of
which is to find out more about the patient.
The COTA might interview to obtain information about the patient's self-care habits
and skills, his academic history, vocational
history, play history, social skills, interpersonal relationships, occupational roles, and
leisure interests and experiences.

Observation is a method of collecting information by watching what a person does.
The COTA may also be assigned to observe the patient as he performs activities,
in order to help collect information about
his:

1. Activities of daily living skills (grooming, eating, dressing, travel, communication, and ability to use common objects like keys)
2. Work skills (task skills such as neatness,
   attention to detail, rate of performance,
   etc.)
3. Sensorimotor skills (including coordination and sensory awareness)
4. Cognitive skills (orientation, concentration, attention span, memory, etc.)
5. Psychosocial skills (self-expression and
   self-control, and ability to relate to others individually or in a group).

The COTA might also be directed to administer standardized or criterion-referenced
evaluations and tests to assess the patient's
daily living skills, gross and fine coordination, tactile awareness, and orientation (3).
Such evaluations and tests are designed to
be given in a highly specific way; the instructions are spelled out, and the person
administering the evaluation is expected to
follow them exactly. Procedures for admin-

istering and scoring this type of evaluation will be discussed later in this chapter.

REVIEW OF MEDICAL RECORDS

The occupational therapy assistant may be asked to collect some or all of the following information about the patient: age, sex, family situation, education, occupation, work history, leisure habits and history, self-care habits, social relationships, cultural background, diagnosis, medical history, psychiatric history, current medications, and medication history. Looking in the patient's medical record is one quick and reasonably accurate way to obtain this information. In inpatient settings the patient's chart is usually kept at the nurse's station. Many people use the charts, and so the assistant may find that they are not always available when she wants them, especially in short-term settings. She will also need to cooperate in sharing charts with other staff. Charts should not be removed from the nursing station unless specific permission is given by the nurse in charge.

Many medical charts are divided into sections; this is helpful in locating specific records about the patient, since the reader can ignore lab results and other sections that are not relevant. The information an assistant is assigned to collect is often found in the admitting note and the social worker's history on the patient. The admitting note is written by the person who admits the patient to the hospital; it includes facts about why the patient was admitted, what she was acting like at the time of admission, her tentative diagnosis, any known medical or psychiatric history, and her age, sex, occupation, and family background. The social worker's history will include more details about the patient's family and occupation, her education, cultural background, financial situation, and habits. The nurses' notes over the past few days give information about how the patient has

been functioning in the hospital and how she has adjusted to hospitalization (whether she is sleeping, eating, socializing with others, etc.). The doctor's notes may indicate changes in diagnosis or medication. Records from past hospitalizations, if available, will often yield more detail about the patient's history and the success of various treatments that have been attempted. Reports on psychological and neurological testing, if available, can be valuable also, but may contain complex scientific information and thus should be read by the registered therapist rather than the assistant. Finally, any occupational therapy notes or goals or evaluation information from previous admissions may provide details that will prevent needless repetition of past procedures.

The OTR who assigns the assistant to gather data from the patient's chart will specify what kinds of information she wants. For example, she might want to know only the education, work history, and previous living situation. In general, when assigned to find specific information, the assistant should ignore everything else, regardless of how interesting it is (e.g., that the patient believes he is a special agent of the KGB). However, she should stay alert for information that might help the OTR with the patient's evaluation and treatment plan (e.g., that the patient's four most recent admissions occurred after he ran out of his medication). Any information about precautions (dietary, medical, suicide, or elopement risk) should always be noted.

INTERVIEWING

Besides looking in the medical record, the other way to gather information about the patient is to interview her or someone who is close to her. The idea of learning how to interview from reading a book is like trying to learn to swim by listening to a radio talk show about it. The best ways to learn interviewing are to watch someone who is good at it, analyze the process, and try it yourself. It helps to practice in school, with your classmates and friends, and to have yourself videotaped so that you can see how you come across. Some concepts of communication in the therapeutic relationship were discussed in Chapter 10. These are meant to be a foundation for all phases of the treatment process, starting with screening and evaluation. It will help to review these concepts before attempting your first interview.

All of the interviews the assistant will be assigned to conduct are structured or semistructured. Both types of interviews consist of sets of questions, which are to be asked in a given order. In a structured interview, the interviewer is supposed to stick to the questions as they are given. In a semistructured interview, the questions may be rephrased and more questions added. The purpose of this is to get more details and more information. During the training phase in which you establish service competency, you will learn whether you can change the wording, or add or skip questions.

You may be asked to give the interview to the patient, a member of his family, or someone else who is very familiar with his daily activities (e.g., the operator of the community residence where he lives). The patient himself may not give accurate information; he may not be able to assess his own behavior objectively, or remember necessary facts, or be willing to tell you the truth. Someone else may be a more reliable informant. A *reliable informant* is someone who knows the situation, can think and communicate, and is willing to talk. It obviously makes sense to get the information from someone who is able to give it.

Prepare for the interview by selecting a comfortable environment in which to conduct it. The room should be private, quiet, and well ventilated, have comfortable seating, and be free of distracting stimuli. Do not neglect general safety precautions about being alone with patients and having help available. The interviewer should have the necessary interview form, pencils or pens, and a watch or clock, and should set aside enough time to cover the information in the interview. The amount of time needed depends on the number of questions and the attention span of the person being interviewed. The interviewer should review the patient's medical record to find any facts that pertain to the interview. The patient should not be asked to provide the same information twice, unless there is a good reason for this.

The interviewer should pay attention to what the patient is saying, and his behavior should communicate this listening attitude. If the interviewer is physically relaxed, seated comfortably, and able to move freely, he will be more comfortable and thus more receptive to the patient. Making eye contact with the patient and leaning forward to show interest will also convey receptivity. Eye contact should be varied and one should avoid staring, however.

One of the hardest skills to acquire is knowing when to comment, and what to say. It helps to think of the patient as telling a story that you are interested in. Then your comments and questions will flow naturally. Try not to change the subject or interrupt the patient when he is speaking. Remember that periods of silence may help the patient collect his thoughts.

Being aware of yourself is very important for good interviewing. You have to be in touch with what you are communicating and what you are feeling about the patient. Any prejudices you have about the patient will impair your ability to really listen. If, for example, you believe that the patient is a derelict who will never amount to anything, you are probably not going to be too receptive to any strengths he might have. Or if you think the patient is too smart and good-looking to have any problems, then you might not recognize some that he does have.

Start any interview by saying hello, and introducing yourself if you do not already know the patient. Always explain the purpose of the interview. Think of it from the patient's point of view. Why should he tell you anything, especially some of the painful or shameful or difficult things you might ask him about? Make the patient comfortable before you start asking him questions. Shaw presents the following contrasting situations at the beginning of an interview:

1. The client enters the office: you remain seated, nonverbally indicating where the client should sit. You then begin to question him about his work history.
2. The client is waiting in the clinic; the therapist approaches and introduces himself. The therapist invites the client into the office and suggests that he might be comfortable in a particular chair. The interview is formally opened with an explanatory statement regarding the purpose of the interview (37, p. 28).

Obviously, the second situation will make most patients more comfortable and help them talk. Putting yourself in the patient's position can help you figure out what you need to do to make him comfortable.

The next stage in the interview involves asking questions in order to obtain specific information. This part of the interview is most successful if the interviewer embodies the techniques and qualities described in Chapter 10. He should be especially observant of the patient's behavior, facial expression, tone of voice, and body language. More detail on what and how to observe will be given later in this chapter.

During the interview you will need to take notes; try to keep them to a minimum, jotting down only key facts and phrases. Allot some time for yourself after the interview to go back and fill in the missing information. Discuss with the patient the fact that you need to write notes in order to be accurate about important details.

Peloquin (34) recommends that the interviewer use part of the time to help the patient develop a *therapy set*, an understanding of occupational therapy generally and how it will benefit the patient specifically. For example, the depressed homemaker who has had difficulty getting things done might be told that the activity program in the hospital will help her become accustomed to a routine and give her opportunities to learn new ways of doing things or to practice old ones. The COTA should follow the direction of the registered therapist with regard to helping patients develop a therapy set.

End the interview by indicating that it is over; this is easiest if you prepare the patient at the beginning of the interview by telling him how long the interview will take. It is not always easy to bring an interview to a close, especially if you are afraid of insulting the patient by cutting him off. Let the patient know that he has given you the information you need (if this is so). Encourage the patient to ask you any questions he may have, and try to answer them. Do not try to interpret or analyze the interview for him; tell him that you and the OTR need time to review what he has told you. Set a time for your next meeting, if there is to be one, or inform the patient about what will happen next (that he will see the OTR, or that he will attend an evaluation group, for example).

One of the semistructured interviews the assistant might be asked to conduct is the *Occupational History* developed by Linda Moorhead (31). As adapted here (Fig. 14–1), the Occupational History consists of 74 questions divided into sections corresponding to major occupational roles (worker, student, homemaker, playing child, etc.). The patient is asked only those questions that pertain to his life situation. For example, if the patient is a student, the section on the homemaker role would be omitted (unless the student is also a homemaker), and if the patient had no living relatives nearby, questions 60 and 66 would not be asked. Moorhead suggests that the interviewer rephrase questions and probe for

---

The Occupational History Interview

A. Occupational Role—Career Pattern and Satisfaction
  1. What kind of work do you do? What kind of duties does that include?
  2. Do you have special training for this job?** How did you get your training?
  3. Where do you work? How do you get there?**
  4. How long have you worked there? Have your assignments been the same or have they changed during that time?
  5. How and why did you choose your present job?
  6. What things do you particularly like about your work?
  7. What things do you not like about your work?
  8. In doing your job, do you work alone or with other people?
  9. What are the people like that you work with? Are you friendly with them? Do you socialize with them outside your work?**
 10. Is there someone directly in charge of your work? Does he/she supervise you closely? What kind of a person is he/she to work for?
 11. How is your work organized? Do you decide when and how to do things, or does your supervisor?
 12. Is your salary adequate? What do you do with the money you earn?**
 13. How do you feel about your chances of getting ahead (advancement) in your job?
 14. What other kinds of work have you done? Will you tell me what those jobs were like?
 15. What were your reasons for each change in job?

B. School Roles
 16. What is your education? What was your major area of study?
 17. What kind of grades did you get in school?**
 18. What did you like best about school?
 19. Are there things you disliked about school? What?
 20. What did you think of your teachers? Did you have any favorites?

C. Peer Group Roles
 21. What were your spare time interests during your school years?
 22. What kinds of things did you do with friends while in school?
 23. Did you prefer to do things alone, with one or two friends, or with a large group of friends?

D. Family Roles
 24. What did you want to be when you were a child?
 25. What education did your parents have?
 26. What are (were) your parents occupations? What sorts of jobs are they? Did your father like his work? Did your mother like her work?
 27. Did your parents have any influence on your choice of career?

E. For Student—as a Major Life Role (Follow this sequence for asking questions: ask this section first, then go back to questions 21–27, then continue with questions 57–74.)
 28. What school do you attend?
 29. Have you changed schools much? Have you moved much from school to school or have you stayed in the same geographical area?
 30. What is your major field of study?
 31. What are the things you like best about school?
 32. Are there things you dislike about school? What are they?
 33. What kinds of grades do you get in school?
 34. Do you have any favorite teachers? Why are they your favorites? Can you describe them?
 35. Are there teachers you dislike? Can you describe them?
 36. What kinds of things do you do with your classmates who are friends outside of school?

FIG. 14–1. The Occupational History Interview. Questions are based on Moorhead's (31) original instrument. Questions marked with asterisks are suggested by Cynkin's (16) version of the occupational history. Copyright © 1969 by the American Occupational Therapy Association, Inc. Reprinted with permission.

37. What are your interests in your spare time?
38. What are you most interested in now? What are you good at?
39. What are your plans for further education?
40. What do you want to do when you finish school?
41. What are your responsibilities at home? Do you have certain chores to do?
42. Do you have enough spending money? How do you get your spending money (allowance, job, etc.)?
43. What ideas have you had about what you want to do when you are an adult?

F. For Housewife or Homemaker—as a Major Life Role (Follow this sequence in asking questions: ask this section first, followed by questions 16–27, then questions 57–74.)

44. Describe your average day's activities. What time does work begin? What is your schedule? Do you have children? How many? What ages?
45. What part of your work as a homemaker do you enjoy most?
46. Does your family seem to appreciate your efforts?
47. Are there things that you dislike about your work? What?
48. Do you receive any help with your work?
49. Do you visit with other homemakers in your neighborhood?
50. How did you learn to do your job? Who taught you? Would you say your mother was a good homemaker?
51. Do you think homemakers in general have a happy life? If not, why not?
52. If you could choose between being a homemaker and doing something else, what would you choose?
53. Have you ever been employed? What kind of job did you have? When was this? And how did you like it?
54. What are your plans for the future? (If applicable: What will you do when your children are grown and you have more spare time?)
55. Describe an average day (a recent day before hospitalization or onset of disability):
    a. What time do you get up?
    b. What do you do in the morning?
    c. What do you do in the afternoon?
    d. What do you do in the evening?
    e. What time do you go to bed?
56. What do you do about meals? Do you prepare them yourself? What kinds of food do you serve?

G. General Questions

57. Where do you live? Do you live with others, alone, in a boarding house, etc.? (Omit question if answer is known. Instead ask about neighborhood.)
58. Do you have time to do things that are fun?
59. What kinds of things are fun to you?
60. What kinds of things do you and your family do together?
61. Are there things you would like to do in your spare time that you don't do now?
62. Do you attend any sports events or enjoy observing them?
63. Are there any sports you particularly enjoy participating in?
64. Do you look forward to vacations?
65. How do you spend your vacations?
66. Do you have relatives you get together with fairly often?
67. Do you have any especially good friends you see often? How often?
68. How did you meet them?
69. What kinds of things do you do together?
70. Do you enjoy reading? What do you read?
71. Do you enjoy watching television? What kinds of things do you watch? How much time do you spend watching TV?
72. Do you have any hobbies or other special interests?
73. Do you belong to any clubs, church groups, or other organizations? What kinds of things do you do there?
74. How do you spend your weekends?

FIG. 14–1. *(Continued)*

more information to obtain sufficiently detailed answers.

Many of the questions in the interview are designed to help the patient identify and express his feelings about activities he has performed now and in the past. For example, questions 5, 6, 7, 13, and 15 focus on the patient's feelings about his work. Questions 18, 19, 20, and 23 ask about the patient's childhood and early schooling. These feelings and attitudes help in analyzing the patient's strengths and weaknesses as he perceives them. For example, he may state that he dislikes his work because he does not have enough contact with other people.

The Occupational History is designed to obtain information about the patient's occupational role development, about the experiences he has had that led him to his present occupational roles and daily activities. One of the reasons so many questions are asked about the patient's childhood is that early life experiences influence later life patterns. Interpreting the Occupational History successfully requires knowledge of the theories of occupational role development. Since these are not covered in depth in occupational therapy assistant programs, only the registered therapist is expected to interpret the Occupational History.

Florey and Michelman (17) developed a much shorter version of the Occupational History, called the *Occupational Role Screening Interview,* based on Moorhead's original interview design. Their instrument focuses on the occupational role of the patient (worker/homemaker or student). It is used to determine how well the patient is functioning in his occupational role, and to estimate the balance between occupational and leisure activities. Another variant of this type of interview is the *Occupational Performance History Interview* (22) developed by Kielhofner and Henry.

The *Role Checklist,* developed by Oakley (1982) and described by Barris, Oakley, and Kielhofner (5), is also based on the *Occupational History Interview.* The *Role*

Checklist is a short, written inventory that can be completed by higher functioning patients. It lists ten major life roles (and an unspecified eleventh that can be added by the patient). The patient is asked to indicate whether he has performed or will perform each role in the past, present, or future. In the second part of the checklist, the patient is asked to rate the value of each role to him. Service competency for administration of the *Role Checklist* could be easily developed, as the directions are simple and most of the task is completed by the patient. This checklist is valuable for quickly assessing roles important to the patient so that priorities for treatment can be established.

Another structured interview that the COTA might be asked to administer is the *Routine Task Inventory* (Fig. 14–2), developed by Claudia Allen (2). The Routine Task Inventory is a list of behaviors in independent living skills and is designed to assess how well the patient is able to function in the community, and the degree to which his functioning is impaired. It can be used by an occupational therapy assistant as a structured guide to interview a patient or his caregiver about the patient's skills in 14 task areas, including (for example) grooming, toileting, food preparation, and taking medication. A family member or caregiver should be interviewed if the patient is not a reliable informant (and for all patients below level 4). For each of the 14 areas, behaviors are listed that are believed to be characteristic of persons functioning at Allen's six cognitive levels (see Chapter 3). The interviewer should ask about behaviors in the order in which they are listed, starting in each section with the highest level. You can see, in Fig. 14–2, that cognitive level 5 is sometimes the highest level, rather than level 6. The numbers in the table correspond to Allen's cognitive levels.

The Routine Task Inventory is divided into two sections: the physical scale and the instrumental scale. The tasks on the physical scale (grooming, dressing, bathing,

Routine Task Inventory
Physical Scale

Scoring: Circle the number that best describes your observations of behavior.

A. Grooming (Care of hair and nails; cosmetics)

  5. Initiates and completes grooming without assistance.

  4. Initiates grooming tasks but neglects features that are not clearly visible.
     May not match makeup to skin tones, or
     May not shave all parts of the face and neck for men or underarms and legs for women, or
     May neglect the back of the head or body.

  3. Does daily grooming (brushing teeth, washing hands or face or both).
     May need to be reminded, or
     May not use sharp instruments required for nail trimming safely, or
     May not shave safely with a nonelectric razor.

  2. Needs total grooming care.
     May cooperate with efforts of others by spontaneously moving hands, feet, or head, or
     May resist the caregivers help.

  1. Ignores personal appearance and does not spontaneously cooperate with, or resists, the caregivers help.
Additional comments:

B. Dressing

  5. Selects own clothing and dresses without error.

  4. Dresses self. May have minor errors in selection or method of dressing.
     Colors or patterns of garments may not be coordinated, or
     May disregard the appearance of the back of garments, or
     May require a limited choice of garments.

  3. Dresses self. May have gross errors in selection or method of dressing.
     May ignore weather conditions, social conditions (e.g., dining out, guests), social customs (e.g., underwear on top, garments inside out or backwards, misuse of sex-specific garments), button alignment, or daytime versus nighttime garments.

  2. Spontaneously alters the position of the body to facilitate dressing.
     May be unable to dress self, or
     May resist caregivers help.

  1. Must be dressed by caregivers and does not spontaneously alter position of the body to facilitate dressing.
     May hold still or move body position on command.

  Additional comments:

C. Bathing

  5. Bathes without assistance, using shampoo, deodorant, and other desirable toiletries.
  4. Bathes the front of the body.
     May not bathe the back of the body, or
     May not rinse shampoo from the back of the hair, or
     May not remember to use deodorant, or
     May not obtain a safe water temperature.

FIG. 14–2. The Routine Task Inventory. Reprinted with permission from Fig. 2–22 in Allen CK. *Occupational therapy for psychiatric diseases: measurement and management of cognitive disabilities.* Boston: Little, Brown; 1985: 64–72.

3. Uses soap and washcloth in a repetitive action.
   May not bathe entire body unless given verbal or tactile direction, or
   May refuse to soap the entire body.

2. Stands in the shower or sits in the bathtub.
   May not try to wash self, or
   May move body parts to assist the caregiver, or
   May resist the caregivers help, or
   May refuse to enter the shower or bathtub.

1. Does not try to wash self and is given a sponge bath by another person.
   May move body position on command.

Additional comments:

D. Walking

5. Goes about new grounds or city and finds way home.

4. Walks in familiar surroundings without getting lost.
   May require an escort in unfamiliar surroundings, or
   May refuse to go to unfamiliar places.

3. Initiates walking within a room to do a familiar activity.
   May get lost unless escorted from room to room, or
   May follow the lead of other people to the correct or incorrect location, or
   May pace or wander about and manipulate physical objects that happen to capture attention.

2. Follows the lead or pointed direction of others.
   May not initiate movement to do a familiar activity such as going to the dinner table, or
   May pace or wander about aimlessly without regard for objects unless they obstruct his or her path, or
   May resist the guidance of others.

1. Walks or transfers from bed to chair with physical guidance.
   May be bedridden, or
   May remain in a supportive chair, or
   May not notice objects that obstruct his or her path, or
   May require tactile assistance to bend knees.

Additional comments:

E. Feeding
5. Considers the size of food portions and shares a limited quantity of food with others.
   Usually self-monitors a balanced diet.

4. Everday table manners are consistent with social standards.
   May not share a limited quantity of food with others, or
   May not self-restrict portion size of desirable foods.

3. Uses table utensils.
   May not comply with a restricted diet, or
   May not self-monitor a balanced diet, or
   May not use table manners expected by social standards.

2. Uses a spoon or adapted eating devices (e.g., nonslip or scoop-edge plate).
   May not use utensils correctly, or
   Eating may be untidy.

FIG. 14–2. (*Continued*)

1. Chews and swallows voluntarily.
   May eat food with fingers, or
   May need to be told to chew, or
   May need to be fed.

Additional comments:

F. Toileting

5. Cares for self at toilet completely and locates an unfamiliar bathroom with little or no assistance.

4. Cares for self at toilet completely.
   May need to have the location of an unfamiliar bathroom pointed out, or
   May need to be escorted to an unfamiliar bathroom.

3. Uses the toilet.
   May need to be reminded to go to the bathroom, or
   May not adjust garments correctly (e.g., zipping up zippers), or
   May not wipe the body clean.

2. Uses the toilet inconsistently.
   May void in unacceptable locations, or
   May need to be escorted to the toilet, or
   May need to be positioned on the toilet.

1. Fails to control bowel or bladder.

Additional comments:

Instrumental Scale

Scoring: Circle the number that best describes your observations of behavior.

A. Housekeeping

6. Organizes home environment, plans a schedule for completing chores, and plans for long-term maintenance.

5. Recognizes and completes less visible tasks (e.g., dusting under objects and cleaning corners).
   May not plan for long-term maintenance, or
   May not design a new organization of home environment (e.g, reorganize cupboards and drawers).

4. Completes familiar, simple household tasks at an acceptable level of cleanliness.
   May not recognize the need to do tasks that are not clearly visible (e.g., dusting under furniture, cleaning corners, or washing windows), or
   May not be able to find things that are out of place or in a new location.

3. Uses repetitive familiar actions (e.g., dusting) to be of assistance in housekeeping.
   May not obtain an acceptable level of cleanliness, or
   May not complete the usual procedure for doing a task, or
   May unnecessarily do the same task over and over again.

2. Does not participate in any housekeeping tasks.

Additional comments:

FIG. 14–2. (*Continued*)

B. Preparing Food

6. Plans menus for adequate nutrition and anticipates potential substitutions and problems.

5. Supplies ingredients and utensils and follows a new recipe for food preparation.
    May not anticipate burning, or
    May not coordinate the timing of several dishes, or
    May not plan variations by substituting ingredients.

4. Prepares familiar, simple dishes if supplied with the ingredients.
    May not avoid burning food, or
    May not consistently remember to turn off the stove, or
    May handle a knife or hot food and cooking equipment hazardously.

3. Uses repetitive familiar action to be of assistance to meal preparation (peels potatoes, pours milk, sets the table).
    May not prepare a meal, or
    May not recognize mealtime.

2. Does not participate in food preparation.

Additional comments:

C. Spending Money

6. Anticipates infrequent expenses and plans for financial security.

5. Manages routine weekly and monthly purchases and income.
    May not anticipate infrequent major expenses, or
    May not plan for long-term financial security.

4. Manages day-to-day purchases but is slow at making change, may calculate correct change with paper and pencil, calculator, or by counting cash.
    May not calculate change in his or her head, or
    May not accurately anticipate weekly or monthly purchases, or
    May make errors in calculating cost or change.

3. Hands cash to another person.
    May realize that a caregiver is handling money for him or her, or
    May not consider amount of cash given or received, or
    May forget to pay bills, or
    May run out of money, or
    May not understand why he or she owes money.

2. Does not handle money.
    May not realize that money transactions are occurring.

Additional comments:

D. Taking Medication

6. Complies with new dosages and anticipates drug effects accurately.

5. Is responsible for taking routine medications in correct dosage at correct time. Explains why medication was prescribed and reports individual effects.
    Compliance with complicated dose schedules (such as every 6 hours) may be inaccurate, or
    May have trouble distinguishing concepts such as drug effect, drug side effect, drug synergies, drug tolerance.

FIG. 14–2. (*Continued*)

4. Takes desirable medication in simple dosages at routine times, such as with meals.
   May use a pill dispenser to keep track of medications.
   May not understand why a psychopharmacologic drug was prescribed, or
   May refuse to take psychopharmacologic drugs, or
   May need to be reminded to take medications correctly.

3. Medications are given by a caretaker.
   May refuse to take medications, or
   May not distinguish among types of pills (e.g., vitamins versus psychopharmacologic drugs), or
   May not know what he or she is taking, or
   May not recognize that it is time to take medication.

Additional comments:

E. Doing Laundry

6. Anticipates shrinkage and bleeding of dyes without error.
   Anticipates clothing needs (e.g., takes clothes to the cleaners or does laundry ahead of time).

5. Sorts clothing.
   May not anticipate shrinkage or bleeding of dyes of new garments, or
   May not anticipate clothing needs.

4. Does familiar hand laundry or uses a washing machine to do a load of clothing. Puts dirty clothes in a hamper.
   May not sort clothing, or
   May not consider care instructions for new garments, or
   May not distinguish between machine laundry, hand laundry, and dry cleaning.

3. Does not participate in doing laundry.
   May not place dirty clothes in a hamper, or
   May not realize that clothing is dirty.

Additional comments:

F. Traveling

6. Uses a map to anticipate directions and determine present position.

5. Drives a car or finds way in less frequently traveled or unfamiliar routes.
   May make a wrong turn, or
   May get on a wrong bus, or
   May forget where car is parked.

4. Independently travels familiar routes in vehicles driven by others.
   May get lost on unfamiliar routes, or
   May avoid unfamiliar routes, or
   May not be able to drive a car safely.

3. Gets in and out of a familiar vehicle without tactile assistance.
   May get lost without an escort, or
   May not know, or may be confused about, destination.

2. May ride in a vehicle but is unaware of passing external environment.

Additional comments:

FIG. 14–2. (*Continued*)

G. Shopping

   6. Anticipates and plans for shopping needs.

   5. Does routine shopping
      May not anticipate long-range shopping needs, or
      May not follow a monthly budget.

   4. Shops for small, familiar purchases.
      May not do comparison shopping, or
      May not have enough money for selected purchases, or
      May refuse to purchase items because of an exaggerated concern for lack of funds.

   3. Goes to a store.
      May not recognize correct change, or
      May not remember what he or she went to the store to purchase, or
      May accompany another person without an awareness of, or with confusion about, desired purchases.

   2. Does not go shopping.

Additional comments:

H. Telephoning

   6. Uses a classification system to find a number in the Yellow Pages or in the listing of governmental agencies.

   5. Looks up numbers in the White Pages or in a personal address book.
      May not use the Yellow Pages or consider subclassifications such as governmental agencies, or
      May become confused when calls must be transferred.

   4. Dials familiar numbers and calls information for new numbers. Relays a message.
      May not look up new numbers in the telephone book, or
      May have trouble locating infrequently used numbers in an address book, or
      May be slow in writing down new numbers or messages.

   3. Answers the phone when it rings and may answer even if it does not ring. May dial one or two well-known numbers.
      May not relay a message, or
      May not call a person to the phone, or
      May forget the telephone number he or she was trying to find, or
      May take the receiver off the hook.

   2. Does not use the telephone.

Additional comments:

FIG. 14–2. (*Continued*)

walking, feeding, and toileting) are ones that most people need to be able to perform, regardless of social class and occupational roles. Those on the instrumental scale (housekeeping, preparing food, spending money, taking medication, doing laundry, traveling, shopping, and telephoning) may not be familiar or important to some people, depending on their life space, life-style, and social support. This means that low scores on instrumental tasks may occur for reasons other than disability caused by mental illness.

The occupational therapy assistant may be assigned to carry out other structured interviews. Some are used only for research purposes; others are used only in certain types of hospitals or parts of the country. Regardless of the particular interview instruments, the occupational therapy assistant will have many opportunities to practice and develop his interviewing skills. Students and new graduates may find that some of their first interviews go badly, or that patients refuse to give them certain information. Usually there is a discernible reason for this; by thinking about the attitudes you expressed and the questions you asked and how you asked them, you can become more sensitive to the needs and feelings of the patient, and more competent at interviewing. With attention and practice it is a skill you will find easy to acquire.

OBSERVATION

Observation is inseparable from the treatment process; we are constantly watching and listening to the patient, from the moment we first meet him. Of all the skills the occupational therapy assistant needs to learn, observation is perhaps the most critical. We base our ideas and plans for the patient on what we observe; therefore we must learn to observe as accurately and uncritically as possible.

To observe clearly it is important to know the difference between observation and interpretation or inference. *Observation* is the process of noticing or taking note of behavior or of whatever is happening that we can take in through our senses. We *see* what the patient does, we *hear* what he says; these are observations. *Interpretation* or *inference* is the process of giving meaning to what we have observed. Why the patient did what he did, how what he said relates to other things we know about

him—these are inferences and interpretations.

One way to quickly differentiate between an observation and an inference or interpretation is to examine the words that are used. Observations usually include action words (verbs) that describe what the person did. Inferences and interpretations, on the other hand, usually contain opinion or value words. Keeping this distincion in mind, identify whether the following descriptions are observations:

> She traced the pattern after lifting it up several times and looking underneath.
> She was hostile to the patient who passed her the glue.
> She didn't want to finish the project.

If you paid attention to the words used, you may have realized that only the first is really an observation; it describes what the patient did. Another person watching the patient would be able to agree that this is what happened. The second description contains an opinion word: "hostile." We cannot tell from this description what the patient actually did: Did she glare, clench her teeth, or snatch the bottle away? Can we be sure that the patient was "hostile?" Or was she perhaps indifferent, frightened or suspicious? Can you think of specific behaviors that would be conclusive evidence of hostility?

You can probably recognize what is wrong with the third "observation"; it presumes that we can see inside the patient's mind. How do we know she did not want to finish the project? Did she say so? If so, this behavior should be part of the description. "The patient said she didn't want to finish the project" *is* an observation, because it reports behavior without interpreting it. It is also perfectly accurate to state as an observation that the patient did not finish the project, if that is the case.

Beginners frequently find it difficult to observe because they do not know what to focus on, and there is so much to observe. This feeling is even more overwhelming when the observation is supposed to be *un-*

TABLE 14–1. *Guide to observing and describing behavior*

GENERAL APPEARANCE:
  Clean, neat, appropriately dressed
  Fastidious, meticulous
  Dramatic, theatrical
  Looks younger than stated age
  Bizarre dress or makeup
  Inappropriate dress
  Disheveled, stained clothing
  Has noticeable body odor
  Hair not combed

PHYSICAL BEHAVIORS:
  Relaxed, at ease
  Restless, overactive
  Agitated
  Slow, listless, inactive
  Formal, stiff
  Appears tense or uncomfortable
  Shuffling gait
  Hesitating or uneven gait
  Grimaces or has facial tics
  Postures
  Drools
  Expectorates (Spits)
  Incontinent
  Masturbates
  Smokes incessantly
  Rocks self
  Scratches or rubs self
  Makes repetitive movements
  Makes odd movements
  Bites nails
  Chain smokes
  Always drinking coffee

ATTITUDE TOWARD COTA:
  Seeks assistance when appropriate
  Seeks approval
  Rejects attention from assistant
  Ignores therapy assistant
  Does not follow instruction
  Ingratiates self
  Combative, argumentative
  Tests limits
  Relates to therapist but not peers
  Relates to peers but not therapist

DESCRIBED SENSATIONS:
  Has odd sensations
  Feels familiar things to be new
  Feels new things to be familiar
  Does not feel like himself
  Surroundings don't look real
  Feels numb all over
  Reports distorted sense of time
  Reports body seems strange to him
  Reports hearing things not there
  Reports seeing things not there
  Reports strange odors

ATTITUDE:
  Helpful, cooperative
  Seems pleasant, yet obstructs
  Demands attention or praise
  Makes excuses for his actions
  Blames others for his problems
  Contemptuous
  Rigid, not flexible
  Seems self-centered
  Appears indifferent
  Antagonistic
  Appears bored
  Appears resentful
  Seems suspicious
  Makes negative remarks
  Appears timid
  Seems fearful or apprehensive

COMMUNICATION:
  Logical, clear
  Speaks slowly, hesitatingly
  Speaks rapidly, speech seems pressured
  Initiates conversation
  Repetitive, perseverative
  Rambles
  Uses vulgar language
  Swears, curses
  Uses words oddly
  Makes up words (neologisms)
  Rhymes
  Speaks in low tone of voice
  Mute
  Speaks only when others initiate
  Loud, boisterious, shouts

EXPRESSED THOUGHTS:
  Dwells on illness or symptoms
  Focuses on here and now
  Dwells on past
  Expresses few thoughts
  Can't make up his mind
  Things are hopeless; he is no good
  People are unfair, out to get him
  Reports intrusive, unwanted thoughts

COGNITIVE BEHAVIORS:
  Alert, responsive, concentrates well
  Bewildered, confused
  Forgetful
  Seems not to pay attention
  Learns new steps with difficulty
  Easily distracted
  Repeats errors
  Concentrates on details but misses the main point
  Shows good judgment
  Shows poor judgment
  Plans actions before acting
  Skips from topic to topic
  Seems dull, slow to respond

TABLE 14–1. *(Continued)*

MOOD AND GENERAL DISPOSITION:
   Difficult to ascertain
   Enthusiastic, excited
   Smooth, even disposition
   Easily upset, irritable
   Tearful
   Shows little reaction or emotion
   Seems ill at ease
   Independent, appears aloof
   Positive attitude (toward . . . ?)
   Negative attitude (toward . . . ?)
   Excessively cheerful, euphoric
   Sad
   Angry
   Anxious, worried
   Constricted, restrained
   Gloomy, pessimistic
   Appears preoccupied
   Mood doesn't fit situation
   Manic

BEHAVIOR TOWARDS OTHERS:
   Polite, well-mannered
   Rude, inconsiderate
   Outgoing, enthusiastic
   Isolates self, withdrawn
   Avoids opposite sex
   Seeks opposite sex exclusively
   Teases
   Behaves seductively
   Monopolizes one person's attention
   Hangs back, seems timid
   Is a member of a clique

SKILLS:
   Good eye-hand coordination
   Clumsy, awkward
   Artistically creative
   Good verbal skills
   Skilled with machine or tool (specify)
   Good with spatial relations
   Good social skills
   Good vocabulary
   Good gross motor coordination
   Mechanically skillful

PARTICIPATION:
   Attends regularly
   Often absent
   Arrives late, early
   Remains only a short time
   Leaves and then returns
   Socializes but does not participate in activity
   Observes only
   Participates infrequently

WORK BEHAVIORS:
   Shows initiative, sees work and does it
   Needs explicit instructions on all steps
   Works best alone
   Works directly with others
   Works with one other person
   Accepts criticism
   Rejects criticism
   Seeks out direct supervision
   Seldom completes projects
   Impatient with detail
   Meticulous with detail
   Has realistic view of own efforts and abilities
   Underestimates efforts and abilities
   Overestimates efforts and abilities
   Tenacious, persistent
   Consistent, reliable
   Work shows planning

ROLES PATIENT ASSUMES IN A GROUP:
   Leader
   Follower
   Initiator-contributor
   Information seeker
   Information giver
   Opinion seeker
   Opinion giver
   Evaluator-critic
   Coordinator
   Orienter
   Compromiser
   Harmonizer
   Blocker
   Aggressor
   Observer

Based on and adapted from a list from the student program at Buffalo Psychiatric Center, Buffalo, NY. Roles are based on the classification developed by Benne and Sheats (8).

structured or *naturalistic;* this means that the patient is observed while he is doing something that he would be doing anyway. He is not asked to do something in particular. Table 14–1 provides some categories and descriptive words to help guide such unstructured observations. The list is by no means comprehensive or exhaustive. The careful reader will note that opinion words occur on the list; they should be used cautiously, only when the observer is certain they are valid.

The question of whether to take notes while observing has been debated countless times; notes can capture details that might otherwise be forgotten, but other details may be missed while the observer is writing. The role of the observer during an ob-

Comprehensive Occupational Therapy Evaluation Scale

	DATE	1	2	3	4	5	6	7	8	9	10	11	12	13	14	15
I.	**GENERAL BEHAVIOR**															
A.	APPEARANCE															
B.	NON-PRODUCTIVE BEHAVIOR															
C.	ACTIVITY LEVEL (a or b)															
D.	EXPRESSION															
E.	RESPONSIBILITY															
F.	PUNCTUALITY															
G.	REALITY ORIENTATION															
	SUB-TOTAL															
II.	**INTERPERSONAL BEHAVIOR**															
A.	INDEPENDENCE															
B.	COOPERATION															
C.	SELF-ASSERTION (a or b)															
D.	SOCIABILITY															
E.	ATTENTION-GETTING BEHAVIOR															
F.	NEGATIVE RESPONSE FROM OTHERS															
	SUB-TOTAL															
III.	**TASK BEHAVIOR**															
A.	ENGAGEMENT															
B.	CONCENTRATION															
C.	COORDINATION															
D.	FOLLOW DIRECTIONS															
E.	ACTIVITY NEATNESS OR ATTENTION TO DETAIL															
F.	PROBLEM SOLVING															
G.	COMPLEXITY AND ORGANIZATION OF TASK															
H.	INITIAL LEARNING															
I.	INTEREST IN ACTIVITY															
J.	INTEREST IN ACCOMPLISHMENT															
K.	DECISION MAKING															
L.	FRUSTRATION TOLERANCE															
	SUB-TOTAL															
	TOTAL															

SCALE 0—NORMAL, 1—MINIMAL, 2—MILD, 3—MODERATE, 4—SEVERE

COMMENTS:

_____

(THERAPIST'S SIGNATURE)

FIG. 14–3. Comprehensive Occupational Therapy Evaluation Scale. From Table 1 of Brayman SJ, Kirby TF, Misenheimer AM, Short MJ. Comprehensive occupational therapy evaluation scale. *Am J Occup Ther* 1976; 30:94–100. Copyright © 1976 by the American Occupational Therapy Association, Inc. Reprinted with permission.

PART I. GENERAL BEHAVIOR

A. APPEARANCE

The following six factors are involved: (1) clean skin, (2) clean hair, (3) hair combed, (4) clean clothes, (5) clothes ironed, and (6) clothes suitable for the occasion.

0—No problems in any area.
1—Problems in 1 area.
2—Problems in 2 areas.
3—Problems in 3 or 4 areas.
4—Problems in 5 or 6 areas.

B. NONPRODUCTIVE BEHAVIOR

(Rocking, playing with hands, repetitive statements, appears to be talking to self, preoccupied with own thoughts, etc.)

0—No nonproductive behavior during session.
1—Nonproductive behavior occasionally during session.
2—Nonproductive behavior for half of session.
3—Nonproductive behavior for three-fourths of session.
4—Nonproductive behavior for the entire session.

C. ACTIVITY LEVEL (a or b)

(a) 0—No hypoactivity.
1—Occasional hypoactivity.
2—Hypoactivity attracts the attention of other patients and therapists but participates.
3—Hypoactivity level such that can participate but with great difficulty.
4—So hypoactive that patient cannot participate in activity.

(b) 0—No hyperactivity.
1—Occasional spurts of hyperactivity.
2—Hyperactivity attracts the attention of other patients and therapists but participates.
3—Hyperactivity level such that can participate but with great difficulty.
4—So hyperactive that patient cannot participate in activity.

D. EXPRESSION

0—Expression consistent with situation and setting.
1—Communicates with expression, occasionally inappropriate.
2—Shows inappropriate expression several times during session.
3—Show of expression but inconsistent with situation.
4—Extremes of expression-bizarre, uncontrolled or no expression.

E. RESPONSIBILITY

0—Takes responsibility for own actions.
1—Denies responsibility for 1 or 2 actions.
2—Denies responsibility for several actions.
3—Denies responsibility for most actions.
4—Denial of all responsibility—messes up project and blames therapist or others.

F. PUNCTUALITY

0—On time.
1—5–10 minutes late.
2—10–20 minutes late.
3—20–30 minutes late.
4—30 minutes or more late.

G. REALITY ORIENTATION

0—Complete awareness of person, place, time, and situation.
1—General awareness but inconsistency in one area.
2—Awareness of 2 areas.
3—Awareness of 1 area.
4—Lack of awareness of person, place, time, and situation (who, where, what, and why).

FIG. 14–4. Comprehensive Occupational Therapy Evaluation Scale definitions. From Table 2 of Brayman SJ, Kirby TF, Misenheimer AM, Short MJ. Comprehensive occupational therapy evaluation scale. *Am J Occup Ther* 1976; 30:94–100. Copyright © 1976 by the American Occupational Therapy Association, Inc. Reprinted with permission.

PART II. INTERPERSONAL

A. INDEPENDENCE
0—Independent functioning.
1—Only 1 or 2 dependent actions.
2—Half independent and half dependent actions.
3—Only 1 or 2 independent actions.
4—No independent actions.

B. COOPERATION
0—Cooperates with program.
1—Follows most directions, opposes less than one half.
2—Follows half, opposes half.
3—Opposes three-fourths of directions.
4—Opposes all directions and suggestions.

C. SELF-ASSERTION (a or b)
(a) 0—Assertive when necessary.
1—Compliant less than half of the session.
2—Compliant half of the session.
3—Compliant three-fourths of the session.
4—Totally passive and compliant.

(b) 0—Assertive when necessary.
1—Dominant less than half of the session.
2—Dominant half of the session.
3—Dominant three-fourths of the session.
4—Totally dominates the session.

D. SOCIABILITY
0—Socializes with staff and patients.
1—Socializes with staff and occasionally with other patients or vice-versa.
2—Socializes only with staff or with patients.
3—Socializes only if approached.
4—Does not join others in activities, unable to carry on casual conversation even if approached.

E. ATTENTION-GETTING BEHAVIOR
0—No unreasonable attention-getting behavior.
1—Less than one-half time spent in attention-getting behavior.
2—Half-time spent in attention-getting behavior.
3—Three-fourths of time spent in attention-getting behavior.
4—Verbally or nonverbally demands constant attention.

F. NEGATIVE RESPONSE FROM OTHERS
0—Evokes no negative responses.
1—Evokes 1 negative response.
2—Evokes 2 negative responses.
3—Evokes 3 or more negative responses during session.
4—Evokes numerous negative responses from others and therapist must take some action.

PART III. TASK BEHAVIOR

A. ENGAGEMENT
0—Needs no encouragement to begin task.
1—Encourage once to begin activity.
2—Encourage 2 or 3 times to engage in activity.
3—Engages in activity only after much encouragement.
4—Does not engage in activity.

B. CONCENTRATION
0—No difficulty concentrating during full session.
1—Off task less than one-fourth time.
2—Off task half the time.
3—Off task three-fourths time.
4—Loses concentration on task in less than 1 minute.

C. COORDINATION
0—No problems with coordination.
1—Occasionally has trouble with fine detail, manipulating tools or materials.
2—Occasional trouble manipulating tools and materials but has frequent trouble with fine detail.
3—Some difficulty in gross movement—unable to manipulate some tools and materials.
4—Great difficulty in movement (gross motor); virtually unable to manipulate tools and materials (fine motor).

D. FOLLOW DIRECTIONS
0—Carries out directions without problems.
1—Occasional trouble with more than 3 step directions.
2—Carries out simple directions—has trouble with 2.
3—Can carry out only very simple one step directions (demonstrated, written, or oral).
4—Unable to carry out any directions.

FIG. 14–4. (*Continued*)

*E. ACTIVITY NEATNESS
0—Activity neatly done.
1—Occasionally ignores fine detail.
2—Often ignores fine detail and materials are scattered.
3—Ignores fine detail and work habits disturbing to those around.
4—Unaware of fine detail, so sloppy that therapist has to intervene.

*F. ATTENTION TO DETAIL
0—Pays attention to detail appropriately.
1—Occasionally too concise.
2—More attention to several details than is required.
3—So concise that project will take twice as long as expected.
4—So concerned that project will never get finished.

G. PROBLEM SOLVING
0—Solves problems without assistance.
1—Solves problems after assistance given once.
2—Can solve only after repeated instructions.
3—Recognizes a problem but cannot solve it.
4—Unable to recognize or solve a problem.

H. COMPLEXITY AND ORGANIZATION OF TASK
0—Organizes and performs all tasks given.
1—Occasionally has trouble with organization of complex activities that should be able to do.
2—Can organize simple but not complex activities.
3—Can do only very simple activities with organization imposed by therapists.
4—Unable to organize or carry out an activity when all tools, materials, and directions are available.

I. INITIAL LEARNING
0—Learns a new activity quickly and without difficulty.
1—Occasionally has difficulty learning a complex activity.
2—Has frequent difficulty learning a complex activity, but can learn a simple activity.
3—Unable to learn complex activities; occasional difficulty learning simple activities.
4—Unable to learn a new activity.

J. INTEREST IN ACTIVITIES
0—Interested in a variety of activities.
1—Occasionally not interested in new activity.
2—Shows occasional interest in a part of an activity.
3—Engages in activities but shows no interest.
4—Does not participate.

K. INTEREST IN ACCOMPLISHMENT
0—Interested in finishing activities.
1—Occasional lack of interest or pleasure in finishing a long-term activity.
2—Interest or pleasure in accomplishment of a short-term activity—lack of interest in a long-term activity.
3—Only occasional interest in finishing any activity.
4—No interest or pleasure in finishing an activity.

L. DECISION MAKING
0—Makes own decisions.
1—Makes decisions but occasionally seeks therapist approval.
2—Makes decisions but often seeks therapist approval.
3—Makes decision when given only 2 choices.
4—Cannot make any decisions or refuses to make a decision.

M. FRUSTRATION TOLERANCE
0—Handles all tasks without becoming overly frustrated.
1—Occasionally becomes frustrated with more complex tasks; can handle simple tasks.
2—Often becomes frustrated with more complex tasks but is able to handle simple tasks.
3—Often becomes frustrated with any tasks but attempts to continue.
4—Becomes so frustrated with simple tasks that he refuses or is unable to function.

*Rate either Activity Neatness or Attention to Detail, not both.

FIG. 14–4. (*Continued*)

servation is to observe—to watch, listen, and sense what is going on. Preparation, paperwork, and note taking should be done after or before the observation, not during it. It is impossible to observe well when your attention is elsewhere.

It is wise to write brief notes for yourself as soon as the observation is over. These notes need not be grammatical or even make sense to anyone but you; their purpose is to jog your memory when you record or report them formally later on.

Sometimes a checklist or other structured format is used to record observations. Of these, the *Comprehensive Occupational Therapy Evaluation Scale* (11, 12) is perhaps the most widely used. The COTE Scale (Fig. 14–3) may be used for a single observation or a series of observations of a patient performing a task. It lists 25 behaviors and provides a scale for rating them. Behaviors are divided into three areas: General Behavior (7 items), Interpersonal Behavior (6 items), and Task Behaviors (12 items). Each can be rated on a scale of 0 (normal) to 4 (extreme or grossly abnormal). Some items, activity level (1C) for example, have two rating scales, reflecting the possibility of abnormal behaviors in either direction. The observer chooses *either* hyperactive (overactive) or hypoactive (underactive), depending on the patient's behavior. Fig. 14–4 lists the definitions used in rating the 25 behaviors.

Notice that the COTE scale contains 15 columns, so that the patient's behavior during up to 15 sessions can be noted on the same page; this is helpful in measuring progress during treatment and documenting effects of medication and ECT. Some therapists use the 15 columns in a different way, to rate several patients during the same group session; each patient is rated in a different column. The ratings can then be transferred to each patient's individual form.

Whether the COTE or another observational scale is used, when observing a patient for purposes of evaluation the assistant must maintain her position as an observer, and not interfere with what the patient is doing. She cannot give help, advice, or encouragement, or recommend that the patient try a different technique, or even smile approvingly. All of these behaviors may change what the patient does, and what then ends up on the rating form is how the patient performs with advice and support rather than how he performs on his own. Administering an evaluation and performing treatment are different tasks and require different behaviors from the occupational therapist or assistant.

STRUCTURED EVALUATIONS

In addition to observing the patient under both naturalistic and structured conditions, the occupational therapy assistant can administer various structured evaluations. During a structured evaluation the assistant engages the patient in an activity or series of activities, while following highly specific directions for administration and scoring. Many of these evaluations have been or are in the process of being normed. This means that many people (patients and nonpatients) have been given the evaluation, and their scores have been recorded. Working from the scores of this large group, the developers of the evaluation try to predict what the normal range of scores is like. Once the normal range has been identified, the score of a particular patient can be compared to it.

When administering a structured evaluation, the assistant must follow the directions exactly as they are written. If she changes the directions, the patient's score cannot reliably be compared to the norms. A simple analogy illustrates this point: An oral thermometer will not give an accurate reading when the patient has been outside, or exercising, or had anything to eat or drink within the past half-hour. A "temperature" of 101° obtained five minutes after drinking a cup of tea is meaningless.

Have everything prepared before the patient arrives; this allows for better use of your time with the patient and prevents his becoming upset with the delay or skeptical of your competence (either of which might prejudice the results). Make sure you have recorded all necessary identifying information (e.g., time and date) and that you or the patient fill out any required information about her (age, sex, medical records number, etc.). Then begin the evaluation, the first part of which is usually a brief statement that you make to the patient about the purpose of the evaluation.

It is not possible to discuss here each of the evaluations the occupational therapy assistant might be called on to administer; only a few of the more widely used evaluations are presented.

The *Activity Configuration* (39) is a two-part evaluation that examines the patient's use of time and his feelings about the activities he performs in a typical week. The first part is a schedule or chart with seven columns (representing the seven days of the week), and three horizontal rows (representing morning, afternoon, and evening hours). The hours are further broken down into two-hour segments (e.g., 7 A.M. to 9 A.M.). The patient records his activities for the previous week on the chart; patients whose previous week's activity was atypical because of illness may be instructed to fill out the chart with a typical week before the illness.

In the second part of the evaluation the patient uses the chart he has made to generate a list of all of the activities done during the week. He then classifies each activity according to which of 10 functions it serves (e.g., work, recreation, rest, chore), and rates it as to whether he has to do it or wants to do it (or both). He also answers questions about how adequately he thinks he performs each activity, and whether he does it because he wants to or someone else wants him to.

The Activity Configuration may easily take two or three hours to complete even if the patient fills it out on her own time. Because many patients do not have sufficient attention span for such a lengthy task, some therapists have adapted the Activity Configuration to eliminate all but one weekday and one weekend day; the second part of the evaluation is sometimes conducted as an interview. The Activity Configuration requires that the patient be able to read and write, but many psychiatric patients cannot read and write well enough to complete this kind of form (9, 15).

The *Barth Time Construction* or BTC (6, 7) is a variation on the Activity Configuration that requires less literacy from the patient. The chart is divided into 24 rows, representing the hours of the day. Color-coded paper is used to represent 12 different categories of activities (e.g., blue for sleeping, black for watching television, pink for grooming and dressing). The paper is precut to the width of the column, so the patient need only cut it to size and glue it in the appropriate place. The patient selects each color in turn, and continues to cut and paste until the entire chart is filled. The evaluator uses a *BTC Summary Form* to record any unsolicited comments made by the patient, and afterward totals the hours spent in each of the 12 activity categories. These totals are then converted to percentages of time per week spent in each activity.

Instructions and materials for the BTC are quite specific; for example, cylindrical glue bottles were selected so that patients with weak grasp would be able to use them easily. The BTC has several advantages over the original Activity Configuration. It can be administered in a group, to as many as four patients at a time. The 12 categories include several in which some patients spend many hours but that were not in the Activity Configuration: shopping, television, meetings and groups, and drinking and drugs. The instructions are very brief, simply worded, and presented in large print. The patient does not have to write a single word; therefore the instrument can be used with less literate patients. Finally, the end-product, the colored chart, depicts the patient's use of time so vividly that the patient can see it for himself; the chart is easily understood by other staff for the same reason.

The *Bay Area Functional Performance Evaluation* or BaFPE (10, 20)[2] is a standardized instrument that assesses some of the general skills needed for independent activities of daily living. It begins with a brief interview to orient the patient to the purpose of the evaluation and to collect basic information. This is followed by a task-oriented assessment (TOA) consisting of five tasks: sorting shells, a money and marketing task, drawing a house floor plan, constructing nine block designs from memory, and drawing a person. The evaluator rates the patient's performance of these tasks using a rating guide included in the evaluation; decision making, motivation, and organization of time and materials are some of the items rated. The evaluator also observes and records perceptual motor behaviors such as use of both hands in sorting shells. Finally, the way the patient relates to other people is rated on a separate Social Interaction Scale (SIS).

Normative data are available for the BaFPE, and research seems to show that it is reliable (gives comparable results every time it is given) and has construct validity (measures what it says it measures).

There are several structured evaluations designed to assess self-care and independent living skills. Psychiatric patients, especially those with chronic disorders, frequently have problems with such areas as hygiene and grooming, housekeeping, money management, and other skills basic to independent community living. Because occupational therapy assistants are often given major responsibility for assessing the self-care and daily living skills of psychiatric patients, three different evaluations for this area will be discussed.

The *Comprehensive Evaluation of Basic Living Skills* or CEBLS (13) has three sections: a Personal Care and Hygiene Checklist, a Practical Evaluation and Checklist, and a Written Evaluation. Nursing staff might complete the first section, since they generally have more direct experience of the patient's behavior during dressing and grooming. Whoever completes the Personal Care and Hygiene Checklist must rate the patient on such details as proper motions in brushing teeth and whether the toilet is flushed. Behaviors are rated on a four-point scale, with 4 signifying independent correct performance and 1 inability to perform independently or correctly.

The Practical Evaluation is administered by the occupational therapist or assistant. The evaluator uses the Practical Evaluation Checklist and the four-point scale to rate the patient's performance during menu planning, making a shopping list, telephoning, use of public transportation, grocery shopping, meal preparation, serving and eating, and cleaning up. The patient completes the Written Evaluation by himself; it tests his ability to read and write, understand time, and manage numbers and money. The assistant or therapist scores the Written Evaluation using a separate score sheet. Parts of the CEBLS can be administered separately, depending upon the occupational roles and needs of the patient.

Two other independent living skills evaluations that are quite similar to each other are the *Kohlman Evaluation of Living Skills* (29, 30) and the *Scorable Self Care Evaluation* (14). Each aseseses skills in personal care, safety and health, money management, transportation, use of the telephone, and work and leisure. In addition, the Scorable Self Care Evaluation has a section on housekeeping skills. Several different tasks are presented in each skill area on both evaluations. The Kohlman is preceded by a

---

[2]Discussion is based on the 2nd edition of the Bay Area Functional Performance Evaluation (1987), available from Consulting Psychologists Press, Palo Alto, Calif.

brief reading and writing test, which, like the written evaluation on the CEBLS, is intended to supplement the rest of the evaluation.

Administration of the two evaluations is similar; generally the patient must perform a task or respond to questions from the evaluator. As an example, for the task on making change the evaluator presents the patient with an item (magazine or bar of soap) marked with a price. The patient must pretend to purchase the item (with play money) and is scored on whether he is able to identify if the evaluator has given him the correct change.

Both evaluations give very specific directions for administering the items and rating the patient's responses. The rating systems are different for each, however. The patient is rated as "independent" or "needs assistance" for items on the Kohlman Evaluation, but is given only a numerical score for items on the Scorable Self Care; these scores are totaled and transferred to a record sheet, which lists ratings of "functional," "needs skill development," and "dysfunctional." Both of these evaluations seem to be widely used and are often administered by occupational therapy assistants. A videotape is available that demonstrates how the Kohlman Evaluation of Living Skills is administered (21).

The *Milwaukee Evaluation of Daily Living Skills* or MEDLS (24) is another standardized evaluation for this area. A screening form is used to determine which areas (of 21 subtests) need to be tested. The evaluation is administered individually, using equipment that may be provided by the patient; this creates a context in which the patient's performance is most likely to approximate her natural performance.

In addition to using any of the structured evaluations discussed above, the occupational therapy assistant may be asked to administer the *Allen Cognitive Level Test* (ACL) and the *Lower Cognitive Level Test* (LCL) (2). These are the evaluations used

to asseses Allen's cognitive levels discussed in Chapter 3. The assistant should practice until she is proficient and has achieved service competency before administering either test. Directions for materials, administration and scoring of the ACL are given in Fig. 14–5, and those for the LCL in Fig. 14–6.

The ACL uses the patient's performance of progressively more difficult leather lacing stitches to assess his cognitive level. The test includes the running stitch, the whip stitch, and the single cordovan stitch. Allen (2) believes it is possible that women might do better on the test than men, because of previous experience with sewing; the running stitch and the whip stitch are used in sewing, and the single cordovan is similar to the blanket stitch. She also warns that visual problems, blurred vision as a side effect of medication, and hand impairment or motor incoordination can result in a score that is lower than the patient's real cognitive abilities. On the other hand, previous experience doing leather lacing may falsely raise a patient's score.

Allen recommends that the leather lacing material be replaced after several administrations of the test, as it becomes twisted more easily as it becomes worn. She recommends that Life-Eye needles not be substituted for the Golka tip unless the evaluator knows how to secure the lace to the Life-Eye so that it will not come off; the trick is to cut a very long diagonal on the tip of the lace.[3] It is important not to add to or change the directions; telling the patient to stop and think may falsely raise a Level 5 to a Level 6, for example.

The LCL was designed for patients who are at cognitive levels 1, 2, and 3. The patient is asked to imitate the therapist, who claps three times. Clapping was chosen because it is a familiar motor behavior in most

---

[3]Allen CK. "Cognitive Disabilities. 1: Measurement and Management." Workshop given by Advanced Rehabilitation Institutes, New York, 1985.

Allen Cognitive Level Test

Materials:

1   natural cowhide carving weight Tom Thumb purse kit. #4109, Tandy Co. (Do not use zippered piece included in kit.)

2   30-inch-long 3/32-inch English calf lace, #5004, Tandy Co.

2   Golka needle tips

1   pair Golka needle pliers

1   15-inch-long 5-cord linen thread, beeswaxed, dark brown

(Items described are available from Tandy Leather Co., P.O. Box 791, Fort Worth, TX 76101 and Robert J. Golka Co., P.O. Box 676, Brockton, MA 02403.)

Preparation:

1. The therapist divides the leather into thirds and attaches the two pieces of leather lacing, completing at least two whip stitches with one piece of lacing and at least two single cordovan stitches with the other piece of lacing. The linen thread is attached, and two running stitches are completed.

2. The therapist selects a relatively distraction-free setting with adequate lighting and sits beside the patient at a slight angle. The therapist shows the patient the leather lacing stitches and asks if he or she knows how to do leather lacing. The response (yes or no) is recorded.

Administration:

Running Stitch (Levels 2 and 3)

The therapist says:

I AM INTERESTED IN SEEING HOW YOU LEARN. THIS WILL HELP ME PLACE YOU IN OCCUPATIONAL THERAPY GROUPS. I WILL SHOW YOU HOW TO DO A STITCH NOW, SO WATCH WHAT I DO CAREFULLY.

This explanation of purpose can, of course, be changed according to the treatment setting. I recommend keeping the explanation brief. The therapist then holds the leather project so that it is facing both the therapist and the patient and both sides of the leather's edge are visible. Therapists should practice holding their hands in a manner that affords the patient a clear view of the stitching process.

TAKE THE NEEDLE AND PUSH IT THROUGH THE HOLE, THEN PULL THE THREAD THROUGH THE HOLE. NOW PUSH THE NEEDLE BACK UP THROUGH THE NEXT HOLE. PULL THE THREAD THROUGH THE HOLE AND TIGHTEN IT. DON'T SKIP ANY HOLES. NOW YOU DO IT.

These directions may be repeated once if the patient cannot complete the stitch on the first attempt.

The individual is scored at level 2 if unable to complete two running stitches and at least level 3 if able to complete two running stitches.

Whip Stitch (Level 4)

If the patient is able to complete the running stitch, the therapist proceeds to the whip stitch. These directions may be repeated once if the subject cannot complete the stitch on the first attempt.

FIG. 14–5. Allen Cognitive Level Test. Reprinted with permission from Tables 4–1 and 4–2 and pp. 110–111 in Allen CK. *Occupational therapy for psychiatric diseases: measurement and management of cognitive disabilities.* Boston: Little, Brown; 1985.

SEE HOW THIS LEATHER LACE HAS ONE ROUGH SIDE AND ONE SMOOTH SIDE. ALWAYS KEEP THE SMOOTH SIDE UP AS YOU DO EACH STITCH, BEING CAREFUL NOT TO TWIST THE LACE. NOW I WILL SHOW YOU ANOTHER STITCH. WATCH ME CAREFULLY.

TAKE THE LACE AND BRING IT AROUND TO THE FRONT, OVER THE EDGE OF THE LEATHER. PUSH THE NEEDLE THROUGH THE HOLE, AND TIGHTEN IT. MAKE SURE THE LACE ISN'T TWISTED. DON'T SKIP ANY HOLES. NOW YOU DO IT.

The individual is scored at least at level 4 if he or she is able to complete two whip stitches, that is, twice bringing the lacing over the edge and pushing the needle from front to back. A score of level 3 is assigned to those who are able to do the stitch but cannot untwist the lacing. (Clinically we have noticed that people who score at level 4 usually stop after two stitches have been done, whereas the level 3 patients continue. Although this difference has not been empirically tested, it might prove to be an important differential between levels 3 and 4.)

Single Cordovan Stitch (Levels 5 and 6)

If the individual is able to complete the whip stitch, the therapist gives the following directions, which may repeated once if the patient cannot complete the stitch on the first attempt.

NOW I WILL SHOW YOU ANOTHER STITCH. WATCH ME CAREFULLY. BRING THE NEEDLE AROUND TO THE FRONT OF THE LEATHER. PUSH THE NEEDLE THROUGH THE NEXT HOLE, TOWARD THE BACK OF THE LEATHER. DON'T PULL THE LACE TIGHT, BUT LEAVE A SMALL LOOP IN IT. BRING THE LACE AROUND TO THE FRONT OF THE LEATHER AGAIN. THIS TIME PUT THE NEEDLE THROUGH THE LOOP YOU HAVE MADE, AND PULL THE LACE THROUGH IT TOWARD THE BACK OF THE LEATHER. KEEP THE LACE TO THE LEFT SIDE OF THE LOOP. TIGHTEN THE LOOP FROM THE BACK, THEN TIGHTEN THE LONG LACE END. MAKE SURE THE LACE ISN'T TWISTED. NOW YOU DO IT.

A score of level 5 is given if inductive reasoning is used (physically trying out various ways of completing the stitch) or if the patient requests a second demonstration after noting an error. A score of level 6 is given if deductive reasoning is used (mentally trying out various ways of correcting an error or pausing to think and select the best course of action) and one demonstration is all that is required. Two stitches must be completed correctly at level 5 and 6; twists in the leather lacing are scored as errors that must be corrected. If the errors are not corrected, the score is level 4. The final score is the highest level achieved on the test. Any unusual circumstances, events, behaviors, or reactions occurring during testing are noted by the therapist.

SCORING CRITERIA

Level	Criterion
2	Unable to imitate the running stitch
3	Able to imitate the running stitch, two stitches
4	Able to imitate the whip stitch, two stitches
5	Able to imitate the single cordovan stitch using overt trial-and-error methods (physically trying out various ways of completing the stitch), two stitches, two demonstrations
6	Able to imitate the single cordovan stitch using covert trial-and-error methods (mentally trying out various ways of completing the stitch before physically completing it), two stitches, one demonstration

FIG. 14–5. (*Continued*)

Lower Cognitive Level Test

Verbal Directions:

I'D LIKE TO SEE HOW WELL YOU CAN FOLLOW DIRECTIONS. PLEASE CLAP YOUR HANDS LOUDLY THREE TIMES. WATCH ME.

Demonstration:

At the midline, the therapist claps three evenly spaced beats that are distinguishable and clearly audible. The direcions may be repeated one time. The therapist may say, "I DID NOT HEAR YOU," when there is some doubt about the claps being audible. The therapist may also help to initiate the action by placing the palmar surfaces of the hands together.

Setting:

The test should be given in a setting where the patient and the therapist can hear the clapping.

SCORING CRITERIA

Level	Criterion
3	Three audible, consecutive, evenly spaced claps: contact at the palmar surface (may be more than three)
2	One or two claps, claps not audible Other movements between claps Clapping initiated by therapist Attempts to clap, but contact with other than palmar surface (e.g., fist into palm, pads of digits)
1	No response
No score	Refusal

FIG. 14–6. Lower Cognitive Level Test. Reprinted with permission from Table 4–3 and p. 113 in Allen CK. *Occupational therapy for psychiatric diseases: measurement and management of cognitive disabilities.* Boston: Little, Brown; 1985.

---

cultures and does not involve crossing the midline of the body with either hand. Patients who achieve a score at Level 3 on the LCL may be unable to imitate two running stitches on the ACL; these patients should be considered to be at Level 2, and their Level 3 score on the LCL should be disregarded.

Another, very different kind of structured evaluation that the occupational therapy assistant might be asked to administer is the human figure drawing. Occupational therapists (and psychologists) have been using this kind of evaluation for decades. The patient is asked to draw a picture of a person; the therapist later examines the drawing, looking for specific details that may indicate various problems. For example, those who follow psychoanalytic theory may look for evidence of unconscious feelings; a large mouth is believed to indicate problems in the oral stage of development. Large or reinforced ears or eyes are associated with auditory and visual hallucinations.

Figure drawings are also used to estimate mental maturity; the number of details and the complexity of the image are believed to be related to intelligence and mental development. Recently, King has begun to use

---

Person Symbol Assessment procedure

Materials and Equipment: A table and two chairs are needed. White, unlined paper, 8-1/2 by 11 inches of typing paper grade (not onion skin), and two or three pencils, #2, fairly long, with usable erasers, completes the equipment.

Directions: Seat the subject comfortably at the table. Place the paper directly in front of the subject and lay the pencils above the top of the paper, erasers toward the subject so that he can easily pick a pencil up with either hand.

Say, I'D LIKE YOU TO TRY A PENCIL AND PAPER TASK. TAKE A PENCIL PLEASE, AND MAKE A PERSON, A WHOLE PERSON. If the subject responds that he can't draw, say, IT DOESN'T REALLY MATTER HOW WELL YOU CAN DRAW. WE ARE JUST INTERESTED IN HOW YOU HANDLE PENCIL AND PAPER TASKS.

Any further questions should be answered casually and noncommitally. For example, if the subject asks, "Male or female?" reply, WHICHEVER YOU WANT. If the subject asks, "With or without clothes?" respond IT DOESN'T MATTER, etc.

The therapist should sit in the other chair and look busy, so as not to appear to be watching the subject too closely. Nevertheless, observe such things as great pressure (breaking the lead), signs of discomfort with the task, such as frequent erasures, fidgeting, overflow, tongue thrust, or lip biting. Exaggerated speed and carelessness, flushing, perspiration, or other signs of stress should be noted. Note also such things as turning the paper so that the subject is drawing sideways, frequent turning of the paper, covering or closing one eye while drawing, etc. When the subject is finished, return overt attention to him and say, GOOD, THAT'S FINE, or THANK YOU. Put the paper away without further comment and go on to other assessment tasks, or else chat casually with the subject for a few moments. It is important not to ask questions about the figure as that is, in effect, teaching the subject what you are looking for in a drawing, and to a degree would invalidate the subsequent use of the task as a posttreatment evaluation measure.

As soon as possible after the subject leaves, record on the back of the drawing the date, name, sex, age, and hand used for drawing. All this information is absolutely vital for research purposes, and failure to record it will likely render the drawing useless for scientific purposes. Diagnosis and length of hospitalization should also be included if known. Other information which might be recorded is educational level, any physical handicaps such as visual problems, glasses, tremors, history of seizures, etc. A separate sheet should be used for clinical observations, and it should be attached to the drawing.

If the subject indicates that he is finished but has only drawn a head, say, THAT'S FINE. Lay down another sheet of paper and say, NOW MAKE A WHOLE PERSON, PLEASE. Whether or not the second attempt produces a complete figure, it should be accepted without further comment and the subject thanked pleasantly.

Scoring: If a quantifiable score is desired, it is suggested that the Goodenough-Harris rating scale be used. It is important to establish the sex of the person symbol drawn, since the scoring is different for male and female figures. If there is doubt as to which sex is intended, assume that the drawing is the same sex as the subject. The most reliable use of the numerical score is to compare the subject with himself. Before and after drawings can reveal substantial changes in score.

FIG. 14–7. Person Symbol Assessment procedure. Reprinted with permission from King LJ. The person symbol as an assessment tool. In: Hemphill BJ, ed. *The evaluative process in psychiatric occupational therapy.* Thorofare, NJ: SLACK; 1982: 174–175.

figure drawings to assess body concept and to obtain clues as to possible physical and/or sensory integrative dysfunction. She has named her evaluation the *Person Symbol Assessment* (23). Directions for administering it are given in Fig. 14–7.

The Person Symbol Assessment is used to assess the patient's body concept—his understanding of body parts and their relationship to each other. A person's ability to perform skilled actions depends to a great extent on body concept. King cites many examples of patients who omitted or misdrew body parts on their Person Symbol Assessments, only later to reveal an actual physical problem in that body part. Because the drawing is used to investigate the possibility of other neuromotor problems, it is important for the observer to watch the subject carefully and note any unusual body postures, movements, or manipulations of the paper or pencil.

When the drawing is completed, the assistant gives it to the registered therapist for interpretation. The therapist will look for such features as reinforced lines, broken lines, erasures, and vague, hesitating lines; any of these might suggest a problem in body concept or sensory processing. He will also look at the placement of the figure on the page, its relationship to the vertical axis, and its symmetry and movement.

Other structured evaluations using the human figure drawing are the *House-Tree-Person* (sometimes referred to as the H-T-P), the *Kinetic Self Image,* and the *Kinetic Family Drawing.* These assessments are used primarily by psychologists. In the H-T-P the patient is asked to draw three pictures: one each of a house, a tree, and a person; all of these are believed to represent the self. The Kinetic Self Image requires the patient to draw a picture of himself doing something, and in the Kinetic Family Drawing he draws a picture of himself doing something together with his family.

All of these and the Person Symbol Assessment are examples of *projective* evaluations. These drawings are believed to represent projections from the patient's unconscious; in other words, the patient expresses, on the paper, feelings that he is not consciously aware of. In King's Person Symbol Assessment the projections assessed are of perceptions about the body, its parts, and their relationships. In the other drawing evaluations, the projections assessed are of feelings about the self, one's ability to affect the environment, and one's relationship with one's family.

Another evaluation with projective content is the *Magazine Picture Collage.* Collage is the French word for pasting or gluing, and the Magazine Picture Collage is a glued arrangement of pictures from magazines. The patient selects and cuts out the pictures, and glues and arranges them as he wishes. Lerner (25) has designed a scoring system that focuses on aspects of the Magazine Picture Collage that may indicate pathology. She found, for example, that collages made by patients had fewer pictures on them, and often did not have a central theme (26). The occupational therapy assistant might administer the Magazine Picture Collage, under supervision; the resulting collages should be interpreted by the registered therapist, perhaps in collaboration with the assistant. Directions for administering the evaluation are given in the references cited.

While projective evaluation techniques such as the Magazine Picture Collage and the various human figure drawings provide fascinating data, these data are not as measurable or quantifiable as data from standardized or criterion-referenced evaluations. Different evaluators may disagree on the meanings assigned to the patient's productions, and the relationship between a figure drawing and the patient's ability to function is not entirely clear. In today's atmosphere of reimbursement-driven health care, such evaluation procedures are rarely used and should always be backed up by more objective measures.

Another type of structured evaluation is a questionnaire or checklist that the patient completes on his own and later discusses with the therapist. The occupational therapy assistant is often assigned to give out questionnaires and collect finished ones from patients. The assistant should treat questionnaires just like any other structured evaluation, and should not add to or change the directions, or help the patient interpret them (unless this is part of the standard procedure). The *NPI Interest Checklist* (28, 36) is an example of a questionnaire the patient can complete on his own. Shown as Fig. 14–8, it lists 80 activities; the patient is asked to check off in the appropriate column whether his interest in each activity is casual, strong, or non-

NPI INTEREST CHECK LIST

Name: .... Unit: .... Date:........

Please check each item below according to your interest.

ACTIVITY	INTEREST CASUAL	STRONG	NO
1. Gardening			
2. Sewing			
3. Poker			
4. Languages			
5. Social Clubs			
6. Radio			
7. Bridge			
8. Car Repair			
9. Writing			
10. Dancing			
11. Needlework			
12. Golf			
13. Football			
14. Popular Music			
15. Puzzles			
16. Holidays			
17. Solitaire			
18. Movies			
19. Lectures			
20. Swimming			
21. Bowling			
22. Visiting			
23. Mending			
24. Chess			
25. Barbeques			
26. Reading			
27. Traveling			
28. Manual Arts			
29. Parties			
30. Dramatics			
31. Shuffleboard			
32. Ironing			
33. Social Studies			
34. Classical Music			
35. Floor Mopping			
36. Model Building			
37. Baseball			
38. Checkers			
39. Singing			
40. Home Repairs			

ACTIVITY	INTEREST CASUAL	STRONG	NO
41. Exercise			
42. Volleyball			
43. Woodworking			
44. Billiards			
45. Driving			
46. Dusting			
47. Jewelry Making			
48. Tennis			
49. Cooking			
50. Basketball			
51. History			
52. Guitar			
53. Science			
54. Collecting			
55. Ping Pong			
56. Leatherwork			
57. Shopping			
58. Photography			
59. Painting			
60. Television			
61. Concerts			
62. Ceramics			
63. Camping			
64. Laundry			
65. Dating			
66. Mosaics			
67. Politics			
68. Scrabble			
69. Decorating			
70. Math			
71. Service Groups			
72. Piano			
73. Scouting			
74. Plays			
75. Clothes			
76. Knitting			
77. Hairstyling			
78. Religion			
79. Drums			
80. Conversation			

Please list other special interests:

FIG. 14–8. NPI Interest Checklist. Reprinted with permission of the University of California at Los Angeles, from Fig. 1 in Matsutsuyu JS. The interest checklist. *Am J Occup Ther* 1969; 23:323–328.

existent. The assistant may encounter other versions of the interest checklist in the clinic; Hemphill indicates that "there are almost as many interest checklists as there are therapists" (19). Perhaps this reflects changing cultural patterns and therapists' desire to incorporate activities that are currently popular.

The original NPI Interest Checklist was intended to be used to identify areas that the patient was most interested in. The 80 activities were sorted into categories of manual skills, physical sports, social rec-

reation, activities of daily living, and cultural/educational. Matsutsuyu (28) suggested that the therapist could infer the patient's interests from the distribution of his scores in these five categories. Rogers, Weinstein, and Figone (36) showed, however, that individuals' scores in these categories did not always accurately reflect their interests. They suggested that the number of categories may need to be expanded in order to, for example, separate activities that reflect traditional sexual roles. Despite these problems, the Interest

Checklist (or variations of it) is used in almost one-fourth of psychiatric occupational therapy departments (18). Often it is used as a starting point for a discussion of how the patient spends his leisure time, whether he enjoys the leisure activities he does, and whether there are others he has done in the past that he might like to renew, or new ones that he would like to try for the first time.

To summarize, all of the structured (standardized or criterion-referenced) evaluations discussed in this section are designed to be administered according to the directions given, using the same tools, materials, setup, and directions each time. This rule applies to other structured evaluations as well. Obviously, because of space limitations, not all of the structured evaluations used by psychiatric occupational therapists across the country are presented here. We have selected those that the occupational therapy assistant is most likely to encounter, and have emphasized those for which the COTA might be asked at entry level to develop service competency in administration and scoring.

Many unstandardized evaluations have been and continue to be used in mental health clinics. Some of these involve tasks like constructing a mosaic tile ashtray or a paper mobile; some are paper and pencil tasks that may require measuring, or following directions; still others are questionnaires about the patient's occupational history and interests. The assistant may anticipate that he will encounter others in the clinic and that he will observe the registered therapist administering still others. Wherever an evaluation lacks a set procedure for administration and scoring, its usefulness must be questioned. What is the evaluation measuring? Would another evaluator agree with the results? If the patient were tested again, would the results be similar? If not, does this indicate a change in the patient or a weakness in the test? How can service competency be developed and assured, if the evaluation gives unreliable results?

The use of unstandardized evaluations is questionable practice. An evaluation that does not give reliable information that can be used to plan treatment and to measure change is most likely a waste of time.

DOCUMENTATION AND COMMUNICATION OF EVALUATION DATA

Once the assistant has observed the patient, there yet remains one of the most important steps in the data gathering and evaluation process: that of reporting the information to those who need to know it. There are two ways in which this is usually done: by writing in the medical record, or by making an oral report. The two processes will be discussed separately.

An evaluation note is written into the chart, generally by the OTR. The COTA may contribute information in writing or orally, which the OTR then incorporates. Detailed suggestions for writing evaluation and observation data into note form will be given in Chapter 16, along with sample notes.

The occupational therapy assistant should also be prepared to present her observations orally to her supervisor, other members of the occupational therapy department, or other staff. Sometimes the presentation happens spontaneously, in the hallway or the nurses' station; these presentations are casual and informal. Other, more formal presentations are made in team meetings, rounds, and department meetings. Regardless of the context, standard English and correct pronunciation should always be used.

Watching and listening to another occupational therapy staff member make a presentation is a good way to learn what is expected. Oral presentations should be loud enough to be heard by everyone present (try directing your speech to the person farthest away). Try to make eye contact with people you are comfortable with. It may help to rehearse your presentation in advance, perhaps using a tape recorder.

The most important thing to consider when making any presentation is the audience that will be listening to it. Who are these people? What do they want to hear about? Doctors, for example, may want to know about how the medication is affecting the patient. What terminology and vocabulary are they comfortable with? As discussed previously, occupational therapy jargon, although appropriate for department meetings, will probably not be understood by other staff. Choose words that your audience will understand.

Students and new graduates often suffer perfectly normal fears about speaking in large groups. Their fears are legion: Will I say the wrong thing? Will they think I'm stupid? Will they notice that I'm nervous? What if my voice cracks? What if I forget what to say? It may not help to hear that almost everyone has these fears in the beginning, but whether or not it helps, it *is* true. Public speaking, like many other desirable professional skills (e.g., interviewing), is only mastered by doing it, and doing it again. Practice helps.

SUMMARY

Data gathering and evaluation are the foundation of the treatment process, providing essential information about who the patient is, what his life is like, the kinds of things he wants and needs to do, and the problems that stand in his way. The occupational therapy assistant contributes to data gathering and evaluation by collecting information from medical records and interviews and by performing observations and structured evaluations as directed by the registered therapist. The assistant also records and reports her observations to the therapist and to other professionals working with the patient.

The ability to observe dispassionately, free from personal bias or preconceived ideas, is an essential skill. The observations and evaluations performed by the assistant and others become the basis of the patient's treatment plan; the patient's future depends on them. For this reason, service competency must be established before the occupatinal therapy assistant evaluates the patient. Being involved in any part of a patient's evaluation is a serious responsibility, but also a wonderful opportunity to explore and come to better understand the unique and sometimes perplexing world of another human being.

REFERENCES

1. Adler F. Sisters in crime (1972). In: Maggio R, compiler. *The Beacon book of quotations by women.* Boston: Beacon Press; 1992: 179.
2. Allen CK. *Occupational therapy for psychiatric diseases: measurement and management of cognitive disabilities.* Boston: Little, Brown; 1985.
3. American Occupational Therapy Association Entry-Level Role Delineation Task Force. Entry-level role delineation for registered occupational therapists (OTRs) and certified occupational therapy assistants (COTAs). *Am J Occup Ther* 1990; 44:1091–1102.
4. American Occupational Therapy Association Uniform Terminology Task Force. Uniform terminology for occupational therapy, second edition. *Am J Occup Ther* 1989; 43:808–815.
5. Barris R, Oakley F, Kielhofner G. The role checklist. In: Hemphill BJ, ed. *Mental health assessment in occupational therapy: an integrative approach to the evaluative process.* Thorofare, NJ: SLACK; 1988.
6. Barth T. Barth time construction. In: Hemphill BJ, ed. *Mental health assessment in occupational therapy: an integrative approach to the evaluative process.* Thorofare, NJ: SLACK; 1988.
7. Barth T. A new variation on an old theme: the Barth Time Construction. *Am Occup Ther Assoc Mental Health Special Interest Section Newsletter* 1986; 9(1):4.
8. Benne KD, Sheats P. Functional roles of group members. *J Social Issues* 1948; 4(2):42–47.
9. Berg A, Hammitt KB. Assessing the psychiatric patient's ability to meet the literacy demands of hospitalization. *Hosp Commun Psychiatry* 1980; 31:266–268.

10. Bloomer J, Williams S. The Bay Area Functional Performance Evaluation. In: Hemphill BJ, ed. *The evaluation process in psychiatric occupational therapy.* Thorofare, NJ: SLACK; 1982.
11. Brayman SJ, Kirby T. The comprehensive occupational therapy evaluation. In: Hemphill BJ, ed. *The evaluative process in psychiatric occupational therapy.* Thorofare, NJ: SLACK; 1982.
12. Brayman SJ, Kirby TF, Misenheimer AM, Short MJ. Comprehensive occupational therapy evaluation scale. *Am J Occup Ther* 1976; 30:94–100.
13. Casanova JS, Ferber J. Comprehensive evaluation of basic living skills. *Am J Occup Ther* 1976; 30:101–105.
14. Clark EN, Peters M. *Scorable self care evaluation.* Thorofare, NJ: SLACK; 1984.
15. Coles GS, Roth L, Pollack IW. Literacy skills of long-term hospitalized mental patients. *Hosp Commun Psychiatry* 1978; 29:512–516.
16. Cynkin S. *Occupational therapy: toward health through activities.* Boston: Little, Brown; 1979.
17. Florey L, Michelman SM. Occupational role history: a screening tool for psychiatric occupational therapy. *Am J Occup Ther* 1982; 36:301–308.
18. Hemphill BJ. Mental health evaluations used in occupational therapy. *Am J Occup Ther* 1980; 34:721–726.
19. Hemphill BJ. In: Hemphill BJ, ed. *The evaluative process in psychiatric occupational therapy.* Thorofare, NJ: SLACK; 1982.
20. Houston D, Williams SL, Bloomer J, Mann WC. The Bay Area functional performance evaluation: development and standardization. *Am J Occup Ther* 1989; 43:170–183.
21. Kanny EM, Kohlman L. *An occupational therapist evaluating functional living skills in psychiatry* (videocassette and study guide). University of Washington, Seattle: Health Sciences Center of Educational Resources; 1978.
22. Kielhofner G, Henry AD. Development and investigation of the occupational performance history interview. *Am J Occup Ther* 1988; 42:489–498.
23. King LJ. The person symbol as an assessment tool. In Hemphill BJ, ed. *The evaluative process in psychiatric occupational therapy.* Thorofare, NJ: SLACK; 1982.
24. Leonardelli CA. The Milwaukee evaluation of daily living skills (MEDLS). In: Hemphill BJ, ed. *Mental health assessment in occupational therapy: an integrative approach to the evaluative process.* Thorofare, NJ: SLACK; 1988.
25. Lerner C. The magazine picture collage. In: Hemphill BJ, ed. *The evaluative process in psychiatric occupational therapy.* Thorofare, NJ: SLACK; 1982.
26. Lerner C. The magazine picture collage: development of an objective scoring system. *Am J Occup Ther* 1977; 31:156–161.
27. Maurer P, Barris R, Bonder B, Gillette N. Hierarchy of competencies relating to the use of standardized instruments and evaluation techniques by occupational therapists. *Am J Occup Ther* 1984; 38:803–804.
28. Matsutsuyu JS. The interest checklist. *Am J Occup Ther* 1969; 23:323–328.
29. McGourty LK. *Kohlman evaluation of living skills.* Seattle, Wash: KELS Research; 1979.
30. McGourty LK. Kohlman evaluation of living skills (KELS). In: Hemphill BJ, ed. *Mental health assessment in occupational therapy: an integrative approach to the evaluative process.* Thorofare, NJ: SLACK; 1988.
31. Moorhead L. The occupational history. *Am J Occup Ther* 1969; 23:329–334.
32. Mosey AC. *Three frames of reference for mental health.* Thorofare, NJ: SLACK; 1970.
33. Oakley F. Role checklist, parts 1 and 2 (Appendices A and B). In: Hemphill BJ, ed. *Mental health assessment in occupational therapy: an integrative approach to the evaluative process.* Thorofare, NJ: SLACK; 1988.
34. Peloquin SM. The development of an occupational therapy interview/therapy set procedure. *Am J Occup Ther* 1983; 37:457–461.
35. Rogers JC. The NPI interest checklist. In: Hemphill BJ, ed. *Mental health assessment in occupational therapy: an integrative approach to the evaluative process.* Thorofare, NJ: SLACK; 1988.
36. Rogers JC, Weinstein JM, Figone JJ. The interest check list: an empirical assessment. *Am J Occup Ther* 1978; 32:628–630.
37. Shaw C. The interview process. In: Hemphill BJ, ed. *The evaluative process in psychiatric occupational therapy.* Thorofare, NJ: SLACK; 1982: 15–42.
38. Watanabe S. Four concepts basic to the occupational therapy process. *Am J Occup Ther* 1968; 23:439–445.
39. Watanabe S. 1968 Regional Institute on the Evaluation Process, New York Report RAS-123-T-68. Rockvill, Md: American Occupational Therapy Association.

ADDITIONAL REFERENCES AND SUGGESTED READINGS

Allen CK, Kehrberg K, Burns T. Evaluation instruments. In: Allen CK, Earhart CA, Blue T. *Occupational therapy goals for the physically and cognitively disabled.* Rockville, Md: American Occupational Therapy Association; 1992.
Allen CK. *Occupational therapy for psychiatric diseases: measurement and management of cognitive disabilities.* Boston: Little, Brown; 1985.
Barris R, Kielhofner G, Watts JH. *Psychosocial occupational therapy: practice in a pluralistic arena.* Laurel, Md: RAMSCO; 1983.
Cynkin S. *Occupational therapy: toward health through activities.* Boston: Little, Brown; 1979.
David SK, Riley WT. The relationship of the Allen

cognitive level test to cognitive abilities and psychopathology. *Am J Occup Ther* 1990; 44:493–497.

Fidler G, Fidler J. *Occupational therapy: a communication process in psychiatry.* New York: Macmillan; 1963.

Froelich RE, Bishop FM. *Clinical interviewing skills.* St Louis: Mosby; 1977.

Hasselkus BR, Maguire GH. Functional assessments used with older adults. In: Hemphill BJ, ed. *Mental health assessment in occupational therapy: an integrative approach to the evaluative process.* Thorofare, NJ: SLACK; 1988.

Hemphill BJ. Listening as an evaluative tool in the interviewing process. In: Hemphill BJ, ed. *Mental health assessment in occupational therapy: an integrative approach to the evaluative process.* Thorofare, NJ: SLACK; 1988.

Josman N, Katz N. A problem-solving version of the Allen cognitive level test. *Am J Occup Ther* 1991; 45:331–338.

Katz N, Heimann N. Review of research conducted in Israel on cognitive disability instrumentation. *Occup Ther Mental Health* 1990; 10(4):1–15.

Katz N, Josman N, Steinmetz N. Relationship between cognitive disability theory and the model of human occupation in the assessment of psychiat-

ric and nonpsychiatric adolescents. *Occup Ther Mental Health* 1988; 8(1):31–43.

Kielhofner G, Henry AH. Use of an occupational history interview in occupational therapy. In: Hemphill BJ, ed. *Mental health assessment in occupational therapy: an integrative approach to the evaluative process.* Thorofare, NJ: SLACK; 1988.

Mosey AC. *Activities therapy.* New York: Raven Press; 1973.

Peterson CQ. Pre-vocational assessment in mental health. In: Hemphill BJ, ed. *Mental health assessment in occupational therapy: an integrative approach to the evaluative process.* Thorofare, NJ: SLACK; 1988.

Shapiro M. Application of the Allen cognitive level test in assessing cognitive level functioning of emotionally disturbed boys. *Am J Occup Ther* 1992; 46:514–520.

Shaw C. The interviewing process in occupational therapy. In: Hemphill BJ, ed. *Mental health assessment in occupational therapy: an integrative approach to the evaluative process.* Thorofare, NJ: SLACK; 1988.

Willson M. *Occupational therapy in long-term psychiatry.* Edinburgh: Churchill Livingstone; 1983.

15

Treatment Planning

The art of practice includes the ability to establish rapport, to empathize, and to facilitate choices about occupational and human potential within a community of others. Engaging in the art of practice commits the therapist to an encounter with an individual who is a collaborator in his or her plan for treatment.

SUZANNE M. PELOQUIN (14)

Occupational therapy treatment is a planned process for creating change so that the patient will be able to carry out his chosen daily life activities as independently and comfortably as possible. The patient is the final authority as to which goals are most important. Occupational therapists have at their disposal a variety of treatment activities and methods that can be used to create change in the direction of the goal, but the methods must be chosen carefully, depending on the patient's needs. By its nature, treatment is individual and must be planned so that it meets the needs of the particular patient.

The registered occupational therapist is responsible for the treatment plan (2,6,16). The occupational therapy assistant assists the therapist in developing treatment goals and selecting treatment methods. With experience, the assistant may become more practiced and independent, but the final responsibility for treatment planning and management still rests with the registered therapist. In practice, this most often means that the therapist will determine a general treatment goal and the major steps

within it, and will make the final decision about the treatment methods. The assistant contributes to the plan as it is being developed by sharing her observations of the patient, giving her opinion about what the patient needs and is capable of, and suggesting treatment methods.

This chapter will present an overview of the treatment planning process. It will discuss some of the problems occupational therapists encounter in planning treatment for psychiatric patients that they do not encounter as often in planning treatment for patients with other kinds of problems. It will relate clinical reasoning to the planning process, and will delineate the steps. Since occupational therapy assistants may be asked to contribute to the writing of treatment goals, this chapter will explain how a goal is selected. Since occupational therapy assistants work directly with patients, carrying out treatment, it will explain how treatment methods are selected (how we determine how to try to reach the goal). Finally, it will describe how to monitor the success of treatment and modify the treatment plan.

TREATMENT PLANNING
IN PSYCHIATRY

Planning treatment for a psychiatric patient is like trying to assemble a complex puzzle from which several pieces are missing. Our scientific and clinical understanding of mental illness is not yet well enough developed for us to know for sure what is the real cause of the patient's problems, and because of this, it is hard to identify the correct solution. To appreciate what a serious obstacle this is, let us look first at the situation of a patient with a *physical* disability.

Mark is an 18-year-old high school senior who sustained a severe crushing injury to his right (dominant) hand as a result of a motorcycle accident. His middle, ring, and index fingers were amputated just distal to the PIP (proximal interphalangeal joint). When the cast was removed it was noted that all motions of the thumb and fingers were severely limited. There is severe pain on movement. Mark has a girlfriend and several close friends. He belongs to the math and science club, the computer club, and the track team. He had been planning to attend college and major in computer science.

We know enough about this patient to plan his treatment, in general terms at least. First, we can anticipate that, because of his injury, he will have problems performing bilateral activities such as dressing, grooming, and using a computer keyboard. We know that the immediate causes of Mark's difficulty are limited motion, weakness, and pain, and we know what caused them: a crushing injury. We can see the effects of the injury physically, by examining the patient and looking at his X-rays. We know treatment methods that will increase range of motion and strength in the hand, and we know ways to reduce pain. We can suggest adaptive equipment and adapted methods for performing activities. In short, we know that occupational therapy can help Mark learn new ways to do the things he needs to do now, and help him regain his physical

functions and previous level of activity for the future.

Contrast this with the following case of a psychiatric patient of similar age and background:

Drew is a 19-year-old college freshman who has been living at home with his parents while attending school. During Thanksgiving weekend he ran away from home; after 24 hours his parents notified the police. He was found two days later wandering on the street, wearing only his underwear. He had not eaten since he left home. His parents reported that he had been growing more isolated over the past 18 months, staying in his room for days at a time and refusing to come downstairs even for meals. He had been a good student, receiving As and Bs in his courses for the first three years of high school, but his grades fell to Cs and Ds in his senior year. He says that he needs to be left alone because he "ruins other people's lives." Drew's diagnosis is schizophrenia, type unknown.

What, exactly, do we know about *this* patient? We know he "has schizophrenia" and that he has been having increasing difficulty functioning in his role as a student over the past year and a half. His grooming and hygiene skills seem marginal at best; his ability to obtain a proper diet seems questionable; he is socially isolated. What can we do to help him? And where should we begin? Unlike physical disabilities, the causes of which can be seen on X-rays, physical examinations, and laboratory tests, the causes of the psychiatric disability associated with schizophrenia elude us. Psychiatrists know some medications that help relieve the symptoms for some patients, but they are still trying to understand why and how these medications work. They do not know the *cause* of schizophrenia and its functional disability any better than we do or the patient does. Perhaps research will give us an answer within our lifetimes.

In the meantime, however, how are we to help the patient? We first have to decide what we can reasonably expect this patient

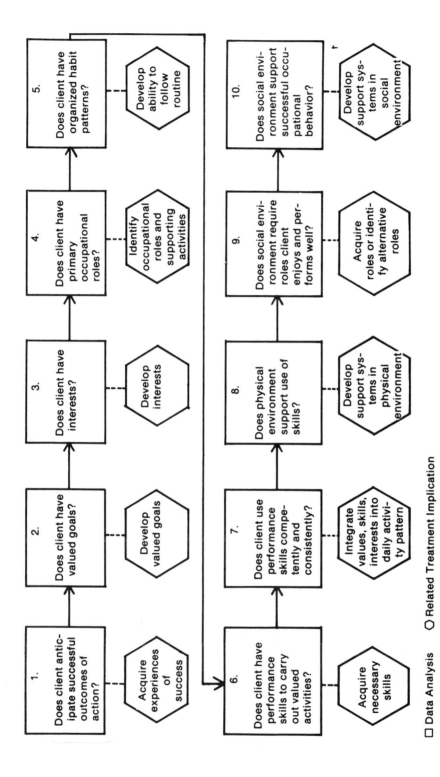

□ Data Analysis   ○ Related Treatment Implication

FIG. 15–1. Model of human occupation: data analysis and treatment implications. Reprinted from Fig. 2 of Cubie SH, Kaplan K. A case analysis method for the model of human occupation. *Am J Occup Ther* 1982; 36:645–656. Copyright © 1982 by the American Occupational Therapy Association, Inc. Reprinted with permission.

to achieve. It is not clear what our immediate and long-term goals should be for him, although we can identify areas that need attention: self-care, other independent daily living skills, nutrition, academic and study skills, leisure and social skills. But which one shall we tackle first, and why?

And once the goals are chosen, how shall we address them? As occupational therapists and assistants we are proficient in analyzing, teaching, and adapting activities of daily living and a wide range of work and leisure activities. We know how to break new learning into manageable small steps so that a patient can master a complex skill one step at a time. We have many techniques and methods at our disposal. But how shall we choose which ones to use?

Part of our uncertainty about how to answer all of these questions stems from our ignorance of exactly how schizophrenia works to undermine the patient's ability to function in daily life. Another source of uncertainty for beginners (students and new therapists) is inexperience with patients such as this one, and the lack of a mental file of treatment attempts and outcomes.

When a therapist plans treatment, she is taking the patient's life in her hands. Perhaps she does not have the same life-or-death responsibility as the surgeon at the operating table, but the decisions she makes *will* affect his life. People with severe psychiatric disabilities have many fewer choices and in some senses less freedom than the rest of us; their disabilities limit what they can do, and even how they can think about what they can do; social pressures limit them still further. Therapists and other professionals are asked to make recommendations about where the patient should live, what he should do during the day, how much supervision he should receive, and so forth. This is a weighty responsibility and requires clinical reasoning.

APPLYING CLINICAL REASONING TO TREATMENT PLANNING WITHIN THE MODEL OF HUMAN OCCUPATION

In planning treatment, it is essential to work from a practice model. Let's look at the questions the occupational therapist might derive from the model of human occupation. Cubie and Kaplan (5) have formulated a series of assessment questions and treatment implications based on the model. Their data analysis sequence, shown as Fig. 15–1, shows assessment questions and the order in which they should be approached; the numbered questions appear in the square boxes. For each assessment question there is a related treatment implication (hexagonal box); if the patient has a deficit in the assessed area, these provide a focus for intervention. The flow of the questions is determined by the hierarchical nature of the subsystems within the model. As described further in Chapter 4, these are the volition subsystem at the highest level (questions 1, 2, and 3), the habituation subsystem next (questions 4, 5, and 6), and the performance subsystem at the lowest level (questions 7 through 10). This diagram is included so that the occupational therapy assistant can appreciate how his contribution to treatment planning fits into the overall plan designed by the occupational therapist.

STEPS IN TREATMENT PLANNING

Let us break this clinical reasoning process down still further, into discrete steps. Using these steps the occupational therapy assistant can help formulate treatment plans in areas such as independent daily living skills. Table 15–1 highlights the steps in treatment planning.

The first step, reviewing the results of the evaluation (or evaluations), should be executed with an open mind but at the same time with a clear idea of what kinds of in-

TABLE 15–1. *Steps in planning treatment*

1. Review the results of the evaluation(s).
2. Identify problems (and their causes, if possible).
3. Identify the patient's strengths and assess his motivation for treatment.
4. Set goals (long and short term, in order of priority).
5. Identify treatment principles.
6. Select treatment methods.

formation one is seeking. The occupational therapy assistant will be assigned a specific area in which to plan treatment; independent living skills is one example. Obviously, evaluation results that relate directly to this area would be the most important, but other information may also be valuable. For example, the patient's relationship with other family members in the household may give some clues about why he has deficits in independent living skills. It is important not to confine your search to what you expect to find, and to maintain a curious and alert perspective. Try not to be too influenced by the patient's diagnosis or by the opinions of other staff. Stereotyped thinking can stand in the way of seeing the patient's strengths and his individual potential. Who knows? The diagnosis might even be wrong.

The purpose of reviewing the evaluation is to obtain the answers to steps two and three, to learn as much as you can about the patient's problems (or deficits), his strengths (or assets), and his motivation for treatment. This will require combining information from many sources; you cannot expect to find the answers in one place, and you may need to combine what you know to come up with an answer. Try to define as clearly as you can the causes of the patient's problems as well as the problems themselves. An understanding of the causes is often the key to the correct treatment approach.

For example, a patient may have very poor hygiene, as evidenced by greasy hair, stained teeth, and body odor, for a variety of reasons: He may never have developed good hygiene skills, or he may have gotten out of the habit of using the skills he once had, or his usual environment may make it difficult for him to perform hygiene and grooming tasks (e.g., if he is homeless). There may be cultural reasons; daily bathing and frequent shampooing are Western values; personal hygiene standards elsewhere vary. There may be reasons that derive from the disease process: the patient may not remember to bathe and care for his body, or his sense of time may be so distorted that he does not realize he should, or he may be so frightened of other people that he deliberately ignores his hygiene in order to drive others away. You can see that these various causes for the patient's poor hygiene will lead to very different ideas about what kind of treatment is needed and where it should begin.

The patient himself can often tell you what is wrong and help to define the problem. Involving the patient in planning his treatment, to the extent he is capable, ensures that the patient understands and agrees with the plan, a first step in motivating him to work on these goals. Even patients who have limited ability to verbalize their concerns can be guided to participate. In such cases, the therapist may need to present limited choices from which the patient can make a selection. The patient might choose which goal or area is most important for him to work on, for example (13).

The patient's strengths must also be considered. Although the main focus of our energies will be on finding solutions to the patient's problems, we, as well as he, need to appreciate his endurance and persistence and courage in carrying on with his life despite his disability. The skills and habits he has developed and maintained, and his resolve to work hard and succeed in treatment, can only be strengthened by our recognition and support.

Questions sometimes arise about the patient's motivation for treatment. The patient may be labeled as unmotivated when he fails to work toward goals that the therapist and assistant feel are appropriate and necessary. Although it may be true that he is not motivated toward those goals, this is often only because the goals do not reflect his real concerns. An example is the 27-year-old legal secretary with a diagnosis of paranoid schizophrenia who says she would rather collect public assistance and stay home and watch television than go back to work. Rather than force her to accept a work adjustment training program, the occupational therapist or assistant might do better to explore the thinking behind this decision. The treatment cannot succeed unless the patient is actively involved.

Where disagreements exist between the patient and the treatment staff about the best course of treatment, it is important to discuss the question at length. If the staff has identified problems that they believe the patient should work on, they need to explain them to the patient so that the patient understands them. They must listen and respond to the patient's questions, concerns, and preferences. In presenting recommendations the staff should stress the tangible benefits that will result. If the patient cannot accept the staff's recommendations, then the staff must modify its expectations, and work with the patient to reach agreement about what should be done.

It must be noted, however, that it is not always possible to obtain the patient's cooperation and participation in planning treatment. It is very difficult to engage the attention or even the awareness of a patient who is psychotic and out of touch with reality; therefore, in acute settings the staff may develop a treatment plan on behalf of the patient, sometimes in consultation with members of the patient's family.

Once the staff and the patient have decided on a general direction for treatment, the next step is to set specific goals. A goal is a statement about what the patient will achieve. Goals can be classified as long-term or short-term. A short-term goal is one that depends on the length of time available for treatment as well as on the patient's sense of time and ability to visualize the future. What makes a goal long-term rather than short-term is either that it involves completing several smaller (short-term) goals or that it can only be accomplished over a period of time that is long by the patient's standards. Breaking long-term goals down into a series of short-term goals can make it easier for the patient to tackle them.

Goals should be organized in order of priority. Priority means the importance or urgency of the goal. In many cases, especially with severely disabled patients, it is possible to come up with a list of 20 or 30 goals. Not all of them would be equally important, however, and the therapist would have to choose the goals of greater urgency or highest priority as the ones to be tackled first. Some goals by their nature must be achieved before others; for example, a patient who needs to learn basic cooking so that he can live on his own must first learn elementary kitchen safety. Usually only a few (not more than three or four) goals are attempted at one time; sometimes only one goal is selected at first. Decisions about how many goals to choose should be based on the patient's ability to divide his energies effectively among the different goals and on the amount of effort needed to reach a particular goal.

Regardless of which goals are chosen as the first ones to work on, there should be an overall plan that describes the ultimate goals of the patient's program. Although it may take him months or years to reach these goals (or he may never reach them), having a clear objective helps unify the smaller goals. Otherwise the program may become fragmented and the purpose obscured. In other words, short-term goals such as "learning to follow a schedule" or "arriving on time for activity groups" should be part of a larger plan, the ultimate goal of which might be (as an example) for the patient to get a job and be able to support himself.

These first steps in treatment planning (identification of problems, strengths, and motivation, and setting of treatment priorities) should be done in consultation with other treatment personnel who are working with the patient. If the other staff do not agree with the occupational therapist's or assistant's assessment of the patient's problems, they are not likely to cooperate with the occupational therapy plan. Plans that the patient, his family, and all staff agree on have the best chance of success, because everyone will support them.

GENERAL GOALS OF PSYCHIATRIC OCCUPATIONAL THERAPY

Let us start with the understanding that the overall aim of occupational therapy (regardless of area of specialization) is to help the patient function as independently as possible within the limits of his disability. Thus, whether the occupational therapy assistant is helping the arthritic patient learn to use energy conservation and joint protection techniques in cooking, or the occupational therapist is providing tactile stimulation to the tactilely defensive autistic child, the final purpose is the same: to make it possible for that person to function as best he can within his chosen activities and occupational roles.

It is traditional to classify occupational therapy intervention as fitting into one of four broad categories: treatment (sometimes called functional restoration), maintenance of function, rehabilitation, and prevention (19). The focus of intervention differs, depending on the category.

Treatment or *functional restoration* aims to alter the underlying disease process; the principles and techniques of sensory integration fit into this category. It is not really clear whether occupational therapy interventions (even those of sensory integration) really affect the underlying disease process

in most psychiatric disorders. We do not yet know enough about the underlying disease process to say one way or the other.

Maintenance of function is aimed at assisting the patient to use whatever remaining capabilities he has. This is often the focus of programs for patients with chronic or progressive disorders such as schizophrenia and organic mental disorders. Within this approach, the occupational therapist or assistant focuses on creating an environment that supports and encourages the patient to care for his own needs and to take charge of his own life, in whatever way he can, for as long as possible. Despite the best efforts of patient and therapist, the long-term outlook in some cases is that the patient will function less and less well as time goes by. Without occupational therapy, however, he will lose the ability to function more rapidly.

Rehabilitation focuses on restoring the patient's ability to function after the disease process has been medically treated. The patient has lost his ability to function as a result of the disease; this loss of function is sometimes called a residual disability. Even though the disease process has been cured (or, more typically in psychiatry, stabilized with medication), the patient still may not perform his daily activities and carry out his occupational roles as well as he could before he became ill. The word *habilitation* is used to distinguish intervention for those patients who never developed these functional abilities, because they became ill at a younger age. Rehabilitation (or habilitation) is a major focus within psychiatric occupational therapy. It is important to recognize, however, that this approach is appropriate only for patients who are able to change their habits and learn new skills. This is difficult to judge since some patients may resist changing for many months (perhaps because they are frightened of the responsibility this might imply), but then suddenly seem to begin applying themselves to their own rehabilitation. Cognitive level should be considered here. Patients at Level 4 and

TABLE 15–2. *General goals of psychiatric occupational therapy*

Skill area	Goals (to develop, improve, or maintain ability to . . .)
Activities of daily living	Initiate and effectively perform to a level that is socially acceptable such activities as grooming, oral hygiene, bathing, toilet hygiene, dressing, eating, medication routine, using telephone and other communication devices.
ADL—socialization	Interact in ways that are socially appropriate to culture and context.
ADL—transportation	Travel within the community on foot and by mechanical transport (car, bus).
ADL—sexual expression	Meet sexual needs in ways that are socially appropriate and safe for self and others.
Work—home management	Organize and carry out tasks related to clothing care, cleaning, meal preparation and cleanup, shopping, money management, household maintenance, and safety procedures.
Work—care of others	Provide physical care, psychosocial nurturance, and appropriate activities for children and others under one's care.
Work—education	Plan and carry out tasks related to schooling, such as homework, study, preparation for tests, extracurricular activities.
Work—vocational exploration	Identify aptitudes and interests, identify and pursue vocational training and job opportunities suited to ones' aptitude, interests, and skills.
Work—job search	Search, identify, and select work opportunities. Carry out application and interview process. Evaluate results of application and interview process.
Work—job performance	Follow directions. Perform job tasks effectively, within the context. Work neatly and with attention to detail that is reasonable for the situation. Follow a schedule, maintain attendance, adhere to time standards of the job. Demonstrate appropriate behaviors for the work situation, in the areas of grooming, interpersonal communication, and safety.
Work—retirement	Determine valued goals and interests, and pursue them.
Play and leisure	Identify interests and skills and locate appropriate opportunities to pursue them. Schedule time and actually follow through on using leisure to pursue interests.
Sensory motor components	Attend to sensory input. Correctly interpret sensory input. Organize information received through the senses. Integrate body parts in reaction to sensory input.
Cognitive skills	Demonstrate alertness and responsiveness to situations in the environment. Locate self with regard to time, place, and person. Concentrate and attend to a task long enough to complete it. Remember important information and skills. Place information, steps, concepts in order. Generalize learning to new situations. Make decisions. Solve problems as they arise.
Psychological skills—roles	Identify, value, and carry out roles within a social context (e.g., worker, student, neighbor).
Psychological skills—values	Identify and enact ideas and beliefs important to the self.
Psychological skills—interests	Identify and pursue activities that bring pleasure to the self.
Psychological skills—engagement	Initiate and maintain performance and attention in an activity.

TABLE 15–2. (*Continued*)

Skill area	Goals (to develop, improve, or maintain ability to . . .)
Psychological skills—disengagement	Cease an activity when it is appropriate or desirable to do so.
Psychological skills—self-concept	Accept and embrace the self as having value. Identify one's assets and limitations. Perceive, understand, accept, and enact the direction of the self.
Social skills—behaving in context	Identify and carry out socially appropriate behaviors in context, in relation to manners, personal space, eye contact, gestures, etc. Compromise, negotiate, cooperate, and compete with others. Interact comfortably with one other person and within a group.
Social skills—communicating	Convey and receive information and feelings through words and gestures in a manner appropriate to the situation.
Social skills—self-expression	Use facial and bodily gestures, voice tone and volume, to express feelings and ideas. Assert self.
Self-management—coping skills	Identify stress, stress reaction, stressors. Identify, select, and apply stress management strategies.
Self-management—time management	Balance work, leisure, and self-care. Budget and schedule use of time.
Self-management—self-control	Recognize one's own behavior and its causes (internal and external). Control feelings and impulses. Take responsibility for one's own behavior. Modify one's behavior as appropriate for the situation.

lower are not likely to learn new skills, even with great motivation and effort.

Prevention aims to intervene before dysfunction occurs. It is usually applied where a dysfunction is predicted. An example of this is a supportive activity group for children of alcoholic parents. Prevention overlaps with the other areas already discussed; for example, maintenance of function is in some senses a form of prevention since it aims to prevent a deterioration that is otherwise inevitable.

Keeping these important categories in mind, look now at the skills listed in Table 15–2. The skills are derived from the Uniform Terminology, Mosey's adaptive skills, and other practice models. Several goals are listed for some skill areas; each goal may be phrased in such a way as to focus on either rehabilitation/habilitation, maintenance of function, or prevention. Beginning the goal statement with verbs like "to develop, to restore, or to improve . . ." indicates emphasis on rehabilitation or habil-

itation. Maintenance of function is the indicated focus of goals that begin with the words "to maintain ability to," and prevention is the focus of goals that begin "to prevent dysfunction of ability to."

The list in Table 15–2 is by no means exhaustive, and the reader should remember three important cautions in using this list. First, not every possible goal is listed; do not be discouraged if a goal you think is important is missing from the list. Second, other occupational therapy goals (such as those that relate to physical functions) may need to be addressed even for patients whose primary diagnosis is psychiatric; for example, the patient with depression who is recovering from a tendon repair following a wrist-slashing will need physical restoration as well. Third, many of the goals listed are themselves dependent on smaller goals or subskills. The needs of the individual patient must be considered, because for many the place to begin is with the subskills. The goals listed in Table 15–2 are an overview of the general objectives of psychiatric occupational therapy; they are only a reference point and are not meant to substitute for the highly specific treatment goals that are developed for each patient. Writing more specific, individualized, and measurable treatment goals (derived from these general goals) is the subject of the next section.

HOW TO WRITE A TREATMENT GOAL

Goals in a patient's treatment plan should be written so that they describe very clearly what the patient will do. Goals should follow logically from problems that have been identified by assessment and selected by the patient and staff as important. The more specific the description of the problem, the easier it is to write the corresponding goal. Consider the following:

a. Mr. Peters has low self-esteem.
b. Ms. Danford has poor reality testing.

These problem statements are confusing because they describe not the patient's behavior (or indeed anything measurable or observable) but rather some unverifiable internal state. Each could be converted into a specific behavioral problem statement by the addition of some observable evidence. For example, "Mr. Peters has poor self-esteem as evidenced by greasy hair, rumpled clothing, and stained teeth," is a more behaviorally oriented statement. However, one is left with questions about whether these behaviors reflect poor self-esteem or perhaps something else. Therefore, problem statements that contain observable behaviors are preferred to those that refer to intrapsychic phenomena or other intangibles. Here are some problem statements that meet this criterion:

c. Ms. Flint has very poor hygiene, as evidenced by greasy hair, stained teeth, and body odor.
d. Mr. Mills has no regular leisure interests except watching television and drinking.

e. Ms. Woolworth has been fired from many jobs as a result of arguments with supervisors.

Once the problems have been adequately described, the goals that correspond to them can be written. Goals also must be phrased in terms of how the patient will behave or what he will do once the goal is reached. Examples of goals for the three problems described above could be:

c. Ms. Flint will wash her hair twice a week, bathe daily, and brush her teeth twice every day.
d. Mr. Mills will attend the activity center two evenings a week and will have dinner with a friend once a week.
e. Ms. Woolworth will, for a period of three weeks, refrain from arguing with the therapists and group leaders in her activity programs.

These goals have been written in behavioral terms so that all concerned (therapist, patient, and other staff) will know when the goal has been reached. By contrast, it is impossible to agree on when or whether a goal such as "Mr. Peters will have increased self-esteem" has been reached; there is no way to measure success.

Some therapists use the mnemonic "RUMBA" to evaluate the goal statements they write. RUMBA stands for:

RELEVANT
UNDERSTANDABLE
MEASURABLE
BEHAVIORAL
ACHIEVABLE

A goal is *relevant* when it reflects the patient's life situation and future goals. As discussed previously, both the patient and the therapist should agree that the goal is important, and the other treatment team members such as the social worker, the psychiatrist, and the nurse should support these goals. Making sure that everyone involved agrees that the goals are relevant helps to prevent conflicts during treatment. For example, a 24-year-old man may describe his main goal as "having a girl-friend." The therapist or assistant might explain that socialization groups at the day treatment center will help the patient learn how to meet people and develop relationships with them.

A goal is *understandable* when it is stated in plain language and observable terms. Professional jargon should be eliminated, and the goal should be phrased so that the patient and his family can understand it. A goal is *measurable* when it contains a criterion for success. It is best if the criterion is stated in quantifiable terms (numbers) rather than qualitative ones. For example, "bathing once a day" is more easily measured than "having adequate hygiene." Similarly, it is important to include an estimated date of completion, a time by which the goal should be reached.

A goal is *behavioral* when it focuses on what the patient must *do* to accomplish the goal. It is *achievable* when it is something that the patient is likely to be able to accomplish within a reasonably short period of time (as defined by the patient and the therapist together). For instance, assume the patient is a very isolated 24-year-old man who has always lived with his parents and who has never held a job. Getting a job and moving into his own apartment *might* be future goals, but certainly not immediate ones; *achievable* goals might be limited to traveling back and forth to the day treatment center on his own and arriving on time.

The follow are some goals, developed from those in Table 15–2, using the RUMBA criteria:

Psychological skills—roles

1. The patient will be able to identify the primary functions and tasks of her role as mother of a preschooler, by the end of six weeks.
2. The patient will be able to identify the ways in which her disability interferes with her functioning effectively in the role of mother of a preschooler, and will

identify ways to compensate, within six weeks.

Psychological skills—interests

1. Given the opportunity, the patient will be able to identify and discuss at least three interests that are important to him, by the end of two weeks.
2. The patient will be able to identify at least three ways to pursue his interest in watercolor painting, by the end of the next treatment session.

Activities of daily living

1. The patient will be able to locate the telephone number and address of a pharmacy near his home, using the Yellow Pages, by the end of the next treatment session.
2. The patient will visit the pharmacy near his home and locate the counter for dropping off and picking up prescriptions, within the next week.
3. The patient will drop off and pick up his prescription medication at a pharmacy near his home, within two days of receiving the prescription.

Social skills—behaving in context

1. The patient will consistently stand *at least two and a half feet* from another person when engaged in a work-related conversation, by the end of four weeks.
2. The patient will make and maintain eye contact with another person in the group, for at least 30 seconds, at least once in the three-hour session.

Despite application of the RUMBA criteria, the therapist or assistant may find that some goals appropriate for patients with psychiatric disabilities are hard to measure. Abilities such as self-assertion, self-control, and independence cannot, unlike range of motion or muscle strength, be physically measured and quantified. One way around this problem is to develop a rating scale for each goal. Goal attainment scaling (GAS) (8,10,12) identifies five levels of possible achievement for a goal. Two of the levels are higher than what is expected, two are lower than what is expected, and the middle level defines the expected outcome. Table 15–3 gives two examples of how this might be done. Goal attainment scaling provides the patient (and the team and the reimburser) with a clear understanding of what the patient is expected to achieve.

Scott and Haggerty (17) used GAS concepts in a partial hospitalization (outpatient) setting to help patients set their own goals and define their own criteria for success in meeting them. With the use of a paper-and-pencil form, the patient was asked to select a goal based on problems identified through evaluation. Next, the patient was encouraged to explore and discuss why he chose that particular goal, and how it related to his immediate and future concerns. Then the patient was asked to state what outcome he would *expect* to achieve. (Scott and Haggerty give the example of a patient who is chronically 15 minutes late; the ex-

pected outcome is that he will be 10 minutes late.) Working from this expected outcome, the patient then describes a least favorable outcome and a most favorable one. Finally, outcomes intermediate between the expected one and the extreme ones are described (less favorable, more favorable). Of course, it is really not necessary to identify five different points on the rating scale; three points (expected, more than expected, and less than expected) are sufficient.

Involving patients directly in selecting goals and measuring success can help them feel and become more independent and assertive; it can also give the staff (and the patient) some sense of how the patient sees his needs and what kinds of goals he believes are possible. Scott and Haggerty point out that not all patients are capable of generating their own goals and attainment scales, and that patients with organic disorders and cognitive disabilities need assistance from the therapist. Acutely ill patients seem to have more difficulty mon-

TABLE 15–3. *Goal attainment scale for two goals*

Predicted attainment	Score	Goals	
		Social interactions	Weight loss
Most unfavorable outcome	−2	Speaks to no one except therapist during 3-hr session	Gains 5 lb within 1 month
Less than expected outcome	−1	Says "hello" or other greeting to fellow workers during 3-hr training session	Maintains weight over 1-month period
Expected level of outcome	0	Holds sustained, interactive conversaion of 200 words (or 10 min) with one other worker during 3-hr session	Loses 5 lb within 1 month
Greater than expected outcome	+1	Holds interactive conversation of more than 200 words (or 10 min) with two or more workers (independently or simultaneously) during 3-hr session	Loses 10 lb within 1 month
Most favorable outcome likely	+2	Holds interactive conversation of 500 words (or 20 min) with three or more workers during 3-hr session	Loses 15 lb within 1 month

From Table 1 in Ottenbacher KJ, Cusick A. Goal attainment scaling as a method of clinical service evaluation. *Am J Occup Ther* 1990; 44:519–25. Copyright © 1990 by the American Occupational Therapy Association, Inc. Reprinted with permission.

itoring themselves once they have set up the attainment scales, and this may be due to their fluctuating symptoms; the approach seems to work better with chronically ill patients.

To summarize, treatment goals may be written by the OTR or the supervised assistant. The patient's involvement in selecting and refining goals for his own treatment may be limited to varying degrees by cognitive impairments or psychotic symptoms. Nonetheless, occupational therapy staff must try to involve him as much as possible. Goals for treatment should be relevant to the patient's needs and values and stated in terms that he can understand. They should contain some criterion against which success can be measured, and they must indicate the behavior the patient is to perform. Finally, they must be achievable, that is, realistic for this patient at this time in his life.

IDENTIFYING TREATMENT PRINCIPLES

Once the goals are written, the next task is to figure out how to reach them. At the beginning of this chapter we emphasized the importance of identifying the causes of the patient's problems as well as the problems themselves. In other words, we try to choose a theory or principle that we believe best explains the patient's problems to guide us in selecting treatment methods. To return to our example, a patient may have poor hygiene for many different reasons. It makes a difference whether the reason is that he never learned the necessary hygiene and grooming routines, or he just forgets, or he does not wash because his skin feels funny when he touches it. Or perhaps he is afraid of washing away part of this body. Each of these reasons leads to different notions about how to approach the problem.

If the reason for the patient's poor hygiene is that he never learned proper grooming and hygiene, then the most logi-

cal approach would be to teach him the skills; but we must first determine whether there are any sociocultural or personal reasons that might interfere with his wanting to learn.

If the reason is that he forgets, then we need to know more about why he forgets (organic memory loss, disorganization, or having too many things to do, or lack of a reinforcing environment are just a few possible reasons), and then we can figure out a way to help him remember.

If the reason is that his skin "feels funny," then we will suspect a sensory integrative problem and recommend to the OTR that this be evaluated. The point is that the more we know about the cause of the patient's problem, the easier it will be to select a practice model and treatment methods.

The different treatment theories and practice models discussed in Chapters 2, 3, and 4 contain principles for organizing our thinking about the patient's problems and how to approach them. We choose a theory on the basis of how well it explains the patient's problems and how effectively it helps us solve them. A theory like Allen's theory of cognitive disabilities is very useful for evaluating how well a chronic schizophrenic can function in an independent living situation, and for pinpointing how to modify his environment so that it supports his functioning better. However, this theory helps little in designing a work adjustment program for an intelligent but depressed middle-aged woman whose children have grown up and left home. For this situation the model of human occupation or the role acquisition model is a better guide for planning treatment. No one theory seems adequate to address every problem, and so it is important to choose the best one for the particular situation.

Intangible factors such as self-esteem can, and often should, be considered in this stage of treatment planning. Several of the theories covered in this text are based at least in part on ideas about the individual's feelings and internal psychodynamics. The patient's sense of personal causation (model of human occupation) or his narcissistic needs (object relations) may provide clues about what principles we should follow. Although these intangibles cannot be directly measured, and should not (for this reason) be written into the treatment goals, they can guide our selection of treatment methods. If we believe, for example, that the patient is neglecting his hygiene because his self-esteem is low, as a result of being laid off from work for the second time in 18 months, then we will direct our energies toward raising his self-esteem, assuming that the hygiene will follow.

HOW TO SELECT TREATMENT METHODS

Once we have chosen the theory and the principles we believe best explain the patient's problems, we can choose treatment methods based on them. The method specifies the activity to be used, the environment in which it will be performed, and the approach the therapist will use to present the activity. Each of these—activity, environment, and therapeutic approach—will be examined separately.

Activity

Activities are chosen on the basis of the stated principles identified in the plan. Activities are selected primarily for their ability to address the treatment goal. We determine this through activity analysis. Analysis and adaptation of activities for treatment of psychosocial problems is the subject of Chapter 23. Knowledgeable analysis must be the basis of activity selection if we expect to produce the desired therapeutic effect. For example, if we suspect that the patient has trouble making decisions because other people have always made his decisions for him, then we will look for an activity that involves making

choices (rather than one that requires absolute adherence to a sequence of rules or directions); ceramics and leathercraft could be adapted to fit this principle. On the other hand, if the patient has been fired from many jobs because she did not follow the rules, then perhaps an activity with lots of rules and restrictions (and serious consequences for ignoring them) will help her explore her feelings about following them. Working in wood (a notoriously unforgiving medium) might be appropriate for this.

Although occupational therapists and assistants use other therapeutic tools such as counseling and environmental modification, activity should always be their primary treatment tool. Activity, or occupation, has the power to heal and to create change in a way that verbal therapies simply cannot. When the patient actually *does* something, he explores and experiences his own effect on the world; when he talks he only imagines it. By participating in activities people learn about themselves, about their abilities to use tools and materials, about the pleasure of working directly with their hands and bodies and minds, about the reactions of others to what they have done. They discover, refine, and shape their images of themselves; they discover what they can and cannot do.

It is essential that the activities chosen for therapy provide the patient with experiences that are pleasurable and that reinforce and enhance his sense of competence and mastery (1,4). This does not mean that the activities should be easy; they cannot engage the patient's interest and drive toward competency unless they provide a reasonable challenge. Activities themselves will be discussed in detail in Chapters 18 through 22.

Environment

The setting in which the activity takes place influences the patient's response. The patient's home environment and general life space (see Chapter 14) and the treatment setting (see Chapter 7) must be considered. Environments produce both demands and supports for activity performance. An *environmental demand* is an expectation for a certain kind of behavior or action that is evoked by something in the environment. Allen (1) gives the example of the American flag causing a patient to salute.

An *environmental support* is a feature of the environment that encourages and assists the individual to perform a particular behavior. A machine that dispenses premeasured packets of detergent and fabric softeners is an example of an environmental support in a laundromat. Occupational therapists and assistants can alter the demands and supports within the environment by adding or removing objects or people, by changing the arrangement of the furniture or the lighting, or by other factors. The purpose of this environmental manipulation is to stimulate patients to perform activities, develop skills, acquire habits, and enhance their sense of personal causation by succeeding at what they attempt. How to modify the environment and choose the proper level of stimulation will be discussed within the context of activity analysis and adaptation in Chapter 23.

Therapeutic Approach

The basic principles of the therapeutic approach were covered in considerable detail in Chapters 3, 4, 10, and 11 and will be discussed further in Chapter 17. When selecting which approach to use with a particular patient, the therapist must consider the patient's values, learning style and preferences, and motivation for treatment.

MONITORING TREATMENT AND MODIFYING THE PLAN

Once developed, the treatment plan must be carried out; the patient engages in activities or exercises using the chosen methods.

Often the occupational therapy assistant is responsible for this part of the treatment process, known as *treatment implementation*. After explaining to the patient what will be happening and why, the assistant conducts the treatment, which typically involves engaging the patient in an activity or series of activities in a rather specific way. Once the treatment has been implemented, the important questions become how well it is working, and whether it needs to be changed.

Monitoring the treatment to determine how effective it has been is relatively straightforward if there are clearly stated objectives. Unless the objectives are stated in terms of what is observable and what is realistic to achieve during the time provided, measuring their achievement is next to impossible. There are two ways in which treatment effectiveness is monitored: informal assessment and formal evaluation.

Informal assessment occurs almost automatically, as the assistant or therapist observes the patient's reaction to the treatment. The patient's behavior and remarks will provide clues if the treatment is too easy or too difficult for her, or just off the mark for her needs. Once the assistant notes that the patient can easily accomplish the treatment activity, he should consult with the therapist about how to change the treatment plan; similarly, if he observes that the patient is leaving early, or not coming on time, or finding excuses to avoid treatment, he should also consult with the therapist, as these behaviors may signify a need to change the plan.

Formal evaluation is the responsibility of the registered therapist. It occurs on two levels: One is the evaluation of the progress of an individual patient in treatment, and the other is the evaluation of the effectiveness of the occupational therapy program as a whole (or of specific treatment programs, such as particular groups). Evaluation of the progress of an individual patient is best measured by readministering the same evaluations that were used in the original assessment. Improvements in the patient's performance since the time of the initial evaluation may be considered evidence of treatment effectiveness; however, medications and spontaneous remission of symptoms and many other causes can also account for these changes. Depending on the results of the formal evaluation, the therapist may decide to continue with the plan or to change it in some way, or to discharge the patient from treatment.

QUALITY ASSURANCE

Evaluation of the occupational therapy program, or of treatment activities or groups within the program, is also the responsibility of the registered therapist, and is usually designed and supervised by the chief of the occupational therapy service. Often this is part of a larger *quality assurance* program, which may involve other clinical departments. Quality assurance (QA) is a "systematic approach to the evaluation of patient care that enables the identification, assessment, and resolution of problems in order to improve health care benefits for patients" (11). In other words, quality assurance is a way of measuring how well we are doing, so that we can improve what we are doing for our patients. Rather than focusing on an individual patient, quality assurance looks at the entire program. Quality assurance seeks to identify problems in patient care, and to resolve them.

One of the obstacles to implementing quality assurance in psychiatric settings has been the vague and highly subjective nature of mental illness and the difficulty of

TABLE 15–4. *Quality assurance examples for occupational therapy mental health patients*

Occupational therapy monitoring indicator	Measure	Applied to	Threshold/criteria
Prompt patient assessment	Time lag between occupational therapy referral and assessment	All psychiatric patients	90% of patients will be assessed within 24 hours of referral to occupational therapy
Patient participation in goal-directed activities	Time per day spent in occupational therapy/unit activities that have specific treatment goals	All patients in acute care psychiatric unit	75% will spend three hours daily in goal-directed activity
Increased independent functioning by patients	Mean difference between admission and discharge on Comprehensive Occupational Therapy Evaluation (COTE)[a] Scale	All psychiatric patients	80% of patients will decrease score by 10 or more points
Improvement in successful placement in independent living	Scorable Self-Care Evaluation (SSCE)[b] administered before discharge	Psychiatric patients going into independent living	100% of patients will have overall score of 30 or less before being considered for independent living

[a]From Brayman SJ, Kirby TF, Misenheimer AM, Short MJ. Comprehensive Occupational Therapy Evaluation Scale. *Am J Occup Ther* 1976; 30:94–100.
[b]From Clark N, Peters M. *The Scorable Self-Care Evaluation (SSCE)*. Thorofare, NJ: SLACK; 1984.
From Appendix B in Joe BE, ed. *Quality assurance in occupational therapy*. Rockville, Md: American Occupational Therapy Association; 1991: xvii. Copyright © 1991 by the American Occupational Therapy Association, Inc. Reprinted with permission.

measuring improvements in mental health. Nonetheless, very specific and measurable criteria can be established to assess some aspects of occupational therapy patient care in mental health settings, as shown in Table 15–4.

Thien (18) notes three major areas that should be assessed in quality assurance programs for mental health occupational therapy: progress toward goals, patient satisfaction with care, and behavior rating scores. Progress toward goals is most easily measured when the goals are behaviorally observable and measurable. In other words, if the criterion is a five-point improvement on the Scorable Self Care Scale, this is far easier to measure than "the patient will improve in recognition of common safety hazards." Patient satisfaction with care can be measured through exit interviews, but the most objective and easily assessed measures are surveys with rating scales. Figure 15–2 gives an example of such a scale. Behavior rating can be achieved by using numerical rating scales such as the COTE (Comprehensive Occupational Therapy Evaluation Scale, see Chapter 14).

While not responsible for designing a quality assurance program, the occupational therapy assistant will be expected to contribute in various ways. The first is in collecting data for quality assurance by reviewing medical records. The assistant might be directed to search the charts of all patients who participated in a given program (e.g., independent living skills) and to compile a list of ratings (for example, on the Scorable Self Care Scale) for these patients before and after participation in the pro-

	Strongly Disagree	Disagree	Undecided	Agree	Strongly Agree
I felt I was treated with courtesy and respect in occupational therapy.	1	2	3	4	5
Occupational therapy treatment was helpful to me in working on my problems.	1	2	3	4	5
My occupational therapist involved me in developing my goals.	1	2	3	4	5
I felt my occupational therapist understood my problems.	1	2	3	4	5
The time spent in learning relaxation techniques was adequate.	1	2	3	4	5
My participation in living skills group was helpful to me.	1	2	3	4	5
I understood my occupational therapy treatment plan.	1	2	3	4	5

FIG. 15–2. Examples of questionnaire statements related to patient satisfaction with the delivery of occupational therapy care. From Fig. 4–4 of Thien M. Assessing occupational therapy care in mental health. In: Joe BE, ed. *Quality assurance in occupational therapy.* Rockville, Md: American Occupational Therapy Association; 1991: 4–10. Copyright © 1991 by the American Occupational Therapy Association, Inc. Reprinted with permission.

gram. Data collection must be done accurately and completely if it is to have meaning. All of the charts must be reviewed, including those that seem deficient. Another area for COTA participation in quality assurance is as a member of the occupational therapy staff, in selecting measures for quality assurance, and developing plans for actions to respond to areas that need improvement. The assistant often brings a unique practical perspective to the planning process.

Despite its intended purpose as a patient care improvement scheme, the very mention of quality assurance may strike fear in the hearts of staff. One of the reasons is concern about repercussions to themselves or to fellow workers. Staff may suspect that if a program is found lacking, someone will be blamed for it. But quality assurance is not about fault-finding and blaming; it is about patient care improvement. Only by looking realistically at what has happened can improvements be made. Most likely, deficiencies will be greeted sympathetically by senior staff, who will recognize their own responsibility for improvement of care. Other reasons for avoiding quality assurance activities include fears of increased documentation and demands on already limited time. It is important to trust and believe that quality assurance, in the long run, leads to better time use and decreased documentation. Time spent on learning how to write measurable objectives and criteria pays off in time saved documenting the effectiveness of care.

CONTINUOUS QUALITY IMPROVEMENT

Continuous quality improvement (CQI) is another quality management process. Continuous quality improvement monitoring is ongoing (constant) rather than retrospective (looking back). It is more interdisciplinary than quality assurance, and looks at outcomes (results) rather than problems. For example, a CQI program might monitor patient satisfaction through daily response surveys. If patient satisfaction is lower than expected, CQI would seek to identify the sources and correct them. If, for example, patients felt that what they learned in the clinic was not carried over into their lives in the community, then the staff might plan more patient education or community outreach activities. CQI can give feedback to treatment planning by providing quicker assessment of the results of interventions. Interventions that are ineffective can be more quickly identified and adjustments can then be made.

SUMMARY

Treatment planning for patients with psychiatric problems requires careful thought. The causes of most psychiatric problems are not yet clearly understood, and therefore it is often difficult to figure out exactly how to help a patient function better in his life, and feel better about himself and what he can do.

Treatment planning involves identifying specific problems that the patient and the staff charged with his care agree are important to work on. Goals are written to address these problems; both problems and goals must be stated in terms that are relevant to the patient's needs, understandable, measurable, behavioral, and achievable. Above all, goals should be observable and reasonable to accomplish within the time allotted. There are many ways to approach a given treatment goal; different treatment theories and practice models contain principles for selecting and modifying treatment methods. Methods must take into account the activity used, the environment, and the therapeutic approach that will be most effective for engaging the patient. Once treatment has begun, it should be monitored to determine whether it is effective or needs to be changed. This may be done by informal assessment or formal evaluation. A quality assurance program may be used to monitor the effectiveness of patient care within a setting or service.

REFERENCES

1. Allen CK. *Occupational therapy for psychiatric diseases: measurement and management of cognitive disabilities.* Boston: Little, Brown; 1985.
2. American Occupational Therapy Association (1989): *Entry-level role delineation for OTRs and COTAs.* Rockville, Md: American Occupational Therapy Association; 1989.
3. American Occupational Therapy Association. Uniform terminology for occupational therapy, second edition. *Am J Occup Ther* 1989;43:808–815.
4. Barris R, Kielhofner G, Watts JH. *Psychosocial occupational therapy: practice in a pluralistic arena.* Laurel, Md: RAMSCO; 1983.
5. Cubie SH, Kaplan K. A case analysis method for the model of human occupation. *Am J Occup Ther* 1982;36:645–656.
6. Evans A. Roles and functions of occupational therapy in mental health (American Occupational Therapy Association position paper approved by the Representative Assembly, April 1985). *Am J Occup Ther* 1985;39:799–802.
7. Fidler GS, Fidler JW. Doing and becoming: purposeful action and self-actualization. *Am J Occup Ther* 1978;32:305–310.
8. Gaines BJ. Goal-oriented treatment plans and behavioral analysis. *Am J Occup Ther* 1978;32:512–516.
9. Joe BE, ed. *Quality assurance in occupational therapy.* Rockville, Md: American Occupational Therapy Association; 1991.
10. Kiresuk TJ, Sherman RE. Goal attainment scaling: a general method for evaluation of comprehensive mental health programs. *Community Ment Health J* 1968;4:443–453.
11. Lawlor MC. A conceptual framework for quality assurance. In: Joe BE, ed. *Quality assurance in occupational therapy.* Rockville, Md: American Occupational Therapy Association; 1991.
12. Maloney FP, Mirrett P, Brooks C, Johannes K. Use of the Goal Attainment Scale in the treatment and ongoing evaluation of neurologically handicapped children. *Am J Occup Ther* 1978; 32:505–510.
13. Payton OD, Ozer MN, Nelson CE. *Patient participation in program planning: a manual for therapists.* Philadelphia: FA Davis; 1971.
14. Peloquin SM. Sustaining the art of practice in occupational therapy. *Am J Occup Ther* 1989; 43:219–226.
15. Rogers JC. Eleanor Clarke Slagle lectureship—1983. Clinical reasoning: the ethics, science, and art. *Am J Occup Ther* 1983;37:601–616.
16. Schell BAB. Guide to classification of occupational therapy personnel (American Occupational Therapy Association position paper approved by the Representative Assembly, April 1985). *Am J Occup Ther* 1985;39:803–810.
17. Scott AH, Haggarty EJ. Structuring goals via goal attainment scaling in occupational therapy groups in a partial hospitalization setting. *Occup Ther Mental Health* 1984;4(2):39–58.
18. Thien M. Assessing occupational therapy care in mental health. In: Joe BE, ed. *Quality assurance in occupational therapy.* Rockville, Md: American Occupational Therapy Association; 1991.
19. Tiffany EG. Psychiatry and mental health. In: Hopkins HL, Smith HD, eds. *Willard and Spackman's occupational therapy.* 6th ed. Philadelphia: JB Lippincott; 1983.

ADDITIONAL REFERENCES AND SUGGESTED READINGS

Day DJ. A systems diagram for teaching treatment planning. *Am J Occup Ther* 1973;27:239–243.

Foto M. Nationally speaking—managing changes in reimbursement patterns, part 1. *Am J Occup Ther* 1988;42:563–565.

Kielhofner G, Burke JP, Igi CH. A model of human occupation. 4: Assessment and intervention. *Am J Occup Ther* 1980;34:777–788.

Law M, Ryan B, Townsend E, O'Shea B. Criteria mapping: a method of quality assurance. *Am J Occup Ther* 1989;43:104–109.

Line J. Case method as a scientific form of clinical thinking. *Am J Occup Ther* 1969;23:308–313.

Llorens LA. Changing balance: environment and individual. *Am J Occup Ther* 1984;38:29–34.

Lloyd C. The process of goal setting using goal attainment scaling in a therapeutic community. *Occup Ther Mental Health* 1986;6(3):19–30.

Maslen D. Rehabilitation training for community living skills: concepts and techniques. *Am J Occup Ther* 1982;2(1):49.

Mosey AC. *Activities therapy.* New York; Raven Press; 1973.

Nelson CE, Payton OD. The issue is—a system for involving patients in program planning. *Am J Occup Ther* 1991;45:753–755.

Ottenbacher KJ, Cusick A. Goal attainment scaling as a method of clinical service evaluation. *Am J Occup Ther* 1990;44:519–525.

Pelland MJ. A conceptual model for the instruction and supervision of treatment planning. *Am J Occup Ther* 1987;41:351–359.

Peloquin SM. Linking purpose to procedure during interactions with patients. *Am J Occup Ther* 1988;42:775–781.

Peloquin SM. Uniform terminology as a basis for goal formulation. *Occup Ther Mental Health* 1986;6(4):49–62.

Peloquin SM. The development of an occupational

therapy interview/therapy set procedure. *Am J Occup Ther* 1983;37:457–461.

Sperman DM, Wilson SM, Hill MA. The development and validation of the psychiatric OT evaluation of needs and treatment instrument. *Occup Ther Mental Health* 1986;11(4):91–110.

Weed LL. *Medical records, medical evaluations and patient care.* Chicago: Case Western University Press; 1971.

Willson M. *Occupational therapy in long-term psychiatry.* Edinburgh: Churchill Livingstone; 1983.

Willson M. *Occupational therapy in short-term psychiatry.* Edinburgh: Churchill Livingstone; 1984.

Wilson SM, Sperman DM, Hill AM. Quality assurance in occupational therapy: a case study. *Occup Ther Mental Health* 1986;11(1);93–107.

16

Medical Records and Documentation

Omit needless words. A sentence should contain no unnecessary words, a paragraph no unnecessary sentences, for the same reason that a drawing should have no unnecessary lines and a machine no unnecessary parts. This requires not that the writer make all his sentences short, or that he avoid all detail and treat his subjects only in outline, but that every word tell.

WILLIAM STRUNK, JR. AND E.B. WHITE (5, p.17)

The medical record is a legal document. It can be subpoenaed by the court, and it testifies to the appropriateness and effectiveness of treatment. It is used to justify reimbursement, to monitor health care quality, and to communicate with others involved in the patient's care. It is impossible to overstate the importance of accurate and timely documentation. Other than direct service to patients, documentation is *the* most important task of the occupational therapist and assistant. Without proper documentation, it is impossible to receive reimbursement, to justify the need for additional services, or to defend against a malpractice suit. More fundamentally, there is no way to be sure that the treatment worked, or why, or whether it even occurred, unless the treatment is accurately documented.

Although the registered therapist has the overall responsibility for maintaining accurate and complete records on patient services, the occupational therapy assistant is responsible for recording the results of her own services to patients. This chapter will discuss some of the kinds of medical records a COTA might encounter in different psychiatric facilities, and will delineate the roles of the registered therapist and the assistant in documentation of service. The guidelines (as to who is to document various aspects of the occupational therapy process) change often in response to new laws, federal guidelines, certification requirements, and reimbursement policies and procedures. The assistant is legally and ethically responsible to stay informed of these changes and to practice within them. Specific guidelines for writing notes and examples of different kinds of notes will be provided later in this chapter.

PURPOSES OF PSYCHIATRIC RECORDS

The patient's chart tells the story of his care in the medical system. It chronicles why he sought treatment in the first place, what the various health professionals determined his problems were and how they determined this, the kinds of treatments or interventions they attempted, and how well these interventions worked. All medical personnel who work with a patient and record information in his chart are held accountable for the quality of treatment he receives; this applies equally to the psychiatrist and the occupational therapy assistant. Each is responsible to provide services that reflect current practice standards in their respective fields, and to document these services and their effects on the patient.

The purposes of the psychiatric medical record[1] are to:

1. Provide a sequential record of the patient's condition and the evaluations and treatments he received from admission to discharge. This record can be used as evidence in a court of law.
2. Provide information that will assist in the patient's treatment.
3. Allow different professionals working with the patient to communicate with each other, and facilitate a free flow of communication among all personnel.
4. Provide objective information that can be used in research, education, utilization review, quality assurance studies, and reimbursement procedures.

SOURCE-ORIENTED OR NARRATIVE PSYCHIATRIC RECORDS

In this traditional approach, each source (or clinical discipline such as nursing or occupational therapy) records information in a separate section of the chart. Typically, a section of progress notes is used by all disciplines for daily or other periodic notes, which appear sequentially. The first part of the chart contains the patient's name, case number, identifying information, and admission records. This section may also include legal documents such as court orders for involuntary hospitalization. Next there are assessment reports (sometimes called evaluation summaries) and treatment plans from each of the different services that are

concerned with the patient's care; these may be psychiatry, nursing, psychology, social work, occupational therapy, and recreation therapy. A section for laboratory reports and records of medical and other consultations may follow this, or may be placed at the back of the chart. There is also a section for doctor's orders and medication records.

All of these take up only a minor fraction of the chart, however, the bulk of which consists of sequential notes written by all of the different services involved in the patient's care. Each staff member writes notes at assigned intervals, according to the standards that apply to the facility. For example, nurses may be required to write a note on each patient every day; this might apply to all three shifts. Occupational therapists, on the other hand, might be required to write notes only every two weeks. Frequency varies with the setting; some require daily notes, or notes every time a service is rendered.

There are two different approaches to organizing this material. One is to divide the notes into smaller sections, each for a different discipline, so that (for example) all of the occupational therapy notes are in one place, between the social work and psychology notes. A variant on this format uses color-coded pages to indicate progress notes of each discipline (green for nursing, orange for occupational therapy, for example). The other method is to combine all of the notes from different disciplines into one section; the notes are written one after the other, so that a given page in the chart might contain two nursing notes, a medication order from the physician, and an occupational therapy progress note.

One of the problems with this format of psychiatric record, regardless of how the sequential notes are organized, has been that it is difficult to locate specific information about a patient's progress without reading *all* of the sequential notes, most of which probably have none of the desired information. Consider the case of a patient

---

[1]Summarized and adapted from (2).

who has been hospitalized repeatedly over many years, and whose record is correspondingly lengthy. Suppose, for example, that the physician wanted to know the effects of various medications the patient has received. He would have to read all of the notes from occupational therapy and nursing to see how the patient functioned, and whether the staff noticed any side effects. Only a few of those notes would contain information related to medication. As another example, suppose that the occupational therapy assistant wanted to know what kinds of independent daily living skills programs the patient has been involved in, and what the results were. She would have to start at the beginning of the chart and read every occupational therapy note.

It was largely in response to this problem that a different kind of medical record, called the problem-oriented medical record, was developed. Although the majority of psychiatric settings seem not to have changed over to the problem-oriented record, it is important to know how its format differs from that of the traditional record.

PROBLEM-ORIENTED MEDICAL RECORDS IN PSYCHIATRY

The *problem-oriented medical record* or POMR, was introduced in 1969 by Dr. Lawrence Weed as a possible solution to the problems of the source-oriented record. The POMR is organized into three major sections: the data base, the problem list, and the reports of plans and progress. The data base contains the same sorts of information that might be included in the admission report, the psychiatrist's evaluation, and the social history. The data base is developed within the first 48 hours of hospitalization or outpatient treatment, and is usually written by the patient's primary therapist.

The problem list is developed from the data base. It identifies all of the patient's problems. The primary therapist may write the problem list, usually with recommendations from other disciplines, or the treatment team might develop the list together. The occupational therapy assistant can suggest problems to the primary therapist, to the occupational therapy supervisor, or to the treatment team. Some problems that might appear on the list in a psychiatric record are: difficulty expressing feelings, suicidal ideation, poor self-care, and lack of employment. Each problem is given a number, and the date the problem was entered in the chart is recorded.

The reports section includes all of the notes from different disciplines. The problem to which each note refers is indicated in a separate column next to the note. For instance, when the occupational therapy assistant writes a note about the patient's progress in an activities of daily living group, she writes the number of the problem (poor self-care) next to the note. If the note refers to more than one problem, she records all the relevant problem numbers. Organizing the chart in this way enables someone who is interested in the treatment of a particular problem to find all of the notes that pertain to that problem without reading all the ones that do not. The notes in the problem-oriented record are generally written in "SOAP" format, which will be discussed later in this chapter.

DOCUMENTATION OF OCCUPATIONAL THERAPY SERVICES

The different kinds of occupational therapy documentation that are included in the patient's permanent record are classified as follows (2):

1. Initial notes
2. Assessment plans and notes
3. Treatment plans and goals
4. Progress notes
5. Treatment records
6. Discharge summaries
7. Consultation reports

8. Special reports
9. Critical incident reports and notes

Initial notes record the first contact between the occupational therapist or assistant and the patient. *Assessment notes* identify the evaluation procedures that were used, the results of evaluations, and the therapist's interpretation of the results. *Treatment plans and goals* spell out the goals established by the patient and the therapist, the methods to be used, the frequency of treatment, and the time by which the therapist expects the goals to be reached. It is common at present for the initial note to include the assessment data and the treatment plan; this saves time and space and gives a more coherent explanation of the relationship between the assessment and the plan. *Progress notes* document treatment since the last note; this includes a record of the patient's attendance and participation, any change that has occurred since the last note and the probable causes of the change, and any modification of the treatment plan. *Treatment records* are statistics about how many treatments the patient has received; these records are usually *not* filed in the patient's charts, but instead are given to the occupational therapy supervisor. A *discharge summary* gives a concise description of the entire course of occupational therapy treatment, from admission to discharge.

When a professional does not have sufficient expertise to understand a patient's problem and recommend treatment, he will request a consultation with someone who does. Occupational therapists may receive consultation requests from physicians and others, and a *consultation report* records the therapist's assessment of the patient's problems, including recommendations for treatment or other interventions. The entry-level COTA is not qualified to serve as a consultant and therefore does not need to know how to write consultation reports; this is a role reserved for OTRs and for COTAs with considerable experience and

expertise. *Special reports* include various records that legally need to become part of the permanent chart. Examples are referrals to other programs and agencies, summary reports for legal reasons, home programs, and correspondence (2).

A *critical incident report* or *note* documents the facts of an emergency situation in which, for example, a patient was injured or eloped while in the care of an occupational therapy staff member. Specific legal requirements govern the way such reports are written, and the staff member is given precise instructions by a supervisor about how to write up the incident.

DOCUMENTATION RESPONSIBILITIES OF THE OTR AND THE COTA

The registered therapist oversees the documentation of patient treatment, writing some of the notes herself and countersigning all notes written by COTAs and students (2,3). The OTR writes the assessment notes and reports, which summarize the findings from evaluation and data collection. The COTA may be directed to write up the results of a structured evaluation she has performed.

In most cases, the OTR also writes the overall treatment plan; the COTA may contribute to the total plan and even write sections of it (for example, on self-care), but documentation of the treatment plan is ultimately the OTR's responsibility. The OTR is also generally responsible for the discharge summary, although the COTA may be required to write a summary when a patient is discharged from her own program, as, for example, would occur when the patient completes a 10-week money management group led by the COTA.

Each staff member who sees patients must keep treatment records on every service she provides; this applies, of course, to the occupational therapy assistant. An attendance record is kept for each group and must be completed daily. In addition, records of evaluations, interviews, and other services must be maintained on each patient. These may be combined in a monthly report, which tabulates all patient service sessions for the month. Each staff member's monthly report is given to the occupational therapy supervisor or director, who then compiles a report on the entire department.

The entry-level occupational therapy assistant is usually expected to write *simple summary notes,* which concisely describe either a single patient service or a course of treatment over a period of time. The purpose of these notes is to present a clear picture of the service provided, the patient's response, and the assistant's plans and recommendations for the future. These notes are classified according to their content, which may be the initial contact with the patient, an evaluation that was performed, the patient's progress in treatment since the last note, or a summary of treatment and progress from admission to discharge. Each type of note will be discussed separately.

GUIDELINES FOR NOTE WRITING

Writing a simple summary note is not usually a simple task for the beginner. Because it becomes part of the patient's permanent record it is important that it be accurate and complete; future decisions about the patient may be based on what is in the chart. Although the note should be accurate and complete, it should also be concise, brief and to the point; otherwise, given human nature and the busy schedules of most health professionals, no one (except possibly the supervisor) will read the whole thing. Simple observation notes are intended to convey an accurate picture of what happened, so that someone who was not present can understand it almost as well as if he were there. The novice note-writer may benefit from the following *stylistic* advice:

Record observations, not interpretations. Let the reader draw his own conclusions based on the facts you present.

Avoid judgmental language. Judgments are open to varying interpretations. What is a "good job" to one person may not meet the standards of another, for example. Moorhouse and Doenges (4) cite five types of judgmental statements that should be avoided:

Undefined periods of time: Words like "often," "frequently," and "seldom" should be replaced by measurable and defined periods, such as "five times per hour" or "two times during a six-hour work session."

Undefined quantities: Words like "some," "many," and "enough" should be replaced by numerical quantities, as, for example, "five," "ten," or "one."

Qualities: Adjectives that convey opinions, such as "hostile," "spacey," or "bored" should be replaced by actual observations. "Patient clenched his fists and said to COTA, 'I'll knock your teeth down your throat'" is an observation. So is "Patient stared out the window for 3/4 of the activity session, did not participate in discussion, and responded to her own name only after two calls."

Failure to provide an objective basis for judgment: A statement such as "Patient likes trains" does not give evidence to support it. A more effective statement would be "Patient stated that he likes trains and that he will read anything on the subject."

Inappropriate use of clinical terminology: Only the physician can diagnose the patient. Similarly, the assistant should not use medical terms to describe behavior or symptoms unless she is absolutely certain the usage is correct. Even when certain, the assistant must place the description within the context of what she observed. For example, it is incorrect to state that "the patient was hallucinating." This should instead be recorded as "the patient appeared to be hallucinating; she was conversing when no one was there."

Avoid jargon. Your note will be seen (and one hopes, read) by many people, most of them not occupational therapy personnel. Other mental health professionals and paraprofessionals cannot be expected to understand OT jargon like "sensory integration," "habit dysfunction," or "Activity Configuration." Unless these terms are well understood by all staff they should not be used in material for the chart unless a brief explanation of their meaning is included.

Omit extraneous detail. Many of the things that patients do they do more than once. By grouping like observations together, the note-writer can reduce the total length of the note. The reader does not have to know everything that happened, in the exact order it happened, but only needs a general sense. Therefore, rather than writing a process note, which records every behavior in sequence, the assistant should write a summary note.

Be brief. This, more than anything else, will ensure that your notes will be read by the doctors, nurses, social workers, and other professionals working with the patient. And that is the point of writing the note in the first place.

It is normal and expected to have to write several versions of a note when one is first learning this skill. Figure 16–1 gives three versions of a note documenting an observation of a patient making a mosaic ashtray; the third version is similar to what the occupational therapy assistant might write into the chart. Can you see why this is the preferred version?

The first version is written in an informal style. The writer refers to himself as "I," something which is never done in the chart. The information is poorly organized, but the writer has captured some details that are very descriptive of the patient's behavior. The reader understands immediately how the patient behaved in the group. With rewriting this has the potential to become a very useful note!

But look what happened in version two: the writer introduced medical jargon, added his interpretations, and omitted some of the descriptive details that had made version one so compelling and convincing. The reader no longer has a clear picture of what happened. The note is shorter but less useful.

Version three, while almost twice as long as version two, is still shorter than version one. More importantly, it retains many of the details contained in version one. The writer has saved space by grouping like observations (e.g., of gluing tiles to the wrong side) and by choosing more descriptive single words, instead of longer phrases (e.g., regarding the patient's conversations with others). And, interestingly, on this version the writer included new details that had been omitted from version one.

Although narrative-style notes for the medical chart should be written in the style of version three, less formal notes are sometimes written into a communication book, kept in the nurses' station (in inpatient settings) or a central office (outpatient settings). The purpose of these notes is to communicate important information to staff coming onto the ward (or into the center) later in the day or evening. An example might be that the patient got a paper cut in occupational therapy; while this may sound trivial it might be very important for a patient who had diabetes or a circulatory disorder, who was HIV-positive, or whose hygiene habits were poor.

In addition to these stylistic requirements, the following rules and guidelines apply to notes written by the COTA:

1. The note should be organized in a logical fashion. Similar ideas should be grouped together; for example, all statements

---

Three versions of an observation note

These are three versions of a note on a single observation of a patient making a mosaic ashtray. Version three is the final rewrite and is suitable for entering in the medical chart.

Version One:
Marilyn came into the room very slowly. She held on to the chair when she sat down. She didn't know where she was. When I asked her name she knew it but she didn't know the answers to any of the other questions about her age or address. She was willing to make an ashtray when I showed one to her. She wanted to make a checkerboard pattern but she couldn't figure out how to do it so she just did a little bit in one corner and then she turned the tray over and glued a tile to the wrong side. Then she turned it back to the right side and put white tiles over the rest of the tray. Then she glued another tile to the bottom side of the tray. I told her that was wrong and showed her the sample, but she wanted to leave it the way it was. Her tray was a real mess, with glue and gluey fingerprints all over it. She got a lot of glue on the table too, and on her face. She cleaned up though when I told her to, but we had to wait for her because she was so slow. She held onto the sink and the table when she moved around. She didn't talk to any of the other patients at the table except once when someone asked her if she liked snow; she said "Yes." She concentrated totally on her tray. Another patient took her glue bottle when his got stuck, and she let him. I had to get it back or she would have just stopped right there. She didn't say anything at all unless someone asked her a question.

Version Two:
Marilyn participated in an occupational therapy to make a mosaic tile ashtray. She had psychomotor retardation and disorientation. She used good concentration but poor planning. Her work habits were poor. She put some tiles on the wrong side of the tray. She was bored. She let another patient take one of her supplies and didn't say anything.

Version Three:
Patient attended OT group 1X since admission. She was neatly dressed, but her hair was uncombed. She moved slowly and held onto furniture, appeared confused, was able to state her name but not her age or address. Working with apparent concentration, she completed only a few tiles in the checkerboard pattern, and finished with plain tiles. She did not speak to others except to answer questions in one or two words. She stopped working when another patient took her glue bottle (saying nothing to the patient), but resumed work when the therapist retrieved it. She twice glued tiles to the wrong side of the tray, did not recognize this error, and refused to change it when it was pointed out to her. She used more glue than was needed, dripped some on the table, and smeared some on her face. She helped clean up but continued to move very slowly.

FIG. 16–1. Three versions of an observation note

about the patient's self-care and physical appearance should appear in the first paragraph. Each paragraph addresses a different area, and the final paragraph should contain a brief summary and statement about the plan for further treatment; the plan should flow logically from the information that precedes it.

2. Notes must be written neatly so that they are legible, or typewritten or printed if necessary. Correct grammar and spelling are mandatory.

3. The note should be as brief as possible, without omitting essential information or ideas.

4. The note should be precise and factual, providing objective and truthful information about the patient's condition rather than vague generalizations or interpretations.

5. Notes should be written within the deadlines that apply in the particular facility. If notes are to be written every two weeks, then the assistant must make time to complete the notes by the date they are due. If not, one is likely to be

cited for noncompliance. If this happens often enough it can damage one's performance rating.

For legal purposes, each note must contain the patient's name and case number on each page, and the date of the note (including month, day, and year). Without this identifying information notes can be lost or misfiled. Then when the chart is audited the note may be cited as missing, when in fact it was done. The assistant should title the note with the name of the department and the type of note (e.g., Occupational Therapy Biweekly Progress Note); in some facilities, this information may be on the form already. The assistant is required to sign the note with her full name and the professional designation of COTA; the signature must come directly after the note, with no space left between the last line of the note and the signature.

Since it is only human to make mistakes, the assistant should expect a few in the writing of notes. If an error is made and needs to be corrected, the correct and legally required procedure is to draw a line through it (so that it can still be clearly read) and then insert the correction and initial it. Finally, the note must be countersigned by a registered therapist.

FOCUSING ON PERFORMANCE DEFICITS AND FUNCTIONAL GOALS

While version three in Figure 16–1 is clearer, more objective, and more concise than the earlier version, it does not clearly indicate *why* the patient needs occupational therapy or *what benefit* the patient might expect to receive from occupational therapy intervention. These elements are essential to document both the need for occupational therapy services and the results to be expected. We cannot expect that other disciplines or third-party payers such as insurance companies and the federal and state governments will automatically and clairvoyantly understand the point of our observations. The observations have to be connected to problems that will affect the patient's ability to function, and to a plan for addressing these problems. Figure 16–2 shows version four of the note, including the assessment (of deficits in functional performance) and the plan (how these deficits will be addressed). The situation in this note is that the patient has not yet been evaluated, nor has the treatment plan been developed. Both of these tasks are the responsibilities of the OTR. The COTA, in writing this note, is recommending particular evaluation instruments and focuses for

---

Incorporating performance deficits and functional goals into an observation note

Version Four:
Patient attended OT group 1X since admission. She was neatly dressed, but her hair was uncombed. She moved slowly and held onto furniture, appeared confused, was able to state her name but not her age or address. Working with apparent concentration, she completed only a few tiles in the checkerboard pattern, and finished with plain tiles. She did not speak to others except to answer questions in one or two words. She stopped working when another patient took her glue bottle (saying nothing to the patient), but resumed work when the therapist retrieved it. She twice glued tiles to the wrong side of the tray, did not recognize this error, and refused to change it when it was pointed out to her. She used more glue than was needed, dripped some on the table, and smeared some on her face. She helped clean up but continued to move very slowly. ASSESSMENT: Patient demonstrates possible cognitive disability, indicated by grooming errors, errors in task execution with failure to recognize or correct errors, impaired situational awareness. Mobility deficit suggested by using furniture for support. PLAN: Administer cognitive level test and Routine Task Inventory (within one week). Assess mobility deficit (within ten days).

FIG. 16–2. Incorporating performance deficits and functional goals into an observation note

---

Spruce Valley Hospital, Occupational Therapy Department, Initial Note

5/5/93

Case #186302

Pt. referred to OT by Dr. Goodman (5/4/93) for evaluation of task skills and work potential, leisure planning, reaction to stress. Pt. was seen briefly, to schedule and discuss the purpose of the evaluations. Pt. expressed "It won't help" and "I'm not interested," but agreed to eval. at 10 A.M. Wed., 5/6/93.

Jerry Doe COTA

FIG. 16–3. Spruce Valley Hospital, Occupational Therapy Department, initial note

evaluation, based on experience and observation of the patient. The note would be countersigned by the OTR.

INVOLVING THE PATIENT IN PROGRAM PLANNING

Wherever possible, the patient's view of her problems and goals should be included in notes. When asked, patients may give very general goals, "to get out of here" or "to feel better." Skillful questioning based on observation of the patient and some knowledge of the patient's background can elicit more detail, even from less verbal patients. Asking a more concrete question, focusing on a specific observed or known behavior or interest, is most likely to result in a specific response. In the case of the confused patient described in Figure 16–2, one might ask her (diplomatically) if she combed her hair today. She might indicate that she did so, and that her appearance is important to her. This can be restated as a functional goal, "Patient wants to 'look nice.' By the end of one week, patient will recognize completion of essential grooming tasks (hair care)."

Spruce Valley Hospital, Occupational Therapy Department, Evaluation Report

5/6/93

Case #186302

Pt. arrived on time; was neat, clean, dressed appropriately. Her facial and verbal expressions were flat and unresponsive. She appeared oriented to time, place, and person. Task skills were assessed via mosaic tile task.

Patient worked at a reasonable pace, appropriate to the task, and performed independently with minimal assistance from the group leader. She requested instructions twice, but otherwise isolated herself and did not enter into the general conversation. Tiles were neatly and planfully arranged; concentration and coordination appeared excellent. Pt. had some difficulty making simple decisions (e.g., color and pattern) and became agitated when the tiles moved because the glue had not had time to dry. Despite agitation, she stated was not interested in this or any other activity, asked to return to unit early. When request was denied, pt. sat quietly and waited for group to end.

ASSESSMENT: Assets: good task skills. Possible problem areas: task skills lower than expected for educational level, low tolerance of frustration (tendency to abandon tasks that are not immediately successful), difficulty making decisions, impaired interpersonal functioning (isolates self).

PLAN: Continue evaluation by OT to be completed by 5/13/93.

Jerry Doe COTA

FIG. 16–4. Spruce Valley Hospital, Occupational Therapy Department, evaluation report

---

Occupational Therapy Department, Home Arts Program Evaluation Report and Treatment Plan

12/18/92   Page 1 (of 1)
                                                                       Case #291083

Pt. was evaluated for independent daily living skills in six sessions of one hour each (12/7, 12/8, 12/10, 12/14, 12/15, 12/17). Pt. arrived on time, neatly dressed in casual clothes and well groomed. The Comprehensive Evaluation of Daily Living Skills (CEBLS) checklist was used. A score of 135 of possible 176 points was obtained in the Personal Care and Hygiene Section. Pt. scored independent level in toileting, brushing teeth, bathing, hair care, dressing. Pt. needed assistance with shaving, missing areas on the right side of face (probably due to visual deficit). He did not perform any of the personal housekeeping tasks correctly, and could not trim fingernails and toenails using clippers or scissors. Pt. sat with a slouched posture and walked with a shuffling gait.

On the Practical Evaluation, pt. scored 90 of possible 240 points. Pt. independent in use of telephone, but showed poor social behavior on phone. Pt. able to use bus with some assistance in interpreting route and schedule. He did not have any idea of how to plan, shop for, or prepare a meal, and did not know how to serve a meal. Pt. ate appropriately, independently, helped in cleaning up after meal, but needed much assistance (e.g., reminders to wash backs of plates, instruction in how to scrape dishes, etc). Pt. occasionally bumped into objects on his right because he failed to notice them.

When pt. did not know how to proceed he appeared very anxious, began pacing and wringing his hands, and asked to stop the evaluation and be brought back to the unit. This occurred when the correct bus failed to arrive on schedule and was twenty minutes late. Pt. stated that he tends to panic under stress.

ASSESSMENT: Pt. independent in most areas of self-care; unable to perform most housekeeping and cooking tasks correctly unless directly supervised. He fails to compensate for absent vision in the right eye; this is a serious safety risk. Pt. also tends to panic when confronted with a problem he is not immediately able to resolve.

GOALS: 1. Pt. states desire to overcome visual deficit so that he can assume home management tasks.
           a. to learn compensatory techniques for navigating in home environment and for placement of tools and other objects (by two weeks).

           2. Pt. stated desire to be a help to his wife around the house.
           a. to learn to maintain kitchen in clean, safe manner (by two weeks).
           b. to learn to prepare a simple meal (by three weeks)
           c. to learn to plan and shop for weekly groceries (by six weeks)
           d. to learn to keep home clean and tidy (by five weeks)
           e. to learn to launder and care for clothing (by eight weeks)

           3. Pt. verbalized desired to learn to shave face accurately.
           a. to learn compensatory techniques for visual deficit (by one week)

           4. Pt. wants to be able to travel in community and deal with household emergencies without "losing it."
           a. to learn stress management techniques and apply these to situations encountered in daily life (by ten weeks).

PLAN: Enroll pt. in ten-week Home Arts Program, 4 hours per day (9 A.M.–1 P.M.), 4 days per week, beginning 12/28/92 through 3/8/93. Schedule individual half-hour sessions twice weekly to instruct in visual compensatory techniques. Schedule pt. for stress management group one evening per week, with wife. Encourage wife to help patient to practice and reinforce skills taught. Reassess progress in one month (1/18/93).

B White cota

FIG. 16–5. Occupational Therapy Department, Home Arts Program evaluation report and treatment plan

INITIAL NOTES

The purpose of an initial note is to record that the occupational therapist or assistant has received and acted on the referral for service. The minimum content required for the initial note consists of:

1. The patient's name and case number and today's date

2. The source of referral, the reason for referral, and the date referral was received
3. The information obtained and behavior noted at the first contact
4. Plan for further contact
5. The COTA's signature and title
6. The OTR's countersignature.

The sort of initial note the COTA might be asked to write is shown in Fig. 16–3, which refers to Case 1 in Appendix A at the back of the book.

EVALUATION REPORTS

The COTA performs various structured evaluations and from time to time may be required to document them in a simple summary note. This is not to be confused with the assessment notes in which the therapist compiles and interprets the results of all occupational therapy evaluations the patient has received. An evaluation report should contain the following information:

1. The patient's name and case number and today's date
2. Tests and evaluations administered and the results
3. A summary and analysis of the patient's assets and deficits, based on evaluation results and other objective sources
4. Recommendations for occupational therapy services, including what type of service is indicated
5. The COTA's signature and title
6. The OTR's countersignature.

In many settings, particularly those with restrictive reimbursement guidelines, the COTA may not document evaluation data, a task for which the OTR is held responsible. In other settings, such as long-term care or substance abuse or community treatment, the COTA may expect greater involvement in selecting, recommending, or administering evaluations, and documenting the results. Figure 16–4 presents a note documenting the results of a simple task skills evaluation using the Comprehensive Occupational Therapy Evaluation Scale (COTE scale). This note refers to Case 1 in Appendix A.

An example of how the COTA might write up a more complex report on the results of a daily living skills evaluation is shown in Fig. 16–5. This report is based on Case 5 in Appendix A. (The Home Arts evaluation was performed because the patient and his wife decided that he would take on the homemaker role in their household.) This evaluation report incorporates the treatment plan, which focuses primarily on the areas of self-care and homemaking. An entry-level COTA would not typically be responsible to write such a plan. This might be expected of the COTA with a year or more of experience in the particular treatment area, depending on the treatment setting.

TREATMENT PLANS

Less common than the combined evaluation report/treatment plan format is the separate treatment plan. The COTA may be asked to formulate and document the plan for a particular occupational performance area such as self-care. The basic information to be included in a note that documents the treatment plan[2] consists of:

1. The patient's name and case number and today's date
2. Long-term goal or goals as determined

---

[2]Adapted from (2).

by the patient and the therapist or assistant

3. Immediate short-term goals related to the long-term goals
4. Methods to be used, including a general description of activities and treatment procedures
5. The frequency and duration of planned treatment
6. The anticipated completion date
7. The projected outcome, or end result of treatment
8. The COTA's signature and title
9. The OTR's countersignature.

An example of how a treatment plan should be recorded is shown in Fig. 16–6, which relates to Case 5 in Appendix A.

PROGRESS NOTES

The vast majority of notes written by COTAs are progress notes, which document treatment and changes in the patient's condition since the last note. Obviously, the specific content of these notes varies depending on the setting, the patient, and the type of treatment provided by the COTA. At a minimum, however, all progress notes should contain the following information:

1. Patient's name and case number and today's date
2. Record of patient's attendance, including number of sessions and inclusive dates

---

Occupational Therapy Department, Home Arts Program Treatment Plan

12/18/92

Page 1 (of 2)
Case #291083

Long term objectives:
1. Increase pt.'s sense of comfort and confidence in ability to carry out home management role.

2. Improve pt.'s ability to plan, organize, and execute basic household tasks.

3. Develop pt.'s social skills in basic communication, ability to relate to others in small groups, and to assert self appropriately.

4. Pt. to learn and use techniques to compensate for visual deficit.

5. Pt. to learn and use stress management techniques.

6. Pt. to explore leisure interests and develop leisure habits.

Method:
Pt. to attend Home Arts Program (M, T, T, F from 9 A.M. to 1 P.M.) beginning 12/28/92 for ten-weeks' instruction in meal preparation, nutrition, housekeeping, self-care skills, play/leisure skills, sewing, social skills, and use of community resources. Pt. will receive individual training and reinforcement in visual compensation techniques.

Short-term objectives:
1. Pt. will demonstrate ability to plan and prepare a simple meal, including the following steps: preparing shopping list, grocery shopping, food storage, kitchen safety, food preparation and cooking, table setting, meal clean-up, and use of kitchen equipment, utensils, and appliances (by four weeks).

2. Pt. will demonstrate ability to compensate for visual deficit in performance of meal preparation tasks (by four weeks).

B White com (cot)

FIG. 16–6. Occupational Therapy Department, Home Arts Program treatment plan

Short-term objectives (continued):
Pt. will demonstrate ability to identify situations that he finds stressful, and will discuss why.

Plan:
Pt. will receive instruction in basic methods of meal preparation, as a member of a small group, in the kitchen of the Home Arts Center and in the community (e.g., grocery store). COTA will explain purpose of visual compensation, will teach pt. to turn and look to the right before moving any part of the body to the right, and will reinforce use of this technique through praise and verbal encouragement. Through group discussions focusing on recognizing and analyzing stress, pt. will learn to identify his own reactions to stressful situations and will develop awareness of which situations he finds stressful. Reevaluate in one month (1/18/93).

B White COTA

FIG. 16–6. (*Continued*)

Where OT Documents	What the Therapist Thinks!	What the Therapist Does!	What the Therapist Documents!
Daily notations on chart Weekly progress note Monthly summary notes	Constantly re-assessing goals: Are treatment services covered? Are you duplicating services? and Are you providing maintenance care? and Are you changing plans as necessary? and also consider: Should patient be put on hold for a period of time due to illness? Do you need to design a maintenance program for residual deficits?	Chart review Provide treatment Observe performance in requested activities Modify treatment according to patient's response to STG & LTG As patient goals change you modify treatment Verify new short-term and long-term goals with patient/caregivers Discontinue patient temporarily Instruct in-home program	Record briefly: Date, type, length of treatment State change in meeting short-term goals and the effect on long-term goals Record changes in goals in weekly or monthly notes Every 30 days summarize changes in patient's ability to perform functional activities and changes in underlying factors State when patient reaches goals. Explanation if patient does not reach goals and how that affects treatment plan Recertification of Medicare Record temporary discontinuation of treatment and reason Record home program and any follow-up recommendations made

FIG. 16–7. Therapist's short-term goals and changes in goals. From Fig. 5–1 of Allen CK. Clinical reasoning for documentation. In: Acquaviva JD. *Effective documentation.* Rockville, Md: American Occupational Therapy Association; 1992:54. Copyright © 1992 by the American Occupational Therapy Association, Inc. Reprinted with permission.

Spruce Valley Hospital, Occupational Therapy Department, Weekly Progress Note

5/22/92
Hilary Page

Case #186302

Miss Page has been present at six of eight sessions of the Basic Task Skills Group she has been attending for task skills development and further assessment related to discharge planning. Both absences were due to schedule conflicts (lab tests). Hilary has performed adequately at each of the simple clerical tasks offered, but says she is bored. She frequently converses with another female patient (T.M.), but does not join in the general conversation, and relates to the COTA only around the task.

Patient to continue in group until discharge, tentatively scheduled for 5/29, to maintain skills and work habits. Recommendation is that the discharge plan include more challenging activities and assessment of interests so that patient has opportunity to develop decision-making skills and other task behaviors needed for work on further schooling.

Treatment sessions attended: 5/13, 5/14, 5/16, 5/20, 5/21, 5/22

Jerry Doe COTA

FIG. 16–8. Spruce Valley Hospital, Occupational Therapy Department, weekly progress note

3. Summary of media and methods used, and goals addressed
4. Statement of patient's response to therapy (participation, behavior, etc.)
5. Any changes in goals, and explanation for this
6. If treatment has not occurred as planned, state this and explain why
7. A copy of any home program given to patient
8. Plan for continued treatment, including any modifications needed
9. COTA's signature and title
10. OTR's countersignature.

Thoughtfulness and planning are the first steps in preparing a progress note. Allen (1) breaks down the separate processes of thinking, doing, and writing as they apply to the clinical reasoning used to document patient progress. Figure 16–7 shows this breakdown. By taking the steps listed, one by one, and assembling the information in an orderly fashion, the COTA will find that the actual writing of the note is quite straightforward. Examples of different progress notes are contained in Figs. 16–8 through 16–11. These notes refer, respectively, to Cases 1, 2, 3, and 5 in Appendix A.

Progress notes should record what has really happened, not what you wish happened, or what you planned but were not able to do. One of the unfortunate realities

---

Green Manor Nursing Home, Occupational Therapy Department, Biweekly Progress Note

3/12/93
Jenny Anderson

Treatment given: 2/27, 2/28, 3/3, 3/4, 3/5, 3/6, 3/7, 3/10, 3/11, 3/12.
Case #9801

Pt. has been seen individually for the past two weeks on a daily basis. Her condition continues to deteriorate. She is usually found seated in a geri-chair in the dining room. She appears alert and interested in her surroundings, but on approach by COTA is consistently disoriented to time, place, and person. She responds to simple familiar activities like tossing a ball, and will imitate motions (exercises) that are demonstrated. *Plan:* Continue daily visits to provide social and sensory stimulation, and basic movement experiences, in order to orient patient to environment, limit extent of contractures, and encourage as much independent function as possible.

Nelly Cortland COTA

FIG. 16–9. Green Manor Nursing Home, Occupational Therapy Department, biweekly progress note

---

County Hospital, Occupational Therapy Department, Weekly Progress Note

10/7/92
Lucy Lammamoor   Case #082751

Pt. has selectively attended general ward activities over the past week (11 of 18 activity group sessions). She states she does not need the socialization group or the community meeting, and efforts to involve her have been unsuccessful. She participates in the daily crafts group, the senior stretch exercise group, and the semiweekly cooking group. Pt. continues to rely inappropriately on help from group leaders but fails to seek help when she truly needs it. In cooking, she asked for assistance and approval in measuring and mixing ingredients (although she did this correctly and quickly), but then reached for a pot handle without a potholder. Her crafts projects are neat and attractive, but she hoards materials and criticizes other patients. Periodic C/O leg pain (reported to J. Brown, R.N. on 10/2/92). *Plan:* Continue to engage in exercise, craft, and cooking activities, and observe for safety. Continue to encourage participation in social and verbal groups, with one-to-one escort of OTA student. Reassess one week.

M.a. Team COTA

FIG. 16–10. County Hospital, Occupational Therapy Department, weekly progress note

---

Occupational Therapy Department, Home Arts Program, Biweekly Progress Note

(page 1 of 2)

1/8/93   Sessions attended: 12/21, 12/22, 12/23; 12/28, 12/29, 12/30; 1/4, 1/5, 1/7, 18

Dwight Kennedy   Case #291083

Pt. has attended all scheduled sessions over the past two and a half weeks, at first seemed uncomfortable with other members of the group, but has begun to interact spontaneously during the past week. Pt. has mastered all of the meal preparation tasks (see plan 12/18/92), obtained a score of 92 of a possible 100 points on Sections 4, 5, and 6 of the Practical Evaluation, and appears capable to carry out routine cooking safely. Patient still tends to panic in difficult situations; for instance, when he was $1.50 short to pay for groceries he ran out of the store. He was able to discuss this later with the group, and explore other ways he could have handled the problem. Patient says he needs to stop and think before acting; COTA feels this shows insight and growth. COTA contacted patient's wife, who is pleased with his progress and willing to allow him to take over meal preparation responsibilities at home.

New short-term objectives:
1. Patient will demonstrate knowledge of nutrition, as evidenced by ability to plan balanced meals.

2. Patient will demonstrate ability to organize and perform basic household cleaning tasks, including dusting, vacuuming/sweeping, cleaning, and knowledge of household products.

3. Patient will demonstrate ability to compensate for visual deficit in performance of household cleaning.

B White COTA (cont)

FIG. 16–11. Occupational Therapy Department, Home Arts Program, biweekly progress note

(page 2 of 2)

1/8/93
Dwight Kennedy   Case #291083

New short-term objectives (continued):
4. Patient will continue to explore his reactions to stress and to discuss alternative responses.

Method:
Continue group instruction in basic nutrition and methods of household cleaning, in the Home Arts Center and local shops. Continue to teach and reinforce visual compensation techniques. Group discussions on stress and stress management will continue. It is expected that above objectives will be reached by 2/1/93, at which point patient will be able to plan balanced meals and perform housekeeping tasks independently.

B White cota

FIG. 16–11. (*Continued*)

of work with severely disabled people is that they do not always show improvement from session to session. In fact, some patients, like Mrs. Anderson in the note shown in Fig. 16–8, actually get worse despite the best efforts of the staff.

One of the purposes of writing accurate and careful progress notes is to document reasons why treatment should be continued or stopped. If the patient is making progress toward goals that have been established in the treatment plan or in previous notes, it is easy to show why treatment should be continued. Figure 16–10 is an example of a note that documents progress in a measurable way, by including the results of a periodic reevaluation. On the other hand, if the note shows that the patient has been consistently uncooperative, missing treatment sessions for example, then the plan should be reviewed and changed, or perhaps this patient's therapy should be discontinued, and the COTA's resources used to help more receptive patients.

SOAP NOTES

Progress notes are most often written in the narrative form shown in Figs. 16–8 through 16–11, but in a problem-oriented medical record notes are sometimes written in the SOAP format. These initials stand for *Subjective-Objective-Assessment-Plan.*

The *subjective* section of the plan contains what the patient reports he feels or believes, based on what he tells the therapist. This section usually begins with the words, "The patient states (or similar verb of speech). . . ."

The *objective* section describes observable or measurable behavior noted by the therapist. This may include evaluation results and observations of patient performance. This is the section in which most of the information usually contained in a narrative progress note would be written.

The *assessment* section summarizes the therapist's current understanding of the patient's problem. (Remember that everything in the problem-oriented record is organized around the problem list.) Here the therapist draws upon the subjective and objective information contained in the first part of the note, and analyzes whether the plan needs to be modified.

The *plan* section describes the action the therapist will take in response to the patient's problem. Here the therapist records the plan for continued treatment, including modifications to the previous plan, and any new objectives and methods.

The note that appeared as Fig. 16–10 has been rewritten in SOAP format in Fig. 16–12.

County Hospital, S.O.A.P. Note

Note #64

Problem #4—Possible cognitive disability

S: Pt. continues to request assistance from group leaders to perform simple exercises, craft activities, and meal preparation tasks in occupational therapy groups.

O: Pt. performs well in many tasks, as evidenced by her completion of a complicated main dish and her detailed braiding of a basket based on a diagram in a book.
     However, patient also has acted unsafely in kitchen (reaching for pot without potholder to protect hand).

A: Pt. is working in unfamiliar kitchen, with unfamiliar equipment. Pt. seems to know task well. Reasons for errors may be related to unfamiliar environment.

P: COTA will arrange for evaluation of pt.'s cooking behaviors in pt.'s home kitchen.

10/7/92
M. a. Tern COTA

FIG. 16–12. County Hospital, S.O.A.P. note

Because notes in the problem-oriented record are written in response to specific problems, other information unrelated to these problems is omitted in the SOAP note, and would be documented separately.

Some versions of the SOAP note allow for the omission of the S, or subjective, component, which is useful when patients are nonverbal. It is also possible to combine the S and the O, or objective, components into one section, as shown in Fig. 16–13, which restates information found in Fig. 16–2.

DISCHARGE SUMMARIES

The discharge summary reviews the entire course of the patient's treatment. It includes the kinds of evaluation and treatment the patient received, the number of occupational therapy sessions, progress to-

---

Clearview Hospital, S.O.A.P. Note

OT Note #1

Problem #1—Possible cognitive disability

S, O: Pt. arrived for OT group with uncombed hair. Made errors in simple tile task, gluing tiling to wrong side. Dripped glue and did not recognize that she had smeared glue on face. Moved slowly, holding on to furniture.

A: Pt. demonstrates behavior consistent with cognitive level 4.

P: Administer ACL and RTI to further assess cognitive deficit.

2/1/93
C. Sample COTA

FIG. 16–13. Clearview Hospital, S.O.A.P. note

ward goals, and the patient's functional level at discharge. A comparison is made between the patient's condition at the beginning of treatment and at discharge, and recommendations for continued care or referrals to other agencies are included. A discharge summary usually includes:

1. The patient's name and case number and today's date
2. A summary of the occupational therapy process, including the number of sessions, goals achieved, and final outcome
3. A comparison of patient's status at admission to the program with that at discharge
4. Follow-up plans and recommendations

5. The COTA's signature and title
6. The OTR's countersignature.

A COTA might write a discharge summary when a patient is discontinued from or completes a program the COTA supervises. An example of such a discharge summary, relating to Case 5 in Appendix A, is presented in Fig. 16–14.

SPECIAL REPORTS

Occasionally the occupational therapy department may wish to include additional records or reports in the patient's chart, or these may be required for legal reasons. Examples include:

Occupational Therapy Department, Home Arts Program Discharge Summary

3/31/93   (page 1 of 2)

Dwight Kennedy   Case #291083

Mr. Kennedy completed 44 sessions of instruction in the occupational therapy home arts program. Four sessions missed due to illness were made up during the past week. Pt. achieved the following goals during the program:

1. Pt. has learned to plan, organize, and carry out basic household tasks, and states he feels comfortable in role of homemaker.

2. Pt. has learned to participate in and initiate simple social conversations, and to assert self appropriately in social situations.

3. Pt. has learned techniques to compensate for his visual deficit, and uses these techniques consistently.

4. Pt. has learned progressive relaxation and the use of imagery to control the effects of stress.

5. Pt. has identified music as a major leisure interest, and has enrolled in a guitar study course at the local Y.

Pt. is capable of functioning independently in the community in the role of homemaker while his wife continues to work full-time. Wife states that pt. has "really turned his life around," that she looks forward to coming home to a clean house and a hot meal every day. Pt. expresses satisfaction with his accomplishments and his new role. On final reevaluation Mr. Kennedy obtained a score of 173 of 176 possible points on the Personal Care and Hygiene Section and 234 of a possible 240 points on the Practical Evaluation Section of the Comprehensive Evaluation of Basic Living Skills. This compares with scores of 135 and 90, respectively, prior to admission to the program.

B. White COTA (cont)

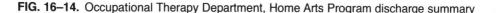

FIG. 16–14. Occupational Therapy Department, Home Arts Program discharge summary

3/31/93   (page 2 of 2)

Dwight Kennedy   Case #291083

Plan: Follow-up visits to the pt.'s home at one-month intervals for three months to ensure pt. continues to carry over learned skills to home environment. Reassess three months (6/93).   *B White cota*

FIG. 16–14. *(Continued)*

1. Referrals to other programs or agencies
2. Letters about or from the patient that relate to his condition and treatment
3. Copies of home programs given to the patient or his family
4. Reports to the court
5. Behavioral counting scales.

Most of these items should be familiar or self-explanatory, with the exception of the *behavioral counting scale*. This is a grid-like chart used to record a specific aspect of a patient's behavior. For instance, the rater might count the number of times an autistic child bangs his head during a one-hour session, or how many ceramic pieces a patient in a work group decorates during a three-hour shift. The rater counts the number of times the behavior occurs during the selected time period and records it on the vertical axis of the chart. The horizontal axis is used to show changes over time, as the behavior is counted day after day. This gives a clear visual picture of whether the behavior is increasing or decreasing as a result of occupational therapy interventions. An example of this kind of record is shown in Fig. 16–15.

The registered therapist makes the final decision about which materials she will recommend be included in the patient's chart. The assistant should therefore bring any correspondence or other special reports to the therapist's attention.

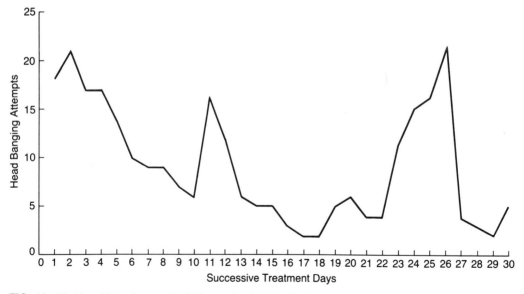

FIG. 16–15. Head Banging per Half-Hour—April 1986. Behavior chart used to record data related to patient change

CRITERIA	WEIGHT	Adequate (1)	Questionable (0)	Not applicable (1)	FOR OFFICE USE ONLY
Therapeutic relationship					
1. Provides positive feedback; reinforces gains	5.00	☐	☐		_____ 41
2. Encourages ventilation of feelings	4.75	☐	☐		_____ 45
Assessment					
3. Functional level	5.00	☐	☐		_____ 49
4. Mental status	4.75	☐	☐		_____ 53
5. Medical history and physical status	4.25	☐	☐		_____ 57
6. Family and social history	4.75	☐	☐		_____ 61
7. Functional and work history	4.75	☐	☐		_____ 65
8. Ongoing reassessment and documentation on change	4.25	☐	☐		_____ 69
Treatment planning					_____ 73
9. Determines achievable goals	4.25	☐	☐		_____ 77
10. Seeks patient consensus on goals	4.25	☐	☐		REV # _____ 2
Treatment					CARD # _____ 3
11. Monitors medical care (medications, appointments)	3.75	☐	☐		_____ 7
12. Promotes discussion of social and interpersonal situations	4.50	☐	☐		_____ 11
13. Promotes social network	4.25	☐	☐		_____ 15
14. Teaches self-care skills	4.50	☐	☐	☐	_____ 19
15. Teaches household management and budgeting	4.00	☐	☐	☐	_____ 23
16. Teaches organizational skills	3.00	☐	☐	☐	_____ 27
17. Teaches leisure time planning	4.00	☐	☐	☐	_____ 31
18. Teaches stress management (relaxation, physical exercise, time management, etc.)	4.25	☐	☐	☐	_____ 35
19. Provides parent effectiveness training	4.00	☐	☐	☐	_____ 39
20. Provides assertiveness training	3.50	☐	☐	☐	_____ 43
21. Provides vocational counseling	3.75	☐	☐	☐	_____ 47
22. Provides counseling with regard to insight	3.25	☐	☐	☐	_____ 51
23. Provides grief counseling	3.25	☐	☐	☐	_____ 55
24. Involves family and significant others	4.00	☐	☐	☐	_____ 59
Consultation and follow-up					
25. Referral made to other agencies as related to treatment goals	3.75	☐	☐	☐	_____ 63
26. Contacts maintained with other involved professionals	4.25	☐	☐	☐	_____ 67
27. Reports serious concerns to appropriate source	4.75	☐	☐	☐	_____ 71
28. Consults with other occupational therapists for supervision when necessary	3.25	☐	☐	☐	_____ 75
29. Makes plans for ongoing follow-up on discharge	3.75	☐	☐	☐	_____ 79

FIG. 16–16. Score sheet for chart audit. From Fig. 3 of McColl M, and Quinn B. A quality assurance method for community occupational therapy. *Am J Occup Ther* 1985; 39:570–577. Copyright © 1985 by the American Occupational Therapy Association, Inc. Reprinted with permission.

In addition to the kinds of notes covered in this chapter, there exist many checklist or grid types of documentation formats, in which information for a number of different sessions can be checked off on one sheet. The COTE Scale (see Chapter 14) is a popular example. Other flow sheets or documentation summaries may be particular to individual facilities.

QUALITY ASSURANCE AND CHART AUDITING

Quality assurance is the name given to methods and programs that try to ensure accountability in health care. Quality assurance programs investigate whether treatment was provided in a timely fashion, in keeping with the accepted standards of practice in the various professional disciplines involved. Another purpose of quality assurance is to demonstrate which interventions were effective and which were not.

Chart audit is one method of quality assurance. The general procedure for chart audit is first to develop a set of criteria or standards for patient care, and then to review patients' charts to see whether they received the care that is required by the criteria. For example, one of the criteria developed by the occupational therapy department is likely to be that every patient must receive an occupational therapy evaluation on referral. When the charts are reviewed (audited), it is easy to demonstrate whether or not this has happened. A sample of a scoring sheet used in a community occupational therapy agency for audit of charts of patients with a diagnosis of depression is shown in Fig. 16–16. The second column of the score sheet shows the weight or relative importance of each item on the list. The third column asks raters to score the chart on whether it adequately meets each of the criteria.

CONCLUSION

Keeping accurate and complete records is an important part of the occupational therapy assistant's job. The patient's chart is a legal document and an important tool for communication among different disciplines involved in the patient's care. Increasingly strict reimbursement guidelines have made it more important than ever before to record measurable objectives and objective signs of progress; written evidence of clear goals and reasonable efforts to achieve them is the only way to convince public and private insurers to continue to pay for occupational therapy services.

REFERENCES

1. Allen CK. Clinical reasoning for documentation. In: Acquaviva JD, ed. *Effective documentation for occupational therapy.* Rockville, Md: American Occupational Therapy Association; 1992.
2. American Occupational Therapy Association. Guidelines for occupational therapy documentation. *Am J Occup Ther* 1986;40:830–832.
3. American Occupational Therapy Association Entry-Level Role Delineation Task Force. Entry-level role delineation for registered occupational therapists (OTRs) and certified occupational therapy assistants (COTAs). *Am J Occup Ther* 1990; 44:1091–1102.
4. Moorhouse MF, Doenges ME. *Nurse's clinical pocket manual: nursing diagnosis, care planning, and documentation.* Philadelphia: FA Davis; 1990.
5. Strunk W, White EB. *The elements of style.* New York: Macmillan; 1959.

ADDITIONAL REFERENCES AND SUGGESTED READINGS

American Occupational Therapy Association Uniform Terminology Task Force. Uniform terminology for occupational therapy, second edition. *Am J Occup Ther* 1989;43:808–815.
Acquaviva JD, ed. *Effective documentation for occupational therapy.* Rockville, Md: American Occupational Therapy Association; 1992.
Baum CM. Management and documentation of occupational therapy services. In: Hopkins HL, Smith HD, eds. *Willard and Spackman's occupa-*

tional therapy. 5th ed. Philadelphia: JB Lippincott; 1978.

Bell J. Sample discharge form. *Am Occup Ther Assoc Mental Health Specialty Section Newsletter* 1980;3(1):4.

Clinical Skillbuilders. *Better documentation.* Springhouse Pa: Springhouse Corporation.

Fidler GS. *Design of rehabilitation services in psychiatric hospital settings.* Laurel, Md: RAMSCO; 1984.

Fischbach FT. *Documenting care: communication, the nursing process and documentation standards.* Philadelphia: FA Davis; 1991.

Hansen S. Documentation simplified in acute psychiatry. *Am Occup Ther Assoc Mental Health Special Interest Section Newsletter.* 1983;6(4):1–4.

Kannenberg K. Special considerations. III: Mental health. In: Acquaviva JD, ed. *Effective documentation for occupational therapy.* Rockville Md: American Occupational Therapy Association; 1992.

Lillie MD, Armstrong HE. Contributions to the development of psychoeducational approaches to mental health service. *Am J Occup Ther* 1982; 36:438–443.

Llorens LA, Shuster JJ. Occupational therapy sequential client care recording system. *Am J Occup Ther* 1977;31:367–371.

McColl M, Quinn B. A quality assurance method for community occupational therapy. *Am J Occup Ther* 1985;39:570–577.

Ort RG. Documentation is the key to good note writing. *Occup Ther News* 1985;39(11):12.

Ottenbacher KJ, Johnson MB, Hojem M. The significance of clinical change and clinical change of significance. *Am J Occup Ther* 1988;42:156–163.

Ottenbacher K, York J. Strategies for evaluating clinical change: implications for practice and research. *Am J Occup Ther* 1984;38:647–659.

Payton OD, Ozer MN, Nelson CE. *Patient participation in program planning: a manual for therapists.* Philadelphia: FA Davis; 1991.

Peloquin SM. Uniform terminology as a basis for goal formulation. *Occup Ther Mental Health* 1986; 6(4):49–62.

Single case reports. *Am Occup Ther Assoc Mental Health Special Interest Section Newsletter* 1985; 8(4):4.

Smith LC, Hawley CJ, Grant RL. Questions frequently asked about the problem-oriented record in psychiatry. *Hosp Commun Psychiatry* 1974; 25:17–22.

Occupational Therapy Methods

17

Group Concepts and Techniques

Our humanity rests upon a series of learned behaviors, woven together into patterns that are infinitely fragile and never directly inherited.

MARGARET MEAD (12)

Much of occupational therapy treatment for patients with mental health problems is carried out in groups. A 1985 survey showed that 100 percent of occupational therapists working in psychiatric hospitals and community mental health centers at that time used groups with their patients, and that groups were used in a wide variety of settings for the physically disabled, and for geriatric patients (4). This chapter will explain why and how group treatment is conducted in occupational therapy in mental health settings. Although a review of some concepts of group dynamics is included, it is assumed that the reader already has a basic knowledge of groups and how people behave in them. People live and work in groups, which makes the skill of relating to others imperative for everyday functioning. Since many psychiatric patients have trouble relating to others, both individually and in groups, it will be important to consider how people generally develop these skills. In addition we need to understand how to analyze, intervene in, and create group environments so as to maximize the individual's ability to relate to others.

The ability to lead groups effectively is one of the most valuable skills the occupational therapy assistant can bring to psychiatric work. An understanding of how ther-apy groups differ from other kinds of groups, and of the role of the leader in the group, is essential. These topics, as well as a procedure for designing a new group, will be covered in some detail. As with so many other clinical skills, however, the ability to run a group well is acquired only through repeated practice and studious self-examination. The material presented in this chapter should prepare the reader to begin this process.

DEFINITION AND PURPOSE OF GROUP TREATMENT

To define *group treatment,* it is first necessary to define what we mean by a *group.* We all experience groups in work, school, social, and family situations. A group is three or more people who are together for some period of time in order to accomplish a common goal or share a common purpose. If this seems a little vague, this is only because there are many different kinds of groups that our definition must include. One important point, however, is that a group, in our definition, is not just a collection of people; it is a collection of people who have a shared purpose in being together. This makes a group different from other collections of people, such as those waiting in line in supermarkets, or riding in an elevator or subway car.

What, then, is group treatment? We stated in a previous chapter that treatment is a planned process for creating change so that the patient will be able to carry out his chosen daily life activities as independently and comfortably as possible. If we add this concept to our definition of a group, we come up with the following: *Group treatment is a planned process for creating changes in individuals by bringing them together for this purpose.*

Treating patients in groups means that several individuals can receive treatment simultaneously. This is usually less expensive than having the therapist treat each patient individually, one at a time. Therefore, group treatment is considered *cost-effective* by administrators, and this is one of the reasons it is so popular. However, cost-effectiveness alone is not a good enough reason for choosing a group treatment; it must also meet the needs of the patient. In most cases, group treatment offers more opportunities for learning, and therefore for change, than a one-on-one situation does. The reason should be obvious: in a group there are more people to learn from. There are also more possibilities for different kinds of interactions, greater potential for problem solving and creativity, more opportunities for reality testing, trying out new roles, and so on. Patients who could benefit from the advantages offered by a group, and who have adequate trust in other human beings, are good candidates for group treatment.

GROUP DYNAMICS: REVIEW OF BASIC CONCEPTS

We have all experienced groups that work well, that reach their goals through the combined efforts of all the members, in a way that is relatively satisfying to the members. Likewise, we have all known groups that never seem to get off the ground, that fail to reach their goals because the members cannot work together; such groups are a dreary experience for all concerned. What accounts for the difference between these two kinds of groups? Why do some groups succeed where others fail? What ingredients are necessary for a group to be successful?

Cohesiveness and Other Therapeutic Factors

Group cohesiveness is the sense of solidarity the members feel toward each other and the group; it is based on a sense of closeness and identification with each other or with the group itself. Cohesiveness serves the same purpose in a group that trust and rapport serve in the individual patient-therapist relationship; it ties people to each other with a sense of "we-ness" or belonging together. Group members feel accepted by each other and accepting toward each other.

Cohesiveness gives a group strength to face its tasks. Individual members feel more comfortable trying out new and unfamiliar roles, because they trust that the group will not reject them if they fail. Similarly, people find it easier to share feelings and concerns in a cohesive atmosphere. Members of cohesive groups are more willing to be influenced by the group and more willing to take the risk of trying something new or disagreeing with the group (18). Because many people will not take risks in situations they perceive to be uncertain, the occupational therapy assistant will need to consider the cohesiveness of a particular group before implementing any treatment activities that require self-disclosure or performance of unfamiliar tasks. Cohesiveness is considered a prerequisite for work in any group (18). Questions to consider include: Do the group members seem to trust one another? Do they work together? Do they support and encourage each other? How much do they reveal about themselves to the other members?

Although cohesiveness occurs spontaneously in many groups, it often must be facilitated in treatment groups. Cohesiveness can be encouraged by adjusting the length and frequency of meetings and by enhancing perceptions of intermember similarity. *Length* refers to the amount of time group meetings run, and *frequency* refers to how often they occur. The more hours a group spends together, the more cohesive it is likely to be; you can verify this by thinking about the amount of time you spend with other occupational therapy students, and how you feel about this group as differentiated from the rest of the students in your school. *Intermember similarity* is the degree to which group members believe they are like each other or share a sense of purpose or reason for being together in the group. The more similar the members feel toward others in the group, the more cohesive the group will be. Again, you can verify this from your own experience. In therapeutic groups the leader may need to point out to the members the ways in which they are like each other; similarities may be based on cultural background, common experiences, shared interests, shared goals, or other factors. A study by Banning and Nelson (2) suggests that activities that elicit humor and laughter may also promote cohesiveness through the shared experience of pleasure.

A study by Falk-Kessler, Momich, and Perel (7) examined the therapeutic factors in occupational therapy groups through a survey of patients in day treatment centers affiliated with a state hospital. According to the survey, the factors rated most helpful by patients were *group cohesiveness, interpersonal learning-output, instillation of hope,* and *universality.* These factors had previously been identified and analyzed by Yalom (18,19) in relation to verbal therapy groups. Group cohesiveness, which was rated by patients as the single most important factor, was discussed earlier in this chapter. *Interpersonal learning-output* refers to learning more successful ways to relate to others. *Instillation of hope* is based on an increased sense of hopefulness from seeing that other group members improve. *Universality* provides a shared experience as the patient learns she is not unique and that others are "in the same boat." Other factors seen as important by those responding to this survey included *guidance* (accepting advice), *family reenactment* (experiencing the group as similar to the family in which the patient grew up), and *altruism* (giving to others).

Group Goals and Norms

Group goals are the purposes for which the group meets. They establish a commonality that supports cohesiveness. Examples range from neighbors who organize to fight crime in their area, to patients who come together to learn money management and daily living skills. Without clear goals and a good reason for being together, a group will often just dissolve. This is an important consideration in treatment groups; the participants need to know why they are meeting and what they can expect to accomplish. Activities should be chosen for their potential to meet the declared goals of the group; these goals must have meaning to the members.

Group norms are the rules or standards for behavior that are expected in the group. They define the limits of permissible and acceptable behavior. Group norms are to a group what laws and etiquette are to a society; they enable social interaction to proceed safely, because the range of things that can happen is predictable. New members may not be aware of the norms; if so, the rest of the group will teach or tell the new member how he is expected to behave. This process, called *socialization,* may take some time, and usually the new member is permitted a grace period to learn the ropes. To preserve their own integrity, groups (like societies) enforce their norms by punishing members who violate them. This punishment, often called a *sanction,* may be as severe as expulsion from the group, or as mild as a verbal chastisement. In therapeutic groups the leader has the major responsibility for enforcing norms, although group members should be enabled to do this wherever possible. It is a good idea to choose norms for the group that reflect the social norms of its community counterpart. For example, in a work group, paying attention to the task rather than to one's emotional needs and those of the other group members is a norm that mirrors work behavior expected on the job.

The clarity of norms and goals affects cohesiveness. If they are unclear or inconsistent, or not really honored by all the members, cohesiveness will suffer. On the other hand, if all the members of the group know why they are in the group and what behavior is expected of them, they are more likely to work together and feel cohesive with the rest of the group. Many people have had the experience of being in a class in which the instructor failed to provide written objectives or assignments or grading criteria, and did not really communicate what or how the students were expected to learn; or one in which some students were allowed to do extra assignments and take makeup exams and others were not, for no apparent reason. Disinterest, anxiety, and rebelliousness are typical reactions in such situations. This illustrates what can happen when the goals and norms are not clearly stated and consistently enforced. Making sure that the goals and norms are clear to all the group members and that they are enforced in a consistent and fair manner is the responsibility of the group leader; when new members enter the group, the leader will need to restate or reclarify the goals and norms. Group members with more highly developed group interaction skills may do this in some groups.

Functional Roles within a Group

If you watch any small group interact for an hour or so, you will see that the individuals within the group behave in very different ways. For example, five students might be studying together for a biology exam. Angie suggests that they ask each other questions; Robert says that it would be better to go over the notes. After a few minutes, Tanya asks if they could settle this dispute by going over the notes and then asking questions. Meanwhile, Mario has gotten coffee for everyone, and Sandra is not really paying much attention because she has been copying Angie's notes from a class that she missed. Each student is playing a different role in the group. As the study group progresses, they may switch roles or take on new ones; for instance, when the group gets cranky and tired, Angie may suggest taking a break to get something to eat, or Sandra may give a pep talk about how important this test is.

Whenever people interact together in groups, individual members take on different functional roles. These roles, which help the group work toward its goals and satisfy the needs of its members, are spelled out in Table 17–1. Examples are given which illustrate how an individual might act in each role. The examples are based on interactions of a student group planning a fund-raiser. The roles fall into three categories: task roles, group maintenance roles, and antigroup or egocentric roles. *Task roles* develop in relationship to the group's goals and the problems it must solve to reach them. *Group maintenance roles* are needed to promote and maintain cohesiveness and closeness among group members; not infrequently the leader takes on several of these roles, depending on the changing needs of the group. For example, the leader may act as gatekeeper and en-

TABLE 17–1. *Roles of group members*

Task roles	Examples
Initiator-contributor: suggests new ideas or new ways of looking at a problem.	Ralph suggests manufacturing and selling silk-screened T-shirts.
Information seeker: asks for facts, and for further explanation of them.	Ginny asks Ralph to explain what's involved in silk-screening.
Opinion seeker: asks for opinions and feelings about issues under discussion.	Nick asks the group whether they think the T-shirts would sell.
Information giver: provides facts, or information from own experience.	Marco says that he saw silk-screened T-shirts at a street fair sell very well, at a good price.
Opinion giver: expresses his feelings or beliefs not necessarily based on facts.	Nick says he believes the T-shirt fad is past, and that no one wants to wear shirts with slogans on them. He suggests a bake sale.
Elaborator: spells out suggestions by giving examples or developing scenarios of how it might work out.	Ralph says that maybe the group could come up with a few designs and show them around to other students. Based on their reactions, the group could then decide whether the T-shirt idea is a good risk.
Coordinator: pulls ideas together by showing the relationship between different ideas expressed.	Ginny says that it should be easy to tell if the T-shirt fad is past, depending on the students' reactions. The bake sale is a good back-up idea.
Orienter: focuses the group on its goals, keeps discussion from wandering off the point, etc.	Michelle reminds the group that they need to decide soon, because the funds are needed in ten weeks.
Evaluator-critic: assesses the accomplishments of the group in relation to some standard.	Jergen says that all of the ideas sound good to him, and that this group seems more harmonious than other student clubs he's been in.
Energizer: prods or arouses the groups to act, stimulates and boosts morale.	Marcia says that "we can pull this off if we all work together, so let's get with it."
Procedural technician: performs routine tasks that help the group accomplish its task.	Gertrude arranged for enough chairs for the meeting, started the coffee and got a portable chalkboard and chalk.
Recorder: writes down main points of the discussion, records group decisions.	Sharons keeps minutes of the meeting and reads her notes back to the group at the end.
Group maintenance roles	Examples
Encourager: praises, accepts, supports others in the group; encourages different points of view.	Rick says that Ralph has a good idea, and that maybe we should think about it seriously.
Harmonizer: settles differences between other members by reconciling disputes, or relieves tension by joking.	After a violent debate between Jergen and Ralph about what price should be charged for the T-shirts, Valeries jokes that "this ain't no fancy boutique, guys!"
Compromiser: gives in to a dispute, and changes his position to preserve group harmony.	Jergen admits that maybe people can't afford to pay $20 for a T-shirt, and says he's willing to compromise at $12.
Gatekeeper: keeps communication going; this may mean asking others to speak, or suggesting ways to give everyone a chance to talk.	Gertrude says there are some people who haven't spoken yet, and that she wonders what they think about the T-shirt prices.
Standard setter: expresses norms or standards for the group.	Valeries says that it will be easier to work together if people would listen to each other and stop shouting.
Group observer: records the communication process of the group; offers this record to the group for its comment and interpretation; provides interpretations where needed.	(This is a role the therapist may play in a therapeutic group. Example: Angela notes that Jergen has snapped at Ralph several times today.)
Follower: goes along with the general mood and decisions of the group.	The student group included 18 people, but not all of these participated in the discussion. The rest listened, and voted by a show of hands on the final plan.

TABLE 17–1. (*Continued*)

Antigroup (egocentric) roles	Examples
Aggressor: belittles or attacks group members, or the group, or its purpose; shows disapproval or tries to take credit for actions of others.	Tricia says that she'd be happy to listen to Ralph's ideas, but since he never follows through on them, she thinks it's a waste of time.
Blocker: prevents the group from progressing by resisting change, opposing decisions, rehashing "dead" issues, etc.	Lenore says she wants to know why the group always has to get involved with "these hair-brained schemes."
Recognition seeker: calls attention to himself by boasting, talking about his own talents, insisting on having a powerful position, etc.	John says that he's got a first-class collection of T-shirts that he'll bring in for the next meeting.
Self-confessor: expresses personal problems, or political ideology, or other concerns to the captive audience of the group.	Gilberto says that he is completely "bummed out" by the "F" he got on the anatomy quiz, and wants to know if anyone else failed.
Playboy: isn't involved with the group; instead, shows disinterest by clowning around, being cynical, etc.	Wanda flirts openly with Marco and Nick, ignoring everyone else.
Dominator: tries to take control by manipulating group or individuals within it; tactics may include interrupting, bossiness, flattery, and seduction.	Frank interrupts Ralph repeatedly, telling him to "get on with it" and "leave out the boring details."
Help-seeker: tries to get sympathy of group by acting helpless, victimized, or insecure.	Leslie says that she isn't sure she can really contribute too much, because she's dyslexic.
Special-interest pleader: pretends to speak on behalf of a particular group, but really is using this group to express his own biases.	John says the group needs to make sure all the money is accounted for, because "some people here aren't too responsible."

Adapted from Benne and Sheats (3).

courager to get the group started and the participants talking to each other, and later perform the roles of harmonizer and group observer. *Antigroup* or *egocentric roles* serve the needs of individuals but interfere with the group's progress. Some individuals will take on these destructive roles in almost any group situation, and need support and training to develop more positive group skills. Some group situations bring out these behaviors in people who have shown the ability to take on productive roles in other groups. This is likely to happen if a group is given a task that is not relevant, or at the right skill level, or if the leader is too dominant or too permissive. For instance, a group of older male patients in a Veterans Administration hospital may take on antigroup roles if they are given a task that they perceive as feminine or childish (e.g., fabric collage).

The occupational therapy assistant can help patients gain awareness and group skill by recognizing which functional group roles they take, and supporting them in their ex-ploration of new roles. Because the central purpose of occupational therapy groups is to help the patient succeed in his chosen occupational role (worker, student, and so on), the COTA must be able to identify which functional group roles are needed for the patient's occupational role. For example, a superintendent of an apartment building needs to use the roles of orienter and energizer in his work. The COTA needs to be able to analyze which roles the patient is able to assume, and design and assign roles in activity groups that enable the patient to practice and become skilled at the functional roles he needs to develop. In addition, the COTA (like any group leader) must be able to recognize what functional roles she herself may need to assume (or delegate) when group members do not have the skill to do so. Getting new groups started may also necessitate the leader's taking a more active role.

Which functional roles are taken by individuals depends on the roles that are needed for the group to accomplish its goals; not every situation calls for every possible role. Groups in the early stages of development may crumble if severe standards are set, but more mature groups can use the same standards as a spur for growth. The roles that individuals undertake in a group depend also on their previous experience. Someone who is used to the role of procedural technician, and who has never really performed in any other group role, may feel threatened and overwhelmed if pushed into a leadership position. Obviously, the highest level of group skills is flexibility and responsiveness in taking on each of the task roles and group maintenance roles, as the situation demands.

Group Process

Many different relationships develop within a group; these relationships shift and change in response to numerous factors. The personality, past experience, and current emotional state of each member affect his relationship with everyone else. For example, sibling rivalry (shown by competition with other group members for the leader's attention and approval) and other transferential reactions[1] have their origins in past family relationships. The reactions of the participants to each other are also a factor; complementary or mutually destructive patterns can develop. Subgroups form within the group as members make alliances with each other; these subgroups may function to exclude others, or to reinforce the status of their members, or to compete with other subgroups. Sometimes the entire group gangs up against one member, incorrectly blaming him for the group's failure to achieve its goals; this is called *scapegoating*.

The following questions may help an observer discover the relationships within the group: Who talks to whom? Who arrives and leaves together? Who seems left out? Do the members talk to each other, or only to the leader? Who talks the most? Who sits where? Which people always sit together? Which people never sit together?

Accurate assessment of group process requires sophisticated analysis based on extensive knowledge of group therapy and group dynamics. Entry level COTAs are not expected to possess this skill, but may develop it through continuing education and supervised clinical practice.

DEVELOPMENT OF GROUP SKILLS

Everyone knows one or two people who are exquisitely skillful in group situations; these rare individuals circulate gracefully at cocktail parties, bring strangers together, and make lonely people feel comfortable. On the job, or in community groups such as the PTA, they can get people organized, give them motivation and direction, take care of uninteresting details, and then step back to let others shine. These people are worth emulating; they have a high level of group skill. If you look around you, it is very likely you will find different degrees of group skill among otherwise mature individuals such as your colleagues, classmates, and peers.

How do human beings develop this ability to interact effectively with others? Anne Mosey, an occupational therapist, analyzed the development of *group interaction skill* (13,14,15). Mosey defines group interaction skill as

. . . the ability to be a productive member of a variety of primary groups. Through acquisition of the various group interaction subskills, the individual learns to take appropriate group membership roles, engage in decision making, communicate effectively, recognize group norms and interact in accordance with these norms, contribute to goal attainment, work towards group cohesiveness, and assist in resolving group conflict. (14, p. 201).

---

[1]Discussed as transference and countertransference in Chapter 10.

Recognizing that we are not just born with these skills, and that psychiatric patients may need help to develop them, Mosey identified five levels of group interaction skill: parallel, project, egocentric-cooperative, cooperative, and mature. She described the subskills learned at each level and estimated the age at which most people learn these skills. She also described what a group leader (or parent or teacher) might do to help people at each level acquire the subskills needed for the next level. The following summarizes Mosey's ideas regarding group interaction skills.

Parallel Level

The skill needed at the parallel level is the ability to work and play in the presence of others, comfortably and with an awareness of their presence. This skill is usually learned between the ages of 18 months and 2 years, when the child becomes gradually more comfortable playing around other children. Most of the play is solitary, although the children interact briefly from time to time, for example to show one another something. In order for this parallel play to continue for long, however, there must be at least one adult available to give each of the children support, encouragement, and attention when they need it. Problems such as taking toys from the other child or throwing a temper tantrum because one cannot have one's own way immediately are common, but must be discouraged if the child is to progress to the next level.

Project Level

The skill learned at the project level is the ability to share a short-term task with one or two other people. This skill develops somewhere between the age of two and four years. The child is interested in the task or the game, and recognizes that he needs other people to do it; therefore he is willing to take turns, to share materials, to cooperate, to ask for help, and to give it. He is not so much interested in the other people as he is in the task. The activities shared at this level last for only a short time, usually not more than a half hour, and the child may engage in a number of different activities in succession; each may have different participants. A parent, teacher, or other adult is needed to provide individual attention and to intervene when children have difficulty sharing.

Egocentric-Cooperative Level

The skill at the egocentric-cooperative level is an awareness of the group's goals and norms and a willingness to abide by them. This skill is based on sensitivity to the rules of the group and the rights of self and others in the group. Because the child now feels a sense that he belongs to the group, and that he is accepted by it, he can carry out long-term activities that allow him to experiment with different roles and levels of participation. Differences among group members become apparent as each "tries on" functional *task* roles (see Table 17–1) needed for the achievement of the various stages of activities; this provides an opportunity to recognize and reward the achievement of others, and to seek recognition for oneself. It is believed that these skills are normally acquired somewhere between five and seven years of age. Supervising adults still need to provide support and encouragement to meet the esteem needs of group members.

Cooperative Level

The skill at the cooperative level is an ability to express feelings within a group, and to be aware of and respond to the feelings of others. Thus, individuals at this level are able to assume group maintenance roles, those roles which support the emotional well-being of the group. This skill usually develops between the ages of 9 and 12, through participation in groups whose members are of the same sex and approximate age. Adults are usually excluded from these groups, which seem to function better on their own. Groups may form spontaneously, with members selected on the basis of their similarity to each other. The group's activities or tasks are not viewed as important; instead the feelings (both positive and negative) of each member on a variety of subjects are the main agenda.

Mature Level

The skill at the mature level is the ability to take on a variety of group roles, both task roles and group maintenance roles, as needed in response to changing conditions in a group. This skill is synonymous with the upper end of the continuum of group interaction skill as defined by Mosey earlier in this chapter. Mosey believes that this skill is learned between the ages of 15 and 18 years, as the adolescent participates in various clubs and groups whose members are of both sexes, come from different backgrounds, and have different interests and skills. It must be acknowledged, however, that exposure to this experience does not in itself guarantee that the adolescent will develop a mature level of group interaction skill; there are many adults whose behavior in groups is restricted to the few membership roles with which they feel comfortable. The development of group interaction skill may continue into middle and even late adulthood, provided the individual is willing to risk trying out new roles.

To summarize, skill in interacting within a group develops gradually throughout childhood and adolescence. Patients with psychiatric problems may function at a level of group interaction skill which is lower than one would expect for someone their age. The COTA must be able to accept

that the patient is probably doing the best he can, and that he will not be able to cope with demands for higher level group interaction. The COTA can structure groups to meet the needs of people at various levels by changing the tasks and by delegating or assuming functional group roles. In this way, the COTA can provide a learning environment for both high and low functioning members.

HOW THERAPY GROUPS ARE DIFFERENT FROM OTHER GROUPS

We have just discussed the developmental process by which people learn to interact effectively in group situations. Daily life presents many opportunities for practicing group interaction skills; work, family, school, and social life all involve participation in groups. To lead a therapy group successfully the occupational therapy assistant needs to understand the difference between a therapy group and other groups that occur naturally.

First of all, all therapy groups are artificial situations, designed to help patients acquire new skills or practice old ones. Second, the group leader is responsible for making sure that learning occurs. In a sense, this makes the therapy group similar to a class in school. Another important difference is that, regardless of the specific activity used or skills taught, the group also acknowledges the emotional experience of each member. In other words, each patient's feelings about what he is doing and what is going on in the group are considered important. For example, in a work group the focus is on acquiring work skills. Therefore, behaviors that would not be acceptable on the job are discouraged. Although discussion of feelings is frowned upon during work time, a period for such discussion is set aside at the end of each session. In this way Molly, who feels that she is always given dull and boring jobs, can air her feelings and the group can help her explore them.

ROLE OF THE LEADER IN AN ACTIVITY GROUP

Activity groups differ from other therapy groups in that "doing" or activity is the medium through which the group members achieve their goals. Thus activity groups can be designed as laboratories in which the patients can experiment with the occupational roles relevant to their daily lives. Thus, the most important function of the group leader is to assign members specific tasks and roles similar to those they may have to assume in real life. For example, in a newspaper group, the leader may assign members to roles as chief editor, copy assistant, and so on. Role assignment is based on similarity of job responsibility of the assigned role to the job responsibility of the patient's real-life occupational role.

The leader is also responsible for making sure that group members feel safe during the group's activities, and that the group focuses its energies on its goals. The group leader may take a very active role, selecting tasks for individual members and intervening in disputes, or the more distant and observing role of a consultant, or may participate as an equal member in the group; this depends on the group interaction skills of individual members and the purpose for which the group is designed.

The leader must assume only those role functions members are not able to assume (because of insufficient group interaction skill) and must delegate those members are able to assume. In addition, the leader must recognize and delegate the role functions that members need to develop in order to increase their group interaction skill to the next level. For example, if one of the goals of the group is to help patients learn to make decisions on their own, the leader cannot assign tasks and responsibilities, as this defeats the entire purpose. On the other hand, patients with very poor attention spans and only parallel level group skills will not be able to carry on a discussion of what activity they should choose.

The relationship between the patient's level of group skill and the role of the therapist or group leader is depicted in Table 17–2, which lists the things a therapist or group leader should do to help patients develop group skills at each level. It is unusual to find a group whose members are all at a single level of group skill. Sometimes, for example in acute short-term settings, there may be individuals at all five levels within the same group. Even in such situations, the information in the table can guide you to help individuals relate to each other and the group. You, as the leader, may step into different roles in order to meet the needs of the members.

When working with any patient, it is important to know his level of group skill and to understand what this means in terms of what he can and cannot do with other people. For example, it is pointless to ask a patient who has only parallel-level group skills to take a leadership role in community meetings; on the other hand, it *is* reasonable to ask him to remain in the meeting and not be disruptive.

In addition to understand the relationship between the patients' group skill levels and the therapist's behavior, there are several other factors to which the group leader should be sensitive. As indicated previously in the section on cohesiveness, an atmosphere in which the members feel accepted and valued is essential if people are to risk themselves by trying new things. New learning is unlikely unless such an atmosphere exists. The leader can promote cohesiveness and create a climate that encourages learning and risk-taking by orienting the group to its goals and activities, by spelling out the norms, and by paying attention to her own behavior. Behaviors of the leader with respect to consistency, autonomy, nurturing, and interpersonal learning have particular effects on the group.

TABLE 17–2. *Role of the therapist in developmental groups*

Indicators of need to develop specified level of group skills	Role of therapist
Parallel group: Patients have limited attention span, and may be quite unaware of others. Unless encouraged to notice others they may ignore them, and isolate themselves.	1. Explain purpose and activities of group to patient. 2. Help patient feel accepted, safe, valued. 3. Support and encourage minimal interaction such as eye contact, casual conversation. 4. Set limits on disruptive behavior. 5. Help patient select simple, short-term activities that are not self-isolating.
Project group: Patients express anxiety about working with others, fearing that they will be unable to complete a task or that the other person will take over. The issue is whether to trust another person enough to share a task with him.	1. Explain purpose and activities of group to patient. 2. Help patient feel accepted, safe, valued. 3. Support and encourage sharing of tasks, cooperation, giving and seeking assistance, etc. 4. Help patients select simple, short-term tasks that can be shared by two or more people. 5. Encourage experimentation with different ways of sharing, members taking different roles.
Egocentric-cooperative-group: Members have trouble engaging in long-term tasks with others. Problems may include concern with competition, indifference to the rights of others, inability to ask for and receive recognition, etc.	1. Takes on group membership roles only as required by the needs of the group. 2. Encourages the group to function as independently as it can, stepping in only when group cannot proceed without help. 3. Models appropriate expression of needs. 4. Assists development and discussion of norms. 5. Helps individuals feel accepted, safe, valued.
Cooperative group: While able to carry out long-term group tasks, people at this level need to expand their ability to express their own feelings and be aware of the feelings of others.	1. Participates in the group *or* provides advice from the sidelines; is *not* an authority figure. 2. May help the group develop initially. 3. May intervene to promote cohesiveness.
Mature group: People at this level need to learn to step into roles as needed, and to maintain a balance between achieving the group task and meeting the emotional needs of group members.	1. Participates as a member. 2. Where necessary, demonstrates group membership roles. 3. Selects members to achieve variety and balance in backgrounds, interests, skills, etc.

Based on ideas and information from Mosey AC. *Activities therapy.* New York: Raven Press; 1973. Groups are designed to help members acquire the named level of group interaction skill. For example, those in the project-level group do not have project-level skills but are trying to develop them.

The first of these behaviors, *consistency,* is essential in most group situations. The leader must show the same degree of respect, interest, and authority toward every group member. Also, the leader should try as much as possible to behave similarly in each meeting of the group. In other words, the leader's behavior should be dependable. The group members should know what to expect from the leader. Some aspects of leader behavior that appear quite subtle can have a profound influence on the group. For example, if the leader one day is preoccupied with personal problems and thus more subdued than usual, group members may wonder why, or feel uneasy—as though the leader were now a different person. If the leader shows favoritism toward one member, others may feel wronged.

The second aspect of leader behavior to consider is the *degree of autonomy* the leader permits among the members. In other words, how much opportunity for independence and decision making does the leader give the group? As a general rule, members should be given as much independence as they can handle, and no more. One way to figure out how much independence is appropriate is to observe. If members seem confused and unable to act, they may have been given too much responsibility, too much independence. If, on the other hand, they refuse to act responsibly, or repeatedly argue with the group leader, or seem not to work to capacity, they probably are not being given enough responsibility. Determining the appropriate level is sometimes a problem for new group leaders, and is an area in which a supervisor who is experienced in working with therapy groups can help. A good supervisor will also be able to help the new group leader learn how to analyze and respond to problems within the group process (interaction among members). The entry level COTA cannot be expected to be able to do this independently, but should be able to develop skills in analyzing group process after several years of supervised group leadership experience.

The third aspect of leader behavior that affects the group is *nurturing behavior,* defined here as any behavior by the leader that supports and promotes the growth of the individual members. Encouragement and praise are the most common examples, but nurturing can take many other forms. It should always be matched to the maturity of the group or the individuals involved. A young mother who is highly skilled at housework but who is depressed for other reasons will probably not be convinced or encouraged by the group leader praising her homemaking skills. It might be more nurturing for the leader to help her find a way to teach these skills to others.

The fourth aspect of leader behavior that needs attention is the leader's skill at promoting *interpersonal learning.* Interpersonal learning consists of all of the processes or relationships between individuals that result in a change in behavior, knowledge, or attitude on the part of any one (or several) of the people involved. In simpler words, interpersonal learning includes all those things a person learns from interactions with other people. Examples of this are learning how one is perceived by oth-

ers, taking on unfamiliar group membership roles, asking for and receiving attention, becoming more aware of how others feel, and learning new skills from another person.

The leader should be able to use the resources of the group to help each member learn more about himself and about the others. The *resources of the group* are all the possibilities for different kinds of interactions and learning among group members, each of whom has different knowledge, skills, feelings, and beliefs to share with the others. The leader cannot assume, however, that these resources will be shared automatically; often the leader has to take charge of the communication process in the group to encourage each member to interact with every other member.

Interactive groups are those in which every member communicates with every other member and with the group leader. By contrast, in *leader-mediated groups* members communicate only with or through the group leader (18). Opportunities for interpersonal learning are greatest where a pattern of interactive communication exists. However, in groups that include persons at lower levels of group interaction skill (parallel or project), the members cannot be expected to interact so freely. Instead, the leader mediates the conversation, asking individuals for their feelings or for a reaction to what another member has said, for example.

The pattern of communication within the group is only one factor in interpersonal learning, which also depends on each member's learning style, or preferred way of learning. The leader facilitates whatever method of learning is most effective for each person. Some of the learning methods that can be used are feedback, reinforcement, trial and error behavior, and imitation or role modeling. These methods were discussed in Chapters 2 and 3. Typically, several methods will be used simultaneously. For example, one person might imitate the behavior of another. Other patients could give him feedback about how well this worked. If the behavior worked well, they might also reinforce it. The group leader may need to facilitate this process by, for example, asking what the group thinks of the way John is dressed today, or what they think about how Ann is dealing with her "shyness."

In summary, the group leader should promote interaction and interpersonal learning among the group members. The group interaction skills of each of the members will define how much interpersonal learning is possible or practical. It is often difficult for students and new therapists to put these elementary principles into practice while running a group. There is always a strong temptation to step in and give one's own opinion, or to provide information, or to show someone how to do something. It may feel strange to sit back and wait for a patient to respond to another patient. Likewise, it may feel awkward to ask patients to share their feelings or opinions, especially when it takes them a long time to respond. Nevertheless, this is what running a group involves. When patients learn from other patients, they learn more than the information or skill imparted. They learn how to talk to other people, and how to listen; they learn that they themselves have value, and that it is possible to learn from many different people, not just those in authority. The skillful group leader knows when to sit on his hands and let the patients do the work.

Preparation for the Group

The success of any group session depends very much on what kind of preparation the leader has made. Four areas need particular attention: knowledge, space, materials, and paperwork.

Knowledge refers to how well the leader understands and can analyze the various factors in groups and how they affect the functioning of the members and the entire group. Knowledge and awareness of one-self and one's impact on others is critical. Equally important is the leader's knowledge of the task or medium that will be the main group activity; it goes without saying that you cannot teach what you do not know. Skills that the group leader has not practiced recently may need to be rehearsed before presenting them to the group.

Space refers to the preparation of the area in which the group will meet. In general, the leader should take care of any special arrangements of furniture or equipment before the group arrives. However, having patients participate in or take charge of preparing the space is appropriate for those who are at a higher level of functioning.

Materials are any tools, supplies, books, sample projects, and so on, that will be needed during the course of the group. These should be prepared in advance by the group leader or an assistant (perhaps a volunteer or a higher functioning patient). The specific requirements depend obviously on the type of group and the functional level of the participants. For example, with lower functioning groups it will be necessary to prepare separate materials for each person, and to set these up so that each has his own work area (although several patients may sit at one table). In higher functioning groups it might make sense to have the patients take out their own projects and obtain and return tools as they need them.

Paperwork is the final item; it consists of attendance sheets, the group protocol and group leader's notebook, and any other forms or documents that the leader might need during the group. With the exception of taking attendance, the leader should try not to write during the group session, but should do so as soon as it is over. Having a notebook handy in which the behavior of each group member can be briefly noted makes it easy to keep track of patients' progress.

Even with all this preparation things can still go awry, but the leader will find it easier to cope with a minor crisis when everything else has been taken care of. The situation to be avoided is one in which the patients arrive at the same time as the group leader, who then must unlock cabinets, hunt for missing items, take attendance, and so forth, all at the same time.

Beginning and Ending a Group Session

The group leader can increase the therapeutic effect of a group by paying particular attention to the beginning and end of each session. The beginning of the session prepares participants for what is to follow. New group members should be introduced, or all members should introduce themselves again; this is especially necessary when the members do not know each other or the group meets infrequently. The leader should state the purpose of the group (or ask a patient to do so) and describe the activity for the day; this may not be necessary in long-running groups where the activities are continuous.

At the end of the group, after patients have enjoyed themselves, or have been involved with an activity and with each other, they need time to reflect on this experience before moving on to the next thing on their schedule. Having patients clean up the room and put things away gives them time to chat informally with each other about what has occurred. It is a good idea to have a discussion at the end, provided at least some of the participants have sufficient group interaction skill (project level or above). The leader can summarize the day's activities and ask participants to reflect on them and share their thoughts. Peloquin (16, p. 780), working with patients who had cognitive problems, used the following four-step approach:

1. Remind patients of the purpose of the group.
2. Set the stage for discussion. Give patients time to think about their experience before asking them to speak.
3. Help patients discuss the skills they have used. Be sure to link the tasks or activities performed by the patients to their individual treatment goals.
4. Summarize what was accomplished and encourage patients to return for the next session.

At the very end of the session, the leader should note the time and day of the next meeting, and the activity and goals for that session. It takes time to carry out these steps at the beginning and end of the group, but it is time well spent.

Record Keeping

As mentioned earlier, it is important to keep track of how patients are progressing in the group; keeping a notebook is one way to do this. A very small notebook or a few pages in one used for other purposes will do. Some observations that should be noted are any progress toward goals, changes in interactions with others, new problems or behaviors seen, and possible side effects of medication. Even though there may be only a few minutes between the end of the group and the next meeting or group that the leader must attend, it is very important to note observations while they are fresh. Writing one or two words about each group member takes little time, but reviewing several days of such notes can yield valuable insights into the process of the group and the progress of its members.

PROGRAM DEVELOPMENT

Starting up a new occupational therapy program for patients with mental health problems requires knowledge, skill, and experience that the entry-level occupational therapy assistant does not possess. Therefore, program development is the responsibility of the registered therapist, generally one with several years' experience in mental health and administration. The assistant can collaborate in program development by planning individual activity groups, which then become part of the overall program.

Planning an Activity Group

One of the biggest challenges new group leaders encounter in their clinical work is planning and running a new activity group. There seem to be so many possibilities that it is hard to focus on just one. Fortunately, there is a logical, step-by-step way of approaching this. The steps are:

1. Identify the patients who need a group.
2. Assess the specific needs and general level of group skills of these patients.
3. Identify rules and resources in your institution.
4. Narrow the focus and outline the main goals.
5. Write a group protocol.

The first step in developing a new group is to identify some people who seem to need one. This involves thinking about the patients you have available, and the kind of groups that already exist. You may notice that some patients are not in any occupational therapy groups, or that they have gaps in their schedules. Or you may perceive that a particular need is not being met by existing groups; for example, patients on a locked ward may not be able to attend sports and exercise groups off the ward, and might benefit from a yoga or calisthenics group. A supervisor or co-worker may identify a particular need or suggest individuals for you to work with.

The second step is to assess the specific needs and general level of group skills of these patients. You may have already begun this during the first step. In other words, you may have noticed a particular need (e.g., exercise). But what if you have identified some patients who seem to need a group, but you don't know what kind of group they need? It may be helpful to think about the general goals of psychiatric occupational therapy, as delineated in Chapter 15; this may give you some ideas. For example, you may have decided that the patients who really need a group are the ones who sit around all day and do not function well enough to participate in task groups or current events and other verbal groups. You observe that they have marginal grooming and hygiene, and show little interest in anything but TV. From these observations you might assume that they could benefit from a group focusing on self-care or leisure skills. Another way to identify their needs is to review the results of the evaluations on each patient.

Besides identifying the needs of these patients, you need to learn how well they can function within a group. Because of other demands it is not always possible to set up a separate evaluation session for this, and you can instead observe each patient informally or interview other staff who know the patient well. Fig. 17–1 shows a checklist developed by Mosey. It lists behaviors for each of the five developmental levels of group interaction skill. The observer checks off any behaviors the patient shows. The level that has the most behaviors checked is probably the patient's current level (although it is common for patients to possess a few behaviors at the next higher level). It is important to assess the patients' group interaction skill so that you know what they will be capable of; for example, those at the project level of skill will not be capable of mutual problem solving through discussion and will find it easier to learn from short-term, concrete activities in pairs or small subgroups.

Other factors that should be considered in addition to group interaction skill include the patients' cognitive skills, in particular their attention span, memory, and capacity for new learning. If these skills are deficient you will have to conduct the group and structure the activities in a way that com-

Level of Group Interaction Skill

Parallel level
Engages in some activity, but acts as if this is an individual task as opposed to a group activity.
Aware of others in the group.
Some verbal or nonverbal interaction with others.
Appears to be relatively comfortable in this situation.

Project level
Occasionally engages in the group activity, moving in and out according to his own whim.
Seeks some assistance from others.
Gives some assistance when directly asked to do so.

Egocentric-cooperative level
Aware of group's goal relative to the task.
Aware of group norms.
Acts as if he belongs in the group.
Willing to participate.
Meets esteem needs of others.
Able to get others to meet his esteem needs.
Recognizes rights of others.
Not overly competitive.

Cooperative level
Makes own wishes, desires, and needs known.
Participates in group activity but seems concerned primarily with his own needs and needs of others.
Able to meet needs other than esteem needs.
Tends to be most responsive to group members who are similar to him in some way.

Mature level
Responsive to all group members.
Takes on a variety of task roles.
Takes on a variety of social-emotional roles.
Able to share leadership.
Promotes a good balance between task accomplishment and satisfaction of group members' needs.

FIG. 17–1. Group interaction skills survey. Reprinted with modifications from Mosey AC. *Activities therapy.* New York: Raven Press; 1973:92.

pensates for this (analyzing and adapting activities is covered in Chapter 23).

The third step is to identify the rules and resources of your institution. These determine the limits of what is possible in a particular treatment setting. Included are the equipment and materials available, the rooms or other environments that can be used as settings for groups, the role of occupational therapy in the setting, and the rules of the particular institution.

If you want to run a group that needs special equipment or materials, you must allow sufficient time to budget money for this and order and receive what you need. You may have to work in a room that does not really suit your purposes, simply because it is the only room available.

The roles of occupational therapy, other activities therapies, and other professional disciplines in your setting may also constrain what kinds of groups you can run. For example, there may be a recreation therapy department that provides all sports and exercise.

Finally, you will have to observe the rules of the institution; there may be rules about what patients can and cannot do, and other rules governing staff. For instance, two staff members may be required to accompany patients on field trips. If you are planning field trips, you will have to make sure another staff member can come. You should therefore think about these things before you actually design the group, to save yourself time and duplication of effort later on. In general you will have to work within these boundaries; if you decide that certain rules are unreasonable and should be changed (and you may be right), remember that changing them can consume time and energy, and prepare yourself for what may be a long (and not necessarily victorious) struggle.

The fourth step is to narrow the focus of the group and outline your main goals for it. You may feel that the patients have needs in several areas, and you may have a number of ideas for activities. You will now have to decide which area to focus on. This is perhaps the most difficult decision in designing a group. You may be tempted to try to meet several different needs in one group; that is, your group could have 15 minutes of self-care activities, followed by 15 minutes of leisure activities, followed by a 30-minute work activity. Or you might consider having the group do a different activity every time it meets. These examples are rather absurd, but they illustrate that trying to meet too many needs at the same time results in a confusing blur of unrelated, and therefore meaningless, activities. It is best to focus on only one area at a time, although incidental learning in other areas may occur simultaneously; for example, self-care groups may provide opportunities for minimal socialization and learning of communication skills.

Once you have chosen the focus of the group, you can begin to outline the goals. These goals should be developed from the evaluation results and individual treatment goals of the patients who will be in the group. They should express in general behavioral terms what you hope the patients will achieve, goals that the patients feel are

important and that are possible for them to reach. Fig. 17–2 presents an example of how the occupational therapy assistant might follow the first four steps in developing a new group. The fifth step is to write a group protocol.

Writing a Group Protocol

A group protocol is a written document that describes the goals of a group and the methods by which these goals will be achieved. It is an outline of what will be happening in the group. It is, practically speaking, a treatment plan for the group.

Writing a group protocol has several purposes. The first is to communicate with other staff who might refer patients to the group. By reading the group protocol other staff members can decide whether or not a particular patient is suited for, or might benefit from, the group.

The second purpose is to define the type of patient who might benefit from the group. This gives you some control over who the members will be, and helps screen out those whose needs and level of group skill are too limited or too advanced for the group.

The third purpose is clarify your goals, your methods, and your own role as leader of the group. Thinking these issues through on paper, before you actually start the group, helps you be more clear and effective in your leadership once the group actually begins.

A fourth purpose of writing the group protocol is that it helps you identify how you will know when a group member has achieved the goals you have set. In other words, it helps you describe how a patient will act when she is ready to "graduate" from the group.

Many different formats are used for writing group protocols, but most contain similar information. The elements typically written into a group protocol are shown in Figure 17–3. These elements may be com-

Identifying a focus for the group	
Steps	*Example*
1. Identify the patients who need a group.	There seem to be eight patients who sit around watching TV all day and don't attend any groups.
2. Identify specific needs,	Review of evaluation results and treatment plans, and informal observation of patients revealed very poor hygiene and grooming. None of these patients seems to be able to relate to other people, except when they want a cigarette. They never get any exercise and seem to have no interests or skills.
and general level of group skills.	It's unlikely that these patients will interact with anyone, unless the group leader structures the situation so that they are forced to. All have very short attention spans (less than fifteen minutes). I can't imagine them giving feedback to each other, or even noticing the others.
3. Identify institutional parameters.	This is a large state hospital. The wards in this building are locked.
Space available	Some activities are held in a separate building, the Activities Center. Most groups are on the ward and can be held either in the day room or in a small (8′ × 10′) OT room.
Equipment and materials available	There are tables and chairs available, and a few craft supplies. A lot of the therapists use donations of scraps from factories for craft groups. You have to be inventive.
Role of occupational therapy	In this hospital occupational therapy staff isn't allowed to lead discussion groups. The psychiatric director says they don't have the necessary training. They are supposed to do only activity groups.
Rules of the institution	Students are not allowed to take groups off the grounds of the hospital or to lead groups by themselves in the activity center, although they can do this on the ward.
4. Narrow the focus and outline the main goals.	The focus of this group will be mainly self-care, with minimal opportunities for socialization. The goals for the patients are: a. to brush teeth, bathe, comb hair, and shave daily b. to change clothes daily c. to wash hands before each meal and after using toilet d. to wash hair at least once a week

FIG. 17–2. Identifying a focus for the group. Reprinted from Early MB. *T.A.R. introductory course workbook: occupational therapy—psychosocial dysfunction.* Long Island City, NY: LaGuardia Community College; 1981:401–403.

bined and may have different titles depending on the style of the treatment center, but all the information is generally included. The *name of the group* should reflect the main goals of the group. Alternatively, it may reflect the task or activity and general level of the group. However, naming the group after the activity used may have un-desirable consequences. If the group is named after the activity (for example, Basic Woodworking Group), people may think of the group as "arts and crafts." However, the therapist running the group may actually be teaching work skills and habits. It is usually easier for staff and patients to understand the purpose of the group if the

Typical elements of the group protocol	
Name	. . . should convey therapeutic purpose if possible.
Description	. . . brief, clear, conveying purpose and accurate sense of what happens in group.
Structure	. . . time, place, size, leader characteristics.
Goals or behavioral objectives	. . . may be multiple and extensive. Should be clear and behavioral and as specific as possible.
Referral criteria	. . . describes the kind of patient who might benefit from the group. May include intake procedure.
Methodology	. . . includes both media (activity) and method (how the activity or media is used). This section includes more detail on the flow of activities within the time period of the group meeting.
Curriculum or agenda	. . . for groups that have an educational or topical focus, this section gives detail on specific items of instruction to be covered in each of a number of successive sessions.
Leader roles	. . . states what the leader will and will not do within the group. Addresses the functional roles to be taken by the group leader.
Evaluation	. . . indicates how the achievement of the group goals will be assessed (through patient survey, therapist observation, peer supervision, etc.).

FIG. 17–3. Typical elements of the group protocol

name reflects its goals rather than the task or activity. Examples of names for groups that reflect the goals are Independent Living Skills Group and Community Socialization Group. Earhart (5), however, contends that patients are concerned about what they will be doing in the group, and that including the task content or the name of the activity in the title meets this need.

The *description* of the group should include its purpose and a brief and clearly written statement of what happens in the group. Technical language should be avoided unless essential to the description.

The section on the *structure* of the group is used to convey information about the time, place and size of the group. For example, a meal planning group might include four to six patients, and meet four mornings a week for one and a half hours in the community room. The qualifications (e.g., COTA) or professional or social character-istics (a male staff member) of the group leader can be stated in this section.

The *goals* or *behavioral objectives* of the group should be stated behaviorally and with as much specificity as possible. They should be relevant to the patients' needs and should be set at a level that they can achieve. Some examples of behavioral objectives that meet these requirements are:

• to tolerate the presence of others while working on a task as evidenced by staying in the room and refraining from derogatory or hostile comments
• to initiate social conversation with others
• to perform simple assembly tasks accurately using written or demonstrated two-step instructions

Some groups may have goals that involve changes in awareness or attitudes or values; such goals are very difficult to state in behavioral terms because they focus not on behavior but on internal psychological or cognitive states. Nevertheless, if these are among the main purposes of the group, they should be included. Examples of such goals are:

- to increase awareness of one's own safety and that of others, as evidenced by following shop rules and reminding others to do so
- to develop a feeling of personal competence, as evidenced by spontaneous or elicited comments about one's achievements or skills
- to improve awareness of one's effect on others, as evidenced by cooperation in cleanup and sharing of space.

Referral criteria describe what kind of patient should be referred to the group. The description may include specific skill deficits and prerequisite behaviors. Skill deficits identify the kinds of problems that will be addressed (e.g., poor hygiene and grooming). Prerequisite behaviors state minimum skills needed to participate successfully in the group (e.g., able to tolerate the presence of others, or not actively assaultive or suicidal). Other entrance criteria may restrict the group by age or sex or cultural background or special interest; this is appropriate in most grooming groups or in groups that focus around cultural identity (e.g., Caribbean Culture Group) or special interest (Creative Writing Group). In some settings and for some groups, each patient should be interviewed before he enters the group. This may be done by the group leader, or by the occupational therapist or assistant who is managing the patient's OT program. These intake procedures can help determine how well the patient meets the referral criteria and at the same time provide an opportunity to introduce him to the purpose of the group and to engage his commitment or interest. The referral criteria should spell out the intake procedure if one is required.

Often, several referral criteria are used to define the population for which a group is designed. Writing clear criteria allows you to define the limits of the group. The following is an example of how such criteria might be written for a low-level task skills group:

> Male and female patients
> Ages 17 to 65+
> Those who are able to attend to a task for 5 to 15 minutes
> Those who have task skill deficits (e.g., poor concentration, inattention to detail, poor rate of production)
> Those who are not actively assaultive or suicidal

A patient would have to meet all of these criteria in order to be placed in the group. This ensures that all of the group members have similar problems and skill levels, which generally makes the group easier to run.

The *methodology* section is one of the most important sections, giving detail on how the time of the group will be used to achieve the stated objectives. Within this section are commonly included both the media (activity) and method (how the activity or media is used). *Media* refers to the activities or tasks that will be used to help the patients meet their goals within the group. Sometimes only one activity, or medium, is used. For our purposes, media means the same thing as activity. Almost all of the activities described in Chapters 18 through 23 can be used in groups.

Method describes how the medium or media will be used to work toward the goals. The method includes the general plan of what will happen in the group. The following excerpt illustrates one way the method section for a low-level task skills group might be written:

> The group will be making small leather projects. The therapist will assign a specific job to each patient. Jobs will be graded from simple to complex, depending upon the patient's current level of functioning or need for challenge. Patients will be encouraged to move from completing a simple task to completing a more complex one.
> Patients will relate primarily to the therapist. Interaction with other group members may also occur. This, however, is not

the primary focus of the group. The therapist will be supportive and set standards for each patient.

When a patient is able to work consistently, maintain set work standards, and show some initiative and minimal interaction with peers, he or she will be referred to another group.

Some groups, such as independent living skills, or men's sexual identity group, lend themselves to multiple topics or units of instruction. Independent living skills may include the use of public transportation, basic cooking and nutrition, care of clothing, etc. Men's sexual identity may include topics such as men's roles in society, sexual orientation and homosexuality, meeting and dating women, developing nonsexual relationships with women, etc. A section on *curriculum* or *agenda/topics* for such groups can elaborate the specific items of instruction to be covered in each of a number of successive sessions.

It is also a good idea to develop *session plans,* which spell out in detail what will happen in each meeting of the group. A session plan identifies the goals for the session, the sequence of activities, and the materials needed. Several books give such session plans (also called lesson plans or modules of instruction) for consecutive group meetings. These can help the group leader sequence instruction in (for example) independent living skills (10) or work skills (11).

The *role of the leader* may be stated within the method section or separately. Wherever it is addressed, the role of the leader should spell out the functional group roles (task roles and group maintenance roles as detailed in Table 17–1) that the leader will undertake to support the group. This section may be brief or highly detailed, depending on the nature of the group. Some examples are:

For a parallel level task group: The therapist will assign specific tasks to each patient. The therapist will support and encourage task completion and will set standards for each patient.

For a community safety discussion group: The therapist will open the discussion and will facilitate participation by members. The therapist will not offer opinions but will encourage members to reach their own.

Defining the role of the therapist in the group protocol helps the therapist analyze how to relate to the patients in the group. Patients at different levels of group interaction skill require different levels of involvement from the group leader. Patients at the parallel and project levels need much more assistance and supervision than patients at higher levels. Table 17–2 earlier in the chapter gives more detail on this point. The *evaluation* section is not always included, but should be. This section provides for measuring the achievement of the stated purposes of the group. To what extent does it "improve patient self-esteem" or "increase consistent application of safety procedures"? The choice of evaluation procedure depends on the content of the group, the skills of the members, and the overall quality management plan of the facility or of the occupational therapy department. Evaluation may be done by surveying the patients' satisfaction with the group, or by having a peer therapist make independent ratings of patient behavior. See the section on program evaluation at the end of this chapter for more detail on this element of the group protocol.

Additional sections not listed in Fig. 17–3 but occasionally included in a group protocol are *exit criteria, reasons for discontinuation, resources* and *references.*

Exit criteria describes the behaviors or skills a patient will demonstrate when she has successfully achieved the goals of the group. These should be quite specific and stated in behavioral terms. In fact, the exit criteria actually restate the goals of the group in an observable or measurable form. The exit criteria should be so clear that any observer could determine whether or not a particular patient has met them. Exit criteria for the low-level task skills group might be:

1. The patient works consistently for a 40-minute work period.
2. The patient works at an acceptable rate.
3. The patient maintains given work standards.

4. The patient shows minimal initiative by asking the therapist questions and spontaneously interacting with peers.

Reasons for discontinuation are the various factors that might cause the leader to discharge a patient from the group before

---

Men's unit-based self-care group

Description: This is a self-care group for male patients who require assistance with personal hygiene.

Structure: The group will meet every week day for forty five minutes, from 8:30 to 9:15 A.M. The group will be held on the ward using bathrooms, day room and patients' rooms. The group is limited to six patients at one time. A male staff member (COTA, OT aide or member of nursing staff) will lead the group.

Goals: Through participation in this group, patients will learn to:

      1. brush teeth, bathe, comb hair, and shave daily
      2. change clothes daily
      3. wash hands before each meal and after using toilet
      4. wash hair at least once a week

Referral criteria: In order to be considered for admission to the group, a patient must meet all of the following criteria:

      1. male
      2. ages 19 to 65 +
      3. deficient self-care skills, as evidenced by body odor, etc.
      4. able to tolerate the presence of others

Methodology: Activities will include grooming and hygiene activities, such as bathing, shaving, hair care, tooth care. The therapist will teach self-care skills to the group and the individual patients. Patients will be encouraged to carry out the tasks on their own. In general, one task at a time will be taught. Once some patients have mastered that task, another will be introduced, but the therapist will continue to teach the first task until all patients have learned it.

The therapist will set individual goals for each patient and will reinforce performance by giving patients praise or tangible rewards when they reach them. The therapist will provide feedback to individuals and will encourage independent performance of self-care tasks.

Once a patient demonstrates consistent self-initiated performance of the skills taught in this group, he will be referred to other groups. Some patients with chronic conditions may need to remain in the group indefinitely.

Role of the leader: The therapist will select and teach skills, and will provide feedback and reinforcement during performance of tasks. The therapist will encourage and support the gradual development of independent self-care habits, and will help patients make the transition to leave the group upon completion of goals.

Evaluation: Regular evaluation is made by the treatment team relative to the goals and prognosis of each patient. Patient satisfaction surveys are administered at intervals determined by the CQI leader.

FIG. 17–4. Sample group protocol

he has achieved the goals set in the exit criteria. There are many different reasons why a particular patient may be eliminated from a group, including:

1. The patient has been discharged from the treatment setting.
2. The patient displays uncontrollable assaultive or suicidal behavior.
3. The patient fails to attend the group on a regular basis.

Resources and *references* refer to items that may be used to help the group reach its goals. For example, if the main purpose of the group is to teach safe sex practices, resources might include condom samples, videotapes on AIDS and other sexually transmitted diseases (STDs), and a list of guest speakers. References would include written material to be used as background information by the group leader, as well as for distribution to group members. Materials in the first language of the patients (if other than English) would be included. Listing the resources and references in some detail makes it easy for another staff member to take over the group in the absence of the original leader.

In summary, writing the group protocol is the final step in designing a group. The protocol describes the goals of the group and the methods by which these goals will be achieved. Fig. 17–4 illustrates how the elements of the group protocol can be combined into a clear description of a group. It describes a self-care group for male inpatients on a locked ward in a state hospital, and is a continuation of the example begun in Fig. 17–2. Other group protocols can be found in Appendix B. There are several other group protocol formats in addition to the one used here; the reader may wish to look at other examples in Arbesman et al. (1). Some of the elements in the group protocol can be combined so that a protocol might include, at a minimum: name, goals, methods, and referral information. In a sense, however, writing the group protocol is only the beginning; getting the group off

to a good start and keeping it running is the real challenge.

STARTING A NEW GROUP

Getting a new group started can be more difficult than picking up a group that has already been running for some time. The first problem is that all of the patients are new to the group. They may not know each other, and if so several sessions may be needed just to help them feel comfortable. They will not be in the habit of coming to the group, and the leader may need to make a special effort to round them up and encourage them to attend.

The second problem is that because the group is new, its goals and activities have not been tested; only the experience of trying the activities with patients will reveal whether the goals are achievable and whether the activities and method are effective. The group leader needs to keep objective records of what happens in each group, and analyze these observations thoughtfully.

ADAPTATIONS OF GROUPS FOR VERY REGRESSED PATIENTS

As has been stated many times already, occupational therapists and assistants often provide treatment to patients who have very severe psychiatric disabilities. These severely regressed patients may be mute, sit for long hours in one position, have postural and sensory-integrative deficits (described in Chapter 3), and appear unresponsive to most efforts of staff. Attempting to treat these patients in the kinds of groups described thus far in this chapter would be an exercise in futility.

Ross and Burdick (17) developed a group approach for regressed patients that is based on principles from sensory integration. A central assumption is that patients can learn by receiving, processing and responding to sensory stimulation. Their approach uses a system of five stages or components that are included in every treatment session. These stages and some sample activities for each stage are shown in Fig. 17–5.

Because of their limited attention spans, very regressed patients can tolerate a group situation for only a half-hour or so. Therefore, the group leader must be very active and provide the momentum to move the group through the five stages. In addition, the leader needs to use touch, eye contact, voice control, and sometimes hand-over-hand techniques to get very regressed patients to respond. Not all the stages need be of equal length; for example, the leader may need to spend 50% of the session in stage 1 in order to arouse some patients.

Kaplan (8,9) advocates the use of *directive groups* with those patients who are se-

verely functionally impaired. These patients cannot generally be scheduled into existing groups as they are disruptive to the other members and obtain little benefit themselves. The purpose of the directive group is to prepare patients to function in other groups that are more readily available, but that require a higher level of task and social functioning than the patient can currently demonstrate. The "directive" aspect of the group refers to the group leaders' active involvement in nurturing, supporting, and facilitating behaviors that lead to understanding the purpose of the group, being able to be present for 45 minutes, concentrating enough to participate, and tolerating the presence of others. The protocols and procedures for such directive groups have been well outlined by Kaplan (8), and the interested reader should consult that reference.

STAGES	REPRESENTATIVE ACTIVITIES
Stage 1: This is the opening of the session, and serves to get the patients' attention and arouse their interest.	Say hello by touching feet or elbows. Pass bell or other unusual object.
Stage 2: Movement is used to increase nonverbal communication, expression of feelings.	Shake hands. Clapping.
Stage 3: Perceptual-motor activities are used to promote integration between sensory stimulation, movement, and cognition.	Dance to music. Ball play (catching, rolling, passing ball). Mat exercises. Large floor dominoes.
Stage 4: Verbal or symbolic activities are used to enhance cognitive functioning.	Make fruit salad (each member contributes). Build a tower of cardboard bricks. Read a poem. Counting games.
Stage 5: Closing the program provides opportunities to emphasize the positive qualities of the experience.	Shake hands or hold hands. Pass out candy or refreshments. Say good-bye to each person.

FIG. 17–5. Five stages of group process for regressed patients. Loosely adapted, based on information from Ross M, Burdick D. *Sensory integration: a training manual for therapists and teachers for regressed psychiatric and geriatric patient groups.* Thorofare, NJ: SLACK; 1981:7–8; and on notes from Ross M, McClean V. "Group Process in Activity Groups for the Severely Physically and Mentally Disabled" (workshop sponsored by SUNY-Downstate at New York Psychiatric Institute, November 23, 1985).

PROGRAM EVALUATION

Program evaluation is a procedure for measuring whether a program is achieving its objectives. Program evaluation is part of the total quality management (TQM) approach, which includes quality assurance (QA) and continuous quality improvement (CQI), discussed in previous chapters. Although program evaluation may be applied to any part of the occupational therapy program, it is discussed here because the assistant may encounter it in the context of measuring the effectiveness of a given occupational therapy group. In the case of a therapy group, evaluation focuses on whether the members' participation in the group has resulted in the behavioral changes specified in the goals. Designing or selecting appropriate program evaluation instruments requires knowledge of evaluation procedures and methodology, and is therefore the responsibility of the registered therapist. However, if the assistant is the group leader, he may administer or participate in the development of the evaluations and should therefore understand their purpose.

Program evaluation is designed to examine the effect of a treatment regimen on those who received it. One way of doing this is to collect evaluation data before patients receive the treatment, and then repeat the evaluation after they have received treatment for some time. This is called a *pretest-posttest design;* for this design to be meaningful, the particular evaluation must be free of practice effects, meaning that it should not be possible for someone to perform better the second time because of having had the experience of doing it the first time. Evaluations used in physical medicine (for example, measures of hand strength or range of motion) are usually free of practice effects, but this is not always true of evaluations of social interaction and psychological factors.

Another method of program evaluation is the *posttest design.* Participants are evalu-ated after they have received treatment, and the results are compared to what normally might have been expected without treatment. Another method is to collect data from hospital records. For example, in an outpatient program measures used might be length of time between hospitalizations or total number of days without hospitalization per year. Other measures used to evaluate the effectiveness of occupational therapy groups include surveys of patient satisfaction (what patients say about what they got out of the group) and evaluation checklists in which patient performance can be rated by the leader or, preferably, a staff member not directly involved with the group.

A significant problem with all program evaluation in mental health is that it is often difficult to demonstrate conclusively that the improvement in the patient's condition is due to the treatment program or therapy group, and not some other factor. These other factors, known as *intervening variables,* may include medication, other therapies, and other life experiences.

Program evaluation is absolutely essential if occupational therapy is to retain its position in the mental health field. It is certainly much more difficult to show that a patient's behavior has been changed by an occupational therapy group than it is to prove that the same patient has improved because of a particular medication. Nevertheless, if we as a profession cannot do this, there is no reason why anyone should continue to pay for our services. The challenge for the next decade will be to design and carry out careful program evaluations that will demonstrate the effectiveness of our interventions.

SUMMARY

The material presented in this chapter should provide the entry-level occupational therapy assistant or student with the basic concepts and methods for developing a new group or leading one that has already been developed. Groups are used in occupational therapy not only because they are cost-effective, but also because they provide more varied and extensive learning opportunities than are available in individual treatment. Effective group leadership consists in being able to identify and help members make use of the opportunities available in the group.

REFERENCES

1. Arbesman F, Armacost P, Hays C, Rauschl M, Swindle S, eds. *Occupational therapy: protocols in mental health.* Baltimore: Betty Cox Associates; 1984.
2. Banning MR, Nelson DL. The effects of activity-elicited humor and group structure on group cohesion and affective responses. *Am J Occup Ther* 1987;41:510–514.
3. Benne KD, Sheats P. Functional roles of group members. *J Social Issues* 1948;4(2):42–47.
4. Duncombe LW, Howe MC. Group work in occupational therapy: a survey of practice. *Am J Occup Ther* 1985;39:163–170.
5. Earhart CA. Occupational therapy groups. In: Allen CA, ed. *Occupational therapy for psychiatric diseases: measurement and management of cognitive disabilities.* Boston: Little, Brown; 1985.
6. Early MB. *T.A.R. introductory course workbook: occupational therapy—psychosocial dysfunction.* Long Island City, NY: LaGuardia Community College; 1981.
7. Falk-Kessler J, Momich C, Perel S. Therapeutic factors in occupational therapy groups. *Am J Occup Ther* 1991;45:59–66.
8. Kaplan KL. *Directive group therapy.* Thorofare, NJ: SLACK; 1988.
9. Kaplan KL. The directive group: short-term treatment for psychiatric patients with a minimal level of functioning. *Am J Occup Ther* 1986; 40:474–481.
10. Kartin NJ, Van Schroeder C. *Adult psychiatric life skills manual.* Kailua, Hawaii: Schroeder Publishing and Consulting; 1982.
11. Kramer LW. SCORE: solving community obstacles and restoring employment. *Occup Ther Mental Health* 1984;4(1):1–135 (entire issue).
12. Mead M. Male and female (1949). In: Maggio R, compiler. *The Beacon book of quotations by women.* Boston: Beacon Press; 1992:29.
13. Mosey AC. The concept and use of developmental groups. *Am J Occup Ther* 1970;24:272–275.
14. Mosey AC. *Three frames of reference for mental health.* Thorofare, NJ: SLACK; 1970.
15. Mosey AC. *Activities therapy.* New York: Raven Press; 1973.
16. Peloquin SM. Linking purpose to procedure during interactions with patients. *Am J Occup Ther* 1988;42:775–781.
17. Ross M, Burdick D. *Sensory integration: a training manual for therapists and teachers for regressed psychiatric and geriatric patient groups.* Thorofare, NJ: SLACK; 1981.
18. Yalom ID. *The theory and practice of group psychotherapy.* New York: Basic Books; 1970.
19. Yalom I. *The theory and practice of group psychotherapy.* 3rd ed. New York: Basic Books; 1985.

ADDITIONAL REFERENCES AND SUGGESTED READINGS

Bradlee L. The use of groups in short-term psychiatric settings. *Occup Ther Mental Health* 1984; 4(3):47–57.
Brown T, Harwood K, Heckman J, Short JE, eds. *Mental health protocols for occupational therapy.* Baltimore Md: CHESS; 1989.
Fidler GS. The task-oriented group as a context for treatment. *Am J Occup Ther* 1969;23:43–48.
Fidler G, Fidler J. *Occupational therapy: a communication process in psychiatry.* New York: Macmillan; 1963.
Gibson D, ed. *Group process and structure in psychosocial occupational therapy.* Binghamton, NY: Haworth Press; 1988.
Gibson D, ed. *Group protocols: a psychosocial compendium.* Binghamton, NY: Haworth Press; 1989.
Howe MC, Schwartzberg SL. *A functional approach to group work in occupational therapy.* Philadelphia: JB Lippincott; 1986.
Keenan B. Essentials of methodology for mental health evaluation. *Hosp Commun Psychiatry* 1975; 26:730–733.
Kuenstler G. A planning group for psychiatric outpatients. *Am J Occup Ther* 1976;30:634–639.
Markson EW. Basic concepts in mental health evaluation: evaluation in mental health: why and how. *Hosp Commun Psychiatry* 1975;26:727–730.
Posthuma BW. *Small groups in therapy settings: process and leadership.* Austin, Tex: Pro-Ed; 1988.
Remocker AJ, Storch ET. *Action speaks louder: a handbook of nonverbal group techniques.* 3rd ed. Edinburgh: Churchill Livingstone; 1982.
Versluys H. The remediation of role disorders through focused group work. *Am J Occup Ther* 1980;34:609–614.
Yalom ID. *Inpatient group psychotherapy.* New York: Basic Books; 1983.

18

Daily Living Skills

If you could make a pudding wi' thinking o' the batter, it 'ud be easy getting dinner.

GEORGE ELIOT (1)

This chapter is the first of five that will present an overview of the activities most frequently used by occupational therapists and assistants working in psychiatry. It is crucial to remember that activities are the core experience of occupational therapy for patients. The use of activities to create change in people is what makes occupational therapy unique among the health professions. It is through participation and involvement in activities that patients develop and practice skills, learn about themselves and other people, increase their sense of competence, express their feelings and ideas, and develop confidence in their own ability to have an effect on the world.

The activities used most often by occupational therapy assistants are presented here; there are many other excellent activities that, because of space limitations, cannot be discussed. This chapter will describe activities in the area of daily life skills. Chapter 19 will give an overview of work skills and work habits, and homemaking and child-care skills. Chapter 20 will discuss leisure activities and expressive skills, Chapter 21 will describe activities to develop expressive and coping skills, and Chapter 22 will briefly introduce cognitive and sensorimotor activities. There is considerable overlap among these categories. Work, for example, requires expressive,

cognitive, and sensorimotor skills. Leisure also requires all of these skills. Occupational therapists use activities as broad instruments of practice and must avoid classifying them too rigidly.

In each category and, where needed, for individual activities within the category, the following information will be covered: general purposes of the activity, prerequisite skills, and precautions. The reader may find helpful the additional references and other resources that are indicated.

Before discussing the activities themselves, we should examine why and how these activities can be used to improve the lives of patients. At first glance, it might appear that all that is needed is for the therapist or assistant to teach the patient whatever skills he lacks, and then he should be able to function on his own. However, while many patients need to participate in activities in order to learn specific skills, there are others who already possess the necessary skills but who fail to use them for various reasons. Even more tragically, there are those who go through the motions of everyday life, with a high degree of skill in the activities they attempt, but who feel miserable and disconnected from any meaning or purpose. To understand why these problems can exist, it is helpful to think about the three basic categories of learning: knowledge, skills, and attitudes.

Knowledge is the acquisition of *information* or facts about reality. For instance, patients preparing to live on their own for the first time may not understand the basic facts and methods of homemaking. They probably do not know what tasks are involved, what tools and supplies they will need, or how often and how thoroughly various tasks should be done. If a patient has spent the past 20 years in hospitals and supervised board-and-care homes, he probably will not know, for example, that sheets should be changed regularly.

Skills are *actions* or behaviors that are learned. For example, the patient described above may not know how to change a bed, and perhaps not even how to make a bed. He probably will not know how to wash sheets, or how to wash dishes, wring out a mop, or clean a toilet either. Skills are the "doing" part of the activity.

Attitudes are learned *feelings,* values, and beliefs. Schwartzenberg (12) suggests that patients may have difficulty staying motivated to use skills they already possess because of various intrapsychic and emotional factors. For instance, low self-esteem or a feeling that one is a failure generally can undermine success and motivation. In other words, the patient lacks the basic energy even to get started, and his previous failures have convinced him there is little point in trying. A related problem is that impaired ability to express feelings may lead to anger and frustration. Schwartzenberg quotes one patient:

> I have recently, since I got sick, for the first time been able to get angry. I have never been able to get angry before. I know I have a lot of anger in me. When I let go of some of it I usually get an anxiety attack after it. Perhaps, I feel, it is not the way one should act. You should act nice. Anger is something that I feel is evil. I should be a good girl. 'Cause of the neck tightening and the phobias I can't go to the store, I can't buy groceries, I can't do any-

thing to take care of myself. I'm not able to walk anywhere. (12, p. 15)

Schwartzenberg also notes the positive effect of social contact on healthy occupational behavior and maintenance of habits. She suggests that people who become socially isolated are deprived of an important environmental stimulus, and because of this may find normal activities much less gratifying. In addition, whereas good habits depend on following a routine, too much of the same thing can lead to boredom and diminished motivation. She quotes another patient:

> I'd get up at 8:30 in the morning, make the beds, and I'd do the dishes. This is all after I ate breakfast, of course, and washed up, put on my makeup and put my dentures in. Then I'd dust around, if it needed to be dusted, and then I'd spend most of my time watching T.V. I prepared breakfast and lunch for myself and I was always alone. That's how I became very depressed. When my husband came home from work I'd prepare his supper and then he would go and listen to his C.B. while I went into the living room and watched T.V. Then around 8:00 or so I'd go in my room, I mean our room, and watch the colored T.V. in there because I got tired of watching black and white all day. So I'd watch the colored T.V. until around 10:00 and then shut the light off and go to bed. It became very depressing for me. I was very lonely. I had anxiety attacks. I live in a younger neighborhood and they work. They are in their thirties and I am left alone. There is no neighbor to come in and talk to me or anything. I don't even have anyone to talk to on the phone because my children work too. I'd say, Oh God the same thing tomorrow and the next day and the next day! (12, pp. 16–17)

In addition, roles and patterns and values learned from one's parents can influence one's willingness to attempt and maintain certain skills. For instance, a patient who was brought up in an upper-class household would be accustomed to having his personal and housekeeping needs taken care of by paid servants, and might have to work through his feelings about having to learn and use basic housekeeping skills. Similarly, a woman whose mother was obsessively tidy in her housework may find it hard to break the habit of spending most of her waking hours cleaning. Schwartzenberg proposes that people may have difficulty sustaining activities that were not approved of or just not done by their parents. Values and beliefs that arise in one's cultural and ethnic heritage may have a similar effect on motivation for activities.

Similarly, personal learning preferences and habits can affect new learning. For example, some individuals possess a lifelong pattern of finding it easy to help or advise other people while avoiding situations where one must demonstrate one's own ability. A difficulty in asking for and receiving help can seriously interfere with learning new skills from a therapist or other patients. Feeling inadequate or unworthy of help or unwilling to reveal inadequacy are all possible reasons for this kind of behavior. There may be a feeling that having to rely on another person is a big risk, and too frightening to attempt. Underlying beliefs and feelings such as these can impair both a person's ability to function and his general feeling of well-being and mental health.

Thus, a careful analysis of the knowledge, skills, and attitudes that a patient possesses is necessary in order to make any activity work for a particular patient. The therapist or assistant must ask: How important is it for this patient to be involved in this activity? What will it do for him? Does the patient know when, where, why, and with whom he might use this activity? Does he know how to do it, and has he practiced it enough to remember how to do it on his own? Does *he* think it is important to do this activity, and *why* does he think it is important? (What does it mean to him?) Chapter 23 will describe further how to analyze and adapt activities for use with different patient groups, or to meet the needs of individuals.

DAILY LIVING SKILLS

Daily living skills form a broad category that includes all of the skills the average adult needs to manage his life on a daily basis. Sometimes these are referred to as *activities of daily living*. Specific skills usually classified as daily living skills are personal care (grooming and hygiene), clothing selection and maintenance, nutrition, medication and health maintenance, exercise, communication, transportation, money management, and time management. (Personal care is sometimes also called *self-care*.)

Not all patients with mental health problems seen by occupational therapists need help with these skills. Higher functioning patients frequently demonstrate adequate to excellent personal care and daily living skills. Diagnostically, the main groups of patients who need help with daily living skills are those with chronic schizophrenia and organic mental disorders. In a review of the literature, Hayes (3) indicated that living skills taught to such patients carried over well to community life, provided opportunity was given for transfer to the new situation and for generalization of learning.

Many psychiatric patients have problems in the area of *personal care*. This is particularly true of those with chronic conditions or severe psychotic disorders; such patients may appear indifferent to their personal hygiene, bathing so infrequently that they have a strong body odor, combing and washing their hair rarely if at all, and dressing bizarrely in clothes that are out of date, ill matched, or inappropriate for the season or the occasion. Patients who have acceptable skills in grooming and hygiene may have other problems that, although less immediately obvious, present serious impediments to carrying out a normal daily routine. Inadequate knowledge of nutrition, poor eating habits, and excessive use of cigarettes, drugs and alcohol, caffeinated beverages, and over-the-counter medications (antacids, diet pills, laxatives, sleeping pills) contribute to malnutrition and chemically induced anxiety. Many chronic patients have serious problems managing money, and are often caught short before they have paid for basics like food, rent, and utilities. Without the knowledge of how to get around their communities on foot or on public transportation, many patients remain isolated in impoverished environments. These are only a few of the problems encountered by those whose daily living skills are deficient. Increasing patients' skills in these areas can dramatically enhance the quality of their lives and in many instances prevent future hospitalizations.

Personal Care: Hygiene and Grooming

This subcategory of daily living skills covers basic grooming and health habits and personal appearance. The needs of individuals within this category vary depending on current functional level, length of illness and hospitalization, previous knowledge and skills, and the social support available. At one extreme, the very regressed chronic patient who has been hospitalized for long periods may need training and reinforcement in basic hygiene habits such as proper use of the toilet, use of toilet tissue, washing of hands and face, and so on. Some individuals whose illnesses are equally severe but who come from middle-class backgrounds may have adequate skills or sufficient social support from their families, so that they always appear presentable (even though they may need reminders or actual physical assistance from family members). At another extreme, some patients may have reasonable personal care skills but low self-esteem, and may benefit from the experience of pampering themselves in a grooming group, experimenting with samples of new self-care products, and receiving praise from their peers.

Personal care skills may be taught on a one-to-one basis. This is appropriate for patients with very poor skills or those who wish or need to learn a skill that is not of general interest. Most commonly, however, personal care skills are taught in groups; these groups are often restricted to patients of one sex or the other, depending upon the specific skill content.

Skills that may be covered include bathing, toilet skills, skin care, use of deodorant, hair care (including when to get a haircut), care of the teeth and use of mouthwash, and shaving or use of depilatories. Following the principle that skills should be taught in the environment where they will be practiced, all of these skills should be taught in the bathroom or an area that simulates it. Ideally, skills should be taught in the patient's home environment, using the tools and equipment to which he is accustomed. Lower functioning patients may need to be reminded to pay attention to parts of the body that are not immediately visible, such as the back of the head or body, the underarms, the soles of the feet. The use of a full-length mirror, a three-part folding mirror, and various hand-held mirrors is helpful. Shatterproof mirrors may be required in some settings, and are safer generally. An important precaution should be mentioned. Since health problems can be transmitted via shared personal care products, each patient should have his own items, or disposable sample sizes should be used.

In addition to these basic personal care skills, occupational therapists or assistants may also teach the use of makeup and nail care. Some female patients use excessive amounts of makeup or apply it in old-fashioned or bizarre ways; skill development often focuses on matching makeup color to complexion, choice of flattering shades, and methods of application and removal. The goal is to help these patients learn to use makeup in an attractive and socially acceptable way. The use of mirrors (including magnifying mirrors) and feedback from peers can reinforce what is appropriate and what is not. Fashion and beauty magazines can be helpful, but those that picture extreme makeups sometimes used in high-fashion modeling should be avoided.

Nail care at its most simple involves cleaning and trimming the nails wherever they need it, and pushing back the cuticles. Teaching patients these skills and reinforcing their continued use will contribute greatly to their making a positive impression on other people. The use of cuticle removers and colored nail polish, on the other hand, are optional practices that are sometimes overused as activities in self-care groups. It seems ridiculous to have patients apply nail polish when they have other self-care problems that are more serious, and when their nails will be dirty again and the polish chipped within one day's time. However, applying nail polish seems appropriate for patients who have done so in the past, or who may get a needed boost to their self-esteem from doing it.

Clothing Selection and Maintenance

A large part of the impression one makes on others depends on being dressed in clean, well-fitting clothes that are appropriate for the season and the occasion. A brief perusal of magazine covers at the supermarket checkout will testify that people in general have a more than casual interest in how they look. Those with mental health problems often lack even the basic skills necessary to present a good personal appearance. Patients who are indigent may be used to wearing clothes selected for them by others or donated to charity; these clothes are rarely in fashion and often appear bizarre because they are too out of date. Patients may wear ill-fitting clothes because they do not know what size they wear, or because they did not adjust their wardrobes when they gained or lost weight. They may not know how to care for their clothing, with shrinkage, wrinkling, and

run colors the result. They may not know to repair ripped seams and missing buttons.

Clothing selection and maintenance activities focus on how to select clothes for a given occasion, how to shop for clothing, and how to maintain it. Specific activities may include those directed at learning about what clothes are appropriate and flattering. Patients may start by taking their measurements and figuring out sizes. This may be followed by a trip to see what is locally available in a clothing store or thrift shop, as a part of learning to budget and comparison shop. Another approach is for patients to bring in garments from their own wardrobes and use a mannequin for the group to assemble and discuss appropriate outfits. Alternatively, the assistant can create visual aids from photographs in magazines to illustrate appropriate clothing for different occasions. Attention should be given to seasonal differences and to the differences between casual, dressy, and work attire.

Learning to shop for clothing requires that patients know their sizes for all garments, including shoes and underwear. Instruction in how to recognize whether a garment is well made and easy to care for is especially important, since patients may have limited funds to replace damaged clothing. Patients may need help in planning their purchases to fit in with other clothing they already own, and in selecting styles and colors that are flattering.

In addition to being able to select and shop for clothing, one needs to know how to maintain it, how to clean it, and how to repair it. Clothing care requires knowledge of how to read care labels, and how to recognize when something needs special care such as handwashing or dry cleaning, or drip drying as opposed to machine drying. The laundry skills needed vary depending upon where the patient lives, whether he or someone else is responsible for his laundry, and whether he has access to a home washing machine or must use a laundromat. Knowing how to control water temperature and use different laundry products is important. All patients should know the rudiments of mending if they are to live on their own; being able to repair a hem or a ripped seam, or sew on a button or a snap, can make the difference between looking relatively normal or "looking like a patient." Shoe care includes matching polish color to shoes, knowing when to polish shoes, and knowing when and where to take them for repairs. All of these skills can be taught by a combination of verbal instruction, demonstration, and actual practice; photographs and written guidelines that can later be used as reminders are often helpful.

Nutrition and Weight Control

Basic nutrition and weight control are of concern both for those patients who have weight problems—anorexia and bulimia (2) as well as obesity—and for those whose eating habits result in a diet that is far from balanced. Nutrition may be taught either as part of a cooking program or within the general area of self-care. Methods of teaching may include the use of flashcards and other commercially available educational aids (companies that supply primary and secondary school teachers are good sources); therapist-created educational aids such as posters and collages; group discussion; and actual practice. Another activity is making a file of recipes that are nutritious, inexpensive, and uncomplicated. Patients can practice by planning and preparing a meal, or by going out to eat and ordering a balanced meal in a restaurant.

A nutrition program provides an opportunity to educate patients to the psychotropic effects of caffeine and cigarette consumption. Both caffeine and nicotine are drugs, and are classified as such by the American Medical Association. The *DSM-III-R* category of substance use disorders includes both of these drugs. Research evidence conclusively shows that ingestion of large amounts of caffeine (in coffee, soft drinks, and chocolate) is associated with increased anxiety, irritability, aggression, and psychomotor agitation, and that it may counteract the effects of prescribed sedative medication (14). Nicotine has similar stimulating effects, and its other negative health effects are well known.

Weight control activities should educate patients to the relationships between calorie consumption, exercise, and weight. Since high-protein, low-carbohydrate diets are known to cause increased fatigue, dehydration, and mental depression, patients should be taught to avoid fad diets. Instead, they should be encouraged to follow diets that are high in complex carbohydrates but low in fat and calories, or just to eat reduced portions at regular meals. A good educational activity is planning a weekly calorie-conscious menu within budget limitations. Skills can be reinforced and monitored through weekly weigh-ins and by requiring patients to keep daily records of food consumption and exercise.

It must be recognized, however, that the issue of weight control is a very sensitive one and very difficult for many people to resolve. Weight control is related to *body image,* which is one's sense of one's own body and how it looks to other people. Body image includes feelings about physical coordination and sexual attractiveness. It takes a very long time to change body image, which may remain constant despite weight loss or weight gain. A change in the way one looks may mean that members of the opposite sex may suddenly become interested, and this unaccustomed social pressure may feel threatening.

Medication Management, Health Maintenance, Sexuality

One of the least obvious but potentially most damaging problems faced by a psychiatric patient living in the community is his mismanagement of his own medication. Some psychiatric disorders appear to be controllable only with continued use of medication; if a patient stops taking his pills he will become ill as soon as the drugs wear off, and this often results in rehospitalization. There are many reasons why a patient might not take his prescribed medication; these range from forgetting to do so, or running out of pills, to deliberately stopping. One reason some patients give for stopping deliberately is that the side effects of psychotropic medication can be uncomfortable; these side effects and how to help patients manage them are discussed in Chapter 8. Individual patients may give different reasons, including a belief that they were "getting better" or a desire to "see if I could get along without the pills."

Any effort to help a patient manage his medication independently should begin with a discussion of his feelings about it; group discussion with peers can provide feedback based on the direct experience of others. Some patients will need instruction and practice in specific skills such as where to go or whom to call when they run out of medication or are about to. Patients whose problem is that they cannot remember to take their medication, or whether they have already taken it, can be taught to use various environmental supports and memory aids such as compartmentalized pillboxes, signs, lists, and timers. Injectable medications that last for as long as two weeks can sometimes be used for patients who are unable to manage their own medication. In any medication management program the occupational therapy assistant should work closely with the prescribing physician, and should *never* give the patient advice that contradicts or countermands the doctor.

Health maintenance consists of the skills needed to respond to the minor and major health problems that occur in daily life. It includes the important skills of knowing where to go to obtain medical care and how to respond to emergencies; these have already been discussed in Chapter 12. In addition, patients should be taught how to deal with minor health problems such as splinters, blisters, colds, burns, cuts, fever, indigestion, sprains and bruises, and headaches. Information should also be available on how over-the-counter medications can impair motor ability and judgment (important for driving) and interact with prescribed medication.

Skills related to sexuality include, for women, care of menstruation and breast self-examination. For both sexes, knowledge of the basic mechanisms of sexual reproduction, the use of contraception, methods for avoiding and recognizing sexually transmitted diseases, the use of condoms, the dangers of unprotected sexual relations, and awareness of socially acceptable behaviors are important. Strange as it may seem, women have occasionally gotten pregnant because they did not know that sexual intercourse had anything to do with having a baby; therefore it is especially important for psychiatric patients (who may have more difficulty raising a child than the average person does) to learn the basic facts. Instruction is directed at the patient's level of understanding, and the use of detailed anatomical vocabulary or elaborate diagrams is not necessary.

Helping patients acquire knowledge about sexually transmitted diseases is extremely important, since some patients may be promiscuous or sexually impulsive, or so passive and submissive that they have sexual relations with anyone who asks them to. Topics that should be covered include what to look for and how to examine a potential sexual partner, and why, when, and how to use condoms. Male homosexuals may need instruction in which sexual practices to abstain from to avoid transmission of AIDS. Therapists and assistants who feel uncomfortable or unknowledgeable in these areas might seek the assistance of a nurse as a co-instructor. In some settings, instruction in issues relating to sexuality may be the responsibility of the nurse or the social worker, and not the occupational therapist.

Finally, individual patients may need instruction and training in basic social standards such as not exposing oneself or masturbating in public, or talking in public about masturbation, or soliciting sexual acts from others.

Exercise

Exercise is part of health maintenance and has many documented health benefits. It reduces the effects of stress and tension, provides outlets for frustration and anxiety and aggression, speeds up metabolism, burns calories, reduces appetite, improves cardiovascular health, and increases strength, flexibility, and stamina. It improves balance, coordination, and other sensory integrative functions. Finally, it enhances self-satisfaction and creates a feeling of well-being. Patients need to learn about these benefits of exercise and to develop the habit of regular exercise three to four times weekly, at a minimum.

A variety of approaches can help patients learn to meet their exercise needs. One is to provide instruction in the basic facts of physical health and fitness; knowing and understanding the value of exercise will motivate some patients to attempt it. Another is to assist patients in working out a schedule for exercise. Other approaches include actually providing instruction in a sport or physical fitness activity, or arranging for a volunteer or fitness instructor to teach an exercise activity to patients.

Exercise and physical fitness activities must be selected carefully. The goal is for the patient to enjoy and value exercise sufficiently that he will follow through on it on his own. The exercise must be inexpensive and convenient enough for him to practice without turning his life upside down. Running, doing calisthenics or yoga, swimming (at a public or YMCA pool), bicycling, and brisk walking are examples of exercises that require little investment of money, equipment, or space. Selection of exercise must also take into account any medical precautions or drug side effects that may impair a patient's ability to perform certain exercises safely.

Communication

The area of communication includes three major skills: basic conversational skills, use of the telephone system, and use of the postal system. Basic conversational skills can be taught by a four-step method: coaching (or motivation), behavior modeling (or demonstration), behavior rehearsal (or practice), and feedback. This approach was discussed in the social skills section of Chapter 3. Instruction should focus on the basic skills of starting and ending conversations, asking for or giving help, listening, and responding (5). Patients may need instruction and feedback about the nuances of nonverbal behavior such as eye contact, minimal response, body language, and maintaining appropriate body distance. A number of excellent resources are available for sequencing instruction in social and conversational skills (5,13) and for developing nonverbal communication skills (10, 11). In any program that aims to develop patients' social and self-expressive skills, the occupational therapy assistant works under the supervision and guidance of the registered therapist.

Use of the telephone can be overwhelming and disturbing to mentally disabled people. Those who have difficulty conversing with others face to face are even more disconcerted by the prospect of carrying on a conversation with a disembodied voice.

Also, those who have been hospitalized for long periods or whose lives have been regulated by family members or professional staff may have little experience in using the telephone. Basic telephone skills needed for independent community living include answering and making telephone calls, taking messages accurately, using the telephone book (White Pages and Yellow Pages), using a pay telephone, and knowing how to make an emergency call. Each of these skills consists of several subskills; recognizing the difference between a dial tone and a busy signal is just one example. Several exercises that teach telephone communication skills are included in Kartin and Van Schroeder (5). Examples of other exercises that might be attempted include calling the telephone number for time, weather, or other information and reporting the information to the group; calling a store and asking for information; and finding the correct number and phoning for bus information. It is a good idea to create an index card file of such exercises for patient use.

Because using the telephone requires a combination of social skills, cognitive skills, and manual skills, actual practice is an essential part of telephone training. Although patients can try out their telephone skills on any phone that is available in the treatment setting, this has some problems. First, the therapist working with the patient can hear only one half of the conversation, and therefore may not be able to give accurate feedback. Second, the patient may feel more anxious because the situation is a real one. Finally, phones in treatment centers are used and needed by many people, and cannot be monopolized by telephone training. One alternative is to use disconnected telephones to practice dialing and conversational skills. A commercially available program, Teletrainer, developed by the telephone company, is another option. It was originally designed to teach school children and the mentally retarded how to use the telephone, and it consists of two telephones (one rotary, one touch-tone), a speaker phone and central control monitor, a 25-foot line cord, and a carrying case. Although expensive, Teletrainer provides several features of interest to therapists, as it can be used to develop skills in recognizing different electronic tones, making emergency calls, telephone manners, and using various information services. More importantly, it allows the trainer (or an entire group) to listen in on a call and hear both parties.

Patients may also need some instruction about various aspects of the postal system. In particular, since they may receive registered or certified mail from various government agencies or from their landlord, they need to know something of the legal implications of this. In addition, they may need to purchase stamps and recognize when a letter needs extra postage. If they wish to send packages they need to know how to wrap them, whether to insure them and for how much, and what options are available for sending them through the post office or other package delivery services. They should be able to locate mailboxes and the post office in their own neighborhoods. Finally, patients need to learn to refuse unsolicited packages and to recognize and avoid solicitations and "rip-offs" in the mail and over the phone.

Transportation

Being able to get around in one's local community considerably enhances the range of resources and experiences that one can use. Without specific training, some patients may be reluctant to venture beyond a one- or two-block radius of their homes. Depending on the geographical area where the patient lives and the extent of the patient's disability, transportation skills (sometimes called *functional mobility skills*) may focus on either public or private transportation, or a combination of the two. Some patients may be able to drive a car, and may benefit from practice in reading maps and planning routes in advance. Others who are unable to drive or who do not have a car available will need to use the public bus or subway system, or a private car service or taxi. Subskills that may be important include knowing where the bus or subway stop is located, knowing how to obtain and read the bus schedule, knowing the correct fare and how to use bus transfers, and identifying how long one must allow to reach the bus stop from one's home or the treatment center. Some patients with severe cognitive disabilities or memory impairment may need repeated supervised practice to learn how to get from their homes to some other location (e.g., the treatment center) and back. Those who cannot master this will need to use a private car service or rely on rides from others.

One aspect of functional mobility that should not be neglected is getting around on foot. Some patients may have no idea of what is available in their immediate neighborhoods; activities that can be used to develop awareness of the immediate environment include walking around and reading or making maps. It is especially important to include safety when walking at night. In the country, where there are no sidewalks, this means wearing light-colored clothing and walking facing the traffic; in the city, it means being "street-smart" and wary of unlit areas and potentially dangerous people.

Money Management

Being able to use money to make purchases and provide for one's basic needs is absolutely essential if a patient is to survive on his own in the community for any length of time. Yet it is not unusual for someone with a chronic mental disorder to run out of money long before his next disability check is due to arrive. Without money the patient may become desperate, perhaps so anxious that he actually becomes psychotic and needs to be rehospitalized. Or he may resort to panhandling and become a public nuisance.

Patients have many different kinds of problems dealing with money. They may loan or give it away, or be swindled out of it in con games. They may have no concept of budgeting money, and no awareness that overspending today will mean going without tomorrow. They may make impulsive or extravagant purchases, take taxis instead of

public transportation, eat in restaurants too frequently, or gamble their money away. Some people may be able to give correct answers on a written evaluation, but fail to make or recognize the correct change in a store. Kaseman (6) reports that it may take as long as three to six months of supervised practice for these patients to learn to budget their money to meet their needs. Individuals with memory impairments or severe cognitive disabilities may never be able to handle their money independently, and will need to rely on family members or court-appointed custodians. Allen's Cognitive Levels as shown in Section C of the instrumental scale of Fig. 14-2 seem to show that independent money management is not possible at Level 4 and below.

Kaseman (6) developed a program for training psychiatric outpatients to manage their money. The first step is assessment of the patient's cognitive and money management skills. Figure 18-1 shows the written questionnaire that is used together with an Asset Information Sheet (not shown) to evaluate the patient's skills before entering the program. The program consists of a 12-week course of modular instruction which is summarized in Table 18-1.

Some of the issues that need to be addressed in a money management training program are awareness of how much money is available, what the priorities are for spending it, and how it is currently being spent.[1] Once these basic facts are established, patients may need help to develop a budget and stick to it; patients with schizophrenic and organic disorders may not be able to adhere to a budget because they become distracted or forget. Keeping a daily record of expenditures can help some of these individuals become more aware of the need to conserve their funds. There are many levels at which budgeting can be

---

[1]Exercises designed to develop awareness of spending habits and budget priorities can be found in Hughes and Mullins (4).

Name _____ Date _____

1. Your checkbook balance is $70.00. If you write a check for $32.25, how much will you have left in your account? _____ ($37.75)**

2. If you want to make a deposit into your checking account, which of the following do you have to do? (Circle the correct answers.) (b, c, & e)**
    a. Drop the check into a night deposit box.
    b. Endorse the check.
    c. Fill out a deposit slip.
    d. The teller will know what to do, so give the check to her.
       (Client may also follow this procedure, but should be encouraged to do it for himself.)
    e. Add the amount to your previous balance in your checkbook.

3. You have received a $485.00 paycheck this month. You want to deposit half into your savings account and the other half into your checking account. Please fill out the appropriate slips necessary to make these deposits. (Banking slips are provided.)

4. Your checking account balance is low due to your unexpected auto repair bill. You need to transfer $100.00 from your savings account into your checking account. Please fill out the necessary slips for this transfer. (The necessary bank slips are provided.)

5. Your checkbook balance is currently $450.00. You need to have your car repairs done and the expected bill comes to $128.50. Please make a check payable to Ray's Auto Repair for the given amount. (A sample check is provided.) After subtracting your expenses for this auto repair, how much do you have left. _____ ($321.50)**

6. Add:	135	158	215	172	795
	+286	+187	+ 15	204	209
				+ 84	912
					+ 16

7. Subtract:	82	61	48	139	579
	−35	−37	−16	− 65	−212

8. Multiply:	6 × 7=	7 × 10=	18 × 3=
	4 × 9=	6 × 5=	10 × 14=
	2 × 15=	8 × 9=	15 × 9=

9. Divide:	14 ÷ 2=	9 ÷ 3=	15 ÷ 5=
	28 ÷ 14=	102 ÷ 2=	182 ÷ 4=

10. Bus fare is 60¢ and you have $1.00. How much will you have after paying the bus fare? _____ (40¢)**

You purchase food for the week; your bill is $25.07 and you have $40.25. How much will you have left: _____ ($15.18)**

In your pocket you have two quarters, five pennies, three dimes, and four one dollar bills. How much money do you have? _____ ($4.85)**

** Answers in parentheses at the end of each question are included here for your information.

FIG. 18–1. Assessment of money management. Reprinted with the permission of Haworth Press from Kaseman BM. Teaching money management skills to psychiatric outpatients. *Occup Ther Mental Health* 1980; 1(3), p. 64.

TABLE 18–1. *Lesson plan for 12 sessions: money management*

Session 1	Give general information and introduction to course. Have client fill out the Assessment of Money Management form.
Session 2	Have client fill out the Asset Information sheet and discuss assets and liabilities. Ask each client: What do you wish to learn in this class? The answers and their ability to learn will set the pace of the course. Homework for the week should be to keep an account of expenditures. Give each client a weekly budget record sheet.
Session 3	Discuss budgeting and examine present use of funds and possible changes in expenditures which will better meet needs of each client. Homework: continue budget-keeping records but use the revised record. Visit a bank and bring to class literature that is available from the bank.
Session 4	Discuss banking; share information literature brought in.
Session 5	Practice using banking forms.
Session 6	Discuss and practice balancing checkbook. Review banking procedures.
Session 7	Review balancing checkbook. Homework: each client should bring to class a list of two things he/she would like to do if he/she had enough funds to make it possible.
Session 8	Discuss savings plans and the items the clients included on the lists they brought to class.
Session 9	Review budget in an attempt to include some kind of savings plan. Homework: draw up a new budget plan.
Session 10	Discuss and examine the new budget plan.
Session 11	Discuss methods of keeping to a budget. Provide encouragement. Review budgets and banking.
Session 12	Again have clients fill out the Assessment of Money Management form. Question/Answer period.

Reprinted with permission of Haworth Press from Table 4 in Kaseman BM. Teaching money management skills to psychiatric outpatients. *Occup Ther Mental Health* 1980; 1(3), p. 66.

taught. Patients with severe disabilities may need to keep daily records, as discussed above; those with good cognitive skills may benefit more from monthly or yearly or long-range planning. Paper-and-pencil exercises are more concrete and therefore more effective for actual budgeting than are group discussions.

Although some patients may say that they would rather not keep their money in a bank, they should be encouraged to do so because it is obviously much safer. Savings accounts have fewer procedures and, since they do not generate transaction fees, require less scrupulous bookkeeping than checking accounts and are therefore easier to learn. Patients will need instruction in how to fill out various deposit and withdrawal and application forms; banks are usually quite willing to provide blank forms for practice. It helps to role-play situations in which a patient might interact with bank personnel to, for instance, open an account or withdraw money. Obviously, trips to the bank and supervised practice in a real situation should be included.[2]

Another aspect of money management is concerned with the ability to judge where and how to spend money; this includes knowledge of comparison shopping and consumer rights, and understanding the pros and cons of using credit cards. Information about how and where to shop for bargains, and where and how to complain about a defective product should be covered. Group discussions of how to handle difficult situations involving money can help patients focus on why they sometimes have trouble sticking to their budgets. Some of the situations[3] that might be considered are:

---

[2]Additional banking and budgeting exercises for patients at all levels can be found in Kartin and Van Schroeder (5).

[3]Additional discussion topics can be found in Hughes and Mullins (4).

1. You receive a circular in the mail that says you have been selected to receive a check for $250 if you purchase a particular sewing machine by mail.
2. You have been invited to a dinner dance and have nothing to wear. You are considering buying a dress and shoes, but the ones you have chosen would use up all your spending money for two months.
3. Your child is constantly begging you for a new bicycle. The old one was stolen.
4. A missionary comes to your door asking for a contribution for children starving in Africa. He shows you pictures that make you want to cry.
5. You have always had trouble losing weight and are considering investing in a reduction plan advertised in the newspaper. It costs only $39.98 and promises a 10-pound weight loss in one week.

Depending on a patient's judgment and experience, situations like these can present real dilemmas and temptations. Willson (14) emphasizes that we cannot realistically expect to prepare patients for every situation they might encounter, but that we can help them develop general skills in identifying the real issues, generating alternatives, and selecting realistic solutions.

Time Management

It was Benjamin Franklin who coined the phrase, "Time is money." Although time may not translate into money for those patients who are not gainfully employed, nonetheless time *is* like money in that there is a fixed amount of it in each day, and in each person's life. However we spend it, once spent it is gone forever; understanding the value of time and knowing how to make the best use of it is an important aspect of mental health.

Time management refers to the skills used to organize and control the way one spends one's time. Among these skills are recognizing values and priorities, structuring a daily routine, scheduling one's time, and organizing tasks efficiently. Patients with mental health problems may need help with these skills for a variety of reasons. One is that the sense of time itself is sometimes distorted by psychiatric illness, especially one with an organic basis. Patients may experience time as very long and stretched out, seemingly endless. The future may seem bleak, empty, or incomprehensible. Another reason is that having one's daily habits disrupted by a long illness or hospitalization or retirement or the death of a spouse may make previously familiar routines feel odd and awkward. Another problem some patients have is in their time habits; they may be chronically late for things, or never have time for leisure, or spend long hours in unproductive activity (taking drugs, drinking, gambling, watching television).

When working with patients around their use of time, it is critically important to remember that time use is based on personal values, and that the values of the patient may be different from those of the therapist. Another consideration is that some individuals may have such severe cognitive disabilities that they cannot be expected to manage their own time. Any time management program should begin with an assessment of how the patient uses his time; the Barth Time Construction (described in Chapter 14) is probably the best instrument for doing this, since the contrasting colors give patients direct feedback about how they allocate their time among various activities. Other areas that should be assessed include the patient's values and goals, and how these are (or, more frequently, are not) reflected in his use of time.[4] Patients who have trouble identifying values and goals might be asked to write a "future biogra-

---

[4]Exercises for this can be modified from those in Lakein (9).

phy" in which they describe what they will be doing at some point in the future.

Patients can be helped to structure their time through the use of daily schedules, monthly calendars, and flowcharts. Lower functioning patients may need to post their daily schedules prominently in their homes; even higher functioning patients may find this is a relatively stress-free way of keeping family members informed of their schedules. Monthly calendars should be chosen according to need; large wall calendars can serve as general reminders in the treatment setting or in the patient's home; patients whose daily activities require traveling to different locations may find a pocket calendar more helpful.

Flowcharts are plans that show the steps that need to be taken to reach a goal, and the time frame for each step. For example, if one of your goals is to travel to the Amazon, you could make a flowchart showing the dates by which you expect to have saved enough money, secured your passport and your inoculations, made your plane and hotel reservations, and so on. For a patient with the goal of getting a job, the charted activities might include writing a résumé, responding to advertisements, practicing interviewing, planning what to wear to an interview, and so forth. Using a flowchart serves the purpose of organizing time around a desired goal while simultaneously clarifying what needs to be done to reach it. It is important to remember that time management aids by themselves will not change a person's time behaviors; patients need to learn to use them, and to get in the habit of referring to them and updating them.

Worksheets and exercises on time management activities can be found in Korb, Azok, and Leutenberg (7,8) and Hughes and Mullins (4).

CONCLUSION

This chapter has presented activities in the broad category of daily living skills. The same activities may be used in various other ways in practice. Each activity has other benefits and potentials besides the obvious ones. Exercise, for example, is not only a health maintenance activity, but can be a leisure activity or a rehabilitative activity structured to develop sensorimotor skills or even social skills. A simple daily living activity such as sweeping the floor can be structured to promote postural balance, or to develop concentration and attention span. Thus, it is not so much the activity itself that is the therapy, but its skillful application by the trained occupational therapist or assistant. This will be explored further in Chapters 19 through 23.

REFERENCES

1. Eliot G. Adam Bede (1859). In: Maggio R, compiler. *The Beacon book of quotations by women.* Boston: Beacon Press, 1992:2.
2. Giles GM. Anorexia nervosa and bulimia: an activity-oriented approach. *Am J Occup Ther* 1985;39:510-517.
3. Hayes R. Occupational therapy in the treatment of schizophrenia. *Occup Ther Mental Health* 1989;9(3):51–68.
4. Hughes PL, Mullins L. *Acute psychiatric care: an occupational therapy guide to exercises in daily living skills.* Thorofare, NJ: SLACK; 1981.
5. Kartin NJ, Van Schroeder C. *Adult psychiatric life skills manual.* Kailua, Hawaii: Schroeder Publishing and Consulting; 1982.
6. Kaseman BM. Teaching money management skills to psychiatric outpatients. *Occup Ther Mental Health* 1980;1(3):59–71.
7. Korb KL, Azok AD, Leutenberg EA. *Life management skills—reproducible activity handouts created for facilitators.* Beachwood, Ohio: Wellness Reproductions; 1989.
8. Korb KL, Azok AD, Leutenberg EA. *Life management skills II—reproducible activity handouts created for facilitators.* Beachwood, Ohio: Wellness Reproductions, 1991.
9. Lakein A. *How to get control of your time and your life.* New York: Peter H Wyden; 1973.
10. Pfeiffer JW, Jones JE, eds. *A handbook of structured experiences for human relations training, volumes I–VL.* La Jolla, Calif: University Associates; 1977.
11. Remocker AJ, Storch ET. *Action speaks louder: a handbook of nonverbal group techniques.* 3rd ed. Edinburgh: Churchill Livingstone; 1982.
12. Schwartzenberg SL. Motivation for activities of daily living: a study of selected psychiatric patients' self-reports. *Occup Ther Mental Health* 1982;2(3):1–26.

13. Weaver RL. *Understanding interpersonal conversation*. Glenview, Ill: Scott, Foresman; 1981.
14. Wells SJ. Caffeine: implications of recent research for clinical practice. *Am J Orthopsychiatry* 1984;54:375–389.
15. Willson M. *Occupational therapy in long-term psychiatry*. Edinburgh: Churchill Livingstone; 1983.

ADDITIONAL REFERENCES AND SUGGESTED READINGS

Allen CK, Earhart CA, Blue T. *Occupational therapy treatment goals for the physically and cognitively disabled*. Rockville, Md: American Occupation Therapy Association; 1992.

Becker RE, Page MS. Psychotherapeutically oriented rehabilitation in chronic mental illness. *Am J Occup Ther* 1973;27:34–38.

Ben-Shlomo LS, Short MA. The effects of physical exercise on self-attitudes. *Occup Ther Mental Health* 1985/86;3(4):11–28.

Ben-Shlomo LS, Short MA. The effects of physical conditioning on selected dimensions of self concept in sedentary females. *Occup Ther Mental Health* 1983;5(4):27–46.

Berland T. *The fitness fact book: the complete guide to diet, exercise and sport*. New York: Signet; 1980.

Broekema MC. Occupational therapy in a community aftercare program. *Am J Occup Ther* 1975; 29:22–27.

Earhart CA. Occupational therapy groups. In: Allen CA, ed. *Occupational therapy for psychiatric diseases: measurement and management of cognitive disabilities*. Boston: Little, Brown; 1985.

Giles GM, Allen ME. Occupational therapy in the rehabilitation of the patient with anorexia nervosa. *Occup Ther Mental Health* 1986;6(1):47–66.

Harris D. *The Woman's Day guide to organizing your life*. New York: Owl (Holt, Rinehart, Winston); 1985.

Hasselkus BR. The meaning of daily activity in family caregiving for the elderly. *Am J Occup Ther* 1989;43:649–656.

Hemphill BJ, Peterson CQ, Werner PC. *Rehabilitation in mental health—goals and objectives for independent living*. Thorofare, NJ: SLACK; 1991.

Katz J. *Swimming for total fitness: a progressive aerobic program*. New York: Dolphin/Doubleday; 1981.

Kramer LW. SCORE: solving community obstacles and restoring employment. *Occup Ther Mental Health* 1984;4(1):1–135.

Maslen DM. Rehabilitation training for community living skills: concepts and techniques. *Occup Ther Mental Health* 1982;2(1):33–49.

Mosey AC. *Activities therapy*. New York: Raven Press; 1973.

Neville A. Temporal adaptation: application with short-term psychiatric patients. *Am J Occup Ther* 1980;34:328–331.

Nochajski SB, Gordon CY. The use of trivial pursuit in teaching community living skills to adults with developmental disabilities. *Am J Occup Ther* 1987;41:10–15.

Ogren K. A living skills program in an acute psychiatric setting. *Am Occup Ther Assoc Mental Health Special Interest Section Newsletter* 1983; 6(4):1–2.

Robinson AM, Avallone J. Occupational therapy in acute inpatient psychiatry: an activities health approach. *Am J Occup Ther* 1990;44:809–814.

Thomes LJ, Bajema SL. The life skills development program: a history, overview and update. *Occup Ther Mental Health* 1983;3(2):35–48.

Trace S, Howell T. Occupational therapy in geriatric mental health. *Am J Occup Ther* 1991;45:833–837.

Vishnudevananda S. *The complete illustrated book of yoga*. New York: Pocket Books; 1960.

Weissenberg R, Giladi N. Home economics day: a program for disturbed adolescents to promote acquisition of habits and skills. *Occup Ther Mental Health* 1989;9(2):89–103.

Willson M. *Occupational Therapy in short-term psychiatry*. Edinburgh: Churchill Livingstone; 1984.

19

Work, Homemaking, and Child Care

To be successfully employed, one must view oneself as employable.

CRIST AND STOFFEL (1, p. 435)

WORK SKILLS

Work is a major life role for the average nondisabled adult; for most people it consumes at least half of their waking hours, and provides a sense of self-worth, identity, and a place in the social structure. By using time in ways that are of value to others, the worker experiences his contribution to the world and affirms his place within it. People who are unable to work, for whatever reason, are therefore deprived of a major source of personal satisfaction and social identity.

Many psychiatric patients have problems with work. Those who have been ill for a long time may have little or no experience of working, and thus no real understanding of the behaviors expected in a work setting. Nonetheless, even among the chronically mentally ill, the desire to work and to have an identity as a worker is quite strong. Others may have cognitive disabilities that prevent their making sense of a typical work environment or of tasks that require even minimal decision making. Still others (this is particularly true of those with character disorders) fail over and over again because they act without thinking, relate hostilely or negatively to others, fail to organize their tasks, or do not take responsibility for their own behavior.

Work-oriented occupational therapy evaluation and treatment is designed to assess the individual's work potential, assist him in developing basic task skills and work behaviors, and help him make the transition to a productive worker role or to further training for a vocation. These programs are obviously appropriate only for those patients with a history of failure at work, or no work history at all, or who need a different kind of work that is more suited to their present interests and functional level.

Work-related programming for psychiatric patients often involves working with other professionals and paraprofessionals. Vocational counselors, rehabilitation counselors, job coaches, work adjustment specialists, work evaluators, and job placement specialists all provide services similar to those that might be provided by occupational therapy. The role of occupational therapy and of the occupational therapy assistant will be affected by the availability of these specialized personnel, the needs of the client population, and the relevant local and federal regulations affecting the service delivery agency. As in any other professional situation, it is important to work cooperatively with other staff, offering services in a manner that is noncompetitive and in the best interests of those to be served.

Prevocational Evaluation

The first step in a work-oriented program is prevocational evaluation, to assess the individual's present work skills and to estimate his potential for work. Sometimes this is called *work potential evaluation.* The areas evaluated include such basic task skills as:

1. *Attendance, punctuality, and productivity* (rate of production)
2. *Work attitudes and social and interpersonal behaviors* such as accepting responsibility for oneself, accepting direction from a supervisor, and relating to peers
3. *Cognitive factors* such as memory, organization, and sequencing of a task
4. *Physical factors* such as standing tolerance, stamina, and eye-hand coordination (which may be impaired by disuse, drug side effects, or the disease process).

Prevocational evaluation is different from *vocational evaluation,* which assesses the individual's interests, talents, and skills for a particular kind of work.

Evaluation methods include the use of job samples (also known as work samples) and work simulation experiences. A *job sample* is a selected piece of the kind of work that is done in a particular job; for example, a job sample for an electrician might involve cutting, stripping, twisting, and taping wire connections. This work would be timed and compared to the average time a "real" electrician would take. Several systems of prepared job samples are commercially available. Although such systems (VALPAR is one example) are expensive, because they are standardized they can provide a normed result. Job samples prepared ad hoc by a therapist may give useful measures of a patient's work potential for an immediate local situation (e.g., a sheltered workshop with specific jobs), but these may not help in comparing the patient's work abilities to those of the nondisabled population. *Work simulation* is a method that involves placing the patient in a work-like setting (work group) on the hospital grounds, in a sheltered workshop, or in the community in order to see how he adapts to it, and thus to predict whether he could succeed in a job.

Prevocational evaluation should be performed by a registered therapist with specific training or experience in selection and design of job samples and other evaluation methods. The occupational therapy assistant may be designated to carry out parts of the evaluation. The purpose of the evaluation is to arrive at a *realistic* assessment of the individual's potential for work; it is important for any evaluator to be objective and to follow standardized procedures exactly in order for the results to be useful.

Several important issues should be considered in any prevocational evaluation or work-related program. One is the question of whether it is realistic or feasible for a particular patient to work now or in the future. At a time of high unemployment one must consider whether disabled mental patients will really be able to compete for jobs. Similarly, the prospect of guaranteed disability income may dampen a patient's motivation to work. Certainly if the likelihood of a patient's obtaining and keeping a job seems insecure, it is unethical for the therapist or assistant to recommend that he seek employment and forfeit his rights to disability assistance. Depending on the answers to these questions, and the results of the evaluation, the patient is then referred to a service that meets his particular needs. If he is eligible for assistance, services may be funded and arranged by the state office of vocational rehabilitation.

Work Adjustment Programs

A work adjustment program (sometimes called *personal adjustment training*) helps patients acquire basic work habits, work attitudes, and social skills. Such programs are directed toward the more functionally impaired client, who needs to reach a socially acceptable level of performance in these skills before competitive employment can be a realistic option. Both inpatient and outpatient programs exist, some permitting or requiring attendance for 30 to 40 hours weekly. Such programs may include training in activities of daily living (especially grooming and hygiene), social skills training, communication skills development, and work behaviors. Work groups, including assembly lines and service groups (e.g., to provide meals to the homebound, or to clean the park), are used to simulate a real work environment and to allow participants to practice work behaviors. Patients are assigned tasks and job responsibilities and are expected to behave and perform as they would be expected to on the job. Behavioral methods such as feedback and reinforcement are widely used in these programs. Videotape is very popular as a feedback medium; clients can critique themselves and their peers at the end of the work day.

The occupational therapy assistant in a work adjustment program may lead discussion groups or work groups, or provide counseling and feedback on an individual case-management basis. For example, the assistant may help a very impulsive patient learn to stop herself, and to think about what she is doing before acting; it may take many separate conversations for this message to get across to the patient. Or the assistant might help someone with limited work tolerance explore why he is so easily bored by the work, and why he avoids work by leaving early. There are many, many issues involved in successful work adjustment that require sensitivity on the part of the assistant. A patient's problems with work may be based on expectations learned from his parents, on personal beliefs, or simply on lack of positive prior experience and lack of knowledge of what is expected.

Successful intervention must be based on accurate assessment of the problem.

Vocational Evaluation and Training

Patients who successfully complete a work adjustment program may then be referred for evaluation of their potential for different kinds of work. Those patients whose basic task skills and work behaviors are adequate but who have no marketable or usable job skills may also enter vocational evaluation directly after prevocational evaluation. Vocational evaluation may be performed by a certified rehabilitation counselor or vocational evaluation specialist, or by a registered occupational therapist, or sometimes by all three. The patient is given paper-and-pencil tests that measure his interests, such as the Kuder or the Strong-Campbell, and other evaluations that measure specific job-related skills (such as the Minnesota Paper-Form Board Test, which measures visual-spatial abilities). The purpose is to assess the patient's potential for and interest in various kinds of work, and to help him, through discussion, to select an area for further training. Helping the patient substitute more realistic choices for interests that are unrealistic (e.g., astronaut, judge, neurologist) occurs at this step. The next step is to arrange for him to enter a training program in, for example, a trade school or community college. Financial, administrative, and advisory support from the state office of vocational rehabilitation is often available.

Role Maintenance Programs

Patients who have jobs already may find hospitalization very disruptive to their work habits and skills; they can be helped to maintain their role responsibilities and skills by participating in a role maintenance group (13). The purpose of such a group is to help the patient identify which responsibilities he can continue during hospitalization, and assist him in communicating and negotiating with his employer and family (important for homemakers). The therapist and the group discuss ways in which the worker's tasks can be redesigned, or if necessary delegated to others.

Later, the patient and the therapist arrange for a gradual transition back to the worker role, by gradually increasing the amount of time the patient spends out in the community doing his job. For example, a secretary might go back to work first on a part-time basis.

Richert (12) described a vocational transition group co-led by an occupational therapist and a vocational counselor. The purpose of this group was to assist psychiatric inpatients to make the transition back to work after discharge. Activities and focuses of this group included identifying personal goals, discussing and problem-solving job stressors, and exploring fears of stigma and prejudice from coworkers.

Job Search Skills and Job Placement

Those who already have adequate and marketable job skills but who do not have a job may be referred to a job search skills group in which they work toward obtaining a job. Patients with good job skills sometimes have trouble getting work because their social skills are poor and they behave oddly during telephone inquiries or job interviews. Still others do not know how to find job leads or write résumés or complete job application forms. Another problem is the difficulty many have in explaining why they have not worked for long periods during hospitalization. (A patient might be counseled to say that she was caring for a sick relative, for example.) All of these problems are compounded by feelings of insecurity and anxiety.

There are several ways to approach the task of teaching patients job search skills. Discussion groups by themselves have limited value, unless they include expectations and opportunities to practice skills both within and outside of the group meeting. Groups that use an educational (classroom) format seem more effective. Kramer and Beidel (9) developed a series of 10 classroom lessons designed to teach interviewing, finding and following up on job leads, résumé writing, and other skills; interviews of group members by hospital staff who were simulating the roles of employers were videotaped and reviewed to improve performance. Homework was assigned in each session, to be completed before the next lesson; exercises included filling out job application forms and coming up with answers to difficult questions an interviewer might ask.[1]

A similar classroom or seminar format was used in the Altrusa Work Readiness Seminar (10). This program was designed for female patients with chronic psychiatric disorders and consisted of five seminars on work readiness and community living. Community leaders and businesspeople provided the instruction, which focused not so much on job search skills as on self-awareness, consumerism, and money management.

Even with a highly structured format that requires member involvement and participation, some patients will not follow through with the skills they learn and actually obtain a job. Some may need more practice, and others may not really be motivated to work.

One approach that has been used with some success is that of placing the client temporarily in a job within the treatment setting or in a volunteer job in the community. Some community employers have been willing to allow a part-time position to be filled by a series of patients each of whom rotates through it for a short period; once the patient becomes comfortable with the idea of working, he is encouraged to move on to a regular job.

---

[1]The exercises and corresponding homework sheets can be found in Kramer (8).

The Americans with Disabilities Act of 1990

Title I of the Americans with Disabilities Act (ADA) of 1990 protects persons with physical and mental impairments from discrimination in employment due to disability. For the ADA to be effective, occupational therapists and assistants may be called upon to assist the individual to fit the work environment or vice versa. Crist and Stoffel (1) described three tasks for occupational therapy in assisting persons with mental disabilities to enter and remain in the work force. The first is to provide advocacy training for patients as well as for employers and coworkers. Advocacy training promotes the acceptance of persons with disabilities, encourages alliance with the value that work is a right for all, and teaches strategies that assist the nondisabled to work effectively with persons with mental impairments. The second is to increase, through training, the mentally disabled worker's *self-efficacy,* or belief about his skills and competence. The third is to work with employers to analyze jobs, identify their essential functions, and work out accommodations so that they can be performed by disabled individuals. Such accommodations might include, for example, flexible or part-time scheduling.

Task Groups and Work Groups

Groups in which participants work on simple tasks are often used as a setting for prevocational evaluation and for work adjustment. The underlying assumption is that basic task skills such as attention span, neatness, speed, and attention to detail are needed for all kinds of jobs; in other words, these skills affect the quality of the work whether the patient is sewing a pincushion, typing a letter, or transplanting seedlings. Therefore, any task that is structured and that has recognizable standards can be used to evaluate and teach these basic task skills. These simple, humble activities may

be less threatening initially for a psychiatric patient who would be overwhelmed by the idea of having a real job or by being assessed for one.

Traditionally, task groups and work groups were different names for the same kind of group; today, however, it appears that therapists generally use the term *task group* to mean a highly structured group in which very low functioning patients learn basic task skills. Among the basic task skills taught or reinforced in task groups are the ability to attend to a task long enough to complete it, the ability to use tools and materials safely and without waste, the ability to work at a consistent and productive rate, the ability to recognize errors and problems, and the ability to work neatly and with attention to detail. Such task skills are basic to successful completion of most tasks across many life roles—student, worker, homemaker, hobbyist, etc. In such a group each patient works independently, on his own project, and receives individual attention from the therapist or assistant leading the group. Patients may all do similar projects or different ones; projects are designed to be completed in a relatively short period.

Although patients in such groups are encouraged to work on neatness and attention span and other basic skills, they are not expected to perform complex tasks, or to work for long periods, or to interact much with others. The task skills that they develop or relearn in these groups are a foundation for more complex work behavior, just as the work habits acquired by the preschool child are the same skills she will need later to succeed in school and ultimately on the job.

Helping a patient develop task skills requires intense concentration from the therapist working with him. It is important first of all to analyze exactly what the patient needs to do to improve his performance, and to communicate this clearly to him. For example, someone who fails to notice errors in his work must be taught how to check his work, and to understand what an error looks like and how to correct it. Close supervision and immediate feedback are essential. Some patients may become distracted, confused, or overwhelmed if asked to work on more than one problem at a time, and so the therapist should design the learning experiences in steps or stages.

Work groups are designed to simulate a work environment; the group actually produces a product or provides a service. Patients who have at least parallel-level group interaction skills and some basic task skills are generally eligible (11). Participants are assigned specific job tasks and different levels of responsibility; behavior appropriate in a work setting is expected, and acting-out is discouraged. The group leader designs and analyzes the tasks the group will perform, and divides and assigns them to members. Patients are expected to do the jobs they are assigned and to work for the full time, just as they would in paid employment. These groups generally meet at least three times a week, and for relatively long periods (two hours or more). Activities that are suitable for a work group are those that can be structured into clear tasks and work roles. Among the many possible tasks might be refinishing furniture, cleaning the treatment center, preparing food for others, or doing office work.

One popular format is the *production line,* in which a product is manufactured by dividing the task into steps that are performed by different members; each person does only a part of the process, and then passes the item along to the person who does the next step. For example, in a jewelry production line, one member might design the beading sequence for two or three different necklaces. Another patient might be assigned to attach the jump rings to the cords; others would actually string the beads, following the designed samples; and one or two others would finish the necklaces by knotting the cords and attaching the catches. Other jobs in this group might include acting as foreman or work supervisor, counting supplies and finished neck-

laces, and boxing or packaging them. A problem that often arises in this type of group is that many of the members want the glamorous jobs of designer or foreman; discussion of this issue after the group's work is finished for the day gives members a chance to work through their feelings about this and about equivalent situations in the work world.

Production lines may employ many different media, including woodwork, ceramics, leathercraft, horticulture, printed matter, and assembly, sorting, or packaging of items produced elsewhere. Some production lines sell their products through hospital gift shops or concessions or bazaars; other provide services through contracts with departments in the treatment setting or with outside companies. Members are often paid for their work. For a production line to work well, the jobs within it must be designed so that each worker has enough work; it may be necessary to assign several jobs to one person, or to give several individuals the same job. Producing a saleable product, or one that is of value to others (e.g., assembling a mailing for the hospital) is also important. The staff member in charge of the group is responsible for ordering and obtaining supplies, for maintaining the environment and equipment used by the group, and for monitoring the quality of the product. At times a higher functioning patient may take over these duties, which are similar to those of an administrator, supervisor, foreman, or manager.

Safety is a concern in production lines that employ power tools, heat, or toxic substances. Safety equipment that complies with OSHA regulations should be used, and patients must be instructed in safety guidelines and emergency procedures. Patients who have visual disturbances, seizures, or motor incoordination should be watched closely and not assigned to work where they might injure themselves. Similar precautions should be taken for patients who have poor judgment or other cognitive deficits, or who are potentially violent or suicidal.

Clerical groups focus on office skills and may be designed around a division of labor similar to a production line (in fact, they are sometimes called office production lines). The activity is the production of printed matter; tasks might include typing or word processing, taking dictation or transcribing from a machine, using a computer for numerical entry or data base work, using duplicating equipment, collating, stuffing envelopes, or sorting outgoing mail by zip code. It is becoming increasingly necessary to have electronic typewriters, word processing equipment, and computers available if patients are actually to be trained to provide secretarial services in the business world. Patients who already have word processing skills also need opportunities to practice and maintain them.

A *newspaper* or *journal group* is a variation on the clerical group, but one that requires more initiative, creativity, and decision making from its members. The group's major activity is to write, edit, type, print, and distribute a newsletter or similar publication. Although many different job functions and levels of responsibility can be designated within the group, it is often left up to the members to decide who does what on a day-to-day basis. In some senses this type of group may be more effective for teaching interpersonal skills than work behaviors. Nonetheless, negotiations among members about what to report, what to print, and what to censor provide opportunities to practice group interaction skills needed for some kinds of jobs. This sort of group is feasible only in long-term or community settings, where membership can remain constant for some time.

Service concessions for the treatment center or for the community are yet another type of work group. A *food service* or *coffee shop* work group provides food and beverages, usually for only a few hours a day. The staff member in charge of this type of group is responsible for making sure that

proper health and sanitary precautions are followed with regard to food storage and handling and maintenance of the equipment and the food preparation area. Accounting and managing of the proceeds from sales is finally the group leader's responsibility, although patients may be assigned these tasks and then supervised. Other service concessions that are sometimes used as work groups in psychiatric settings are a patient *library* and a *child care service* (the latter is possible only where legal requirements permit). Other work groups may be based on the sale in a *boutique* or *thrift shop* of goods made in production lines or items gotten through donations. These groups provide an opportunity for members to practice interpersonal skills needed to relate to the public.

In summary, all of these different kinds of work groups provide a milieu in which patients can practice behaviors appropriate for the work world. Although the same basic work behaviors are reinforced in all of these groups, there are also opportunities for different kinds of learning in different groups. Placement of patients in groups and assignment of patients to particular jobs within groups should be based not on the patient's preference for the particular medium or activity used in that group, but on the group's ability to provide experiences that will help him learn how to succeed at a job. Detailed examples of goals and objectives for work behavior can be found in Hemphill, Peterson, and Werner (2).

Task Groups and the Role of Work for Children and Adolescents

As was discussed in Chapter 6, skills and habits learned during childhood and adolescence lay a foundation for the role of worker in adult life. Therefore, occupational therapy programs for young people with mental health problems generally include activities that provide opportunities to learn and practice these skills. Young children and grade school students can acquire work habits by being made responsible for household chores and school assignments. Within an inpatient treatment setting it is sometimes difficult to create opportunities for every child to perform a task that contributes to the family or the community, but requiring children to clean up after themselves, to put away toys and games and materials, and to wipe the tables and sweep the floor after an activity is a start. Children also need opportunities to fantasize about various adult roles. One way to address this is through costume play and games that involve imitation of adult worker roles. Films, field trips, and visits by adults in different occupations also increase children's awareness of the role of the adult worker.

The adolescent is faced with important decisions about his future occupational role. To choose a career that suits his interests and abilities the adolescent needs to know what his interests and abilities are; this knowledge can be developed through participation in a wide range of activities. It is very important to allow the adolescent to explore areas that interest him, and to expose him to other activities of which he may not be aware, since he will choose his career on the basis of what he knows.

In addition, since the main occupational role of children and adolescents is that of student, occupational therapy task groups can be used to reinforce basic task skills and study habits that support this role. For example, a teenager whose attention span is only about 15 minutes long cannot possibly succeed in a regular school program; by participating in a basic task skills group, he could work on concentrating for longer periods while enjoying an activity that is probably less stressful than school. At the same time, if hospitalized he would attend classes taught by special education teachers within the hospital; if an outpatient, he might attend a regular public school but be in a special class or go to a resource room for extra help during certain class periods each day. The occupational therapist or assistant might provide individual help by providing an environment where he can do his homework, and sometimes by teaching study, note-taking, and test-taking skills.

Sheltered Work Programs

Sheltered work programs provide a work-like experience for persons whose disabilities are so severe that they will never be able, realistically, to enter competitive employment. Such programs help patients achieve a sense of direction, purpose, and productivity by performing simple tasks within a relatively stress-free environment. Long-term placement gives participants a feeling of being productive and making a contribution to the extent they are capable; this is very important for a person's sense of self-worth. Pay is generally based on the amount of work or number of pieces completed, as a fraction of what a nondisabled worker might complete in the same time.

Sheltered work programs are sometimes found within hospital settings, especially in large public institutions, and also in the community; many are operated by charitable organizations such as Goodwill Industries, the Lighthouse, and others. The work itself is usually highly structured and divided into measurable units; assembly and packaging of small items are typical activities. The rates at which workers are paid for their work vary across the country; court decisions have interpreted the Fair Labor Standards Act of 1966 to mean that working patients must be paid when their work benefits the hospital or agency. Generally, payment is below minimum wage and usually based on some measurable criterion such as the number of pieces produced (as compared to workers in competitive employment) or hours worked.

Another model that is sometimes used is *job sharing,* in which several clients share the same job. As a group they may work for more hours (total) than a nondisabled worker, but they are paid (as a group) at the same rate. Their wages are divided according to the relative contributions of each person sharing the job. Typically, a staff member serves as *job coach,* and learns the job, teaches it to the patients, and even fills in when the patient is absent and there is no one else present to do the job. Because the needs of patients in these programs remain relatively constant, occupational therapy assistants can administer sheltered work programs with only modest amounts of supervision from a registered therapist.

Some sheltered work programs are designed so that participants who qualify may graduate into placement in community jobs. Howe, Weaver, and Dulay (4) created a program in which the sheltered work component involved a choice of either house and grounds maintenance work or food services. Classes in daily living skills and various work skills were also included. Patients who consistently demonstrated strong basic task skills and cooperative work attitudes were encouraged to join a transitional employment program, in which they could work first on a volunteer basis and then as a paid employee in an entry-level job at, for example, McDonald's.

HOMEMAKING AND CHILD-CARE SKILLS

Taking care of a home and children is a full-time job, equally as taxing as most paid employment. In fact, the job of homemaker and parent is *more* difficult than many jobs, because the person has to structure and organize the entire process; there is no one to tell her what to do and when. In addition, there are so many different subtasks within the job, and so many possibilities about how to do them, that the homemaker/parent can easily become overwhelmed or discouraged. Programs that help patients learn, practice, and maintain their homemaking and child care skills are usually vocationally oriented, meaning that they view

the job of homemaker as a work role that requires all of the task skills and many of the work behaviors needed for paid employment.

Areas in which the occupational therapy assistant might provide training or practice include meal preparation, housecleaning, and care of children; home decorating and home repair and entertaining may also be included. Skills such as laundry care and money management are considered part of daily living skills but are sometimes taught in a vocationally oriented homemaker training program. Detailed objectives and goals for household management can be found in Hemphill, Peterson, and Werner (2).

A *meal preparation* training program may have an educational or classroom format. Kitchen safety, food storage and handling, nutrition concepts, and meal planning are the first skills taught. Basic cooking skills and use of convenience foods are taught next. Proper mealtime manners and how to set a table and clean up afterward are practiced within the context of actually consuming a meal. Grocery shopping and cost comparison skills and the use of measures (cups, spoons) and weights are often also included. Patients are taught to use a dishwasher and other kitchen appliances (e.g., microwave, food processor) only if they will actually have these appliances in their homes. Obviously it makes sense to teach these skills in the appropriate environments (kitchen, dining area, grocery store). Electrical appliances, knives, and other sharp implements should be used only under close supervision.

Activities covered in a *housekeeping* training sequence include making and changing beds, emptying of ashtrays and trash, airing of rooms and linens, use of a broom and mop and dustrag and other household cleaning tools, storing dangerous products out of reach of children, and procedures such as how to change a light bulb and how to turn off the water if there is a leak. Patients with cognitive impairments may need to be reminded to clean areas that are out of sight, for example underneath the toilet and the bed. Not everyone owns a vacuum cleaner, and so its use should be taught judiciously. Other topics that should be covered in housekeeping are knowing when to repair something yourself and when and where to get help from the superintendent, plumber, or handyman. Patients also need to learn which cleaning products, paper products, and other housekeeping products provide the best value for the money.

In teaching or reinforcing homemaking skills, the occupational therapy assistant must respect the culture and values of the client. Recent immigrants from third-world countries may wish to continue to keep house in the manner to which they have been accustomed. This should be accepted, as long as the particular practices do not violate social norms in a manner that might be offensive to the neighbors. Alternatively, immigrants from rural or poor areas may fail to understand the purpose of technological aids, and for example (in a true case), attempt unsuccessfully to use a dishwasher to do laundry.

Child-care and *parenting skills* cover a wide range of topics. Some parents may need to learn about children's basic needs and how to provide for them. Some parents may have had inadequate parenting themselves, having suffered from neglect, violence, or poverty, and may need time and support to learn new ways to behave. These parents may say, in effect, "*My* parents did okay by me, and they loved me, so I'm going to do things the way *they* did." Such parents may not recognize that their abusive behavior and failure to provide appropriate nurturing may result in developmental deficits in their children (3).

Others may need to learn to talk to their children, or how to praise and nurture them, or how to discipline them effectively, or how to help them structure their time. They may be unaware of community resources where they can receive guidance and ongoing support. Still others may have trouble thinking of things they can do to-

gether with their children. These skills may be taught through group discussion, paper-and-pencil exercises, review of videotaped situations, and role playing, as well as through actual practice with children.

In the area of children's basic needs, some severely disabled psychiatric patients may have trouble keeping their children properly cleaned, clothed, and fed; these patients need supervision on a daily basis, but with enough practice and reinforcement may be able to learn enough to function more independently. A social worker usually works closely with the occupational therapist or assistant in such cases, because of the real possibility that the child may be harmed by the parent's neglect.

A more common problem, shared by parents from all social classes and all levels of disability, is that of how to communicate with children. Parents need to know what a child of a given age is capable of understanding, what he is likely to be interested in, and what his emotional needs are. Discussion groups, augmented by printed reminders with developmental issues listed for each age, are often used. This is also a good way to help parents identify appropriate toys for their children, and to help them think of activities they and their children might do together.

Another problem many parents share is their concern over children's bad behavior and how to discipline them. Discussion with other parents is extremely valuable in helping parents develop a sense of what constitutes a reasonable punishment for a particular misdeed committed by a child of a given age. This is especially important for parents with delinquent adolescent children, who often feel frustrated, overwhelmed, and helpless in dealing with their child's behavior.

Unfortunately, relatively few lesson plans and activities for developing child-care skills have been described in the occupational therapy literature. Those that do exist (5,6,7) provide only a few exercises focusing on limited areas of need. Therefore, the occupational therapist or assistant must create her own materials and activities from the available developmental literature and other sources. The occupational therapy assistant should work under the supervision of, or at the very least in consultation with, a registered occupational therapist with pediatric training and experience.

CONCLUSION

This chapter has focused on the areas of work, homemaking, and child care. Each of these areas of activities provides roles through which a person can contribute to the human community. An adult's self-esteem is deeply rooted in his sense of productivity and his belief about his own contributions and achievements. Occupational therapists and assistants can enhance and maintain their patients' ability to be productive and to see themselves as such, by supporting them as they engage in work-related roles in sheltered or competitive employment or in the home and within the family.

REFERENCES

1. Crist PAH, Stoffel VC. The Americans with Disabilities Act of 1990 and employees with mental impairments: personal efficacy and the environment. *Am J Occup Ther* 1992;46:434–443.
2. Hemphill BJ, Peterson CQ, Werner PC. *Rehabilitation in mental health: goals and objectives for independent living.* Thorofare, NJ: SLACK; 1991.
3. Howard AC. Developmental play ages of physically abused and nonabused children. *Am J Occup Ther* 1986;40:691–695.
4. Howe MC, Weaver CT, Dulay J. The development of a work-oriented day center program. *Am J Occup Ther* 1981;35:711–718.
5. Hughes PL, Mullins L. *Acute psychiatric care: an occupational therapy guide to exercises in daily living skills.* Thorofare, NJ: SLACK, 1981.
6. Korb KL, Azok AD, Leutenberg EA. *Life management skills: reproducible activity handouts created for facilitators.* Beachwood, Ohio: Wellness Reproductions; 1989.
7. Korb KL, Azok AD, Leutenberg EA. *Life management skills II: reproducible activity handouts created for facilitators.* Beachwood, Ohio: Wellness Reproductions; 1991.
8. Kramer LW. SCORE: Solving community obstacles and restoring employment. *Occup Ther Mental Health* 1984;4(1):1–135.
9. Kramer LW, Beidel DC. Job seeking skills groups: a review and application to a chronic population. *Occup Ther Mental Health* 1982; 2(2):37–44.
10. Mauras-Corsino E, Daniewicz CV, Swan LC. The use of community networks for chronic psychiatric patients. *Am J Occup Ther* 1985;39:374–378.
11. Mosey AC. *Activities therapy.* New York: Raven Press; 1973.
12. Richert GZ. Vocational transition in acute care psychiatry. *Occup Ther Mental Health* 1990; 10(4):43–61.
13. Versluys HP. The remediation of role disorders through focused group work. *Am J Occup Ther* 1980;34:609–614.

ADDITIONAL REFERENCES AND SUGGESTED READINGS

Allen CK, Earhart CA, Blue T. *Occupational therapy treatment goals for the physically and cognitively disabled.* Rockville, Md: American Occupational Therapy Association; 1992.
Anderson AP. Work potential evaluation in mental health. *Am J Occup Ther* 1985;39:659–663.
Bettleheim B. *A good enough parent.* New York: Vintage; 1987.
Crary E. *Without spanking or spoiling: a practical approach to toddler and preschool guidance.* Seattle: Parenting Press; 1979.
Custer VL, Wassink KE. Occupational therapy intervention for an adult with depression and suicidal tendencies. *Am J Occup Ther* 1991;45:845–848.
Dooley S. Program description: prevocational assessment center. *Am Occup Ther Assoc Mental Health Special Interest Section Newsletter* 1985; 8(4):3.
Earhart CA. Occupational therapy groups. In: Allen CA, ed. *Occupational therapy for psychiatric diseases: measurement and management of cognitive disabilities.* Boston: Little, Brown; 1985.
Ellsworth P, Davy J, Mitcham M, Parking J, Presseller S. The role of occupational therapy in the vocational rehabilitation process (official position paper). *Am J Occup Ther* 1979;34:881–883.
Faber A, Mazlish E. *How to talk so kids will listen and listen so kids will talk.* New York: Avon; 1980.
Fidler G. The task-oriented group as a context for treatment. *Am J Occup Ther* 1969;23:43–48.
Gordon T. *P.E.T.: parent effectiveness training.* New York: Penguin, New American Library; 1970.
Harris D. *The Woman's Day guide to organizing your life.* New York: Owl (Holt, Rinehart, Winston); 1985;
Harvey-Krefting L. The concept of work in occupa-

tional therapy: a historical review. *Am J Occup Ther* 1985;39:301–307.

Hightower-Vandamm M. The role of occupational therapy in vocational evaluation, part 1. *Am J Occup Ther* 1981;35:563–565.

Hightower-Vandamm M. The role of occupational therapy in vocational evaluation, part 2. *Am J Occup Ther* 1981;35:631–633.

Howe MC, Weaver CT, Dulay J. The development of a work-oriented day center program. *Am J Occup Ther* 1981;35:711–718.

Jacobs K. *Occupational therapy: work-related programs and assessments.* Boston: Little, Brown; 1985.

Kartin NJ, Van Schroeder C. *Adult psychiatric life skills manual.* Kailua, Hawaii: Schroeder Publishing and Consulting; 1982.

Krueger CW. *1001 things to do with your kids.* Nashville: Abingdon; 1988.

Lewin JV, Lewin RA. On treatment integration: psychotherapy and work therapy. *Occup Ther Mental Health* 1987;7(3):21–36.

Loukas KM. The issue is—motherhood, occupational therapy, and feminism: weaving or unraveling the fibers of our lives? *Am J Occup Ther* 1992;46:1039–1041.

Mitchell M, Rourk JD, Schwarz J. A team approach to prevocational services. *Am J Occup Ther* 1989;43:378–383.

Palmer F, Barrows C. Vocational activities for adolescents: a program description. *Occup Ther Assoc Mental Health Special Interest Section Newsletter* 1985;8(4):1–2.

Primeau LA. A woman's place: unpaid work in the home. *Am J Occup Ther* 1992;46:981–988.

Radonsky VE, et al. Occupational therapy in vocational readiness. *Occup Ther Mental Health* 1987;7(3):83–91.

Richert GZ, Merryman MB. The vocational continuum: a model for providing vocational services in a partial hospitalization program. *Occup Ther Mental Health* 1987;7(3):1–20.

Solberg NA, Chueh W. Performance in occupational therapy as a predictor of successful prevocational training. *Am J Occup Ther* 1976;30:481–486.

Stauffer DL. Predicting successful employment in the community for people with a history of chronic mental illness. *Occup Ther Mental Health* 1986;6(2):31–49.

Watts FN. Modification of the employment handicaps of psychiatric patients by behavioral methods. *Am J Occup Ther* 1976;30:487–490.

Willson M. *Occupational therapy in long-term psychiatry.* Edinburgh: Churchill Livingstone; 1983.

20

Leisure Skills

He hath no leisure who useth it not.

GEORGE HERBERT (4)

LEISURE SKILLS

Leisure is the use of time for activities that are personally satisfying and not related to work. In a sense, leisure or recreation actually re-creates the capacity to work, by restoring lost energy and refreshing the spirit. Leisure activities reflect the personal preferences, values, and interests of the individual. Unless these activities are chosen by the patient, there is no reason to believe that he will find them satisfying or refreshing; in fact, staff members may discover that some patients enjoy activities that the staff finds boring, childish, or unpleasant. You need only think about your own family, friends, and acquaintances to realize that not everyone likes listening to rock music, or opera, and that some people prefer playing bingo, collecting stamps, or riding mountain bikes. It should be obvious that in order to improve a patient's use of leisure time you have to help him do the activities that *he* wants to do.

Leisure Planning

Unfortunately, one of the problems some patients experience is that they do not know (or cannot remember) what they enjoy doing in their spare time. Older persons who have recently retired and homemakers whose children are now grown may have difficulty filling the hours that they used to spend in working, and may have little idea of their own interests. There are two approaches to dealing with this problem: One is to review the patient's history, perhaps even back to childhood, or to speak with family members to identify activities that the person engaged in previously. Another approach is to schedule the patient for one or two leisure groups, help him discuss his reaction to the activities, and plan future activities from there. Discussion can focus on which activities were enjoyed, and why. This is perhaps the best approach when the patient really is not familiar with many activities and has no clear sense of his own preferences and competencies. Alternatively, worksheets and exercises such as the one on Leisure Values in Korb, Azok, and Leutenberg (5) can provide a beginning point for planning and selecting leisure activities.

Another, not unrelated, problem is that some people do not manage their time well, as was previously discussed, and therefore appear to have no leisure time even though in fact they may have too much. On the other hand, "workaholics" may actually not have any time for leisure because they spend so much time working. Although there is no magic formula or minimum weekly requirement that we can apply equally to all individuals, it appears that each person should spend enough time relaxing so that he feels restored and refreshed and able to work again. This is an area in which the occupational therapy assistant must be careful not to impose his values on the patient. Activity configurations such as the Barth Time Construction (see Chapter 14) and the Balance Your Life exercise in Korb, Azok, and Leutenberg (6) are useful in promoting self-awareness of poor leisure habits, in that they give a vivid picture of exactly how time is being used.

Yet a third problem is that some individuals who suffer from depression may state that they watch television and read in their leisure time. It may be helpful to supplement these activities with others that provide social contact and the opportunity to experience one's own competence through active doing.

For those patients who need or wish to develop new leisure pursuits, or to work on scheduling more time for leisure, intervention might focus on helping them identify pleasurable activities, discover reasons why pleasurable activities are avoided, and locate community recreation resources. Even though it is possible and sometimes necessary to counsel patients individually, group counseling is probably more effective because patients can get ideas from each other, and no person has to feel put on the spot.

Leisure planning and leisure counseling activities must take into account the patient's ability to make decisions and follow through on them, his financial and time resources, and the recreation and leisure opportunities available locally. One approach is to make a list of possible activities, including classes at the YMCA or the local community college, sports, crafts, games, expressive activities, and domestic activities (cooking, gardening). This helps structure leisure choices for people who have difficulty coming up with ideas; the list can be abbreviated or expanded depending on the patient's age and ability to make decisions. People can be helped to try out new activities through participating in a group

designed to provide a variety of new experiences and leisure-time options.

Because different people have different needs for leisure, the preferred context and style of activity should be explored. For example, does this person want to be alone or to be with others? Would it bring more pleasure to do the activity in one's home, or in a special environment, or a combination of these? Exercises and worksheets to develop these and other aspects of leisure planning and engagement can be found in various of the references (3,5,6,12).

Crafts

Crafts have been used in occupational therapy since the very beginning of the profession. Not everyone perceives crafts as leisure, and in fact some people actively dislike them; other leisure opportunities need to be available to meet their interests. Discussion here will focus on the use of crafts for leisure; the use of crafts to develop task skills and work habits has been discussed separately.

Some factors that should be considered before using any craft as a leisure activity with a patient are the traditional sexual orientation of the craft, the level of difficulty required in manual skills and cognitive skills, the length of time needed to complete the activity, and the likelihood of successful completion. Some crafts, such as needlework, have a strong feminine identification and should be used cautiously, if at all, with males. Leathercraft, woodwork, and metal crafts are more likely to be accepted by men. Some activities require a greater degree of manual dexterity than is immediately obvious; for example, threading a needle, knotting the thread, and making the first stitch are more difficult than continuing a stitch that has already been started. The assistant should practice each activity (including completing a sample) before teaching it to patients; in this way, problems can be identified in advance, and adaptations made (e.g., preparing pre-threaded needles). Other activities require cognitive skills that the patient may not possess; using a ruler is one example. Again, modifications can be made once the problem is recognized; the assistant might teach ruler and measurement skills, or provide premeasured project pieces.

Since the patient will need to be able to carry on with leisure activities in his expected or future environment, the assistant should try to help the patient choose activities that are practical there as well as in the hospital. Obviously crafts that require a special environment or expensive tools or materials, or that are successful only if the patient uses therapist-prepared materials, are poor choices.

Another consideration is that since the purpose of any leisure activity is to refresh and enrich the individual experiencing it, the therapist's opinion is much less important than the patient's. Students and new graduates may wonder how best to respond in a leisure-focused program to patients whose projects have errors in them. The suggested approach is to first say something complimentary about the project or the effort that went into it, and then offer a single suggestion for improvement. Some people may reject this advice; if so, that's fine. They may be more receptive tomorrow or next week. Others may seek further help. The important thing to remember is that the patient should have a pleasurable and (to him) successful experience; too much criticism or advice from staff can totally destroy the value of crafts as a leisure experience.

Hobbies

In addition to crafts, hobbies that involve collecting or creating appeal to many. Model railroading, stamp and coin collecting, baseball card collecting, antiquing, doll collecting, miniatures, bird watching, and other pastimes are not only entertaining but also intellectually challenging. Some of these hobbies provide opportunities to relate to others with similar interests through clubs, exhibitions, competitions, and special events. Specialized magazines addressing these interests may be found in local libraries and used to generate contacts and activities for patients.

The Arts

Painting, music, and literature are major sources of personal pleasure for many. Whether the involvement is receptive (viewing, listening, reading) or creative (making art by painting, playing an instrument or singing, or writing), these pastimes are valued for their capacity to create an alternate reality, in which the day-to-day world recedes as the created world of the artist becomes the focal point of perception. In working with patients for whom these activities have been a source of pleasure in the past, the occupational therapy assistant should first assess why these pastimes have been abandoned. Patients who are or who have been depressed may feel undeserving of the experience of beauty, or may lack the energy to take the first step. The assistant may need to cajole, seduce, or otherwise entice the patient to open a door that has been closed. Interest and willingness can sometimes be facilitated by a trip to a museum, library, or musical performance. Patients with multiple roles and time management problems may need assistance to structure time for pleasure, and will need support to make a personal commitment to the pursuit of such activities. The use of the arts to facilitate self-expression is addressed in Chapter 21.

Gardening and Horticulture

Working with plants and the earth is deeply fulfilling to many people. In inpatient settings and in cities the assistant must use ingenuity to provide these experiences.

A successful program requires that plants be chosen carefully, based on the available light and the size of the pot or container. Gardening is an infinitely diverse activity, with tremendous therapeutic potential. It can provide physical exercise (spading, planting seedlings, weeding) as well as intellectual stimulation (learning the names of plants, their needs for light and water and fertilizer, control of pests, methods of propagation, and so on). Horticulture can be structured as a prevocational experience, with assigned tasks such as transplanting seedlings, cleaning pots, watering, and the like. Helping plants grow can also fulfill a need to nurture and create. McDonald (8) cites infertile couples who addressed their frustration over being childless by raising gloxinias and becoming officers in national horticulture societies.

Games

Like crafts, games have been used in occupational therapy since the beginning. They are seen as a way to learn about the world and how to function in it. Games can be used for relaxation and socialization and to develop physical and cognitive skills. Which particular game should be used for a particular patient and a particular purpose requires an analysis of the characteristics of the game and of the patient's attitudes about play. It may be helpful to use Moore's (9) three categories of games of chance, games of strategy, and puzzles. Moore developed these categories to classify play experiences that help the child acquire knowledge and competency for real-life situations.

Games of chance provide experiences whose outcome is based mostly on luck. Bingo, which is a very popular game with some patients, is an example. Games of chance give everyone an equal shot at winning, and those who lose know that it was not their fault that they lost; varying educational and functional levels among patients cannot influence the outcome. Games of chance simulate real-life events that are random, unpredictable, and beyond the control of the individual. Some games of chance involve an element of skill or strategy; for example, the contestant can improve his chances to succeed at the popular game show Wheel of Fortune by his knowledge of words and spelling, and by choosing the most common letters first.

Games of strategy give participants the opportunity to use skill and planning to influence the outcome of the game. Such games have definite goals and rules, and the players each have a role. The outcome is determined by how the players interact. In this way games of strategy simulate real-life situations that involve interactions with other people. Such games can be used to teach such basic social skills as following the rules, staying in one's role, being aware of the roles of others, negotiation, cooperation, and so on.

Two types of games of strategy often used with psychiatric patients are team sports (such as volleyball, softball, and relay races) and simulation games. Simulation games provide imaginary roles or situations to which the players try to respond. Commercially available simulation games include The Ungame (which encourages sharing of opinions, goals, and ideas), Roll-A-Role (in which players' roles are determined by the roll of large dice that have different roles on each side), and Scruples (in which players must respond to situations requiring tough ethical choices). Many computer games involve simulation; generally these games are for single play and would therefore be socially isolating, but some allow two or more players to play together. For example, playing interactive fiction games can be a team effort; the goal of these games is always to solve a puzzle; for example, finding treasure or unraveling a mystery, and some of them are so difficult that the help of many people is a necessity.

Several role simulation games that teach expressive and interpersonal skills and that require little or no equipment have been published in the social science literature (10,11). A game like Balloon Debate (11), for example, can help develop self-expression; in this game, each player chooses to be a famous person and then must prove to the others why he (rather than they) should be allowed to stay in the basket of a hot air balloon that will crash unless everyone but one person jumps overboard.

Puzzles provide an experience of discovery, exploration, and problem solving. Unlike games of strategy, puzzles have a definite outcome or solution that can be reached only by following a correct procedure. Puzzles thus simulate real-life situations in which the individual (or group) must analyze and deal with a problem like, for example, changing a lock or putting a child's toy or piece of furniture or barbeque grill together.

Another type of game, which evolved during the 1970s, is the noncompetitive game, as exemplified by the "new games" developed by The New Games Foundation (1,2). Most of these games involve some physical activity and strive to develop a community spirit rather than a competitive one. For example, Pile Up (2) is similar to musical chairs, except that the goal is to get everyone on the same chair. The game is played by having people stay where they are or move one seat to the right based on their answers to simple questions (e.g., "Do you have a sister?"). Other "new games" are more difficult (and much more amusing) than they look; in This Is My Nose (2) players touch various body parts while telling their partners that it is a different part (touching one's ear while saying "This is my nose," for example). The partner must then touch a different body part and give it the name of the body part his partner actually touched (touching one's knee while saying "This is my ear.")

Regardless of which type of game is used, it is up to the group leader to structure a therapeutic experience. This may mean, for example, minimizing the importance of winning and losing by stressing sportsmanship or team interaction or fun. In some games it is appropriate to discuss the concept of handicapping the more skilled players so as to give everyone an equal chance. Games can be used to teach skills that are needed for the real-life situations that they imitate. They can also be used to increase one's sense of mastery and competence; winning a game cannot really make up for losing in life, but it does provide a successful experience that can balance minor disappointments and frustrations.

Social Activities

Many people with mental health problems feel lonely, yet are uncomfortable when they are with other people; in some cases, they just do not know how to act, or what is required of them, or how to express what they want. Besides games and the social skills groups described in Chapter 3, many other activities can be used to provide a social experience. Kuenstler (7) developed a format for a planning group for psychiatric patients that helped participants acquire social skills needed to plan and follow through on leisure activities. Behaviors such as asking for help from others and learning what to say (and what not to say) to other people were discussed, rehearsed, and reinforced in weekly meetings.

Other socialization experiences include parties, topical discussions, and community excursions. Planning a party requires the accomplishment of many small tasks that give everyone a chance to participate. Skills in leadership, negotiation, and compromise can also be experienced; this becomes educational and therapeutic when staff involve the group members in a discussion of the interactions that have occurred. Relating to others during a party at the treatment setting can serve as a rehearsal for life outside; it is important for staff to pay attention to patients' behaviors so that they can follow up or give feedback later.

Discussion groups that focus on a general topic are a good way for patients to learn how to converse with other people that they might meet. Generally, such groups are organized around a theme such as sports, current events, or music appreciation. The leader selects topics for each meeting, or arranges for members to bring in topics: appropriate conversational behavior is taught by modeling and reinforcement during the discussion.

Sports and Exercise

In addition to team sports (discussed earlier under games of strategy), other physical activities are used in psychiatric occupational therapy to provide a leisure experience. These activities, which include individual sports, yoga, calisthenics, and aerobics, often have other purposes such as developing body awareness or sensory integrative skills or just maintaining good physical and mental health. Activities may have to be adapted for individuals whenever there are not sufficient numbers for a group (e.g., one-on-one basketball). For those who need to explore exercise options or to understand how to make a commitment to exercise, the worksheets in Korb, Azok, and Leutenberg (5) are useful. In some treatment facilities many physical activities are provided by recreation therapists. The use of physical and sports activities to develop sensorimotor skills will be discussed in Chapter 22.

For many, watching sporting events provides opportunities for release of tension and for socialization with others. The experience of rooting for one's team and sharing an event with friends gives vent to emotions, promotes social identification,

and provides material for post-event discussion.

CONCLUSION

Being able to choose and enjoy leisure activities is essential to health. People with mental health problems sometimes have difficulty using their spare time to meet their leisure needs. Occupational therapists and assistants can help them select meaningful leisure activities, schedule time for leisure, and explore new leisure experiences. These therapeutic services may also be provided by recreation therapists.

REFERENCES

1. Fluegelman A, ed. *The new games book.* Garden City, NY: Dolphin, Doubleday; 1976.
2. Fluegelman A, ed. *More new games.* Garden City, NY: Dolphin, Doubleday; 1981.
3. Hemphill BJ, Peterson CQ, Werner PC. *Rehabilitation in mental health: goals and objectives for independent living.* Thorofare, NJ: SLACK; 1991.
4. Herbert G. Jacula prudentum (1651). In: Bartlett J, ed. *Familiar quotations.* 15th ed. Boston: Little Brown; 1980:268.
5. Korb KL, Azok AD, Leutenberg EA. *Life management skills: reproducible activity handouts created for facilitators.* Beachwood, Ohio: Wellness Reproductions; 1989.
6. Korb KL, Azok AD, Leutenberg EA. *Life management skills II: reproducible activity handouts created for facilitators.* Beachwood, Ohio: Wellness Reproductions; 1991.
7. Kuenstler G. A planning group for psychiatric outpatients. *Am J Occup Ther* 1976;30:634–639.
8. McDonald E. *Plants as therapy.* New York: Praeger; 1976.
9. Moore OK, Anderson AR. Some principles for the design of clarifying educational environments. In: Goslin DA, ed. *Handbook of socialization theory and research.* Chicago: Rand McNally; 1969.
10. Pfeiffer JW, Jones JE, eds. *A handbook of structured experiences for human relations training, volumes I–VL.* La Jolla, Calif: University Associates; 1977.
11. Remocker AJ, Storch ET. *Action speaks louder: a handbook of nonverbal group techniques.* 3rd ed. Edinburgh: Churchill Livingstone; 1982.
12. Simmons PL, Mullins L. *Acute psychiatric care: an occupational therapy guide to exercises in daily living skills.* Thorofare, NJ: SLACK; 1981.

ADDITIONAL REFERENCES AND SUGGESTED READINGS

Anderson WA. *Therapy and the arts: tools of consciousness.* New York: Harper and Row; 1977.

Angel SL. The emotion identification group. *Am J Occup Ther* 1981;35:256–262.

DeCarlo JJ, Mann WC. The effectiveness of verbal versus activity groups in improving self-perceptions of interpersonal communication skills. *Am J Occup Ther* 1985;39:20–27.

Erikson JM. *Activity, recovery, growth: the communal role of planned activities.* New York: WW Norton; 1976.

Hughes PL, Mullins L. *Acute psychiatric care: an occupational therapy guide to exercises in daily living skills.* Thorofare, NJ: SLACK; 1981.

Hurff JM. Gaming technique: an assessment and training tool for individuals with learning deficits. *Am J Occup Ther* 1981;35:728–735.

Kartin NJ, Van Schroeder C. *Adult psychiatric life skills manual.* Kailua, Hawaii: Schroeder Publishing and Consulting 1982.

Kielhofner G, Miyake S. The therapeutic use of games with mentally retarded adults. *Am J Occup Ther* 1981;35:375–382.

McDowell CF. *Leisure counselling: selected lifestyle processes.* Medford: University of Oregon Press; 1976.

Miller KJ. Music for movement. *Am Occup Ther Assoc Mental Health Special Interest Section Newsletter* 1983;6(1):1–2.

Mosey AC. *Activities therapy.* New York: Raven Press; 1973.

Willson M. *Occupational therapy in long-term psychiatry.* Edinburgh: Churchill Livingstone; 1983.

21

Expressive and Coping Skills

Care of the soul is a continuous process that concerns itself not so much with "fixing" a central flaw as with attending to the small details of everyday life, as well as to major decisions and changes.

THOMAS MOORE (13)

The occupational nature of human beings extends beyond the mechanical aspects of carrying out tasks. The feelings with which such activities are done require as much attention as do the details of their execution. There is a world of difference between going through the motions of life and moving joyfully with its rhythms. The aim of this chapter is to present briefly some of the techniques used for identifying and expressing the hidden, often ignored, emotional and innermost aspects of our lives, as they are embodied in our activities. Traditional approaches to self-expression, stress management, time management, and coping strategies will be discussed.

IDENTIFYING, EXPRESSING, AND SATISFYING NEEDS

Many psychiatric patients have difficulty expressing their needs. Some appear not to know that they have needs. This inability to understand, express, and gratify needs results for some in impulsive acting out (sexually or violently) and in many others manifests as a deadness or dullness in their attachment to reality, as if they were living out a sentence on earth. One of the most

useful approaches to understanding needs was developed by Maslow (12). His hierarchy of needs consists of five levels, built upon each other, so that the lower levels must be satisfied before the higher levels (though in some individuals the higher level needs may at times take precedence). The lowest level, physiological, refers to needs for food, shelter, sleep, sex, exercise, light, and air. Safety needs are at the second level; these include psychological as well as physical safety. At the third level are love and belonging needs; these are the needs to be accepted and loved as a unique human being, unconditionally, for what one is. The fourth level is for esteem needs, or the need to be recognized by others. Self-actualization, or the need to accomplish personal goals, is at the fifth level.

White (21) identified a need for mastery or competence, which includes the desire to explore and make sense of the world, to control one's environment, and to make a difference. This may be seen as an aspect of esteem needs and self-actualization needs, or as a separate need.

Intimately connected with needs are feelings and emotions. Frustration of needs results in frustrated emotions (anger, depression, fear, boredom, withdrawal, irritability). Need gratification usually results in positive emotions (happiness, elation, contentment, pride, relief) but may generate more mixed feelings (guilt, indecision, regret, confusion) in persons whose needs are in conflict. The failure to monitor, recognize, accept, and examine one's feelings impoverishes life, and almost always leads to a negative cycle of acting out without understanding the reasons for one's actions.

While the development of self-awareness of needs and emotions is primarily the province of trained psychotherapists, it is also an important aspect of man's occupational nature, and thus is of concern to occupational therapists and assistants, within the context of activities.

Occupational Therapy Interventions

Throughout this chapter we will be examining areas of treatment that overlap with those of other professions. To avoid confusion in presenting our skills and expertise both to patients and to other mental health practitioners, it is useful to review some of the differences between the OT approach and the approach of other professions. First, occupational therapists and assistants are concerned primarily with how people function in their daily life activities. The need gratification and stress management interventions that we use are directed toward improving our patients' ability to function in work, home life, school, leisure, and other occupational areas. Second, ours is a "doing" therapy more than a "talking" therapy. While we do discuss with our patients the problems in their lives, and while we do present much information verbally, the main vehicle for therapeutic intervention in occupational therapy is activities. Third, due to both historical and reimbursement-driven factors, we treat psychiatric patients in groups rather than individually, for the most part. This limits the selection of techniques to those that can be presented in a group format. Often, for specific skills

such as assertiveness training, time management, or stress management, we use a psychoeducational approach, in which we employ a classroom style for delivering information and engaging clients in "classwork" and "homework" to apply it to themselves. We do not, therefore, use techniques that require long-term, one-to-one, verbal interaction. This is not to say that we do not take the individual into account; we individualize therapy by fine-tuning our general approach to the person's presenting problems, and by giving attention to how the approach can be used in activities throughout his life.

Much information has been presented in earlier chapters on activities that gratify physiological needs (see information on homelessness in Chapter 9, on cooking and other activities in Chapters 18 and 19, and on sexuality in Chapter 18). Additionally, for patients having difficulty in specific areas, worksheets and exercises to examine sleep, exercise, and other physiological needs can be found in Korb, Azok, and Leutenberg (9).

Safety needs can be addressed through the information presented in Chapter 12. The psychological aspect of safety may be an issue for patients whose home environment is abusive. While it is helpful to learn coping strategies to distance oneself, it is better to remove oneself from the situation. Intervention in such cases is generally outside the scope of occupational therapy, and the particulars should be communicated to a social worker or other professional better trained to respond.

Psychiatric patients often have difficulty appropriately expressing and gratifying love and belonging needs, which are sometimes acted out in impulsive sexual union or in remarks that are so offensive as to repel the intended object of one's affections. Because the major psychiatric disorders often manifest in adolescence or early adulthood, many patients lack successful dating and relationship experiences, and cannot form intimate relationships without help. Social skills training (see Chapter 3) and role plays can help teach patients to differentiate between behavior that is appropriate (and likely to succeed) and that which is not.

Esteem needs are generally met through work and related activities (see Chapter 19). However, there are other problems in gratifying esteem needs that have to do with a mismatch between the esteem desired and the source from which it is sought. For example, a woman may desire respect from her family for her work as an artist. But if the family places low value on artistic work, preferring scientific or academic or business careers, the desired esteem might not be forthcoming. Thus, sometimes patients have to learn to look elsewhere for esteem. This might involve, for someone who desires praise from a gruff and businesslike boss, recognizing the need to find a new job working for someone who is more effusive and social. Alternatively, a person can learn to give herself praise or to allow herself to be nurtured by the reactions of customers, co-workers, and subordinates. Exercises to explore and bolster self-esteem can be found in Korb, Azok, and Leutenberg (9).

Self-actualization is gratified through individually chosen leisure, expressive, and value-driven activities. Leisure activities were discussed in Chapter 20. Expressive activities will be presented later in this chapter. Value-driven activities are chosen on the basis of values chosen and cherished by the individual. For those who are unaware of their values, exercises can be found in Korb, Azok, and Leutenberg (9). Values that have been identified through such paper-and-pencil activities should be "road-tested" by participation in situations that embody those values. For example, someone who believes he wants to help people should try volunteer work in a variety of settings and with different populations to see if this desire will hold up to the reality of the experience.

Mastery needs are best met through experiences that permit practice, repetition, and experimentation. To learn to do something well requires time and opportunity. Once the preferred activity has been identified, the patient can be helped to achieve a feeling of competence by scheduling repeated and prolonged experiences, assisted by the presence of a therapist or volunteer who can provide feedback and suggestions. It is important for the therapist, assistant, or volunteer to tailor the activity to maintain the experience of challenge without going beyond the patient's limits and endurance to the point of failure. For patients who catastrophize or evaluate experiences in black-and-white, either-or terms, group discussion may be valuable to help the patient to put failure in perspective and to accept occasional setbacks as an inevitable (and not valueless) aspect of the journey toward competence.

EXPRESSIVE SKILLS

Identifying and expressing one's emotions are useful skills, allowing one to release tension, recognize and gratify needs, and communicate with others. For a variety of reasons, many psychiatric patients need help in this area. Some may have experienced extreme emotional deprivation as children, and thus have learned to turn off or ignore their feelings. Others, due to the symptoms of their disease, may tend to extremes of emotion (euphoria and despair) and may lack appreciation of the subtle distinctions of emotions in the middle range (contentment, serenity, satisfaction, confusion, mischievousness, shyness, boredom, etc.). Korb, Azok, and Leutenberg (9) give some paper-and-pencil exercises to develop and expand the ability to identify emotions.

In addition, occupational therapy has always included creative activities that help patients express their inner thoughts, feelings, beliefs, anxieties, and perceptions. Depending upon their purpose and the needs of the patient, these activities may be used to teach basic communication skills or leisure and social skills. More typically, however, they are used to develop the patient's self-concept and self-identity, his awareness of himself and his own feelings and needs. Activities from the arts are most often used, although communication games and exercises are also available. Settings that have large numbers of staff may employ creative arts therapists to run these expressive activities. Creative art therapists have special training in one or more of the arts, such as dance, music, art, or poetry, and in how to use the arts as therapy.

Graphic and fine arts media, such as drawing, painting, collage, and clay, are familiar to most people from experiences in school and during childhood. These media are very unstructured and can be overwhelmingly complex unless the therapist creates structured activities from them. The patient may be totally paralyzed if presented with numerous choices, unfamiliar tools and materials, and a blank canvas or piece of paper. Adults may feel insecure or anxious about engaging in art activities because they feel their work will be seen as childish or unsophisticated, or because they fear it will be analyzed for unconscious content.

One approach that seems to work is to provide structured paired or group activities with a specific procedure, purpose, or theme. For example, in Pass-A-Drawing (16) each participant draws something to represent himself; the drawings are then passed around the room so that everyone has an opportunity to add to everyone else's drawing. Discussion then focuses on why people sometimes see each other differently from the way they see themselves. As another possible activity, each person can trace his hands on a piece of paper, labeling one of them "present" and the other "future"; he then draws in the hands the things that he believes he has now, and the things he would like to have in the future. Each person discusses his drawing with the group.

Creative writing and the study and appreciation of the written word can also be used expressively in occupational therapy groups. Patients can perform plays or write and act out their own, thus learning not only to express ideas but also to identify with the emotions of a particular role. Patients who are too self-conscious to act out a role themselves may enjoy using puppets to express their feelings and ideas (17). Groups that work with poetry may include both poetry appreciation and writing; writing a poem can be an individual or a group project.[1] Keeping a daily journal can give patients a structure to record and explore what happens in their lives and how they react to situations and experiences; when he later reviews what he has written the patient may see patterns that he otherwise might not have recognized. For example, a patient may learn that he usually gets depressed around family holidays, or that his episodes of tension and outbursts at home usually follow disappointments at work.

Another valuable writing exercise is life review (7,15). Most often used with older adults, life review consists of the recording of a personal biography. Going over the events of one's past and thinking about the things one has done can help the depressed older adult resolve the developmental (Erikson) crisis of ego integrity versus despair by revealing that his life did indeed have meaning, purpose, and direction. Volunteers can assist those who are unable to write because they are illiterate or infirm or too depressed and fatigued. Alternatively, tape recorders can be used.

Playing musical instruments or moving to music through dance or exercise can help nonverbal patients express themselves. Keeping the beat or creating one's own beat with a rhythm band instrument is an example. It is not a good idea, however, to make a practice of having music on continuously in the background during all different kinds of occupational therapy groups. Although music can serve as a kind of

---

[1] Ideas on how to structure exercises for a poetry-writing group can be adapted from those in Koch (8).

acoustical wallpaper to create a mood, not everyone enjoys it while they are working. Music and dance are often used in sensorimotor groups, which will be discussed in a later section.

COMMUNICATION OF NEEDS AND EMOTIONS

Once the patient has learned to identify and accept his needs, values, and emotions, it remains to communicate them to others so that they can be understood, and so that one can ask for what one needs. There are many ways to communicate—verbally and nonverbally, clearly or confusedly, directly or obliquely, and effectively or ineffectively. Patients with mental health problems generally need assistance to learn how to communicate effectively to get others to help them meet their needs. Again, it is important to recognize that occupational therapy should be concerned with these skills only where they directly impact the patient's occupational functioning. More general treatment of need expression falls under the scope of psychotherapy rather than occupational therapy.

A variety of media and approaches have been used. Role plays and small group discussions are the most common. Hemphill, Peterson, and Werner (5) provide a list of step-by-step goals for this area. Videotape (4, 6) has become a popular medium for facilitating self-expression and personal awareness. Patients can create and record their own dramas; if done as a group activity this can develop communication and group interaction skills as well as personal expression. Video can also be used to teach social functioning. Patients can watch videotaped models of effective social skills and discuss what is effective about them. More importantly, they can review and analyze their own recorded behaviors to identify their own strengths and weaknesses and select areas for change. Alternatively, Korb, Azok, and Leutenberg (9) provide worksheets for un-

derstanding and communicating verbally and nonverbally. Regardless of the medium used, it is most important to help the patient to analyze his own behavior, to understand what worked and what didn't, and to formulate a plan for the next social encounter.

Assertiveness

Assertiveness is the ability to state one's needs, thoughts, and feelings in an appropriate, direct, and honest way (19). When one reflects on the life experience of psychiatric patients, one quickly appreciates how repeated hospitalization and involvement with the mental health system might diminish any sense of personal assertiveness. Thus, most patients must learn or relearn these skills. Often, assertiveness is taught through a structured set of exercises in assertiveness training (9,10,18). The usual format is to begin by defining assertiveness, usually by illustration in a variety of social encounters. The next step is to help the patient identify his own assertiveness patterns. This may be done through a questionnaire or a diary or logsheet. Next, obstacles to assertiveness (fear, shyness, self-doubt) are identified and tackled. Specific assertive strategies and behaviors are taught and practiced in hypothetical role plays. Then, participants are asked to put these strategies to use in their own lives and to keep records in a diary. Experiences are reported back to the group, which engages in problem-solving and feedback.

Anger Management

Anger is a feeling that most people recognize. The problem for many is that the feeling is recognized only when it is expressed. Recognizing that one is angry *before* the urge to express it is acted out is essential to success in work and social situations. Difficulties in identifying, managing, and appropriately expressing angry feelings are common in patients who had poor role models in their own families or who were never expected to express anger appropriately (due to their illness). Anger management can be taught in a step-by-step format, similar to assertiveness training (10). The first step is to define anger and help the patient to identify his typical patterns of dealing with anger (stuffing, escalating, etc.). Next, strategies for managing anger through techniques such as visualization, empathizing, relaxation, and conflict resolution are taught. Then, the patient is asked to put the strategies to use in his own life and to report back on the results, which are analyzed.

Taylor (20) described the application of an anger intervention model to occupational therapy. This model, initially developed by Novaco (14), proposes a very thorough individual assessment of anger as experienced by the patient. Elements such as his physiological reactions, his specific thoughts, environmental factors that are provocative to the patient, and the patient's behaviors when he is angry must be all documented. The treatment phase focuses on developing in the patient an awareness of the relationship between stress and anger, and on increasing the patient's stress management skills and his actual use of those skills. Taylor advocates the use of activities to divert attention from negative, anger-producing thoughts. Two elements are essential here. First, the patient must recognize that his anger is being aroused and that he needs to shift attention to something else. Second, the activities chosen for this purpose must be pleasurable, and not ones which will lead to other negative thoughts. Taylor specifically mentions that some activities that occupational therapists have traditionally believed to provide outlets for anger (e.g., woodworking, metal hammering) may actually increase anger. Gardening, socializing, watching television, and other more passive activities may actually provide more relief, at least in some indi-

viduals. A study by Larson (11), however, suggests that such passive occupations, particularly if solitary and if used to an extreme, may bring on depression.

Managing Grief and Loss

Sometimes life deals a blow in the loss of something that we never expected to be taken from us. Whether the loss is of a family member or friend, a pet, a job, the possibility of future pregnancies, or a normal lifespan, the response is the same. Grief and loss derail normal activities with turbulent and distracting emotions that demand attention and that interfere with "business as usual." The typical dysfunctional pattern of responding to grief is to deny it or "stuff" it. Since this approach does not remove the pain, grief settles in the body and the spirit and may manifest as physical symptoms, cognitive deficits, and other impairments. Constructive, honest, and self-respecting techniques for responding to loss must often be learned. Korb, Azok, and Leutenberg (10) give some exercises that can be useful. The life review activities suggested earlier in this chapter can also be used to express and relieve feelings of loss.

STRESS MANAGEMENT

Most readers will no doubt recognize the experience of stress, yet the condition is hard to define. Stress occurs when a threat is perceived. The threat, or stressor, may be a life event (marriage, birth of a child, death of a parent), an environmental factor (hurricane, economic recession), a hassle or series of hassles (having to run out to buy milk, a child staying home from school, a parking ticket, a challenging examination or school assignment), or the individual personality style in reaction to normal events (a tendency to catastrophize, a tendency to hypervigilance, etc.). Stress that is not effectively managed will lead in time to a variety of problems—physical illnesses, irritability, depression, mood swings, impulsivity, etc.

Cotton (1) provides a thorough analysis and description of stress and techniques for stress management. She divides these into techniques that are *problem-focused,* that aim to change the stressful situation, and those that are *emotion-focused,* that aim to change the stress response to the situation. For each of these two areas, she further delineates techniques based on whether the focus of intervention is primarily physiological (aimed at the body's stress response), cognitive (aimed at the negative thoughts), or behavioral (aimed at the actions taken by the patient). The attentive reader will immediately recognize that occupational therapy, with its activity orientation, will most likely employ techniques that are behavioral in their focus. Since activities are rarely simple or one-dimensional, we will see that these techniques also affect the physiological and cognitive processes.

Some of these techniques have already been mentioned in this and earlier chapters. Exercise, particularly aerobic exercise, seems to be associated with improved responses to stress. Yoga, meditation, and stretching exercises are also stress-reducing. All of these techniques affect the physiological response, as well as providing an activity focus that diverts attention from cognitive ruminations over stressful events. Assertiveness training and anger management can also mediate stress by increasing skills in recognizing and dealing with feelings and needs.

Psychoeducational Stress Management Groups

A format that seems popular in the occupational therapy literature is the psychoeducational stress management group, in which patients are instructed in the effects of stress and in personal stress analysis and stress management. This approach creates change in a step-by-step manner, by first helping the individual identify what she finds stressful and how her stress manifests itself. Then, techniques for changing one's response to stress, in terms of how one thinks, feels, and acts, can be presented one by one, and can be applied in homework assignments and reported in a diary or log. An outline for such a group can be found in Cotton (1, p. 16) and a more detailed description in Courtney and Escobedo (2). Exercises in Korb, Azok, and Leutenberg (9,10) provide structure for teaching and reinforcing specific aspects of stress management, such as the use of diversional activity, problem solving, and putting things in perspective.

Time Management

A frequent complaint heard from persons who are stressed is that they don't have enough time. This complaint should be taken seriously, since the subjective experience is legitimate. Even if the person appears to be wasting time, this is likely because she hasn't an effective strategy for managing it. Since occupational therapy assistants, like everyone else, need to manage time, many strategies are given in Chapter 25. These strategies can effectively be taught to patients as well. One of the most common approaches to teaching patients time management is the psychoeducational approach described above. A multisession time management group might begin by defining time management and analyzing each person's time use patterns using an activity configuration. Later sessions would focus on developing specific skills such as prioritizing, using lists, organizing one's day, etc. A protocol for a psychoeducational-type time management group can be found in Gibson (3). Exercises in Korb, Azok, and Leutenberg (9,10) also address time management.

Social Support

Another important stress management tool is increasing the use of social supports, of people and institutions that may help by providing feedback, socialization, information, and material support. A single parent may, for example, benefit from meeting with other parents either formally (in a group or self-help format) or informally (at the playground or in the neighborhood). Interaction with other parents provides the opportunity to confirm and validate her own feelings, to become aware of parenting strategies, and to work out play dates and child care swaps. An isolated elderly person may blossom if given the opportunity to meet with peers in a social situation or to work as a volunteer. In addition, people in all sorts of situations may obtain relief from stressful situations by investigating and using resources in their own communities, such as YMCA, YWCA, and other community organizations.

SUMMARY

Activities are not just actions. They are actions driven by needs, feelings, and desires, and they generate feelings as well. Being able to identify, express, and act on one's feelings contributes to a sense of personal identity and improves the quality of one's life. Being able to assert oneself, manage one's feelings with self-control and dignity, and channel stress into successful outcomes are all useful skills. While many mental health professionals teach these skills to patients, occupational therapists and assistants have a unique perspective in their emphasis on functional outcomes in daily life activities. It is important, when addressing these areas, to remain within the scope of occupational therapy practice. Even more important, one should provide a good role model to patients by demonstrating the qualities of self-control and self-expression, satisfaction of needs, and management of stress. Personal experiences, especially those that are immediate and germane to the situation, should be shared with patients to help them understand that we are people too, and that these techniques really do work.

REFERENCES

1. Cotton DHG. *Stress management: an integrated approach to therapy.* New York: Brunner/Mazel; 1990.
2. Courtney C, Escobedo B. A stress management program: inpatient to outpatient continuity. *Am J Occup Ther* 1990;44:306–310.
3. Gibson D, ed. *Group protocols: a psychosocial compendium.* Binghamton, NY: Haworth Press; 1989.
4. Goldstein N, Collins T. Making videotapes: an activity for hospitalized adolescents. *Am J Occup Ther* 1982;36:530–533.
5. Hemphill BJ, Peterson CQ, Werner PC. *Rehabilitation in mental health: goals and objectives for independent living.* Thorofare, NJ: SLACK; 1991.
6. Holm M. Video as a medium in occupational therapy. *Am J Occup Ther* 1983;37:531–534.
7. Kiernat JM. The use of life review activity with confused nursing home residents. *Am J Occup Ther* 1979;33:306–310.
8. Koch K. *Wishes, lies and dreams: teaching children to write poetry.* New York: Random House; 1970.
9. Korb KL, Azok AD, Leutenberg EA. *Life management skills: reproducible activity handouts created for facilitators.* Beachwood, Ohio: Wellness Reproductions; 1989.
10. Korb KL, Azok AD, Leutenberg EA. *Life management skills. II: reproducible activity handouts created for facilitators.* Beachwood, Ohio: Wellness Reproductions; 1991.
11. Larson KB. Activity patterns and life changes in people with depression. *Am J Occup Ther* 1990;44:902–906.
12. Maslow A. *Toward a psychology of being.* Princeton, NJ: Van Nostrand; 1962.
13. Moore T. *Care of the soul: a guide for cultivating depth and sacredness in everyday life.* New York: Harper Collins; 1992.
14. Novaco R. The cognitive regulation of anger and stress. In: Kendall P, Hollen S, eds. *Cognitive-behavioral interventions: theory, research, and procedures.* New York: Academic Press; 1979.
15. Quigley P. *Those were the days: life review therapy for elderly residents in long term care facilities.* Buffalo, NY: Potentials Development for Health and Human Services; 1981.

16. Ryder B, Gramblin J. *Activity card file*. Brookfield, Ill: Fred Sammons; 1981.
17. Schumann SH, Marcus D, Nesse D. Puppetry and the mentally ill. *Am J Occup Ther* 1973; 27:484–486.
18. Simmons PL, Mullins L. *Acute psychiatric care: an occupational therapy guide to exercises in daily living skills*. Thorofare, NJ: SLACK; 1981.
19. Stone EM, ed. *American psychiatric glossary*. 6th ed. Washington, DC: American Psychiatric Association; 1988.
20. Taylor E. Anger intervention. *Am J Occup Ther* 1988;42:147–155.
21. White RW. Motivation reconsidered: the concept of competence. In: Rabkin L, Carr J, eds. *Sourcebook in abnormal psychology*. Boston: Houghton Mifflin; 1967.

ADDITIONAL REFERENCES AND SUGGESTED READINGS

Engel JM. Social validation of relaxation training in pediatric headache control. *Occup Ther Mental Health* 1991;11(4):77–90.

Frye B. Art and multiple personality disorder: an expressive framework for occupational therapy. *Am J Occup Ther* 1990;44:1013–1021.

Gibson D. Theory and strategies for resolving conflict. *Occup Ther Mental Health* 1985;5(4):47–62.

Higdon JF. Expressive therapy in conjunction with psychotherapy in the treatment of patients with dissociative disorders: recommendations for therapists. *Am J Occup Ther* 1990;44:991–993.

Maynard M. Exploring adult day care participants' responses to psychosocial stressors. *Occup Ther Mental Health* 1990;10(2):65–84.

Rance C, Price A. Poetry as a group project. *Am J Occup Ther* 1973;27:252–255.

Sachs RG. The sand tray technique in the treatment of patients with dissociative disorders: recommendations for occupational therapists. *Am J Occup Ther* 1990;44:1045–1047.

Smith TM, Glickstein CS. Art as a therapeutic modality for individuals with alcohol-related problems in a milieu setting. *Occup Ther Mental Health* Winter 1980/1981;1(4):33–44.

Stein F, Nikolic S. Teaching stress management techniques to a schizophrenic patient. *Am J Occup Ther* 1989;43:162–169.

Wade JC. Socialization groups: using the *Book of Questions* as a catalyst for interaction. *Am J Occup Ther* 1992;46:541–545.

22

Cognitive and Sensorimotor Activities

Walking onto a ward of chronic, neurologically and psychiatrically impaired male patients who had seen me often during the past six months, I started a ball throwing activity. Not only did I introduce a large ball, but I requested that the patients stand to participate. Their usual behavior was to sit throughout the group. What a lot I was asking!

MILDRED ROSS (9, p.1)

Almost every activity we undertake requires cognitive and sensorimotor functions of which we are usually quite unaware. Taking notes in class depends on being able to hold the pen with just the right amount of pressure (judged by our proprioceptive feedback mechanisms), to hold our balance without having to think about it, to understand the lecturer's words and emotional expression, and to concentrate despite distractions. And these are just a *few* of the countless internal mechanisms that support our ability to perform everyday activities successfully.

These internal cognitive and sensorimotor functions are often impaired in individuals with psychiatric disorders. These malfunctions are most severe in disorders with a known organic basis or neurological symptoms.[1] Also, psychotropic medications may create additional sensorimotor or cognitive problems. This chapter explores some of the activities occupational therapists and assistants employ in their work with patients who have these problems.

COGNITIVE SKILLS

Cognitive skills are the mental functions needed for thinking. Specific cognitive deficits and recommended strategies for helping patients cope with them were discussed in Chapter 11. We may think of these as *compensatory strategies* (1), which aim to substitute personal assets and environmental supports when cognitive skills are impaired. In addition, the occupational therapy assistant sometimes provides group and individual activities whose purpose is to improve patients' memory, orientation, concentration, and attention span. These are *remedial strategies* (1), as they seek to enhance underlying abilities and support the reintegration of cognitive skills.

Reality orientation is an educational technique designed to reinforce confused patients' sense of personal identity, and help them stay aware of time and place, who they are with, and what they are doing. Reality orientation consists of staff members talking with patients, asking them questions and encouraging them to think about such things as what place this is, what time of year it is, what the next meal

---

[1]For some interesting case examples, see Sacks.

will be, and so on. Reality orientation can be done one-to-one or in groups. It can also be used to organize an entire therapeutic milieu; in this case the environment would be saturated with memory and orientation aids such as calendars, clocks, and signs, and every activity from bathing to eating would include reality orientation. Protocols for these groups can be found in Fidler (4) and Brown et al. (3).

Remotivation is a group discussion technique for helping depressed and confused patients organize and verbalize their thoughts and feelings. Topic selection is based on patients' interests, age, cultural backgrounds, and personal histories. For example, topics that might interest patients in their 70s or 80s include music from past decades, what they remember of their first automobile ride, and what it was like to go swimming when they were young. The leader generally opens the group by showing and then passing around an object that is related to the topic for the day's discussion. The object should be immediately recognizable and interesting. For a discussion of ocean swimming, suitable objects might be an old photograph from a seaside resort, or a seashell. For a discussion of music, a photograph of a singer (e.g., Billie Holiday) or a musical instrument (harmonica or tambourine) might be used. The leader then asks a series of simple questions developed in advance about the topic, calling on each member by name and involving everyone in the discussion. Wherever possible, the leader encourages individual contributions; for example, a participant who shows the slightest interest in doing so may be asked to demonstrate a dance step, or sing a song, or imitate a famous person. Remotivation topics usually draw on patients' long-term memory, which may remain intact and quite sharp despite deterioration of short-term memory and orientation to the present.

Although reality orientation and remotivation discussion groups are the two approaches the occupational therapy assistant is most likely to be expected to know on the job, many other cognitive activities are used by occupational therapists working in psychiatry. These may include puzzles, problem-solving discussions, visual and auditory training exercises, and computer software. The registered therapist may instruct the assistant in how to use these activities to help individuals or members of small groups improve their cognitive functioning, or the therapist may evaluate the patient and identify a specific cognitive deficit, and then rely upon the assistant to select an appropriate activity to build skills.

SENSORIMOTOR SKILLS

The ability to perceive and respond to sensory stimulation underlies almost all daily life activity. As discussed in the sensory integration section of Chapter 3, this ability may be impaired in persons who suffer from mental disorders. Very depressed patients tend to move and respond slowly; those in manic episodes often move quickly and respond rapidly and impulsively. Patients with organic disorders and schizophrenia sometimes have very specific sensorimotor problems, which may include stereotyped movements, S-shaped posture, or shuffling gait. Occupational therapists use sensorimotor activities to stimulate movement and to improve patients' perception of and response to sensory stimuli.

Because assistant-level programs cannot provide in-depth training in neuromuscular facilitation and sensory integration, sensorimotor treatment programs must be designed and supervised by a registered occupational therapist. The assistant can carry out selected aspects of the program and can assist in other ares. Those activities that an entry-level assistant is expected to perform independently will be addressed here. The specific sensorimotor skills that these activities are designed to develop are tactile awareness, postural balance, gross and fine coordination, range of motion, endurance, and strength.[2]

Tactile awareness is the perception of sensation through the skin. Activities that are used to promote tactile awareness involve applying objects with different textures and temperatures to the skin. Examples include rubbing or being rubbed with different textured cloths or lotions, receiving or giving a massage, shampooing, manicuring, putting on makeup, finger painting, and matching paired objects by texture while blindfolded.[3] Certain individuals find some of these activities threatening and unpleasant, and the group leader should *never* force tactile stimulation on a patient who says he does not want it. Tactile stimulation may have a disorganizing effect on some people, causing them to have trouble sleeping or paying attention. A patient who is unwilling to have the therapist touch him may be more willing to apply the stimulation to himself.

Olfactory and gustatory awareness exercises can also be included. These might involve passing around tidbits of food (olives, raisins, etc.) and things to smell (lemon slices, cotton balls perfumed with vanilla or scented oils). The purpose of all of these activities is to alert and arouse the patient to take notice of his environment and become involved in activity. These alerting activities are generally used at the beginning of a sensorimotor treatment session and should be done with the group seated or standing together in a circle. This allows for physical contact and promotes a feeling of cohesiveness without putting anyone on the spot.

Postural balance is the ability to maintain balance and control of the body while seated, standing, or moving. Unless a person has adequate postural balance, he will feel insecure at almost any activity. Dance, movement, and exercise are the modalities most often used to promote postural balance. Patients generally enjoy these activities, but may have difficulty getting started. Music affects the nervous system at a level below conscious awareness, and is therefore a good way to stimulate movement or to change a patient's level of physical activity. Because of its central nervous system effects, music should be used cautiously. Karen Miller (8), an occupational therapist with a degree in music therapy, developed the guidelines summarized below:

1. Match the *tempo* to the patient's ability to move. Start with a slow or moderate tempo and adjust the speed up or down as needed. When patients are able to perform a movement easily, gradually increase the tempo.

2. Use music with a clear, steady *beat,* and keep the movements in time with the rhythm.

3. Adjust the *volume* so that everyone can hear both the music and the group leader's voice.

4. Use *instrumental* music rather than vocal music, as patients are sometimes distracted by the words. Use *vocal* music to set a theme or to establish a mood; for example, the song "You Can Get It If You Really Want" by Jimmy Cliff[4] establishes an optimistic, positive mood.

5. Use good equipment and good recordings, since poor sound quality will interfere with comprehension of the tempo, beat, and rhythm.

6. Choose music that is appropriate for the age, cultural background, and tastes of the patient population.

7. Plan your music in advance. One way to do this is to make several cassette recordings, using different tapes for music of different tempos. Continue to use the same music in successive sessions, in

---

[2]This delineation of responsibility is described in more detail in (2).

[3]Other activities can be found in the gray section of Vander Roest and Clements (12).

[4]Cliff, J. "You Can Get It If You Really Want," on the album *The Harder They Come.* Island Records, Los Angeles; 1972.

keeping with the principle that practice and repetition are necessary for learning.

8. Be alert to how patients react to the music. Watch for signs of depression and retarded movement, which may indicate that the music is too slow. Likewise, agitation and uncontrolled movement may be signs that the music is too fast.

Movements and dance routines must be selected carefully so that they are within the patients' range of ability. With regressed or vegetative patients it may be necessary to start by copying the way one of the patients is moving; for example, the group leader might say, "Let's all rock back and forth in our chairs, like Susan is doing." The next step would be to extend the range of the movement (by rocking to a standing position) or to change the speed or direction of the movement. Gradually other simple movements can be added, always retaining the original pattern. Unfamiliar movements may confuse patients or make them anxious, and should be avoided. Movements in which both sides of the body move the same way are the easiest to imitate.

Gross and fine coordination, range of motion, endurance, and *strength* can all be developed through physical activities, which are described in detail in the literature (7, 10, 12). Other activities can be designed around specialized equipment like the parachute, the balance beam, and T-stools. Many of the "new games" (5, 6) discussed in Chapter 20 can be used for sensorimotor stimulation and skill development.

To obtain the greatest benefit from sensorimotor activities the group leader should create an atmosphere of fun, pleasure, and joy in movement. If the participants pay too much attention to what they are doing, their movements will lose spontaneity. The leader should obtain everyone's attention before demonstrating a new movement, and should repeat movements several times, even using the same activities over and over in different treatment sessions. It is a good idea to end an activity by bringing the participants together in a circle to say goodbye.

Sensorimotor treatment activities can be overstimulating to some individuals, and the assistant is cautioned to be alert to patients' condition and response. Signs like nausea, dizziness, sweating, flushing or blanching, fatigue, and cessation of activity indicate that the patient has had too much stimulation and that the activity should be stopped. People who are ill or who are taking medication may fatigue quickly, and the pace of the activity should be adjusted so that they can participate for longer periods. Patients who are uncoordinated or clumsy in their movements are liable to fall or injure themselves, and because of this it is important to pay attention to the condition of the equipment and the environment. The assistant must obtain the physician's approval and advice on special precautions before initiating sensorimotor activities with patients who have medical conditions that might impair their ability to participate safely (e.g., asthma, seizures, or cardiovascular problems).

CONCLUSION

Cognitive and sensorimotor activities are important therapies for patients who have problems in thinking or moving or being aware of their surroundings. By providing frequent stimulation, the occupational therapy assistant can help the patient maintain her current skills and improve upon them.

Chapters 18 through 22 have described the incredible variety of activities from which the occupational therapy assistant can choose when providing treatment for patients with psychiatric problems. Almost any activity can be applied therapeutically, but in order for an activity to have value as treatment, the assistant must know precisely why and how it is being used. You should be able to explain the purpose of activities to the patients who participate in them, and to state the benefits quite clearly. This can only happen if you know the activity well yourself, have practiced it, have analyzed its effects and demands, and have structured it to meet the needs of patients in your care. Otherwise, what you are doing will be activity, but not occupational therapy. The analysis and structuring of activities in psychiatric practice is the subject of the next chapter.

REFERENCES

1. American Occupational Therapy Association. Statement: occupational therapy services management of persons with cognitive impairments. *Am J Occup Ther* 1991;45:1067–1068.
2. American Occupational Therapy Association Entry-Level Role Delineation Task Force. Entry-level role delineation for registered occupational therapists (OTRs) and certified occupational therapy assistants (COTAs). *Am J Occup Ther* 1990;44:1091–1102.
3. Brown T et al, eds. *Mental health protocols for occupational therapy.* Baltimore, Md: CHESS Publications; 1989.
4. Fidler GS. *Design of rehabilitation services in psychiatric hospital settings.* Rockville, Md: American Occupational Therapy Association; 1991.
5. Fluegelman A, ed. *The new games book.* Garden City, NY: Dolphin, Doubleday; 1976.
6. Fluegelman A, ed. *More new games.* Garden City, NY: Dolphin, Doubleday; 1976.
7. French R, Horvat M. *Parachute movement activities: a complete parachute movement program for elementary grades and beyond.* Bryon, Calif: Front Row Experience; 1983.
8. Miller KJ. Music for movement. *Am Occup Ther Assoc Mental Health Special Interest Section Newsletter* 1983;6(1):1–2.
9. Ross M. *Group process: using therapeutic activities in chronic care.* Thorofare, NJ: SLACK; 1987.
10. Ross M, Burdick D. *Sensory integration: a training manual for therapists and teachers for regressed psychiatric and geriatric patient groups.* Thorofare, NJ: SLACK; 1981.
11. Sacks O. *The man who mistook his wife for a hat.* New York: Summit Books; 1986.
12. Vander Roest LL, Clements ST. *Sensory integration: rationale and treatment activities for groups.* Grand Rapids, Mich: South Kent Mental Health Services; 1983.

ADDITIONAL REFERENCES AND SUGGESTED READINGS

Earhart CA. Occupational therapy groups. In: Allen CA, ed. *Occupational therapy for psychiatric diseases: measurement and management of cognitive disabilities.* Boston: Little, Brown; 1985.

Fowler RH, King LJ, Snow BA. The use of dance in therapy. *Am Occup Ther Assoc Sensory Integration Special Interest Section Newsletter* 1984; 7(2):2–3.

French R, Horvat M. *Parachute movement activities: a complete parachute movement program for elementary grades and beyond.* Bryon, Calif: Front Row Experience; 1983.

Mosey AC. *Activities therapy.* New York: Raven Press; 1973.

Ross M, Burdick D. *Sensory integration: a training manual for therapists and teachers for regressed, psychiatric and geriatric patient groups.* Thorofare, NJ: SLACK; 1981.

Vander Roest LL, Clements ST. *Sensory integration: rationale and treatment activities for groups.* Grand Rapids, Mich: South Kent Mental Health Services; 1983.

Willson M. *Occupational therapy in long-term psychiatry.* Edinburgh: Churchill Livingstone; 1983.

Willson M. *Occupational therapy in short-term psychiatry.* Edinburgh: Churchill Livingstone; 1984.

23

Analyzing, Adapting, and Grading Activities

. . . seemingly small changes in the . . . materials or instructions can cause large changes in performance.

DAVID L. NELSON (11)

To the casual and uninformed observer, psychiatric occupational therapy might appear deceptively natural and easy. What could be simpler than doing everyday activities or arts and crafts with patients? Despite appearances, these seemingly natural activities are possible only because the therapist or assistant has spent many hours in mental and physical preparation. That patients will be willing to do an activity, and are able to do it, cannot be taken for granted. Only by selecting activities carefully, analyzing them thoroughly, and adapting and preparing them to match the needs of the patients can therapists and assistants create a task environment that motivates patients and enables them to succeed.

This chapter will discuss how to select, analyze, adapt, and grade activities to meet treatment goals for patients with mental health problems. Several different methods of activity analysis will be described, along with the rationale for choosing one over the others in a particular situation. General principles for adapting activities will be outlined, and examples will be given. Finally, we will discuss the concept of gradation, and consider some traditional meth-

ods for grading activities to promote a variety of skills and behaviors.

SELECTION OF ACTIVITIES

Whose job is it to select activities for patients—the registered therapist's or the occupational therapy assistant's? The answer is both, with input from the patient. Although the registered therapist may reserve this responsibility for himself in some treatment areas (e.g., sensory integration), more often the therapist will call upon the assistant to choose activities or to collaborate by discussing which activities could and should be used for a particular patient or group.

There are two major factors to consider when selecting an activity. The first is how well it suits the treatment goal. In some cases, the activity may have to be modified or structured by the therapist to meet the needs of the treatment situation. Unless the activity is going to help the patient reach treatment goals, there is no reason to consider it further.

The second factor is the match or fit between the activity and the patient. Is the patient interested in the activity? Is it consistent with his values and personal goals? How does he feel about doing the activity? Is it compatible with his age, sex, and sociocultural background? How does it help him develop or maintain his chosen or predicted occupational roles? Can he *do* the activity now, at his current functional level?

Only those activities that are well matched to the patient should be considered. Although it is often possible to alter the way an activity is performed, or the materials that are used to do it, these changes cannot be expected to compensate for the patient finding the activity irrelevant or uninteresting. There is one clear exception: Work-oriented treatment sometimes uses activities that the patient may find boring or tedious; nonetheless, even these activities must be acceptable within the patient's culture.

ANALYSIS OF ACTIVITIES

It is impossible to judge whether an activity will meet the treatment goals and be acceptable to the patient without analyzing the activity first. To do this, the occupational therapist or assistant must tear the activity apart, examining each piece against a vast number of concepts and theories drawn from his medical, psychological, and sociological background. Every step of the activity, every tool and material used in it, every social interaction it involves—all of these and many other aspects must be examined to determine whether the activity can do what it is meant to do for the patient. (Obviously, the patient must also be evaluated in the same scrupulous fashion.) An activity analysis, therefore, is the systematic breakdown of something complex (the activity) into its smaller, simpler parts.

Many different formats and procedures have been used by occupational therapists to analyze activities for mental health practice. Some of these are based on particular theories or practice models; these activity

analysis formats emphasize specific aspects of the activity that are relevant to a particular theory. For example, an activity analysis based on object relations theory would examine the unconscious meanings associated with the motions and materials used in the activity.[1] On the other hand, an activity analysis based on sensory integration theory would stress the sensory stimulation and neuromuscular involvement provided. Thus, wedging clay can be analyzed in relation to anal conflicts (object relations) or in terms of its tactile properties and its motions of shoulder retraction, abduction, rotation, and forward flexion (sensory integration). Where a particular theory or practice model is used to plan treatment, it is essential to analyze the activity from the same perspective.

If an activity is to be used as part of an evaluation rather than a treatment, it must be analyzed for its ability to measure whatever it is designed to evaluate. For instance, if the activity will be used to evaluate a patient's decision-making skills, not only must it provide choices and decision points, but the therapist must know precisely what outcomes and responses are possible, and what these different outcomes mean about the person's ability to make decisions. The analysis of activities to be used as evaluation is always the responsibility of the registered therapist.

Another type of activity analysis is one that explores all of the possibilities and potentials of an activity, without reference to a particular treatment goal or patient. Although this exercise can help students appreciate the multiple facets of activity and strengthen awareness of how the activity might be used, it is too broad and vague to be of much value in a real clinical situation (9).

The assistant will more often need to analyze activities in order to adapt them to help

---

[1]For an example of an outline based on concepts of object relations and psychodynamic theories, see Fidler and Fidler (5).

a particular patient reach an identified treatment goal. To do this, he must start by identifying and describing the activity as exactly as possible. To illustrate, "making a leather belt" might mean weaving a pre-cut link belt, or stamping designs on a pre-cut belt strip, or cutting a strip from a side of cowhide and carving and tooling it. These are three *different* activities. Thus, the first step in analysis is a complete description of the materials, tools, and procedures used in the activity. Any equipment needed and the kind of environment where the activity will be performed must also be identified.

The second step is to clarify the relationship between the activity and the treatment goals for the patient. Why is this a good activity for this patient? What treatment purposes does it serve?

The third step is to analyze further all the aspects of the activity that might affect the patient's performance, and to modify or design them to match the patient's needs. For example, repairing ripped hems and seams might be selected for a patient who is learning to live on her own in the community. How should this activity be taught, and over how many sessions? Should samples or photographs be used to demonstrate what needs to be done? Is it better for the therapist to teach the activity to the patient individually, or in a small group? These are only a few of the questions that need to be answered.

Table 23-1 gives a general structure for analyzing and designing an activity to meet the needs of a particular patient's treatment situation. This outline can be used as a foundation, and other analyses can be added where needed (e.g., if a specific practice model is used). For those using the model of human occupation, the activity must be analyzed for its environmental and personal factors, as shown in Table 23–2. A more comprehensive version of an occupational analysis format for the model of human occupation can be found in Kielhofner (7, Exercise 8).

To use any activity analysis format effectively, the assistant must understand and know how to apply the principles of adaptation and gradation. *Adaptation* is a word that has many meanings. Used here it means the modification of the activity to meet the needs of the situation. Many aspects of activities can be modified, among them the tools, materials, directions, procedures, rules, environment, and number of people involved. For instance, "basket weaving" is traditionally done with reed, but other materials such as plastic tubing (which is easier to manipulate) can be substituted. Or a game that is usually played by two people might be played by two teams instead.

The assistant may need to adapt an activity to enable a patient to do it. In other words, the patient cannot do the activity in the usual way, but can do it if it is modified. For example, a patient with an organic mental disorder and poor postural balance might not be able to execute traditional calisthenics, but could do less rigorous exercise while seated in a chair. Or someone with hand tremors (a side effect of some medications) would not be able to paint glaze with a brush on a ceramic project, but would be able to dip the project in glaze. Another very common example is that some patients with cognitive deficits find it difficult or impossible to start a stitch in leather lacing or knitting or sewing; however, if the assistant starts the stitch for them, they can continue it.

Another reason why the assistant might adapt an activity is to change the demands it makes on the patient, to make it more effective as a treatment tool. For instance, if the goal is for the patient to assert himself, the assistant might provide fewer tools so that people have to share. In this task environment the patient will have to ask for what he needs.

Of course, activities are not infinitely adaptable. One is unlikely to turn a solitary activity like doing a crossword puzzle into something that can be done by a large

TABLE 23–1. *Activity analysis outline*

I. General information
  A. Name of activity
  B. Environment where this activity *will* occur (within treatment setting)
    1. Special features of environment (equipment, safety requirements, etc.)
    2. Space per person to do this activity
  C. Breakdown of activity
    1. List of material and supplies
    2. List of tools and equipment
    3. Cost of materials and supplies for one project
    4. Steps, and key points of each step
II. Fit or match between patient, activity, and treatment goals
  A. Relationship of activity to treatment goals
  B. Relationship of activity to patient's interests, values, cultural background, age, sex, activity history, occupational roles, current skills and functional level, previous learning, present and future environment
  C. Motivating reasons for this patient to engage in this activity
III. Time and space factors
  A. Time needed for entire activity (estimate for average person and for this patient)
    1. If more than one session is needed, estimate number of sessions to complete activity
  B. Number of steps in the activity, and time needed for each step
    1. Minimum attention span needed to engage in each step
    2. Opportunity or need to repeat steps
    3. Possibilities for skipping, condensing, or rearranging order of steps
  C. Necessary delays (waiting time)
  D. Demands for rate of performance
  E. Therapist modifications of environment to facilitate patient performance of activity
    1. Arrangement of furniture to increase or minimize interaction
    2. Provision for task and general lighting
    3. Control of distracting elements (e.g., posters, sample projects, noise)
    4. Control of potential dangers in environment
    5. Positioning of patient in relation to activity
      a. Placement of activity, tools and materials
      b. Opportunity or need for patient to move about, get up from chair, etc.
IV. Materials and tools
  A. Potential hazards and precautions
  B. Sensory stimulation available (visual, auditory, tactile, olfactory, gustatory, kinesthetic)
  C. Physical properties (evaluate in relation to patient's abilities and preferences)
    1. Resistivity
    2. Pliability
    3. Controllability (ease with which material is controlled)
    4. Messiness
    5. Noisiness
    6. Effects on others present in environment (dust, smells, noise)
V. Processes involved
  A. Degree of difficulty of each step or process
  B. Technical knowledge required
  C. Presence of magical transformations or other phenomena that may be difficult for those with cognitive deficits to understand (e.g., color change of glaze during firing)
  D. Sensory discrimination required (e.g., of colors, textures)
  E. Perceptual demands (e.g., for matching, spatial relationships, etc.)
  F. Physical factors and demands
    1. Coordination, both fine and gross
      a. Muscular control needed
      b. Dexterity and manipulative skill needed
    2. Strength
    3. Endurance
    4. Postural balance and control
    5. Range of motion
  G. Cognitive factors and demands
    1. Attention span and concentration
    2. Orientation to time, place, person, and activity
    3. Memory
      a. Need to retain or transfer learning from one situation to another

TABLE 23–1. (*Continued*)

    4. New learning required
    5. Prerequisite cognitive skills (e.g., literacy, measurement)
    6. Opportunities for reality testing and consensual validation
  H. Social factors and demands
    1. Individual or group activity
    2. Number of people present (staff, patients, others)
    3. Interactions (both possible and necessary)
       a. Level of group interaction skill needed (parallel, project, egocentric-cooperative, cooperative, mature)
       b. Types of interpersonal transactions needed or possible (e.g., giving and receiving help, depending on others, sharing tools or materials, cooperating, competing, providing leadership, etc.)
    4. Communication needed (how much, whether verbal or nonverbal)
  J. Expression opportunities and demands
    1. Expression of feelings, verbally or symbolically
    2. Exploration and discussion of feelings
VI. Design of instruction
  A. Type of directions (demonstration, oral direction, written direction or diagrams)
  B. Unit of learning (number of steps taught at one time)
  C. Provisions for particular learning experiences (e.g., modeling, feedback, trial and error experiences, practice and repetition, reality testing, etc.)
  D. External instructional aids provided (e.g,., stimulation, audiovisual aids, activity sample)
  E. Advance preparation of materials (by someone other than patient)

group. One might argue that you could project the puzzle onto a screen so that everyone can see it, or give each person a copy of the same puzzle, but these adaptations are silly. If a group activity is what is required, then an activity that needs more than one person should be selected.

A therapist or assistant must possess both flexibility and good judgment in order to use the principle of adaptation effectively. He or she needs to be able to appreciate the versatility of the activity and to imagine all the different ways it could be changed. At the same time, however, one

TABLE 23–2. *Activity analysis following the model of human occupation*

1. *Environment:* How does the environment affect the person performing the activity? What are the social and cultural meanings of the activity? What objects are used? What tasks are involved and what is their meaning?
2. *Volitional subsystem:*
   Personal causation: What is the relationship between the activity and the person's sense of personal causation? Does the activity increase or support feelings of personal competence?
   Values: What values are implied in the performance of the activity? How do these values reflect those of the person doing the activity?
   Interests: In what way does the activity reflect or expand the interests of the individual?
3. *Habituation subsystem:*
   Roles: With what important life roles is the activity associated? What is the relationship between these roles and the performer of the activity?
   Habits: In what way do habits organize performance of this activity?
4. *Performance subsystem:*
   Perceptual-motor: Which perceptual-motor skills are used, and in which parts of the activity?
   Planning, process, and cognitive skills: What cognitive skills and planning skills are required in the activity? In which stages?
   Communication skills: Are communication skills required? What kinds of skills? And with whom?

Adapted and greatly condensed from Kielhofner G. *A model of human occupation: theory and application.* Baltimore, Md: Williams & Wilkins; 1985.

needs enough common sense to recognize when the adaptation is excessive or impractical, or one that the patient will find unacceptable.

Gradation is defined in the *Oxford English Dictionary* as "the process of advancing step by step; the course of gradual progress." In other words, a goal that is out of reach today can be attained by steady, stepwise movement, as illustrated in Fig. 23–1. The assistant or therapist designs a graded activity program so that at first the patient is asked to do only what he is capable of doing. Over the course of several or many sessions, the assistant gradually adds new challenges, so that the patient can develop new abilities by building on what he has already done. The example shown in the figure illustrates some of the ways that activities might be structured to provide increasing opportunities to make decisions; although 5 steps are shown, as many as 20 or 30 might actually be needed. In addition,

choices other than those shown could be used to stimulate decisions.

It requires imagination and logic to design a graded program of activities for many of the treatment goals common to psychiatric occupational therapy. Range of motion or strength or other typical treatment goals of physical rehabilitation are concrete, visible, and easy to measure; they can be graded by performing simple physical procedures such as changing the position of the activity in relation to the patient, or adding weights. Not so with some goals of psychiatric rehabilitation; as discussed several times elsewhere in this text, many important psychiatric goals are intangible and difficult to measure. This imposes a certain vagueness and uncertainty about how to approach them, and how to grade activities to make them easier to reach.

The following section addresses some of the ways in which activities can be graded to help patients work toward some of the

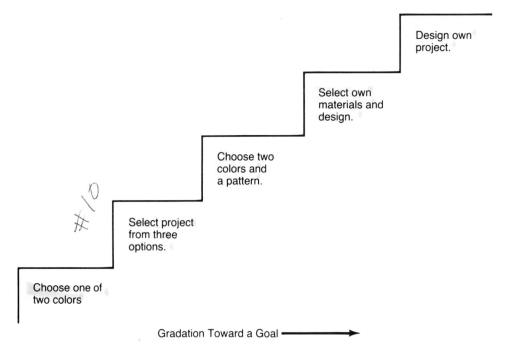

FIG. 23–1. Gradation of decison-making: an example of gradation toward a goal

goals typical of psychiatric occupational therapy programs. These include increased ability and performance in the following areas: attention span, decision making, problem solving, self-awareness, awareness of others, interaction with others, and independence and self-responsibility.

Attention span can be graded by requiring a person to work for increasingly longer periods. For example, if the patient can work for only 15 minutes without being distracted, then the program would begin with 15-minute work periods. Gradually, the patient would be asked to work for longer times without taking a break: 20 minutes, a half-hour, 45 minutes, and so on. The amount by which the time period increases and the rate at which the program progresses are based on the patient's ability to tolerate increased demands. As a general rule, the patient should be expected to do as much as he can, as quickly as he can. One has to assume that the patient is eager to reach his goal of increased attention span, and that he will work toward it diligently. However, the program should also be designed to accommodate day-to-day variations in ability and motivation that may be caused by medication, stress, or other factors.

If a program is designed to help a patient increase his attention span, then other factors that might interfere with this goal need to be eliminated. The task should be one that is meaningful, one that the patient is capable of doing, and one that really does require constant attention over time. If the patient thinks the task is meaningless, it is not reasonable to expect him to want to pay attention to it. If the task is too difficult, the patient is likely to be too frustrated or anxious to try to do it for very long. Finally, tasks that take only a short time (e.g., making coffee) or that people generally approach casually (picking them up and then stopping them to do something else, as in knitting and many other crafts) are not really suitable activities for increasing attention span.

Decision making can be an unfamiliar and difficult process for someone who has had other people taking care of the important details of his life. Two kinds of patients who may find it hard to make even simple decisions are those who have been hospitalized for years and those whose families have controlled their environment and activities. A program to help someone improve his ability to make decisions must logically include many opportunities for him to face real choices and decide among them. It must also take into account the resistance of family members to change, and must provide ways to deal with this.

It is easy to structure the number and kinds of choices presented to a patient in a craft activity. Most crafts can be approached on a very simple level at first, and then made increasingly complex. The assistant can limit or expand choices and possibilities with regard to color, design, tools, size, and amount of detail. For example, a patient can be given no choice ("Make a coaster exactly like this one") or can make a mosaic tile coaster in which he chooses *only* the color of the tile (the assistant would provide squares of tiles prespaced and mounted on mesh and cut to the exact size of the tray). At the other extreme, by providing a choice of different kinds of tile and mounting surfaces, grout colors, tile nippers, and reproductions of elaborate mosaic work from Italy and Greece, the assistant can make the same activity very complex, requiring many choices and decisions.

Although a craft activity may be the easiest place to begin helping a patient learn to make decisions, other real-life decisions that are important to the patient should also be included. As we have already discussed, the patient should be invited to say what he would like to get out of treatment, and how; some may find this overwhelming unless the therapist or assistant gives examples.

If the problem is that the person is really inexperienced and does not know how to make decisions, then instruction about how to generate alternatives and predict outcomes can be combined with simulations and real practice. Once the person begins to make decisions he will not necessarily make sound ones, but with encouragement to try again, discussion of what happened, and acceptance of the outcome, he will have the support to refine his skill.

Problem solving can be graded in a similar fashion. One can begin with activities that have minor problems with relatively obvious solutions and little chance of failure (e.g., leather stamping, with its need to vary the force of the mallet for stamps of different sizes). Gradually, more problematic activities and situations (e.g., attaching buckles, rivets, and snaps) can be introduced. As with decision making, it is important to work also with problems that the patient really faces in his life (e.g., what to do when his older brother asks him for money, or how to get into his apartment if he loses his keys). Again, education about how to analyze a problem and generate solutions should be interwoven with opportunities to practice these skills both in simulations and in real life.

Self-awareness is a skill that has many developmental layers. At its most basic, it is the awareness of the body and its effects on the environment. Patients who have severe deficits may need to begin with sensorimotor activities. Usually, however, when we say that a person needs to develop greater self-awareness, we mean that he has unrealistic ideas about his talents and skills, about what he wants and does not want, and about how he feels about the things that happen to him.

A graded program to develop a person's self-awareness must include both experiences that allow one to explore one's effect on the world and opportunities to discuss these experiences with other people. Activities should be chosen based on the interests and past experience of the patient. Almost any activity can be used, although most people would agree that you can learn more about yourself through an art activity or a game played with other people than you can from doing a crossword puzzle or typing a manuscript. This suggests that suitable activities must provide either an expressive medium or interaction with others (or, if possible, both). The most essential ingredient, however, is the opportunity to verbalize one's ideas and feelings and to receive feedback from others in a safe setting. Thus, it is not the activities that are graded, but the way the therapist structures the activities to encourage self-reflection and feedback.

When we say that someone needs to develop more *awareness of others,* we usually mean that the person acts in a way that shows he does not understand the needs or rights of other people. For the patient to develop this awareness, the therapist provides activities that require interaction with other people and that include opportunities to discuss and analyze what happens between them. Thus, as with awareness of self, a program to develop awareness of others is graded in its demands for reflection, discussion, and analysis, rather than in the activity itself.

Patients who are socially isolated, or who rely on a few rigid patterns of relating to other people, can improve their social skills and comfort through a graded program to increase *interaction with others.* Activities are graded on the basis of how much involvement with other people is required, and the nature of the involvement. Table 17–2 lists ways to grade activities to increase interactions with others. As discussed in Chapter 17, the assistant must be careful not to push patients too quickly to become involved with other people. Interaction skills take a long time to develop, and cannot develop at all if the person is uncomfortable. Among the many factors that the therapist can vary to accommodate the patient's needs are the frequency of involvement, the length of involvement, and the intensity of involvement with others.

Programs to help patients develop a greater sense of *independence and self-responsibility* require activities that can be graded in terms of how much the patient must rely on the therapist or other people for help. In other words, the program begins with an activity in which the patient requires instruction from the therapist. Gradually, as the patient acquires more skills and knowledge, he will need the therapist less. This does not automatically mean that he will ask for less help than at the beginning; often the therapist must help him discuss and explore what he is able to do on his own. Patients who are not accustomed to doing things on their own may not recognize that they are able to do so, or that they have done so. In this case, the therapist encourages the patient to reflect on what he has done, and to think about how little assistance he received. Activities that can be graded to increase independence and self-responsibility must be ones that require some instruction in the beginning, allow for increased mastery with practice over time, and are complex enough that they include opportunities to develop new skills and to make multiple decisions. Woodworking, leathercraft, and cooking are activities that meet these criteria.

ACTIVITY ANALYSIS AND COGNITIVE DISABILITIES

We have discussed in a broad and general way how the principles of adaptation and gradation can be used to tailor an activity to meet the needs of patients at various levels. To match activities more accurately and precisely to the needs and capabilities of patients, however, we need a more rigorous method of analysis. Claudia Allen's theory of cognitive disabilities provides such a method. Table 23–3 delineates the factors that should be assessed to determine whether an activity is one that the patient can perform successfully at his current level of functioning. Using the same method of analysis, the therapist can make an activity less demanding or more demanding. To use this method of task analysis, it is essential to understand what the various terms in Table 23–3 mean, and what they imply about the activity.

Directions are instructions given by another person (most often the therapist or assistant). Verbal directions use words; demonstrated directions do not use words, but instead use actual physical examples of what is to be done. This may involve the therapist touching the patient. *Physical properties of material objects* (which Allen calls "perceptibility") are the kind of sensory information that the patient must respond to in order to perform the activity. The patient can act only upon what he knows and perceives. So it is important to present the activity in a way that he can understand it and act on it. *Motor actions* are behaviors exhibited by patients. The number of actions, both different actions and repetitions of the same action, is considered. *Tool use* means whether or not tools are used and what kind of tools are used to do the activity. *Stimulus for motor action* refers to the kind of stimulation that will catch the patient's attention and interest and motivate him to do the activity. Since what we want is for the patient to *do* something (the activity), we need to know what kind of stimulation will get him started.

Allen (2) explains how to present each of these aspects of the task for each of the six cognitive levels. We can use this information to design activities so that the patient will be able to understand and enjoy them.

Level 1

The patient is only aware of what penetrates the threshold of conscious awareness. Therefore, shouted one- or two-word directions and physical contact are needed to start the action. The patient will be able to do only one action at a time, and may not repeat it unless prompted to. For example, the assistant might get the patient to stand up by tugging on her hand and saying

"Stand up!" in a loud voice. By contrast, the patient probably would not stand up just because everyone else did or because the assistant said "Please stand up" in a normal tone of voice.

Level 2

The patient is aware of his own movements and those of others and is able to perform simple gross motor actions that have been demonstrated by the assistant. Calisthenics and sensorimotor activities can be used. Although the patient will not understand how to use tools, he may respond to simple familiar objects such as balls and jumpropes. The verbal directions can include names of body parts, but the assistant must also demonstrate the desired action. Each demonstration is limited to one action at a time; repetitions or variations on the same action can be introduced.

TABLE 23–3. *Task analysis for Allen's cognitive levels*

	Level 1: automatic actions	Level 2: postural actions	Level 3: manual actions
Directions verbal	verbs ("eat!", "chew!") introjections ("wait") directions may have to be shouted.	pronouns (you, I) and names of body parts ("move your arms")	add names of concrete objects ("peel these carrots with this tool, like this")
demonstrated	physical contact, guiding hands, touching, pushing	gross motor movements, guided movement	action of hands on an object (e.g., stringing beads or peeling carrots)
Physical properties of material objects	subliminal properties,— for example, of food or drink or presence of others	the patient's own body and your body, confining properties of furniture and clothing	exterior surfaces of objects (what is visible and touchable)
Motor actions number	one action (may need prompting to repeat it)	one action (may spontaneously repeat it or do variation)	one action, repetition of same action
tool use	none—may use body parts when stimulated (e.g., puts food in mouth)	uses body parts and may use familiar objects spontaneously (e.g., tosses ball)	uses habitually-used tools but often uses them poorly (e.g., brushes hair incompletely, messily)
stimulus for motor action	alerting stimuli (e.g., touching)	demonstrated action (e.g., hand clapping)	manual action used during task (e.g., sanding wood)

Level 3

The patient at this level is more aware of things around him, particularly what he can see and touch. The patient enjoys hand movements that are repeated, and will participate in activities that have a repetitive manual action. He does the activity not because he wants to make the project or arrive at some end goal but because he enjoys performing the action involved. The directions can include the names of objects used in the action, but the action must also be demonstrated. The same action is repeated over and over.

Level 4

The patient at this level is motivated by a desire to make the project rather than by an interest in the motions involved. The pa-

TABLE 23–3. (*Continued*)

	Level 4: goal-directed actions	Level 5: exploratory actions	Level 6: planned actions
Directions verbal	add adjectives, adverbs ("cut them in smaller pieces" or "sand the wood until it is smooth")	add prepositions and explanations (e.g., "this piece goes under, then over" and "the glaze will melt and turn blue")	add conjunctions and conjectures (e.g., "what if you did this . . . and then that. . . . what do you suppose would happen?")
demonstrated	several actions on an object if demonstrated one at a time	up to three steps demonstrated together, including precautions and options (e.g., not to strike leather stamps too hard, and how to combine them for new designs)	not required—may follow written directions or diagrams
Physical properties of material objects	color and shape (preferred projects are two-dimensional with contrasting colors)	space and depth (e.g., spacing tiles, rotating leather stamps to produce different patterns)	intangible and abstract qualities (e.g., an engineer designs a wall fastener based on type of wall, weight of object, angle of forces, etc.)
Motor actions number	one step at a time (add next when first is finished)	several steps at a time (not more than three if one is new)	unlimited (can sustain action toward goal for extended time)
tool use	uses tools to make projects or produce an effect, but may have trouble with tools that cover up objects (e.g., stapler or hole puncher)	uses tools to produce different effects by varying how they are used (e.g., changes angle of blade, force of hammer blow, grade of sandpaper)	makes own tools, alters existing tools, operates power tools
stimulus for motor action	desire to produce exact match of sample project provided	desire to experiment with or explore how to use materials (e.g., may produce several different leather belts)	ideas, imagination, plans

tient is interested in the color and shape of objects and materials, and prefers contrasting colors and clear shapes. The activity can have several steps, but each must be demonstrated separately and then performed by the patient before the next step is demonstrated. The verbal directions can include adjectives and adverbs that clarify the standards of performance. The patient can use simple tools like scissors and hammers, but may be flustered by tools that hide part of the project (as when a stapler covers the pages).

Level 5

Individuals at this level can perform most activities that can be demonstrated. The demonstrations can include up to three steps at a time. Because the person at this level is aware of space and depth and the relations between objects, the verbal directions can include prepositions and terms about spatial relationships. Activities that require understanding of a spatial pattern (e.g., mosaics) can be introduced. The person can use all hand tools, and will spontaneously experiment with different ways to use them to obtain varying results. New learning may be self-initiated.

Level 6

At this level the individual can understand abstract ideas. Because of this, written directions and diagrams can be used, and demonstrations may not be required. The possible range of activities is unlimited.

Allen's task analysis methods can be used to select, adapt, and grade activities to make it easier for the patient to succeed. For example, it is obvious that spacing mosaics is a poor choice of activity for someone at level 4, but is perfectly suitable for someone at level 5. A level 4 patient who says she is interested in making a mosaic

tile trivet is probably responding to how the project looks rather than the process used to make it. Therefore, the assistant could substitute something that gives a similar appearance but requires less complex thought (e.g., making a trivet but eliminating spacing and grouting from the process).

ANALYSIS IS AN ONGOING PROCESS

Additional tantalizing information about the surprisingly large effects of small adjustments in how activities are presented has come from the research of Nelson and others (1,3,4,6,8,10,11,12,13,14,15). Although the studies were performed with small groups (often very different from psychiatric patients), the results indicate, for example, that having a real purpose or outcome enhances enjoyment (15), participation (6), length of performance (14), and positive perceptions of the experience (8). Being allowed to keep what one has made increases positive feelings toward an activity as well (12). Another study (10) demonstrated that, for the well elderly, socialization and enjoyment were greater in a project group format when contrasted with a parallel group format. Yet another study (13) showed that tool scarcity appeared to increase engagement in the activity, when compared to the same activity with sufficient tools for each member. A study (3) involving college students demonstrated that humorous and silly activities may increase cohesiveness. These findings should suggest to the occupational therapy assistant that much thoughtful planning and some experimentation with how an activity is presented are needed to create the best possible treatment outcome.

CONCLUSION

The format used in Table 23–1, the questions asked in Table 23–2, and the task analysis presented in Table 23–3 may seem highly detailed and complex. But this is the nature of activities, which are themselves very complicated, even though we often do them almost as second nature. The individual parts, though, need to be analyzed, and by looking at the activity part by part and step by step in relation to the patient and his needs, one can assemble a picture that is comprehensive enough to be used in planning treatment.

REFERENCES

1. Adelstein LA, Nelson DL. Effects of sharing versus non-sharing on affective meaning in collage activities. *Occup Ther Mental Health* 1985;5(2):29–45.
2. Allen CK. *Occupational therapy for psychiatric diseases: measurement and management of cognitive disabilities.* Boston: Little, Brown; 1985.
3. Banning MR, Nelson DL. The effects of activity-elicited humor and group structure on group cohesion and affective responses. *Am J Occup Ther* 1987;41:510–514.
4. Boyer J et al. Affective response to activities: a comparative study. *Am J Occup Ther* 1989; 43:81–88.
5. Fidler G, Fidler J. *Occupational therapy: a communication process in psychiatry.* New York: Macmillan; 1963.
6. Hatter JK. Altruism and task participation in the elderly. *Am J Occup Ther* 1987;41:379–381.
7. Kielhofner G. *A model of human occupation: theory and application.* Baltimore, Md: Williams & Wilkins; 1985.
8. Miller L, Nelson DL. Dual-purpose activity versus single-purpose activity in terms of duration on task, exertion level and affect. *Occup Ther Mental Health* 1987;7(1):55–67.
9. Mosey AC. *Occupational therapy: configuration of a profession.* New York: Raven Press; 1981.
10. Nelson DL et al. Effects of project versus parallel groups on social interaction and affective responses in senior citizens. *Am J Occup Ther* 1988;42:23–29.
11. Nelson DL. Occupation: form and performance. *Am J Occup Ther* 1988;42:633–641.
12. Rocker JD, Nelson DL. Affective responses to keeping and not keeping an activity product. *Am J Occup Ther* 1987;41:152–157.
13. Steffan JA, Nelson DL. The effects of tool scarcity on group climate and affective meaning within the context of a stenciling activity. *Am J Occup Ther* 1987;41:449–453.
14. Steinbeck TM. Purposeful activity and performance. *Am J Occup Ther* 1986;40:529–534.
15. Thibodeaux CS, Ludwig FM. Intrinsic motivation in product-oriented and non-product-oriented activities. *Am J Occup Ther* 1988;42: 169–175.

ADDITIONAL REFERENCES AND SUGGESTED READINGS

Allen CK. Activity: occupational therapy's treatment method. *Am J Occup Ther* 1987;41:563–575.
Allen CK. *Occupational therapy for psychiatric diseases: measurement and management of cognitive disabilities.* Boston: Little, Brown; 1985.
Barris R, Kielhofner G, Watts JH. *Psychosocial occupational therapy: practice in a pluralistic arena.* Laurel, Md: RAMSCO; 1983.
Cynkin S. *Occupational therapy: toward health through activities.* Boston: Little, Brown; 1979.
Fidler G, Fidler J. *Occupational therapy: a communication process in psychiatry.* New York: Macmillan; 1963.
Friedland J. The issue is—Diversional activity: does it deserve its bad name? *Am J Occup Ther* 1988;42:603–608.
Hopkins HL, Smith HD, Tiffany EG. The activity process. In: Hopkins HL, Smith HD, eds. *Willard and Spackman's occupational therapy.* 5th ed. Philadelphia: JB Lippincott; 1978.
Levy LL. Activity, social role retention, and the multiply disabled aged: strategies for intervention. *Occup Ther Mental Health* 1990;10(3):2–30.
Mosey AC. *Activities therapy.* New York: Raven Press; 1973.
Mosey AC. *Occupational therapy: configuration of a profession.* New York: Raven Press; 1981.
Mosey AC. *Three frames of reference for mental health.* Thorofare, NJ: SLACK; 1970.
Reed K. *Models of practice in occupational therapy.* Baltimore: Williams & Wilkins; 1984.
Reed KL. Tools of practice: heritage or baggage? 1986 Eleanor Clarke Slagle lecture. *Am J Occup Ther* 1986;40:597–605.
Smith NR, Kielhofner G, Watts JH. The relationships between volition, activity pattern, and life satisfaction in the elderly. *Am J Occup Ther* 1986;40:278–283.
Spackman CS. Methods of instruction. In: Hopkins HL, Smith HD, eds. *Willard and Spackman's occupational therapy.* 4th ed. Philadelphia: JB Lippincott; 1971.
Tiffany EG. Psychiatry and mental health. In: Hopkins HL, Smith HD, eds. *Willard and Spackman's occupational therapy.* 6th ed. Philadelphia: JB Lippincott; 1983.
Willson M. *Occupational therapy in long-term psychiatry.* Edinburgh: Churchill Livingstone; 1983.

Professional Development

24

Supervision

This system is the most difficult, the least common, and the most thorough way to teach. It is most difficult because it demands constant alertness, invariable good humor, complete earnestness, and utter self-surrender to the cause of truth, on the part of both teacher and pupil. It is least common because it is expensive in time, money, and effort.

GILBERT HIGHET (7, p. 108)

Students and new COTAs usually enter mental health practice with a desire to help patients, and to apply what they have learned in school. However, reading about something and actually doing it are different experiences. New practitioners often find that actual clinical practice is more complex than they expected, and that it is difficult to apply the skills they learned in school. It soon becomes clear that new skills need to be developed and previous ones further refined. One of the best ways to enhance one's skills as a fieldwork student, a new practitioner, or really at any time in one's career is through the *active* use of supervision. Chances are that your supervisor will be an experienced clinician, someone with advanced knowledge and skills, or at least someone who knows more about mental health practice than you do. A seasoned clinician is an invaluable guide who can increase your understanding of the role of occupational therapy and help you develop your own abilities, skills, and clinical style.

The main purposes of this chapter are to acquaint students and entry-level COTAs with the goals and limits of supervision, and to help them learn how to use the supervisory relationship effectively to further their own growth and development as mental health practitioners. The following topics will be addressed: the definition and goals of supervision, the responsibilities of the supervisor and the supervisee, factors affecting communication in the supervisory relationship, and the supervisory contract. The chapter will also describe how to prepare yourself for the experience of being supervised, and how to get the most from supervision.[1]

Since occupational therapy assistants may, after a year of practice, become supervisors themselves, an additional purpose of this chapter is to identify some of the issues that concern a beginning supervisor. Readings and other resources that

---

[1]Much of the material in this section is derived from Early (6).

the novice supervisor might consult will be indicated.

DEFINITION AND GOALS OF SUPERVISION

The definition of supervision that will be presented here may seem very different from your past experience and ideas about supervision. You may have thought of a supervisor as someone who tells you what to do and then checks to see whether you have done it, and how well. This *is* one aspect of supervision, the *administrative* function. One of the supervisor's responsibilities is to make sure that the work is done well and on time.

In addition, the occupational therapy supervisor has a second responsibility. The supervisor must evaluate how well the student or employee is performing on the job. In the case of students, the supervisor must decide whether the student has met the criteria of the fieldwork placement, and is ready to go on to the next level. The supervisor must make decisions about whether new employees should be continued on probation, or promoted to permanent status, and may determine whether or not a staff member should be promoted or given different job responsibilities. We will return to this *evaluative* aspect of supervision later in this chapter.

A third aspect of supervision is the *learning process*. In occupational therapy and other health professions, a very important goal of supervision is to help the supervisee (person being supervised) grow and develop in a helping role. Supervisor and supervisee must work together toward this goal; it is a responsibility that both of them share. Combining these three functions of administration, evaluation, and facilitation of learning, Fine has defined supervision as "a mutual undertaking to promote the growth and development of the supervisee

while evaluating performance and maintaining standards."[2]

What can you hope to get out of supervision? In what ways can you grow and develop? What will this "learning process" help you learn? Some specific goals you might wish to work toward in supervision are:

1. To develop a sense of your own role and identity as a COTA, and as a member of the occupational therapy profession.
2. To independently identify questions, problems, issues, and concerns that you are experiencing in your work.
3. To accept responsibility for your own behavior and your personal needs as they affect your work.
4. To solve problems and make decisions with increased confidence and independence.
5. To expand your skills and knowledge about occupational therapy and psychiatry.
6. To develop and maintain good working relationships with members of other disciplines.
7. To become more aware of yourself and your own behavior, feelings, and needs.

Let's explore each of these goals in more detail:

1. *To develop a sense of your own role and identity as a COTA, and as a member of the occupational therapy profession.* This goal focuses on your growth and development as a certified occupational therapy assistant. A COTA is a trained and certified technician who assists and collaborates with the registered occupational therapist in the planning and implementa-

[2]Fine SB. "Using supervision to meet clinical and professional needs." Speech given at the workshop entitled *Focus on Mental Health. II: A Plan for Action,* sponsored by the State University of New York, Downstate Medical Center, College of Health Related Professions, Occupational Therapy Program, at the Payne-Whitney Clinic, New York Hospital, March 21, 1986.

tion of treatment. The COTA also assists the OTR in making the occupational therapy department run smoothly.

On your internship, or in your first job, you may find yourself in a setting where there are no other COTAs employed, or in which COTAs have a different role from what you would want or expect for yourself. The OTR who is supervising you may have extensive knowledge of the COTA's role and considerable experience working with COTAs, or, on the other hand, may have little knowledge or experience of COTAs and what they can do. Together with your supervisor you can explore what your role should be. You can identify what possibilities exist for changes in your role in the future. You can discuss the role and contributions of the COTA to the profession generally, both locally and nationally.

2. *To independently identify questions, problems, issues, and concerns that you are experiencing in your work.* Being able to identify the problems and concerns you are experiencing is a necessary skill if you are to make use of the many learning opportunities available to you on the job. It is important to have the confidence to admit that you do not know something, that you do not have all the answers. Sometimes new graduates and students who have finished their coursework feel that they *should* know everything. If you think about this, you will realize it is a silly position to take. How could *anyone* learn *everything* about occupational therapy in a two-year program? Even clinicians with advanced degrees and years of experience still have questions. This is one of the things that makes our profession exciting. The questions you raise will help you develop your skills and knowledge further, and enable you to identify and discuss the central concerns and issues of our profession. The questions we *all* raise help us identify areas for research and new directions for practice.

Another aspect of this goal involves developing the skill to think through and to verbalize (speak about) the issues and problems you encounter. Although supervisors have many skills, reading minds is not one of them. You will have to let your supervisor know what is on your mind. That is the only way she can help you work on the problem. If you hold back because you are afraid of sounding ignorant, you are wasting a valuable opportunity to learn whatever it is you are afraid you do not know.

3. *To accept responsibility for your own behavior and your personal needs as they affect your work.* There are times when each of us finds it easier to make excuses for our behavior than to admit that we are in some way responsible. "The bus was late," "I left it at home," "You didn't give me enough time," are all excuses we have heard others use. Perhaps we have even used such excuses ourselves. Taking responsibility for yourself is an important aspect of mature behavior. It is an attitude that all of us could develop further.

Sometimes the excuses we make are rather subtle. For example, an occupational therapist or assistant might be faced with a situation in which only two of the eight patients scheduled for a new group actually show up on the first day. This is anxiety provoking and could be handled in several ways:

1. The therapist could dismiss the patients and not hold the group.
2. The therapist could refuse to admit the missing six patients to the next session of the group because they missed the first one.
3. The therapist could give the two patients something to do while she telephoned around to find out why the others were missing.
4. Finally, she might just run the group as planned and inquire later about the whereabouts of the missing patients.

Which do you think is the most responsible way to handle this situation? The first solution deprives two patients of a scheduled treatment. The second deprives six patients of treatment for reasons that are not really very clear. Does either of these solutions seem responsible? Can you think of situations in which they might be justified? The third and fourth solutions seem to be more responsible ones, but deciding which one was better would depend on the type of setting and the kind of patients and group. The key point made by this example is that a mature occupational therapy staff member accepts responsibility for her behavior, and bases her actions on ethical principles. Blaming others or making excuses for not providing patient services does not solve the problem.

4. *To solve problems and make decisions with increased confidence and independence.* This goal is related to others we have just discussed. To solve problems one must first be able to admit that problems exist. One must also accept the responsibility for solving problems and making decisions. There are systematic methods for solving problems and making decisions. You may have learned some of them in school. Your supervisor will be able to help you find ways to develop these skills further.

5. *To expand your skills and knowledge about occupational therapy and psychiatry.* You will first have to identify exactly what you wish to learn about occupational therapy and psychiatry. Once you have done this, your supervisor will be able to point out the resources you can use. These may include books and other printed information, audiovisual programs, discussions with knowledgeable professionals, and field trips and other activities. Being honest about how you prefer to learn and how you learn best will help your supervisor work more effectively with you in selecting resources. (Don't wait a month to tell her you don't understand the articles she gave you to read.)

Your supervisor may identify specific learning goals that she feels are priorities for a particular patient group or program. Your receptiveness to such direction will have a strong impact on your relationship with your supervisor and on the quality and scope of the services you are able to provide.

6. *To develop and maintain good working relationships with members of other disciplines.* Typically, patients with mental health problems are treated by a team of professionals and paraprofessionals, who may include physicians, nurses, psychologists, social workers, occupational therapists and assistants, recreation therapists, other activity therapists, counselors, and aides. In community settings there may be fewer medical personnel but more paraprofessionals such as aides and counselors, and perhaps teachers. Working together with these other people is essential if the patient is to receive the best care. Yet it can be difficult to sort out the roles of these different workers and develop relationships with them that really work. Your supervisor can help you analyze or identify specific problems you may be having in this area, specific goals that you can work on, and ways to achieve these goals.

One of the things that frequently happens in mental health practice that does not happen to the same extent in other practice areas of occupational therapy is role blurring. This occurs when members of different disciplines provide very similar kinds of services. For example, the nurse may work with the patients on their activities of daily living, or the social worker may take this role, or the occupational therapist or assistant. In some settings, teachers and special educators take on this function. Thus the student or new occupational therapy graduate is confronted with the uncomfortable idea that the job he went to school for is being done, and done well or not so well, by someone in another discipline. Unless this feeling is identified and discussed, it will fester, and perhaps be acted out in resentment, withdrawal, or defensiveness. Role blurring *is* a frequent concern of students and new graduates; this is an area in which an experienced supervisor can really help. Keep in mind, however, that the roles different disciplines play in a given setting were established over a long time and are not easily changed.

7. *To become more aware of yourself and your own behavior, feelings, and needs.* As a member of a profession that serves the needs of other people, you will need to be aware of your own behavior and feelings. Many scary feelings can arise as you encounter patients who are your own age and whose problems do not seem all that different from your own. You will need to know how these and other feelings affect your relationships with other people. You will want to learn how others perceive you. This sort of learning can be difficult and threatening at first. It is hard to open yourself to possible criticism. It can be hard to face the fact that others see you differently from the way you see yourself. However, be actively working on this goal, you will gain increased confidence and control over your own behavior and your relationships with others.

We have just discussed the definition and purposes of supervision in its function as a learning process. As stated in our definition of supervision, it is a *mutual* process, requiring the attention and energy of both the person doing the supervising *and* the person being supervised. Let us turn our attention now to the responsibilities of the supervisor in the supervisory relationship.

RESPONSIBILITIES OF THE SUPERVISOR

The supervisor, as the more experienced person, takes the initiative in setting up the supervisory relationship. This involves the following responsibilities:

1. To assign a time for supervision meetings, and to be available to the supervisee at the scheduled time.
2. To identify the specific responsibilities of the supervisee for patient care and indirect services.
3. To set reasonable expectations for the supervisee's performance of these duties.
4. To respond to the supervisee as an individual, and to help the supervisee begin to identify personal learning goals.
5. To explain how and when and by what criteria the supervisee will be evaluated.
6. To clarify for co-workers and patients the roles and responsibilities of the supervisee.
7. To orient the supervisee to the larger institution, its rules and resources.

Once the supervisory relationship has been established (this may take one or two weeks), and the supervisee is more comfortable and oriented to what is expected, the supervisor guides the supervisee in making the best use of supervision as an opportunity for personal and professional growth. This involves additional responsibilities for the supervisor:

8. To help the supervisee identify and focus on specific learning goals.
9. To provide timely, behaviorally focused feedback about the supervisee's progress and any problems she may be having.
10. To perform periodic evaluations of the supervisee's performance and to discuss these with the supervisee.
11. To provide appropriate learning opportunities suited to the goals and learning style of the supervisee.
12. To provide an atmosphere of security, acceptance, recognition, and enthusiasm.
13. To respect the confidences of the supervisee.

Although one of the supervisor's functions is to help the supervisee grow and develop, it is important to remember that patients always come first, and that the growth and development of the supervisee is secondary to the provision of patient services. What this means in practical terms is that the supervisor must first make sure that patients are being served *before* she turns her attention to the needs of the supervisee. In addition, her evaluation of the supervisee's performance is based on how well the supervisee is providing for the patients' needs.

Since we have already stated that supervision is a *mutual* undertaking, let us now look at the supervisee's role and responsibilities.

RESPONSIBILITIES OF THE SUPERVISEE

If you are a student or new graduate, you should be supervised by an experienced OTR or COTA. Since one of the major purposes of supervision is to help you develop and grow as an occupational therapy practitioner in mental health, it is important for you to recognize that *you* have responsibilities in supervision. These are:

1. To meet with your supervisor as scheduled.
2. To follow through with assigned responsibilities to the best of your ability.
3. To ask for clarification of any responsibilities you do not understand.
4. To let your supervisor know when you are not capable of doing something you have been asked to do.
5. To identify problems that you experience in your work.
6. To respond to your supervisor as a person who is trying to help you learn, and to be as honest and open as you can.
7. To take an active role in setting your own learning goals.
8. To follow through on learning opportunities suggested by your supervisor.
9. To ask for assistance when you need it.
10. To accept evaluation as an opportunity for learning more about your own strengths and weaknesses.
11. To respect the confidences and authority of your supervisor.
12. To abide by the administrative chain of command.
13. To abide by the rules of the institution.

It should not be surprising that you, as the supervisee, have as many responsibilities as your supervisor does to make the supervisory relationship a good one. Let us look at the supervisee's responsibilities in more detail:

1. *To meet regularly with your supervisor at the assigned times.* The responsibility is fairly clear. If for any reason you are not able to attend a scheduled supervision meeting, you should let your supervisor know as soon as possible, in advance of the meeting time. If you feel that you need or would like more supervision than is being provided, you have to let your supervisor know. Be prepared to accept the possibility that your supervisor's time is already committed to other priorities, and that she cannot spare any more for you. Nonetheless, she may be able to suggest other routes for you to use to meet your learning needs.

2. *To follow through with assigned responsibilities to the best of your ability.* This needs little explanation. Your supervisor knows that you are just starting out. She will not intentionally assign you any responsibilities that are beyond your abilities.

3. *To ask for clarification of any responsibilities you do not understand.* If you are not sure exactly what your supervisor wants you to do, ask for an explanation. Trying to interpret what your supervisor means without getting any further clarification from her can cause serious problems.

4. *To let your supervisor know when your are not capable of doing something you have been asked to do.* Occasionally your supervisor may ask you to do something you have not been trained to do. For ex-

ample, she might ask you to lead a group in a craft that you have never done yourself. It is your responsibility to identify what you can and cannot do, so that your supervisor can decide how to handle this. In the example we have used, she might give you a few days to learn the craft on your own before working with the group, or she might ask you to use another activity with which you *are* familiar.

5. *To identify problems that you experience in your work.* These might include difficult patients, staff members with whom you disagree, or problems applying techniques and knowledge you have learned.

6. *To respond to your supervisor as a person who is trying to help you learn, and to be as honest and open as you can.* If you have worked in the past under supervisors whose main relationship to you was as overseer, boss, and critic, you may feel reluctant to confide in any supervisor. Try to realize that an occupational therapist does not have to take on the responsibility of supervising students or new therapists, and that she usually does so because she wants to share her knowledge and expertise with a less experienced person.

7. *To take an active role in setting your own learning goals.* As has already been stated, your supervisor cannot read your mind. It might seem easier and less troublesome to let your supervisor set your goals for you, and tell you what you should be learning. But you really know a lot about your own learning needs. Share this information with your supervisor so that you can work together to set meaningful and realistic goals.

8. *To follow through on learning opportunities suggested by your supervisor.* Once you and your supervisor have identified your learning objectives, your supervisor will help you select methods and resources. It is up to you to follow through on them. If the methods do not suit you, or if you would rather approach your learning goals through another method, you should dis-

cuss this with your supervisor immediately, so that the two of you can develop another plan.

9. *To ask for assistance when you need it.* It is natural to want to function independently, without any help from anyone. This is not realistic, however; we all need help occasionally. Be sure to ask for it. Asking for help does not mean that you are incompetent; it means that you are aware of your own limitations and willing to use the resources that are available. Try to keep track, however, of how many times you have asked for help or clarification with the same task.

10. *To accept evaluation as an opportunity for learning more about your own strengths and weaknesses.* This may sound idealistic. There *are* aspects of evaluation that are unpleasant. It is often hard to listen to criticism. But evaluation is an opportunity for you to hear what others think of your performance. Through evaluation, you will become aware of your areas of strength and success, and will be able to identify areas that you need to work on further.

11. *To respect the confidences and authority of your supervisor.* From time to time your supervisor may share important facts, ideas, or feelings with you, and may ask you to keep these confidential. Respect her wishes, as you would have her respect yours. It is possible that your supervisor may even ask or order you to do something, without explaining why. Remember, your supervisor is responsible not just for you, but for the smooth operation of the occupational therapy program. She may have reasons for her decisions that she cannot possibly share with you. This may seem unreasonable, even arrogant, at first, but if you think about it you will see why it is sometimes necessary.

12. *To abide by the administrative chain of command.* Just as you are responsible to your supervisor, she is responsible to someone else in a higher position of authority.

And so it goes, up the chain of command to the chief administrator of the hospital or agency (who, by the way, is responsible to the board of trustees, to consumers, and to government authorities). To abide by the chain of command means not to go over your supervisor's head to a higher authority, not to take actions that will affect your supervisor or her superiors without consulting your supervisor first, and not to accept orders and responsibilities from others without consulting your supervisor.

The only situation in which you might legitimately seek the advice and intervention of a higher authority on your own is when you are having serious problems communicating with your supervisor. Before doing this, though, you should let your supervisor know that you feel a problem exists.

13. *To abide by the rules of the institution.* Rules are the boundaries that define the rights and responsibilities of people within a social system. The rules of the institution cover routine issues such as attendance and sick leave policies, and nonroutine ethical questions such as the rights of patients. You are expected to follow the rules and to question any that you do not understand. Blind obedience is not required; informed compliance is.

The responsibilities of the supervisee just described, and the responsibilities of the supervisor described previously, together provide the rules for a relationship that will help the supervisee grow and develop in clinical skills and knowledge. This can happen only if both parties communicate effectively with each other, and so we need to consider some of the factors that affect communication in clinical supervision.

FACTORS AFFECTING COMMUNICATION IN SUPERVISION

Any relationship that involves two people is affected by the qualities that each of them possesses as individuals. To discuss this fully we should probably examine all of the literature on human relationships in general. Since this is not within the scope of this text, we will highlight four major factors that often affect the interaction of two individuals in supervision. These are emotional needs, ideas about social and professional roles, personal values and beliefs, and communication style.[3]

The first factor is the *emotional needs* of both people, the supervisor and the supervisee. As a student or new graduate, you may want to depend on the guidance and leadership of your supervisor. If your supervisor needs you to be more independent or autonomous, conflicts will arise. On the other hand, your supervisor may enjoy having you somewhat dependent, as this makes her feel important. If you act very independently, she may be disappointed, or you may think she is. Conflicts are bound to arise if a supervisee's desire for independence and autonomy is stronger than the supervisor's perception of her skills and ability. What you do about such situations depends upon how you analyze them. You may decide that it is better to try to change your own behavior, without involving your supervisor. However, it is obviously best to work together with your supervisor to achieve a balanced and mutual perspective, by discussing what each of you thinks is going on.

Related to dependency and autonomy is the issue of self-esteem. Some people can take criticism more easily than others. Some appear to take criticism well, but inwardly feel devastated. Still others welcome criticism as an opportunity for learning and discussion. These variations apply to supervisors as well as to supervisees. If you discuss with your supervisor how *you* feel about criticism, and what kind of criticism is most likely to be acceptable to *you*, this can help set a tone for future evalua-

---

[3]This discussion summarizes ideas expressed by Fidler G. "Five dimensions of the dyad." Speech delivered at Columbia University, November 16, 1979, as part of the forum entitled *The Supervisory Dialogue.*

tions. Be aware that your supervisor has feelings too.

Another factor affecting communication in supervision is each individual's *ideas about social and professional roles*. Both you and your supervisor have definite notions, conscious and unconscious, about how an occupational therapist or assistant should act, and how a supervisor and supervisee should act. For example, your supervisor may think that your blood-red nail enamel or unusual hair style is out of place in a psychiatric clinic. You may feel she is being just another nosy mother figure and should mind her own business. As another example, you may want to have a social relationship with your supervisor, which she may resist because she thinks it would interfere with the supervisory relationship. Or you may think that your supervisor should read and correct the first drafts of all of your written work. She may think that *you* should develop a final draft before showing it to her (or vice versa).

Your ideas about social and professional roles encompass your conception of how a person should act and what she should do in a given role. If a person in that role does not act the way you think she should, you may feel uncomfortable. Discussing your feelings can help and gives both of you a chance to understand each other better.

A third factor affecting communication in supervision is the area of *personal values and beliefs*. Even where these are unrelated to the supervisory relationship, they can affect it. For example, if the supervisor is younger than the supervisee, and both come from cultures in which age is a sign of authority, they may interact as though the older person is the one with the greater authority. Or the supervisee (being older) may expect to be treated more deferentially than the supervisor (who is, after all, young enough to be her daughter) is treating her.

Values and beliefs about the nature of occupational therapy and mental health can also affect what occurs in supervision. For example, one person may believe that it really does not matter what a patient's craft project looks like in the end, as long as he gets something out of the experience of doing the activity. If the other person believes that the beauty of the final product is a reflection of the patient's self-esteem, and that everyone should work toward a perfect final product, there is bound to be some conflict. Resolving these conflicts is not always possible, but identifying them clearly helps limit their influence. You may need to recognize and adjust to the other person's values and beliefs in order to preserve the relationship.

Communication style has a profound effect on relationships. We each have our own individual ways of communicating, our own favorite words and ways of saying things. However, a listener who does not know us well may take a very different meaning from our words than what we actually intended. This can be a special problem for people who have learned English as a second language; they may have problems both in understanding and in being understood, problems that *both* parties in the supervisory relationship need to monitor carefully. Unless we are alert to possible errors in communication, misunderstandings will result. One method for handling this is to ask the other person to reflect back what she understood you to mean, or for you to reflect back what you thought she meant. In this way the received meaning can be checked against the intended meaning.

Obviously, supervision is affected by factors other than those we have discussed, but by attending to the four factors of emotional needs, ideas about social and professional roles, personal values and beliefs, and communication style, the supervisee can begin to analyze and understand the major influences on the relationship.

THE SUPERVISORY CONTRACT

You might wonder what contracts can possibly have to do with supervision. Perhaps you have seen formal contracts such as leases and other legal documents. A contract is an agreement between two people (or among several), which lets each person know what to expect from the other, and what each is responsible for doing. In supervision, both supervisor and supervisee need to agree upon what they expect to happen in the supervisory process. This is why contracts are sometimes used. The contract may be written, or it may be an oral agreement based on discussion. During your initial meetings with your supervisor, she may mention the idea of a supervisory

---

The parties named below agree that they will meet the following responsibilities during the student's three month internship which runs from _____, 19___ to _____, 19___.

Supervisee (Student)

I will meet every _____(day) with my supervisor at _____(time) to discuss issues which concern both of us.

I will follow through with assigned responsibilities, which will include (at a minimum); individual treatment plans on four patients, a group protocol, assisting in four weekly activity groups, running a group three times a week by myself, a written case study which I will present orally to the occupational therapy staff, attendance at OT staff meetings every Tuesday and Thursday from 12 noon to 1 P.M., attendance at team meetings, ordering and maintaining supplies and equipment for my groups.

In addition, I will identify specific areas in which I wish to increase my knowledge and skill, and I will make a separate contract with my supervisor to work on those goals.

I will abide by the rules of this hospital, will respect the rights of patients and staff, and will model my actions on the Principles of Occupational Therapy Ethics, as prescribed by the American Occupational Therapy Association.

Signed on _____, 19___.

_____
Supervisee (Student)

_____
School

Superviser

I will meet with the student at the agreed-upon time.

I will make available to the student all resources needed to carry out assigned responsibilities.

I will notify the student in advance (where possible) of any additional duties.

I will help the student identify specific learning goals and will provide direction and resources to help the student reach these goals.

I will provide ongoing informal feedback on the student's performance, and will discuss my formal evaluation with the student on _____, 19___ (midterm evaluation) and _____, 19___ (final evaluation).

_____
Supervisor

_____
Facility

FIG. 24–1. Sample supervisory contract

contract. If she does not, you may wish to. Setting up a contract with clear expectations helps prevent misunderstandings.

Written contracts have an important advantage over oral ones; they provide concrete evidence of what was agreed upon. Therefore, disputes about who said they would do what, and by when, can be avoided. One way to set up a written contract is to divide a sheet of paper into two columns. One column is headed "supervisor" and the other "supervisee." The expectations for each person are listed in the appropriate column. A sample of part of a supervisory contract is shown in Fig. 24-1. Such a contract need not cover every right and responsibility of supervisor and supervisee. The contract can focus on just one aspect of your work, and can be updated or rewritten to reflect changes in your interests and learning needs.

Whether or not you use a formal supervisory contract is entirely up to you and your supervisor. If you feel that there might be misunderstandings without a contract, or if you have had supervisory problems in the past, it might be a good idea to have a written contract.

GETTING THE MOST FROM SUPERVISION

As a place to learn, the clinic is very different from the classroom. In the classroom, your learning was the most important goal; in the clinic, the health and welfare of patients is the primary goal, and your learning is secondary. On the other hand, learning from a supervisor rather than a classroom instructor can be more individualized, and focused on you as a person, rather than on a group of people like you. This means that you can learn as rapidly as you wish, by practicing the same kinds of skills you used to learn in the classroom: asking questions, reading independently, and following through with available resources. The quality of your learning will depend on the quality of the questions that you ask and your motivation to find the answers.

Succeeding in supervision requires that you recognize that your supervisor has other demands on her time. Your willingness and flexibility to respect her need to sometimes change the schedule, or her inability to meet your needs at a particular time, will go a long way toward building an effective relationship. Supervision is a mutual, two-way undertaking, and you as supervisee must understand that *you* contribute to the process.

RESOLVING CONFLICTS IN SUPERVISION

In the ideal supervisory experience, supervisee and supervisor are an exact match. The supervisor provides the precise support needed by the supervisee, who grows by leaps and bounds under this nurturance. The real world of supervision frequently does not match the ideal. Supervisors and supervisees do not always agree, but these disagreements need not become major conflicts. Assignment of responsibilities, differences in treatment preferences and professional values, and disagreements about ratings on evaluations are some possible sources of conflict, and there are many others. Resolving conflicts is not only the supervisor's burden, but yours as well. Orr (8) suggests the following approach:

First, leave your anger behind you. Don't let hurt and anger and other negative emotions contaminate the situation.

Second, assume that your supervisor is as willing as you are to resolve the problem. Expect a positive outcome.

Third, prepare in advance exactly what you are going to say. Be specific, and focus on observable facts.

Fourth, listen actively, try to understand your supervisor's point of view, and be willing to compromise. A small positive step now can be the first of many to come; you can reach your goal in increments.

BECOMING A SUPERVISOR

Helping less experienced people learn how to work with patients can be one of the most satisfying challenges available to the seasoned clinician. After a year of practice as a COTA, you will be eligible, under American Occupational Therapy Association guidelines (1,2,3), to supervise others. Wanting to do this is one thing; knowing how to do it is another. A study by Christie and others (5) revealed that most occupational therapy supervisors learn by ex-

perience how to be supervisors, and that beginning supervisors feel unprepared and uncertain of their own performance. The purpose of this section is to provide you with some resources and direction, should you wish to undertake the supervision of occupational therapy students and personnel.

The American Occupational Therapy Association has identified the level of experience and expertise needed to supervise other occupational therapy personnel at various levels. These are shown in Table 24-1. As shown in the table, COTAs with one year or more of experience may supervise entry-level COTAs, volunteers, occupational therapy aides, and occupational therapy assistant students at both levels of

TABLE 24–1. *Recommended supervisory patterns for occupational therapy personnel*

Personnel classification	Is supervised by	Supervises
Entry-level OTR (Less than one year as an OTR)	Intermediate- or advanced-level OTR. In some general practice situations may work without supervision.	COTAs, OT aides, and volunteers.
Intermediate-level OTR (One or more years of practice as an OTR)	More experienced intermediate- or advanced-level OTR provides general (less than daily) supervision.	COTAs, OT aides, volunteers, OT and OTA students on Level I and Level II Fieldwork.
Advanced-level OTR (More than three years experience as an OTR, and an advanced degree or equivalent education and certification in a special area of practice)	Occasional supervision or consultation with an OTR qualified to provide this on an advanced level.	COTAs, OT aides, volunteers, OT and OTA students on Level I and Level II Fieldwork.
Entry level COTA (Less than one year as a COTA)	Close supervision by an OTR or intermediate- or advanced-level COTA. (This means daily on-site supervision.)	None
Intermediate-level COTA (One or more years of practice as a COTA)	General (less than daily) supervision by an intermediate- or advanced-level OTR.	Entry-level COTAs, OT aides, volunteers, OTA students on Level I and Level II Fieldwork.
Advanced-level COTA (More than three years experience as COTA, and additional coursework or certification in a special area of practice)	General (less than daily) supervision by an intermediate- or advanced-level OTR.	Entry-level COTAs, OT aides, volunteers, OTA students on Level I and Level II Fieldwork.

Information in this table is based on guidelines from American Occupational Therapy Association Commission on Practice: Guide for supervision of occupational therapy personnel (official position paper of the American Occupational Therapy Association). *Am J Occup Ther* 1981; 35:815–816; and Schell BAB. Guide to classification of occupational therapy personnel. *Am J Occup Ther* 1985; 39:803–10.

fieldwork. Each of these can perform different job tasks and should receive supervision according to his level of responsibility.

You should be well aware that an *entry-level* COTA is one who has been certified for less than one year. The new COTA is usually most interested in learning how to apply and develop her clinical skills, and in acquiring a professional identity as a competent practitioner. Supervision, therefore, focuses on shaping her awareness of what it means to be a certified occupational therapy assistant, and on refining and expanding her techniques for working with patients.

An *occupational therapy aide* (OT aide) is an employee (not a volunteer) who has been taught through on-the-job training how to perform routine maintenance tasks in the OT department, and to assist with some portions of patient-related activities. Some of the functions that might be performed by an OT aide include transporting patients, preparing supplies and setting up equipment for the therapist or assistant, and providing recreational (nontreatment) general activities. In addition, OT aides may be asked to help patients with their personal needs, such as toileting or getting a drink of water. Supervision of OT aides should focus on these specific job tasks and the attitudes and knowledge needed to perform them successfully.

Mental health therapy aides (MHTAs) are technical-level personnel assigned to assist nurses and other staff in general patient care. They are sometimes assigned to the occupational therapy department to assist in escorting patients and to provide security and additional support in situations where patients may become unmanageable. Frequently, MHTAs acquire enough on-the-job experience to function as OT aides in other areas. The focus of supervision for MHTAs is therefore similar to that for OT aides.

The standards of the Joint Commission on Accreditation of Hospitals (JCAH) stipulate that only a qualified OTR or COTA can provide occupational therapy services. Because OT aides have no formal training, certification, or licensure, they are not qualified (and should not be permitted) to perform evaluations or treatments, and should not be involved in recording patient information in the medical chart or reporting to the treatment team (4).

Volunteers are people who have decided to work in the occupational therapy area because they enjoy it and want to help or because they want to learn about the field. Volunteers are usually unpaid, but they may receive a small stipend for lunch or carfare. The knowledge and skills of volunteers are varied; some may be college graduates, others high school students. Some are retired people with years of life experience; others are young people whose lives have not exposed them to the kinds of suffering that many psychiatric patients have encountered. Supervision of a volunteer should focus first of all on that person's motivation for volunteering; when the supervisor knows *why* the volunteer wants to work, then the supervisor will be able to help him best. A high school student who is volunteering in order to get work-study credit has different needs and expectations than a retiree who is volunteering to share his craft skills. Supervision of a volunteer should include a thorough orientation to the facility, to occupational therapy, and to the volunteer's responsibilities. With instruction and direction, volunteers can perform most of the functions of an OT aide.

Occupational therapy assistant students are in training to become certified occupational therapy assistants. Common errors in supervision of students usually lie in one of two areas: expecting too much, or expecting too little. Students on level I Fieldwork know little (or perhaps nothing) of psychiatric occupational therapy practice, and need to observe and shadow you and other staff. The student on Level II Fieldwork is not yet a trained and skilled assistant, but is in the process of becoming one. It is unreasonable to expect a student to perform at the same level as a staff member. On the other hand, the student is more than a volunteer or aide, and needs to be challenged to perform at a higher level. Making excuses for the student's lack of performance is not going to help her acquire entry-level skills.

Many resources are available to guide the beginning supervisor. These include several short papers in Appendix B of the American Occupational Therapy Association's *Guide to Fieldwork Education* (10–13) and an article by Schwartz (9), which gives directions on how to identify and meet the needs of students at different cognitive levels. Workshops and courses on supervision are another possible resource. Your own supervisor should be able and available to give you guidance as well.

In addition, Christie et al. (5) have identified some of the factors that students feel are positive in a fieldwork supervisor. The first is an individual approach at the level of the student's needs. The crucial ingredient seems to be the supervisor's ability to present experiences that the student is ready for and finds challenging. Another factor cited by students as positive is the supervisor's ability to organize the fieldwork experience, and to make the student's responsibilities and the objectives of the fieldwork clear. Students also praised supervisors who made themselves available and who provided constructive, timely, and honest feedback. Supervisors who were enthusiastic and sure of themselves were seen as positive role models whom students wanted to emulate.

The list of additional references and selected readings at the end of this chapter contains resources that would be valuable to the beginning or intermediate-level supervisor.

SUMMARY AND CONCLUSION

Supervision is "a mutual undertaking to promote the growth and development of the supervisee while evaluating performance and maintaining standards."[4] It functions in three ways: as an administrative process for making sure the work gets done, as an evaluative process for ensuring that the work is performed at an acceptable standard, and as a learning process for developing the skills and competencies of those being supervised. Successful supervision requires the active and involved participation of both the supervisor and the supervisee. This chapter has explored the goals of supervision and the responsibilities of supervisor and supervisee, and has addressed some of the factors affecting students and new assistants in the role of supervisee. The process of becoming a supervisor, as many experienced COTAs finally do, was discussed briefly.

REFERENCES

1. American Occupational Therapy Association. Entry-level role delineation for registered occupational therapists (OTRs) and certified occupational therapy assistants (COTAs). *Am J Occup Ther* 1990;44:1091–1102.
2. American Occupational Therapy Association Commission on Practice. Guide for supervision of occupational therapy personnel (official position paper of the American Occupational Therapy Association). *Am J Occup Ther* 1981;35: 815–816.
3. American Occupational Therapy Association. Supervision guidelines for certified occupational therapy assistants. *Am J Occup Ther* 1990; 44:1089–1090.
4. American Occupational Therapy Association Practice Division. I'm glad you asked (second question). *Occup Ther Newspaper* 1985;39(2):4.
5. Christie BA, Joyce PC, Moeller PL. Fieldwork experience. 2: The supervisor's dilemma. *Am J Occup Ther* 1985;39:675–681.
6. Early MB. *T.A.R. introductory course workbook: occupational therapy—psychosocial dysfunction.* Long Island City, NY: LaGuardia Community College; 1981.

[4]Fine SB. "Using supervision to meet clinical and professional needs." Speech given at the workshop entitled *Focus on Mental Health. II: A Plan for Action,* sponsored by the State University of New York, Downstate Medical Center, College of Health Related Professions, Occupational Therapy Program, at the Payne-Whitney Clinic, New York Hospital, March 21, 1986.

7. Highet G. *The art of teaching.* New York: Vintage; 1950.
8. Orr M. COTA share. *Occup Ther Newspaper* 1983;37(8):13.
9. Schwartz KB. An approach to supervision of students on fieldwork. *Am J Occup Ther* 1984; 38:393–397.
10. Wiemer RB. Student transition of academic to fieldwork settings. In: Oberzan K, Baldwin D, eds. *Guide to fieldwork education.* Rockville, Md: American Occupational Therapy Association; 1984.
11. Yerxa EJ. Duties and responsibilities of fieldwork educators in the educational process. In: Oberzan K, Baldwin D, eds. *Guide to fieldwork education.* Rockville, Md: American Occupational Therapy Association; 1984.
12. Yerxa EJ. Problems of evaluating fieldwork students. In: Oberzan K, Baldwin D, eds. *Guide to fieldwork education.* Rockville, Md: American Occupational Therapy Association; 1984.
13. Yerxa EJ. Techniques of supervision. In: Oberzan K, Baldwin D, eds. *Guide to fieldwork education.* Rockville, Md: American Occupational Therapy Association; 1984.

ADDITIONAL REFERENCES AND SUGGESTED READINGS

American Occupational Therapy Association. Member hotline. *Occup Ther Newspaper* 1985;39(7):4.
American Occupational Therapy Association Practice Division. I'm glad you asked. *Occup Ther Newspaper* 1983;37(3):3.
Benson KE, Higgins TE. Issues regarding practice and education for certified occupational therapy assistants. *AOTA Education Special Interest Section Newsletter* June 1992;2(2):3–4.
Blechert TF, Christiansen MF, Kari N. Intraprofessional team building. *Am J Occup Ther* 1987; 41:576–589.
Boyd EM. Contract learning. *Phys Ther* 1979;59: 278–281.
Christie BA, Joyce PC, Moeller PL. Fieldwork experience. 1: Impact on practice preference. *Am J Occup Ther* 1985;39:671–674.
Devereaux EB. Principles of communication. In: Blair J, Gray M, eds. *The occupational therapy manager.* Rockville, Md: American Occupational Therapy Association; 1985.
Fidler G. Five dimensions of the dyad. Speech delivered at Columbia University, November 16, 1979, as part of the forum entitled *The Supervisory Dialogue.*
Fidler G. Supervision of the occupational therapy student. Speech delivered to LaGuardia Community College, November 12, 1980, for the New York Occupational Therapy Education Council.
Gillette N. Occupational therapy and mental health. In: Willard HS, Spackman CS, eds. *Occupational therapy.* 4th ed. Philadelphia: JB Lippincott; 1971.
Jas-Weathers T. Progressive student expectations based on AOTA's fieldwork evaluation. *Am J Occup Ther* 1990;44:848–851.
Kadushin A. Games people play in supervision. *Social Work* 1968;13(3):23–32.
Mitchell MM, Kampfe CM. Coping strategies used by occupational therapy students during fieldwork: an exploratory study. *Am J Occup Ther* 1990;44:543–550.
Rogers JC. Mentoring for career achievement and advancement. *Am J Occup Ther* 1986;40:79–82.
Sabol PS. Student support group intervention. In: Oberzank K, Baldwin D, eds. *Guide to fieldwork education.* Rockville, Md: American Occupational Therapy Association; 1984.
Schell BAB. Guide to classification of occupational therapy personnel. *Am J Occup Ther* 1985;39:803–810.
Slater DY, Cohn ES. Staff development through analysis of practice. *Am J Occup Ther* 1991; 45:1038–1041.
Yuen HK. Fieldwork students under stress. *Am J Occup Ther* 1990;44:80–81.

25

Organizing Yourself

Order and simplification are the first steps toward the mastery of a subject—the actual enemy is the unknown.

THOMAS MANN (4)

The occupational therapy assistant has many duties and demands on his time and energies. It is difficult to perform well at such a complex job without being organized. Being organized makes it easier to fulfill responsibilities, keep up with paperwork, do things on schedule, and carry out long-range projects. When Allen and Cruickshank (1) surveyed 613 newly registered occupational therapists in 1976, they found that out of 96 items on a checklist those rated among the 5 most bothersome were the following:

Finding ways to treat more patients with limited staff and time

Finding time to meet all my work-related responsibilities

Maintaining an uninterrupted treatment schedule

Getting systems (such as patient scheduling, transportation, discharge, and transfer) to be more efficient.

Furthermore, they rated the following item eleventh on the same list:

Budgeting time for nontreatment tasks such as paperwork, clinic clean-up, fabricating equipment, etc.

Allen and Cruickshank concluded that therapists need to improve their ability to develop realistic schedules and to manage their time. Although this survey was restricted to registered therapists, we can assume that at least some of these concerns are shared by newly certified occupational therapy assistants. This chapter provides information and hints on how to manage your time and environment, with the expectation that being organized will make you feel more competent, energetic, and confident in your work.

The following topics will be discussed: priorities, scheduling, paperwork, management of supplies and equipment, and organization of space. For each, typical problems and suggested solutions will be described. Which suggestions to adopt, and to what extent, is an individual choice. Fitting you into a prescribed mold is not the goal of this chapter, but rather helping you become organized in a way that suits you and your style.

PRIORITIES

For occupational therapy assistants who are working in clinical situations, the first priority is patient care. Providing treatment and performing interviews and evaluations as directed are the usual patient care responsibilities. These tasks come before all others, but should not be used as an excuse for ignoring other priorities such as documentation, supervision and meetings, and activity preparation and clinic maintenance. In other words, the occupational therapy assistant needs to manage his time so that he can take care of his patient responsibilities, paperwork, and meetings with other staff, and still leave enough time so that he can get materials ready for patients and make the clinic a clean, orderly, and inviting place to work.

How can you find the time for all of these major responsibilities? The first step is to assess whether you are spending valuable time doing other things that are less important. Typical examples include filing and cataloguing things that may never be used again, chatting with patients and staff (outside of scheduled times), and sharpening pencils and arranging desk supplies. Another time-waster is striving for perfection in things that do not really demand it; examples include rewriting or retyping paperwork to "make it look nicer," deliberating indecisively about how to approach a problem, trying to save money by reusing supplies that really could be discarded, and using detailed but cumbersome filing and record-keeping systems.

Developing the habit of using time efficiently takes only a little effort, but it has to be consistent effort. Lakein (3) suggests making a daily "to do" list. For such a list to work for you, it should include only things that you really plan to do today (you can make another list tomorrow). You can save time by not listing routine tasks that will get done anyway, but only those that might be forgotten without a special reminder. You can prioritize the list, giving the "must do" items a rating of A, the less important ones a rating of B, and the ones that do not matter so much a rating of C. Make time to do the A items, and try not to be distracted by less important tasks during the day. People who use daily "to do" lists

report that they feel satisfied by what they accomplish, and have a clearer and more realistic sense of their goals.

SCHEDULING

Every worker, and every patient for that matter, needs a schedule. Using a schedule is the first step in time management. The occupational therapy assistant's schedule is based on the master schedule for the treatment setting and for the occupational therapy department. In other words, certain hours in his schedule are fixed time slots, representing meetings and groups that occur at times determined by others. These include regular patient groups, supervision meetings, and other staff meetings. Time slots not reserved for these fixed events are called flexible time slots. These flexible time slots are used to meet the other responsibilities of paperwork, preparation, and clinic maintenance.

A common error is to assume that these tasks will automatically get done during these times, and that there is no need to schedule them for any specific hour. However, what happens to many people is that they are interrupted by other staff or patients or telephone calls. These interruptions expand to fill the empty time, and soon there is none left. The only way to avoid this trap is to schedule time for specific tasks, and to *actually do them at the scheduled time.* The first step is to make a list of the things you need to do every week (or every month). These might include:

Writing progress notes
Administering interviews or evaluations to
  new patients
Reading medical records
Making phone calls or writing letters to arrange or confirm details about supply orders, community activities, or equipment repairs
Preparing materials for patients to use
Setting up an area for an activity

Transporting patients
Writing up notes on a group
Inventorying supplies received
Unpacking orders and stocking and arranging the supply room and closets
Cleaning up after activities, and general clinic housekeeping
Writing up monthly statistics.

Just one look at the items on this list (which is by no means exhaustive) should prove that the COTA can accomplish them only if he organizes his time to do so. It is crucially important to recognize that all of these tasks take time. For example, an "empty" hour-long time slot quickly dwindles to 20 minutes or less if the assistant must escort patients back to the ward after a group that just ended, and then has to travel across the hospital grounds to a meeting in another building. A single phone call can easily consume the remaining time.

The point here is that a schedule must be accurate and realistic if it is to be of any use to you. Creating a realistic schedule involves the following steps:

1. Get or make a schedule form that you can duplicate so that you can revise it.
2. Fill in the activities that occur at fixed time slots.
3. Around these fixed activities, fill in the time *you* need to perform any tasks that necessarily occur with them. Examples might include setting up the activity, escorting patients, or jotting down notes on what happened in the activity.
4. List all of your other routine responsibilities.
5. Leaving at least two hours a week for unexpected activities, fill in the rest of your schedule.
6. Live with the schedule for a while, to see if it is accurate. Update it as needed.
7. Give a copy of your schedule to your supervisor. Keep another with you, and *use* it. Revise it as needed.

When you make up your schedule, give some consideration to how much of what kind of activity you can really accomplish in a given time slot. For example, a half-hour slot is next to useless for writing progress notes, especially if you need to gather your records first. But this *is* plenty of time to make a few phone calls, or to begin to write out a supply order.

In addition to the schedule, the assistant should consider using an appointment book. Some prefer one that shows an entire month on a single page, although there are many other format options available. A large stationery or office supply store should have several models to compare. The appointment book is the place to record planned meetings with individual patients and staff, special events, and non-routine tasks.

For example, some of the COTA's responsibilities might involve events that occur only once a month or once a year. Examples include craft fairs, bazaars, bake sales, holiday parties, student fieldwork, inventory of supplies, and sharpening of saws and knives. Each of these involves some preparation in advance, and time must be allotted for this. Listing these tasks and entering them in an appointment book ensures that you will remember to do them at the appropriate time, and that you will not schedule other things that might conflict. You can use last year's appointment book as a guide to setting up reminders in a new book for the coming year. A departmental calendar would be even more efficient; this calendar could be kept or posted in a central location so that all staff, students, and volunteers could be informed of pending events.

PAPERWORK

As much as you might dislike it (and you are not alone in this), paperwork is an inescapable aspect of clinical work. Progress notes and other documentation of patient services are required. Budgets, purchase orders, requisition requests, maintenance requests, inventories, and statistics are also unavoidable. In addition, occupational therapy staff may feel inundated by catalogs, continuing education flyers, memos, and copies of printed matter used in patient activities. The four keys to transforming this chaos into an order you can live with are having a filing system, having a complete set of office supplies, setting aside blocks of time for paperwork, and using the wastebasket.

Filing System

A filing system can be as simple or as complex as your needs require. Avoid making the system too complicated, as it will take more time to use. If you keep copies of patient records you will need a locked file drawer; each patient should have his own file folder. Catalogs should be kept together, in a separate location which could be a shelf, a wall rack, or a file drawer. Important memos and statements about standard operating procedures should be kept together; a looseleaf binder is perhaps the best place, since obsolete material can be removed and new material added.

Printed matter used in patient activities can quickly accumulate unless it is filed. The recommended method is to create a series of folders for these handouts and sheets of directions. Another approach is to use heavy accordion files with internal dividers to sort out materials according to how they are used. For example, you might have an accordion file for your money management group, and another for your laundry skills group. Materials can be divided into sequential sessions, or any other way that makes sense for you. Label everything, though, so that you can find it when you need it.

Keeping track of information that will later go into progress notes can be a problem, unless you create a system for it. One approach is to keep a daily log, with a new page for each day, in which you jot down brief records of the day's events, including a few words on each patient you have seen. Another approach is to use a minicassette recorder.

Office Supplies

It is amazing how much time you can waste looking for paper clips or running to borrow the hole puncher. Considering how little these things cost, every staff member should have the following: scissors, tape, ruler, paper clips, stapler and staples, staple remover, pencils and sharpener, pens, marking pens, letter opener, correction fluid, scratch pad, stationery and forms, envelopes, rubber bands, dictionary, and wastebasket. You should also have immediate access, preferably in the room where you do your paperwork, to the following: three-hole punch, telephone, and file folders.

Blocking Out Time for Paperwork

Unless you are an accomplished writer and already a very organized person, you will probably find it possible to get your paperwork done only if you set aside large (at least two-hour) blocks of time for it. This must be time free of interruptions, and if you find the telephone or your co-workers in the office a distraction you may have to isolate yourself elsewhere.

Using the Wastebasket

Lakein (3) writes that one of his best rules is to "handle each piece of paper only once." Not everything is important, or needs to be saved, or in some cases even read. Throw out everything that you are sure you will not need later. Evaluate each piece of mail or printed matter the first time you see it. Saving things to "read later" makes sense only if you really are interested and will actually do it.

MANAGEMENT OF SUPPLIES AND EQUIPMENT

So much of the pleasure of doing an activity depends on having the necessary supplies and equipment available, prepared, and in working order. In some departments the occupational therapy assistant is responsible for these tasks not only for his own activities, but for those of other staff as well.

Ordering Supplies

Attention should be given to whether supplies should be ordered in bulk or not. Certainly those supplies that are used frequently and repeatedly should be ordered in quantity. Ordering supplies only a few times a year saves a lot of time. Of course, there are items that should be ordered only as needed (food, and to some extent leather and wood). Copies of previous orders are useful reminders of what needs to be reordered, and from where.

Since many days, weeks, and even months can elapse between the placement of an order and its receipt, the occupational therapy assistant should provide time for this, and inform other staff of when they might realistically expect to get their supplies. Bureaucratic procedures such as paperwork and bidding requirements and policies of vendors (e.g., orders must be prepaid) can create delays.

Storing Supplies

This is an area where the individual must create a system to meet the needs of the situation. For example, if supplies are ordered only once or twice a year, in bulk, a separate supply room is needed to contain those that will not be used immediately. Also, the activities done in occupational therapy require a maddening array of tools and supplies of various shapes, sizes, perishability, and potential danger. Storage systems have to be designed to accommodate this vari-

ety. Locked storage must be provided for sharp and other dangerous objects, and separate vented metal cabinets for flammables. These specialized items are described in more detail in Chapter 12. For storage of other materials, many different organizers and kinds of storage equipment are available commercially from office suppliers, art supply stores, hardware stores, closet shops, and furniture stores. The following are suggested items that some occupational therapists have found useful:

Stacking bins. These are made of plastic, stack on top of each other, and have open fronts so that their contents are easily seen. They can be arranged on open shelves.

Sliding wire baskets on metal frames with wheels. These are good for storing lightweight loose materials such as yarn.

Sets of tiny transparent plastic drawers. These are useful for sorting hardware, leather and jewelry findings, and other small items. It helps to label them.

Large flat sets of drawers for large sheets of art paper. These are available from art and architecture supply stores.

Tool racks. These can be purchased from hardware stores, or custom-made by an aide or volunteer or the maintenance staff.

Pegboard. Contact paper tracings of tools can be used to create a shadowboard showing which tools belong where.

Cubbyholes. Each patient can have an assigned slot to store his projects in process.

Flat drawers, easily accessible, with contact paper tool shadows, for storing sharp objects. These, obviously must be locked.

Bright, eye-catching, pressure-sensitive labels. These can be used to identify occupational therapy property, or give instruction to patients or staff.[1]

---

[1]Preprinted occupational therapy labels with a range of messages in black print on various fluorescent colored backgrounds are available from United Ad Label, Inc., 10035 S. Greenleaf Avenue, P.O. Box 2165, Whittier, CA 90610.

Even the best storage system can be defeated by a tendency to save what should be discarded. Occupational therapists enjoy a reputation for being resourceful, for being able to create terrific activities from donations and leftovers. Without discipline, this resourcefulness can expand into squirrel-like behavior, compelling therapists to rescue scrap lumber from the trash, and save odds and ends of fabric and yarn and supplies left over from kits. Getting rid of this accumulated debris is a liberating experience; not letting it accumulate in the first place is even more energizing. The question that should be asked is whether this material is ever going to be used, and if so, when. Anything that does not have a definite purpose or use within a year should be thrown out, or (if this makes you feel too guilty) given to a local scout troop.

Preparing Supplies

Certain supplies cannot be used by patients without some advance preparation by someone else. This does not necessarily have to be the COTA; these tasks can be handled by aides, volunteers, and even higher functioning patients, provided they are given sufficient direction. Examples include cutting lengths of fabric and leather, attaching hardware, threading needles, unplugging or refilling glue bottles, and laying out supplies for an activity. Disposable paper and plastic containers from the cafeteria (e.g., paper bowls, plastic cups) are handy for setting up individual amounts of loose materials such as tiles.

How to Make Supplies Portable

In situations where the COTA must carry out an activity in a location other than the occupational therapy area, he will need a system for getting the supplies from one place to the other. There are several options. One is to use a small rolling cart with shelves; the shelves should have raised lips to prevent things from sliding off. Another is to use a tool box, with internal trays and compartments. Yet another is to use a special enclosed rolling cart with locked drawers and doors; various models are available from office furniture suppliers, school furniture suppliers, and automobile supply stores.

Equipment Maintenance

Only people who are skilled at repairing equipment should be charged with doing it; inadequate or slipshod repairs are a potential source of accidents. Unless the COTA or the maintenance staff of the facility has expertise with the equipment, it should be repaired by an outside expert. Service contracts should be purchased at the same time as new equipment. For older equipment, it may be possible to arrange a blanket service contract with a company that repairs different kinds of machines.

The occupational therapy assistant may be responsible for coordinating equipment repair for the occupational therapy department. This task can be made easier by providing a place (special notebook or message box) for staff to record a problem with equipment, or by giving them a special form to use. Once you are notified of a problem, you should arrange for the repair, and let the staff know when they can expect it to be done.

ORGANIZATION OF SPACE

Entire books have been written on organization of space. This section will not duplicate the contents of these texts, which can be found in any large library, but will indicate some of the basic issues involved in the organization and use of space in occupational therapy areas in psychiatric settings.[2]

The occupational therapy assistant will not necessarily make the final decisions

---

[2]This discussion is summarized in part from Bachner and Cornelius (2).

about how space will be used and organized, but should be able to participate in the planning, especially regarding activities he will be conducting. In some situations, as when a COTA is in charge of a skills program such as homemaking or a prevocational work group, the COTA may have complete responsibility for organizing the environment. Since storage areas and office areas have already been touched on, the discussion here will focus on activity areas. Several different types of spaces are generally needed, and each has separate requirements.

Areas for Large Groups

Space is needed for parties, athletic activities, community meetings, and other large verbal groups, and perhaps movies and other theater presentations. Making space available may mean doubling up by using a room designed for another purpose, for example the dining room or lounge, and may require removing the usual furniture and bringing in folding chairs and tables. If space is used for more than one purpose, time must be allotted to transform it for its next use.

Areas for Small Groups

"Small" is a relative concept. The size of the group and the kind of activity will determine the kind of space needed. The area should be large enough and sufficiently free of clutter to permit people to move easily within it. On the other hand, it should not be so large that a small group seems lost in it. An area of a larger room can be sectioned off with folding screens.

Private Areas

A place is needed for interviews and confidential discussions. This could be an office or an activity room that is not sched-uled for other use. In an inpatient setting it may be possible to use patients' rooms for this purpose. The important factors are privacy and freedom from interruptions.

Areas for Messy Activities

Some activities (ceramics, artwork, woodworking, etc.) create so much clutter and mess that they need their own areas. If possible, separate locations should be permanently set aside for *each* of these major activities. If this is not possible, the occupational therapy department should carefully evaluate whether conducting such a varied range of messy activities is worth the time and effort needed to clean up the area each time an activity is done.

The appearance of a room profoundly (if subliminally) affects the way people feel while they are in it. If you want patients to want to *be* in your activity area, and to *work* in it, it is up to you to make it inviting, comfortable, and appropriate for the particular activity. This is not difficult to achieve. You need only close your eyes and ask yourself, "Would *I* feel like working in a place like this?" When you open your eyes you will know what you have to do to make the place better. Here are some specific suggestions:

Reduce the clutter. Projects that were done "in the year of the flood" belong in the garbage or in a museum.

Send unused equipment to deep storage, or see if it can be auctioned off.

Provide coat racks or wall pegs for patients' outerwear, and for aprons and smocks.

If the place looks drab, get a paint job. If the maintenance staff cannot do it, see if the patients can.

Repaint the furniture, too, if it needs it. This can be a terrific project for a prevocational work group.

Cover old desktops and table tops with contact paper or painted masonite.

Use display cases and corkboard to show

off patients' projects and samples of crafts that are frequently used. Since these can be distracting to patients with limited attention span, place them so that they can be screened off when necessary.

Instead of displaying a sample of every craft available, keep a photo album of Polaroid shots of projects that patients can select from.

Keep wall displays simple, cheerful, and attractive. A felt banner or wall hanging or a large framed poster can set the mood for the room.

Maintaining an inviting therapeutic environment requires constant vigilance. Finished and half-finished projects and scraps of various materials tend to pile up unless you actively prevent this. As in any other place, dust and dirt inevitably accumulate. If the housekeeping staff cannot be relied upon to clean the room properly, you can do it yourself or organize a work group of patients to do routine cleaning chores such as wiping tables, dusting, sweeping, and mopping.

SUMMARY

Nothing makes a person feel more competent than being able to accomplish what he wants and needs to do in the time available. We know this is true of patients, and it is only fair to admit that it applies equally to staff and students. We know also that chaos in the environment can detract from the skill with which an activity is performed. Do not let this happen to you. It is hoped that the suggestions here will spur you to take charge of your time and space, in whatever way makes sense for you in your particular situation.

REFERENCES

1. Allen AS, Cruickshank DR. Perceived problems of occupational therapists: a subset of the professional curriculum. *Am J Occup Ther* 1977;31: 557–564.
2. Bachner JP, Cornelius E. *Activities coordinator's guide: a handbook for activities coordinators in long-term care facilities.* Washington, DC: U.S. Government Printing Office; 1978.
3. Lakein A. *How to get control of your time and your life.* New York: Peter H Wyden; 1973.
4. Mann T. The magic mountain. In: Bartlett J, ed. *Familiar quotations.* 15th ed. Boston: Little, Brown, 1980:754.

ADDITIONAL REFERENCES AND SUGGESTED READINGS

Allen AS, Cruickshank DR. Perceived problems of occupational therapists: a subset of the professional curriculum. *Am J Occup Ther* 1977;31: 557–564.

Bachner JP, Cornelius E. *Activities coordinator's guide: a handbook for activities coordinators in long-term care facilities.* Washington, DC: U.S. Government Printing Office; 1978.

Cotton NS, Geraty RG. Therapeutic space design: planning an inpatient children's unit. *Am J Orthopsychiatry* 1984;54:624–636.

Harris D. *The Woman's Day guide to organizing your life.* New York: Holt, Rinehart and Winston; 1985.

Lakein A. *How to get control of your time and your life.* New York: Peter H Wyden; 1973.

Winston S. *Getting organized: the easy way to put your life in order.* New York: WW Norton; 1978.

Appendix A
Case Examples

CASE 1: A 21-YEAR-OLD WOMAN WITH DEPRESSION[1]

Hilary Page   Case #186302

This 21-year-old single black female with a *DSM-III-R* diagnosis of dysthymia (300.40) on Axis I and passive-aggressive personality disorder (301.84) on Axis II (see Table A–1) was admitted to the acute admissions ward of a state psychiatric hospital after several months of depression, withdrawal, and refusal to leave her mother's house. This is her first hospitalization. Patient is medicated with Ludiomil, 100 mg., h.s.

Miss Page is the oldest of three children, all living with their mother; the patient's father died when she was 13 years old. The patient states that she has no friends, her sole girlfriend having moved to Florida. She has dated some but has never had a serious relationship.

Hilary is a high school graduate and attended college for two years, majoring in psychology; she enrolled briefly in a nursing school but quit this to move to Florida with her girlfriend. She stayed there only a few months and returned home, withdrawn and depressed. She subsequently refused to leave her mother's home, leading to this hospitalization.

Patient has worked as a babysitter and a housekeeper in a private residence, most recently during her stay in Florida. At present she has no income of her own, relying on her mother for economic support. She was referred to occupational therapy for general evaluation of task skills and work potential, leisure planning, and stress assessment.

The following evaluations were administered: Comprehensive Occupational Therapy Evaluation (COTE scale), Occupational History, Interest Checklist, and Stress Assessment.[2]

The COTE scale rating was based on a single performance of a simple mosaic tile task. The patient completed the task easily, requesting instruction from the therapist only twice. She did not interact with others, tended to isolate herself, and did not respond to casual conversation initiated by the therapist. She expressed indifference about the task, stating that she didn't care whether she completed it or not. No problems were noted in cognition, memory, or coordination.

The Occupational History revealed little new information. Most of the patient's experience in occupational roles has been as a student. She stated she enjoyed school and did well there. She expressed no interest in vocational activities, stating that

---

[1]This case example is based on material contributed by Terry Brittell, COTA, ROH. Certain details have been altered for teaching purposes, but this is essentially a real case. The patient's name is fictitious.

[2]The Stress Assessment is a structured interview that collects data on situations that the patient finds stressful and the way she typically reacts to stress.

she is not interested in going to school or getting a job. Patient appeared despondent throughout the interview. She was, however, clean, neat, and appropriately groomed.

Results of the Interest Checklist indicated a strong interest in social recreational activities (conversation, board games), athletic activities (volleyball, exercise, swimming), and manual activities (mending, sewing, manual arts). Patient reported a particular interest in rock collecting, a hobby she has pursued since childhood.

The Stress Assessment revealed that the patient frequently experiences severe stress occasioned by frustration over situations such as fighting (especially among siblings), rules, financial worries, living conditions, and lack of activity. Hilary finds leisure time frustrating and feels she has no real accomplishments. She says living at home is too strict and cites her relationship with her mother as particularly stressful. Patient also reports a strong feeling of loss associated with the death of her father, her own graduation from school, and her separation from her friend who moved to Florida. In addition, Hilary has asthma, allergies, and acne, and says she feels ugly. She feels that others do not understand her.

TABLE A–1. DSM-III-R *diagnosis at admission (case 1)*

Axis I:	300.40 Dysthymia
Axis II:	301.84 Passive-aggressive personality disorder
Axis III:	None
Axis IV:	Severity: 2—Mild (best friend moved away)
Axis V:	Current GAF: 50 Highest GAF past year: 60

Questions for Case 1

1. Assume that you are the COTA on the case. What additional evaluation(s) would you recommend to your supervisor? What additional information would you like to have, and how would you go about obtaining it?
2. Formulate a treatment plan. Assume that the patient can remain for three more weeks as an inpatient and can be discharged to a day treatment center within the state hospital center.

CASE 2: A 72-YEAR-OLD WOMAN WITH ALZHEIMER'S DISEASE[3]

Jenny Anderson   Case #9801

This 72-year-old married white female was admitted to Green Manor Nursing Home, a skilled nursing facility, with an Axis I diagnosis of primary degenerative dementia with depression (290.21) (see Table A–2). The patient, who also has Axis III diagnoses of cerebral atherosclerosis and congestive heart failure, was first diagnosed with Alzheimer's disease three years ago. Until admission she was cared for at home by her husband of 45 years. However, since Mrs. Anderson has become weaker and incontinent, and Mr. Anderson (who is 74 years old) is not strong enough to help his wife transfer from bed to commode, it was necessary to place her in a home.

Mrs. Anderson is of Norwegian ancestry; her religion is Lutheran. She was the fifth of nine children and is the only one still living. She has a high school degree and was employed for 29 years as a bookkeeper in a local manufacturing business. Mr. and Mrs. Anderson have one son, age 51, who lives in another state. According to Mr. Anderson, his wife used to enjoy needlework, canasta, and gardening, activities that she abandoned as her illness became more severe. During the final six months the patient remained at home, and her husband took care of all of the cooking, cleaning, and household management. According to

---

[3]This case is based on actual clinical material, but names and other details have been changed to protect the patient's identity.

him, the patient complained constantly that he wasn't doing a good enough job, that she didn't like his cooking, and so on.

The following evaluations were attempted: structured interview and mental status examination, functional range of motion examination, functional daily living skills evaluation, and Parachek Geriatric Rating Scale.[4]

At interview, Mrs. Anderson was found seated in a wheelchair in her room. It was noted that the wheelchair was the wrong size, causing the patient's shoulders to be elevated. Mrs. Anderson was well groomed and neatly dressed; conference with the nursing staff revealed that her husband comes in early every morning to help. Patient was able to state her name and that she was in some sort of institution. She did not know the correct date, gave a month that was in a different season, and said the year was 1981. When asked how she came to be in the home, she replied that she had come here for a job interview ("They need someone to straighten out the books"). She then said that she decided not to take the job ("Who'd want to work in a place like this?"). Patient incorrectly answered 7 of 10 questions on the mental status examination; recent memory and fund of general information seemed particularly impaired. Patient could follow a one-step command, but not two steps. Her speech was clear and her hearing apparently unimpaired. The patient wears glasses.

Functional range of motion examination revealed that the patient could not ambulate, even with a walker, because of decreased endurance and poor balance. Patient had full range in most motions of the upper extremities but was unable to elevate the arms above the level of the shoulders (range was more impaired on the right). Grasp was very weak. Range in the lower extremities was evaluated separately by a physical therapist, who noted limitations in all motions.

Functional daily living skills evaluation showed that patient had sufficient pinch and coordination to button and unbutton garments with front closures. She was unable to bathe or care for her teeth and hair without assistance, but seemed aware of the need for help and asked for it. She could feed herself if the tray was prepared (meat cut up, etc.). Sitting balance was poor, and patient could not perform transfers unassisted.

Patient received a score of 28 on the Parachek Geriatric Rating Scale. Breakdown of the scores was as follows: Physical Condition, 10; General Self-Care, 11; Social Behaviors, 7.

TABLE A–2. DSM-III-R *diagnosis at admission (case 2)*

Axis I:	290.21 Primary degenerative dementia of the Alzheimer's type, with depression
Axis II:	None
Axis III:	Cerebral atherosclerosis, Congestive heart failure
Axis IV:	Severity: 3—Moderate (recent move to nursing home)
Axis V:	Current GAF: 22 Highest GAF past year: 25

Questions for Case 2

1. Write an occupational therapy treatment plan, including goals and activities. *Hint:* The plan should focus on maintaining rather than improving function, and should allow for deterioration in the patient's condition. State which activities are to be individual and which in a group.

2. Assuming the patient's condition deteriorates, at what point would you recommend that occupational therapy be discontinued? Identify specific behavioral and functional impairments that would indicate that the patient cannot benefit from further treatment. Write a dis-

---

[4]The Parachek Geriatric Rating Scale is described in Chapter 3.

charge plan (discontinuance from occupational therapy), including recommendations and directions for the nursing staff.

CASE 3: A 54-YEAR-OLD WOMAN WITH SCHIZOPHRENIA, PARANOID TYPE[5]

Lucy Lammermoor   Case #082751

This 54-year-old single white female was admitted to the acute admissions ward on court certification following action by her neighbors. Commitment papers state that the patient has been complaining of people doing things against her; she is suspicious of her neighbors and has been breaking windows. Patient has had two previous psychiatric hospitalizations, in 1964 for three months and in 1969 for six months. Diagnosis is schizophrenia, paranoid type, unspecified (295.30) (see Table A–3). Patient also suffers from chronic phlebitis in both legs. Prescribed medication includes Melaril 100 mg, t.i.d.; Sinequan 100 mg, t.i.d.; Colace 100 mg, h.s., and prune juice 8 oz. h.s.

At admission, Miss Lammermoor was poorly groomed and dressed in dirty clothing. She appeared anxious, tense, and somewhat confused. Her speech was coherent but at times irrelevant. She denied hearing voices and denied having said that her food was poisoned. She stated she had no idea why she was hospitalized, other than the ill will of her neighbors.

Patient is the third child in a family of eight, and was raised in a rural section of northern New York state, near the Canadian border. She has never married. She lives alone in her own apartment with two cats. She has a tenth grade education and has held numerous jobs as a domestic in private homes. She states that she is now "retired" and living on SSI and Social Security.

Patient was referred to occupational therapy two weeks after admission for evaluation of functional living skills and assessment of needs in relation to discharge planning. Evaluation instruments included a structured interview, the COTE scale, and a Functional Living Skills Evaluation.

Interview

Miss Lammermoor arrived on time for the interview and each of the subsequent evaluation sessions. Though her hair was often slightly disheveled, she was otherwise clean and neat. She was cooperative in the interview and spoke at length about her apartment, the "things" (she refused to further define what she meant), and her two cats. She expressed sorrow over the death of her mother five years ago and seemed to have some unresolved feelings. She mentioned that she does not see her family; she feels positively about one of her brothers who lives in California, but expressed hostility toward another brother who lives nearby. She spoke angrily of her neighbors, stating that she feels persecuted, that they pick on her, are stealing from her, and say bad things about her. She also mentioned that the neighborhood children harass her.

She stated that she neither has friends nor wants them. She said she is not interested in learning anything new to fill leisure hours, although she does enjoy solitary activities. The only group activity she expressed interest in was bingo. She was unaware of local resources and activity programs for retired people, and said she wasn't interested in them.

<hr/>

[5]This case example is based on material contributed by Terry Brittell, COTA, ROH. Certain details have been altered for teaching purposes, but this is essentially a real case. The patient's name is fictitious.

Comprehensive Occupational Therapy Evaluation

The COTE scale was used to rate the patient's performance of a simple craft activity (magazine picture collage). The patient worked at a moderate speed and acceptable level of activity. She appeared oriented to place, person, and time. She expressed concern about why certain other persons were not present or were late for the evaluation (which was administered in a group).

Patient was responsive and appropriate in her conversation, but most interactions were either dependent or impulsive. For example, she repeatedly asked for help, extra directions, and materials that she could obtain herself. Other patients appeared to view this as an attention-getting device, and several made negative remarks to the effect that she took needed attention from them. She also made comments that were unrelated to the conversation.

Patient needed no encouragement to engage in the activity, and after receiving repeated direction (which she requested) she was able to follow through and complete the task. She worked neatly, in an organized fashion; coordination and concentration were more than adequate for the task. She was able to make decisions and solve minor problems encountered in the activity despite her requests for assistance in other, less difficult areas. She appeared highly motivated by the activity and expressed interest in other crafts displayed in the OT room.

Functional Living Skills Evaluation

Miss Lammermoor demonstrated an ability to function independently in the following areas: use of medication, use of her savings account, organization and cleaning of her home, selection of clothing and laundry and clothing maintenance, and single-serving cooking. She was unable to identify the correct response to several household emergencies, including what to do if the lights go out or if she smells gas. She was able to use a telephone book to locate emergency phone numbers, but she has limited reading and writing skills, which prevent her from writing simple messages or reading a bus schedule. She apparently relies on others to tell her when and where to take the bus, and she has a good knowledge of the public transportation system. She states that she does have a budget and could demonstrate how to break down her monthly income into weekly budgets. However, she was unable to demonstrate or explain how to make correct change from $5, and she could not figure the sales tax.

TABLE A–3. DSM-III-R *diagnosis at admission (case 3)*

Axis I:	295.30 Schizophrenia, paranoid type, unspecified
Axis II:	None
Axis III:	Phlebitis
Axis IV:	Severity: 2—Mild (trouble with neighbors)
Axis V:	Current GAF: 30 Highest GAF past year: 50

Questions for Case 3

1. How do you interpret the patient's interest in bingo? Is this a good activity for developing social and interpersonal skills? Explain.
2. The physician wants to know whether Miss Lammermoor can function well enough on her own to return to her own apartment, or whether she should be placed in a supervised living situation. Formulate a recommendation, and justify it with evidence from the case history. Indicate any further evaluations or information that you feel are needed or believe will help in making this determination. Document your recommendations in the form of a note suitable for the patient's chart.

CASE 4: A 22-YEAR-OLD MAN WITH CHRONIC SCHIZOPHRENIA AND MILD MENTAL RETARDATION[6]

Johnson Velasquez   Case #085562

This 22-year-old Hispanic male with an Axis I diagnosis of chronic undifferentiated schizophrenia (295.92) and mild mental retardation (see Table A–4) was referred to a community day treatment center in a large East Coast city. The referral originated at another mental health clinic in a different part of the city. He had been attending that clinic for medication, and the staff there believed he could benefit from a structured day program and family therapy.

Mr. Velasquez was born in Colombia, South America. His parents were teenagers when he was born and have subsequently divorced (the father is reported to have been a drug addict and alcoholic). The patient has four younger sisters and a younger brother, and he lived with his maternal grandparents in Colombia while his mother emigrated to the United States when he was 10. The rest of the family emigrated six years ago. Immediately after the move the patient became ill, but was never hospitalized. He was followed at an outpatient clinic and stabilized on medication (Haldol and Cogentin). Johnson dropped out of school at age 16, without completing his high school education.

On admission, the social worker obtained the following information from the family. The mother is currently employed in a factory job. Johnson, who speaks no English, stays home and masturbates all day. He sees no one but family members and has not been able to care for his own hygiene. His 14-year-old sister has been washing and dressing him. He appears to be hallucinating, says that he is in the space shuttle, and has frequent loud outbursts of inappropriate laughter. Mr. Velasquez was also seen by the psychiatrist, who increased his medication.

The occupational therapy evaluation was performed three days later by an occupational therapy student under the supervision of the therapist. Evaluation instruments used were the Occupational Role History Interview[7] and the Allen Cognitive Level Test. Results were as follows:

Mr. Velasquez appeared for the interview neatly dressed, but with the back of his hair uncombed and his pants zipper open. He closed the zipper at the student's reminder to do so. In the Occupational Role History Interview Johnson often gave tangential and irrelevant replies to questions asked by the student. He spoke of violent events such as being beaten by a man with a club in school and having been accused by a classmate of killing her grandmother. When asked about school he stated that he was good at drawing but bad at biology and physics. Mr. Velasquez said emphatically that he had no friends and could think of no one whom he had looked up to in the past as a role model.

Mr. Velasquez attended school in Colombia but has not attended since his family moved to this country when he was 16. He has never had a job. He has very limited understanding of the English language (the interview was conducted in Spanish).

In the Allen Cognitive Level Test the patient was able to complete two running stitches first, and then two whip stitches. He was unable to complete the single cordovan stitch, and he recognized that he had made errors but did not attempt to correct them. The student repeated the instructions (the patient did not request this), but Mr. Velasquez was not able to complete the stitch on his second attempt. This performance was scored at cognitive level 4.

---

[6]This case example is loosely based on an actual case. The names and certain other facts have been changed to protect the patient's identity.

[7]An abbreviated version of the Occupational History Interview. See Chapter 14.

TABLE A–4. DSM-III-R *diagnosis at admission (case 4)*

Axis I:	295.92 Schizophrenia, undifferentiated type, chronic
Axis II:	317.00 Mild mental retardation
Axis III:	None
Axis IV:	Severity: 1—None
Axis V:	Current GAF: 20
	Highest GAF past year: 20

Questions for Case 4

1. What additional information would you like to have on this patient and his background?
2. What additional evaluations do you think might be useful?
3. From the available information, list the patient's apparent assets (strengths) and deficits (problems). Include a discussion of the environment. Plan a schedule of daily activities at the treatment center. Choose one activity for each morning and afternoon, except Wednesday morning, which is set aside for community meeting and medication groups. Give reasons for each activity choice. The activities that are available are:

Tools for Living (Daily Living Skills),
Art Workshop
Piano Workshop
Sewing Workshop
Woodworking
Boutique Sales
Cooking School
Work Preparation (pre-voc)
Messenger Training
Basic Crafts
Yoga
Adult Basic Education
Social Skills Training
Assertiveness Training
Anger Management
Aerobic Dancing
Drama Workshop
Basic Sensorimotor Skills (parachute and ball play)

For one of these groups, list two goals, and explain what *specific* activity you would use and how you would structure and present it.

4. The patient performed at level 4 on the Allen Cognitive Level Test. What additional information in the report supports this? Do you think this assessment is accurate, or do you think a different result might be obtained at a different time? Explain your answer.

CASE 5: A 30-YEAR-OLD MAN WITH BIPOLAR AFFECTIVE DISORDER[8]

Dwight Kennedy   Case #291083

This 30-year-old white male with an Axis I diagnosis of bipolar affective disorder, mixed (296.64), with paranoid features (see Table A–5), was referred to occupational therapy for evaluation and development of skills needed to resume community living with his wife of four months. The patient was admitted to a general hospital following an incident on Valentine's Day one year ago, in which he stabbed and enucleated his right eye. Mr. Kennedy cited a Biblical passage as the reason for this self-mutilation.[9] Patient was subsequently transferred to an outpatient mental health clinic, but three and a half years later he could not be maintained in the community and was admitted to a state hospital. This was his first psychiatric hospitalization, although he had a history of psychiatric consultations dating from adolescence, and difficulty functioning at work because of emotional problems since age 23. Patient is currently medicated with lithium carbonate, although he has received Mellaril, Haldol, and Artane in the past (he was initially diagnosed as having

---

[8]This case material was contributed by Beatrice White, COTA, OT Division, Springfield Hospital Center, Sykesville, Md 21784. Certain details have been altered for teaching purposes, but this is essentially a real case. The patient's name is fictitious.
[9]Matthew 5:28–30.

schizophrenia, paranoid type). Patient has no history of drug or alcohol abuse.

Patient's family background is unclear; his parents separated when he was six years old, shortly after a sister (his only sibling) was born. He moved with his mother and sister from Virginia to Maryland, and has had no contact with his father since that time. Patient's mother is described as rigid and controlling, and very religious; church affiliation is Baptist. Patient's emotional problems were recognized during his school years; he was described as a "schizoid child" and received special education to compensate for his social isolation and difficulty with interpersonal relationships. Patient has a high school diploma. Mr. Kennedy worked for seven years as a horse trainer and groomer at a race track, and for five years at his mother's florist's business.

Around his 24th birthday, patient became ill and could no longer function at work. The precipitating incident occurred when a stranger knocked on the door of his home asking for a man with the same name as the patient; patient then became suspicious and concerned about men following him. He attended Bible class regularly with his mother, met his future wife there, and became engaged to her. Subsequently, he became anxious and indecisive about the pending marriage, and it was at this time that he mutilated his eye. After four months in acute care in a general hospital he was discharged and followed on weekly outpatient visits; at this point he was receiving Mellaril. He then married, despite advice from the clinic not to do so. His medication was changed to Haldol and Artane because of problems with rigidity and catatonic posturing. Patient was unable to consummate his marriage because of impotence, and he then became incontinent of urine and feces and was considered unmanageable at home; he was admitted to the state psychiatric hospital four months after his marriage. On admission he was withdrawn and

rigid, showed blunted affect, and exhibited festinating gait. He was delusional, and expressed the idea that someone was gripping his mind and that Jesus was Satan. His medication was reviewed and changed to lithium, which seemed effective and has been continued since then.

Medical care of the right eye during the patient's tenure as an outpatient and during the first two months of his inpatient stay was extensive. Chronic infections, stretching of the eye socket, and poor hygiene and grooming due to carelessness and poor cooperation by patient made it impossible for him to use a prosthesis. He has been wearing an eye patch.

The rehabilitation team in its initial treatment planning conference identified the primary goal as helping the patient make an effective adjustment to resume community living with his wife. Patient's wife was interested in a possible switching of roles; she would continue her work as a rental agent secretary in an apartment complex, and he would take care of the home. It was not clear initially whether this was the best arrangement, or whether patient should return to work at the race track and the florist's shop.

Occupational therapy evaluation included the Kohlman Evaluation of Living Skills (KELS), a sensory-perceptual-motor assessment, and a street survival questionnaire. All of these were administered by the registered therapist. A deficit in patient's standing balance was noted. In addition, patient was unable to perform basic household tasks, was unfamiliar with household situations, did not know proper first aid, was unable to identify household safety problems, had poor laundry skills, and was unfamiliar with budgeting, grocery shopping, paying bills, and banking. Patient was withdrawn and showed poor social skills. He was unable to identify leisure interests, and showed no motivation for using leisure time productively. The registered therapist established the following immediate goals:

1. Improve standing balance.
2. Improve grooming, personal hygiene, and self-care.
3. Assess and develop work skills in preparation for return to full-time employment.

The therapist began a series of one-to-one sensory integration sessions to improve standing balance, and arranged for patient to attend daily OT self-care sessions and a coordinated vocational adjustment program for a six-month work skills assessment and program in horticulture (the area was selected because of the patient's previous experience in a florist's shop). This vocational effort was coordinated by occupational therapy and the vocational rehabilitation counselor.

Patient's progress was reviewed prior to his completion of this program, at which time it seemed that patient would not be able to return to work because of overwhelming anxiety. Although Mr. Kennedy had participated actively in the work skills program, both patient and his wife agreed that it would be best for him to take over the household responsibilities rather than work full-time. Patient's wife located and signed a lease on a suburban efficiency apartment, convenient to public transportation and shopping. Criteria for patient's release were based on his ability to maintain stability of mood and cooperate with daily treatment programs. Because the ultimate objective was to enable Mr. Kennedy to function in a homemaker role in the community, he was referred to the Home Arts Program[10] for evaluation and skills development.

The COTA in the Home Arts program used the Comprehensive Evaluation of Basic Living Skills (CEBLS)[11] to obtain more detailed information on patient's skills and needs. The following additional deficits were noted: unstable and unsafe posture; failure to compensate for loss of vision on the right; no knowledge of nutrition, menu planning, meal preparation, or grocery shopping; and a tendency to panic under stress. The following additional goals were established by the COTA and patient and approved by the OTR:

4. Increase sense of comfort and confidence in ability to carry out the home management role.
5. Improve ability to plan and execute basic household tasks.
6. Develop social skills in basic communication, ability to relate to others in small groups, and to assert oneself appropriately.
7. Teach techniques to compensate for the visual defect.
8. Teach stress management techniques and establish a habit of using them.
9. Explore leisure interests and develop a habit of participating in leisure on a regular basis.

Methods included attendance at the Home Arts program for four hours a day, four times a week for ten weeks. Patient completed a course of instruction in all areas of home management. He became gradually more comfortable in social situations and showed appropriate curiosity and interest in the program and in other patients. He learned stress management techniques using music, progressive relaxation, and imagery, and he became less suspicious and more spontaneous in his interactions with others.

---

[10]A Home Arts program is designed to help participants develop and improve homemaking skills in the following major areas: meal preparation, nutrition, housekeeping, self-care skills, play/leisure skills, sewing, social skills, and community trips. A protocol can be found in Fidler GS. *Design of rehabilitation services in psychiatric hospital settings*. Laurel, Md: RAMSCO; 1984.

[11]Casanova JS, Ferber J. Comprehensive evaluation of basic living skills. *Am J Occup Ther* 1976; 30:101–105.

Patient was discharged from the hospital in the spring, a little more than a year after admission, following his successful completion of the Home Arts Program. He consummated his marriage in 1984 and now lives with his wife in the apartment she rented. He works part-time in a local greenhouse and nursery. He appears stable and is managing his role as homemaker and part-time worker very well. Maintenance check-ups in the community mental health clinic in his neighborhood are continuing.

TABLE A–5. DSM-III-R *diagnosis at admission (case 5)*

Axis I:	296.64 Bipolar disorder, mixed, with psychotic features
Axis II:	None
Axis III:	Blind in right eye after self-inflicted enucleation
Axis IV:	Severity: 5—Extreme (enucleation of eye, recent marriage)
Axis V:	Current GAF: 10 Highest GAF past year: 30

CASE 6: A 22-YEAR-OLD WOMAN WITH POLYSUBSTANCE DEPENDENCE AND DEPENDENT PERSONALITY DISORDER[12]

Lindsay Balthasar   Case #112188

This 22-year-old white female, self-admitted to a detox unit, stated she sought treatment because she's pregnant and abusing drugs (see Table A–6). Her father and maternal grandfather are alcoholic. Her parents were divorced when she was 13 years old, and she began using alcohol at that time. She has used pot since age 15, and over the past six months crack cocaine. She stated she'd tried speed and acid once in

her mid-teens. Lindsay's pattern of substance use is to drink more than a six pack daily, one to two joints daily, and crack on weekends, anywhere from 10 rocks to two eight balls.[13] Patient was transferred to rehabilitation after five days in detox.

Patient has a 10th grade education, having dropped out of school during early years of drug use. She has been living with her mother (who works two jobs) and two younger sisters until this past week, when she went on a binge and stayed at various places. Patient participates minimally in household chores (i.e., washes dishes and folds clothes). On interview by the occupational therapy assistant, she appeared sad, had poor eye contact, and said she has little self-confidence. She has no hobbies and no friends other than her drug-using peers. She stated she would like to get her GED, have a job, live independently, and raise her baby. Patient reported she's uncertain who is the father of her baby, and so will be solely responsible for the child. She admitted that her life lacks structure and that she has no healthy leisure involvements. She stated that she values her family, sees her strengths in being a hard worker and straightforward and her weaknesses in using drugs and alcohol and allowing others to take advantage of her.

OT Discharge Summary (One Month After Admission)

Lindsay was initially resistant to occupational therapy, but as she developed rapport with staff and interacted with peers she began to participate and show motivation. She completed at least one project per week (e.g., painted sweatshirt, wooden carousel, stenciled teddy bear peg rack). In leisure education, she initially argued that she could not have fun without using chemicals. After several community out-trips and

[12]Adapted from a case contributed by Susan Voorhies, COTA/CAODAC, of HCA Regional Hospital Rediscovery Unit, Jackson, Tenn., in consultation with Anne Brown, OTR, MS.

[13]An eight ball is equivalent to 10 to 12 rocks.

Occupational Therapy Treatment Summary

Goals	Objectives	OT Treatment Given
1. To improve independent living skills (i.e., house-hold, child care).	1a. Patient will identify areas of household skills which she needs to learn (within one week).	1a. Individual OT 1 × wk.
	1b. Patient will participate in independent living skills training such as cooking a meal, planning a budget, etc., 2 × wk.	1b. Independent Living Skills Training Group 2 × wk.
	1c. Patient will schedule self to participate in parenting classes in the community (within three weeks).	1c. OT referral to Carl Perkins' parenting classes.
2. To identify leisure activi-ties appropri-ate for a sober life-style.	2a. Patient will identify leisure interests and hobbies (by two weeks).	2a. Leisure Education 1 × wk; OT Craft Clinic 4 × wk; Community Out-Trip 1 × wk.
	2b. Patient will participate in completing one craft project per week while in treatment.	2b. OT Craft Clinic 4 × wk
	2c. Patient will identify specific leisure activities appropriate for herself and her baby (by four weeks).	2c. Leisure Education 1 × wk; Community Out-Trip 1 × wk.
3. To obtain a GED.	3. Patient will contact and schedule appointment with CARE (Center for Adult Reading and Enrichment) re: GED preparation classes (by three weeks).	3. Individual OT referral to CARE.
4. To improve assertiveness skills.	4a. Patient will identify situations where she could be more assertive (by one week).	4a and b. Assertiveness Training Group 2 × wk.
	4b. Patient will role play difficult situations using assertive techniques (by three weeks).	

recreational activities, such as movies, cookouts, and swimming, she began identifying fulfilling leisure activities such as playing recreational games with peers from AA and NA. She identified sweatshirt painting as a possible hobby after discharge, and plans to make clothing for herself and her baby using inexpensive paints, sale items, and clothing from thrift stores.

She continued to have difficulty demonstrating assertive behavior spontaneously. In structured role playing, she was able to use assertive techniques effectively after these were modeled for her. COTA told patient to continue working on assertive responses in daily interactions. Pt. scheduled three meetings a week with Ms. Walker at the CARE program to prepare herself for her GED test. She will be discharged to a halfway house, where she will continue to receive treatment for the remainder of her pregnancy.

Lindsay has begun working on independent living skills such as cooking from a recipe and planning and cooking a meal, developing a budget on her allowance (from her mother), and general house cleaning tasks. She will continue working on this at the halfway house. Lindsay will also be assigned part-time employment and will be referred to vocational rehabilitation for job training after she receives her GED. The halfway house will provide childcare and a place for her to live while she continues her education and job training. She is sched-

uled to attend parenting classes two night per week, and will attend meetings of her 12-step programs nightly. This patient has responded well to treatment, particularly to structure and support. COTA will follow up on referrals post-discharge.

Questions for Case 6

1. Identify the chief enabler in this patient's situation.
2. What occupational roles is the patient in the process of acquiring? What occupational roles can you foresee that she will need to acquire in the future?
3. What additional skills and social supports will the patient need as her baby gets older?
4. The patient's mother would like her to return home to live with her once the baby is born. What are the advantages and disadvantages in terms of Lindsay's maintaining and developing independent living skills and adult occupational roles?

CASE 7: A 37-YEAR-OLD MAN WITH ALCOHOL DEPENDENCE DISORDER[14]

Bryan Jebson   Case #038947

Mr. Jebson is a 37-year-old white married man admitted to detox after his employer confronted him about his poor job performance and absenteeism due to alcohol abuse (see Table A–7). Patient reported his wife has been threatening to leave him over the past year. Patient was transferred to rehab after three days in detox.

TABLE A–6. DSM-III-R *diagnosis at admission (case 6)*

Axis I:	303.90 Alcohol dependence
	304.30 Cannabis dependence
	305.60 Cocaine abuse
	304.90 Polysubstance dependence
Axis II:	301.60 Dependent personality disorder
Axis III:	None
Axis IV:	Severity: 1—None
Axis V:	Current GAF: 60
	Highest GAF past year: 60

[14]Adapted from a case contributed by Susan Voorhies, COTA/CAODAC, of HCA Regional Hospital Rediscovery Unit, Jackson Tenn., in consultation with Anne Brown, OTR, MS.

Patient began drinking alcohol at age 15 and stated that it has been a problem in his life for at least the past 5 years. He has been fired from two jobs during that time and is having difficulty at a local factory job in which he's been employed for almost 18 months. Patient was able to maintain one job for 11 years, but that ended 5 years ago. He and his wife have been married for 10 years and have an eight-year-old daughter and five-year-old son. Patient denied any marital problems other than drinking.

Mr. Jebson has two brothers and one sister and was raised by his parents on a farm. He stated that he's the only one in his immediate family who drinks, but he's heard that his maternal great-grandfather was alcoholic. Patient completed high school and vocational technical training, acquiring a welding certificate. He stated his pattern is to drink at least six to eight beers after work, and on weekends in excess of a case plus several half pints of Jack Daniels. Patient shared he has mainly drunk alone at home in his tool shop. He does very little individual or family leisure activity. He stated that he has difficulty expressing his feelings and drinks especially when he feels angry. Patient admitted to being violent when drunk, throwing things and punching the wall on several occasions. He denies ever hitting his wife or children. Patient shared that he used to go to the local Baptist church with his family but quit due to his drinking. He had one DWI approximately two years ago, and after that quit going to bars to drink.

Patient identified his strengths as loving his family, being a skilled welder, and caring about people. He named his weaknesses as drinking and holding in his feelings. He identified his family and his job as most important to him. Patient was verbal but tearful at times during the interview. He appears motivated to get sober due to pressure from employer and wife.

Occupational Therapy Treatment Summary

Goals	Objectives	OT Treatment Given
1. To improve leisure and social involvement.	1a. Patient will identify at least five leisure activities that will provide socialization and support for his recovery (by two weeks).	1a. Leisure Education 1 × wk; Community Out-Trips 1 × wk.
	1b. Patient will identify a variety of leisure activities to pursue with his family (by two weeks).	1b. Leisure Education 1 × wk; Community Out-Trips 1 × wk; Family Recreation Night biweekly; OT Clinic 4 × wk.
	1c. Patient will introduce himself to at least one male peer at nightly 12-step meetings and will inquire about the group's recreational activities (by three weeks).	1c. 12-Step Meetings nightly; Individual Leisure Assignment.

Goals	Objectives	OT Treatment Given
2. To improve assertive behavior and expression of feelings.	2a. Patient will begin keeping a "feeling log" on a daily basis (within three days).	2a. Individual OT assignment.
	2b. Patient will identify situations where he has withheld angry feelings (by two weeks).	2b. Assertiveness Training 2 × wk.
	2c. Patient will role play specific situations where he's been angry using assertive techniques to express his anger (by three weeks).	2c. Assertiveness Training 2 × wk.

OT Discharge Summary (Three Weeks After Admission)

Mr. Jebson has been compliant throughout treatment. He made several projects in OT for his family and identified woodcraft as a hobby he could pursue and teach to his children. He named the following as family activities he would like to develop: cookouts, camping, movies, vacations, and community park excursions. He named as additional activities for himself hunting, fishing, boating, flea markets, and AA retreats. He has met several men from his community through AA and has asked two of them to be his sponsors in the program. Patient had difficulty labeling his feelings in the log initially and was given a chart with facial expressions[15] to use as a guide. He began appropriately identifying feelings of anger and fear as dominant in his experience. In assertiveness group, he identified himself as passive unless intoxicated, when

he'd become aggressive. He talked openly about things he's "stuffed" his anger over, and role-played effective expression. He reported using assertion in a marital session with his wife with positive results. Patient asked about becoming a volunteer after one year of sobriety. He identified this as a long-term goal for aftercare. Family and employer are expected to support and encourage patient after discharge.

TABLE A–7. DSM-III-R *diagnosis at admission (case 7)*

Axis I:	303.90 Alcohol dependence
Axis II:	None
Axis III:	None
Axis IV:	Severity: 2—Mild (confrontation with employer)
Axis V:	Current GAF: 70
	Highest GAF past year: 80

---

[15]Such a chart can be found as Exercise 7, Emotions, in Korb KL, Azok AD, Leutenberg EA. *Life management skills: reproducible activity handouts created for facilitators.* Beachwood, Ohio: Wellness Reproductions; 1989.

Questions for Case 7

1. What are this patient's occupational roles? How did his substance abuse affect his functioning in these roles?

2. Which aspects of this patient's treatment as described fall specifically within the scope of occupational therapy? Which aspects could be managed equally well by another treatment discipline?
3. What are the elements of this patient's preferred defensive structure or PDS? (Refer to Chapter 9 for discussion of PDS.)
4. Why was the emotions identification guide given to this patient? What other activities could assist this patient to develop knowledge in this area?

CASE 8: A 21-YEAR-OLD WOMAN WITH COCAINE DEPENDENCE, POLYSUBSTANCE ABUSE, BULIMIA, AND BORDERLINE PERSONALITY DISORDER[16]

Tamara Little   Case #10391

Ms. Little is a 21-year-old black female who sought treatment after the Department of Social Services threatened to take her two children, a boy aged 6 and a girl aged 2.

Patient stated that her neighbor reported her for leaving her children alone. Patient is unemployed and is on welfare. She said that she can't make enough money working to pay bills and childcare.

Patient has drunk alcohol and used pot since age 11. She has tried speed and valium and has used cocaine by snorting, injection, and smoking (see Table A–8). Patient stated she has used crack for the past nine months and denies any other drugs since then except an occasional beer. Patient admitted to using her welfare check for drugs and selling her food stamps to obtain money. She was never married and does not receive financial support from the fathers of her children. Patient, who is slightly overweight, was observed purging food in the bathroom of the detox unit and admitted to episodic purging to control weight.

Ms. Little described herself as a good student in high school until her drug use became more important than studying. She has a high school degree but did not attempt college as she felt she could not afford it. Patient's parents both drank and were physically abusive to one another. Ms. Little denies physical or sexual abuse of self or siblings by parents. Patient reported she cooks, cleans, and takes care of all household chores independently. She stated she has been "out of control" since she took up crack nine months ago, smoking approximately $200 worth one to two days per week at friends' homes or crack houses. She admitted to leaving the children alone twice over the last month and was overwhelmed that she would do such a thing. She admitted to having slept with crack dealers to obtain drugs. Patient stated that she knows she has to get clean or she will lose her children. She has never obtained a driver's license but does have a car of her mother's that she drives. She has no friends except other users, and other than drug use her only leisure activity is renting a movie for the children. Ms. Little stated that she feels depressed much of the time and has no energy.

---

[16]Adapted from a case contributed by Susan Voorhies, COTA/CAODAC, of HCA Regional Hospital Rediscovery Unit, Jackson Tenn., in consultation with Anne Brown, OTR, MS.

Occupational Therapy Treatment Summary

Goals	Objectives	OT Treatment Given
1. To obtain a driver's license.	1. Patient will spend one hour a day studying drivers' manual and will take her driver's test before discharge.	1. Individual OT as needed.
2. Destructive lifestyle.	2a. Patient will identify five leisure activities appropriate for a sober lifestyle, to pursue after discharge (by two weeks).	2a. Leisure education 1 × wk; Community Out-Trip 1 × wk.
	2b. Patient will introduce herself to at least two females per night at 12-step meetings.	2b. Nightly 12-step meeting; leisure education assignment.
	2c. Patient will identify at least five activities to pursue with children at home and five in the community (by two weeks).	2c. Same as 2a.
3. To obtain job/educational training.	3a. Patient will meet with vocational rehab counselor (by one week).	3a. OT referral to vocational rehab.
	3b. Patient will identify job and educational training interests (by one week).	3b. Individual OT sessions.
4. To improve energy level and to decrease craving for crack.	4a. Patient will complete exercise assessment (by three days).	4a. Individual OT assessment.
	4b. Patient will participate in daily exercise program for 20 minutes initially (by four days), increasing to 45 minutes (by two weeks).	4b. Daily Structured Exercise Program.

OT Discharge Summary (Three Weeks After Admission)

Ms. Little has been alternately resistant and compliant with treatment throughout the three weeks. She argued that she didn't need a driver's license but became willing after this issue was addressed repeatedly by COTA, along with treatment team. Patient was assigned specific study times and obtained her license two and a half weeks after admission. She expressed pride at this accomplishment.

Patient was resistant to identifying leisure activities for herself, but after several community out-trips began to identify enjoyable leisure interests such as putt putt golf, swimming, movies, hiking, and eating out. Patient selected as family interests board games, making cookies, going to parks and MacDonald's, etc. She met with the vocational rehabilitation counselor and completed the application. COTA sent all records to the counselor, who has confirmed that patient is eligible for assistance. One of her sisters has committed to keeping her children for her so that she can attend school when the time comes. Patient appeared enthusiastic and stated that an opportunity for education/job preparation gives her hope for the future. She identified a list of job interests and strengths and this was communicated to the counselor.

A goal to increase assertive behavior was added to treatment plan after patient shared how much difficulty she has saying no to peers. She role-played situations, was initially too aggressive, but after practice was able to express herself calmly but firmly. She introduced herself to other women at 12-step meetings, and spent time with two female volunteer alumnae who shared recovery experiences with her.

Patient participated in the exercise program only after much encouragement from staff. Treatment team and COTA several times met with her to stress the importance of her following directions and increasing exercise participation. This patient will continue to meet with COTA on an outpatient basis 2 × week to work on leisure, assertiveness, and exercise compliance.

TABLE A–8. DSM-III-R *diagnosis at admission (case 8)*

Axis I:	304.20 Cocaine dependence
	304.90 Polysubstance abuse (past)
	307.51 Bulimia nervosa
Axis II:	301.83 Borderline personality disorder
Axis III:	None
Axis IV:	Severity: 4—Severe (poverty, unemployment, single parent status)
Axis V:	Current GAF: 50
	Highest GAF past year: 70

Questions for Case 8

1. Compare this patient to the patient of similar age in case 6. What are the differences and what are the similarities?
2. What are this patient's occupational roles now? What occupational roles might this patient acquire for the future?
3. What additional community supports or aftercare strategies would be helpful for this patient?

Appendix B
Sample Group Protocols

HOMEMAKER'S MANAGEMENT GROUP

Description. A group for homemakers, focused on management and delegation of tasks, and reduction of stress.

Structure. Meets one afternoon per week, for one hour. Written assignments are given to assist members to practice concepts discussed in group. Group is limited to six members. Leader: OTR or COTA with homemaker responsibilities in addition to regular employment.

Goals. Through participation in this group, members will learn to:

1. Analyze and prioritize their own household and caregiving tasks
2. Identify and report areas of difficulty for self in homemaker role
3. Learn and apply various problem-solving techniques to get household work done with less stress to self
4. Report results of problem-solving efforts to the group and receive feedback
5. Be able to state one's needs and request assistance from others.

Referral Criteria. Patients who are:

1. Homemakers
2. Able to tolerate verbal group for one hour
3. Able, with structure, to discuss their experience of homemaker role.

Methodology. The group will be structured around a lesson or worksheet. After a brief introduction of members and of the group goals, leader will present the lesson or worksheet. Members will work on the lesson for approximately 20 minutes. A group discussion will follow. The meeting will end with an assignment to be done outside of group. The lesson or worksheet will vary, depending on the needs of individuals and the group. Focuses may include: analysis of time use, time-management strategies, problem identification, generation of alternatives, assertiveness role-plays, etc.

Role of the Leader. The leader will:

1. Structure and present group exercises
2. Keep group on task and on time
3. Facilitate discussion, feedback, and problem-solving
4. Contribute own experiences, serving as a role model.

Evaluation. Patients will complete a forced-choice questionnaire on attitudes toward homemaker role as a pre-test and post-test.

Resources. Exercises on job stress, parenting, assertiveness, money management, role satisfaction, stress management, time management, values clarification, goal setting, coping skills, support systems, etc, from:

Korb KL, Azok SD, Leutenberg EA. *Life management skills*. Beachwood, Ohio: Wellness Reproductions; 1989.

448

Korb KL, Azok SD, Leutenberg EA. *Life management skills II*. Beachwood, Ohio: Wellness Reproductions; 1991.
Simmons PL, Mullins L. *Acute psychiatric care*. Thorofare, NJ: SLACK; 1981.

FAMILY RECREATION SKILLS[1]

Description. A group for recovering substance abusers to assist the development or rediscovery of leisure activities in the context of the family.

Structure. Group meets the first Monday of the month, from 7:00 to 8:45 P.M., in the recreation room, OT workshop, or lounge (depending on activity), led by COTA or OT technician.

Goals. Through participation in this group, the patient will learn to:

1. Identify the effects of addiction and recovery on family leisure patterns
2. Interact pleasurably in a leisure situation with family members
3. Identify enjoyable leisure activities appropriate for families.

Referral Criteria. Patients who:

1. Are newly sober or drug-free
2. Have family members who can attend the group.

Methodology. Leader will assist those present to introduce themselves (10 min). Leader will lecture briefly on a leisure topic related to addiction, such as: effects of addiction on family leisure; healing effects of fun and play; learning to enjoy each other again (10–15 min). Activities are then introduced, distributed. Session ends with a summary and comments from participants, facilitated by leader.

Role of the Leader.

1. To provide information and learning opportunities
2. To facilitate pleasurable interaction in the group
3. To assist participants to explore new recreational options.

Evaluation. Pre-test, post-test—Patient asked to list recreational activities that he would like to do with his family.

[1]This protocol adapted, with permission, from one by Susan Voorhies, COTA, CSAC, and Anne Brown, OTR, MS, of ReDiscovery Unit, HCA Hospital, Jackson, Tenn.

Subject Index